Handbook of Health Promotion
and Disease Prevention

THE PLENUM SERIES IN
BEHAVIORAL PSYCHOPHYSIOLOGY AND MEDICINE

Series Editors: William J. Ray
Pennsylvania State University
University Park, Pennsylvania

Recent volumes in the series:

Handbook of Health Promotion and Disease Prevention

Edited by

James M. Raczynski

Schools of Medicine and Public Health
and UAB Center for Health Promotion
University of Alabama at Birmingham
Birmingham, Alabama

and

Ralph J. DiClemente

Rollins School of Public Health
Emory University
Atlanta, Georgia

Kluwer Academic / Plenum Publishers
New York, Boston, Dordrecht, London, Moscow

Library of Congress Cataloging-in-Publication Data

Handbook of health promotion and disease prevention / edited by James
M. Raczynski and Ralph J. DiClemente.
        p.   cm. -- (The Plenum series in behavioral psychophysiology
and medicine)
    Includes bibliographical references and index.
    ISBN 0-306-46140-4
    1. Health promotion Handbooks, manuals, etc. 2. Medicine,
Preventive Handbooks, manuals, etc.   I. Raczynski, James M.
II. DiClemente, Ralph J. III. Series.
    [DNLM: 1. Preventive Medicine. 2. Health Promotion.   WA 108
H23558 1999]
RA427.8.H36   1999
613--dc21
DNLM/DLC
for Library of Congress   99-37316
                                                              CIP

ISBN: 0-306-46140-4

© 1999 Kluwer Academic / Plenum Publishers
233 Spring Street, New York, N.Y. 10013

10 9 8 7 6 5 4 3 2 1

Printed in the United States of America

To my parents who raised me and Martha who sustains me,
for their continued love.

—J. M. R.

To Gina and my family for their love and support.

—R. J. D.

Contributors

Leslie Aaron, Department of Health Behavior, School of Public Health, UAB Center for Health Promotion, University of Alabama at Birmingham, Birmingham, Alabama 35294

Lynn M. Artz, Department of Epidemiology, School of Public Health, University of Alabama at Birmingham, Birmingham, Alabama 35294

Jason B. Avery, Department of Health Behavior, School of Public Health, UAB Center for Health Promotion, University of Alabama at Birmingham, Birmingham, Alabama 35294

William C. Bailey, Department of Pulmonary and Critical Care, School of Medicine, University of Alabama at Birmingham, Birmingham, Alabama 35294

Vera Bittner, Division of Cardiovascular Disease, School of Medicine, UAB Center for Health Promotion, University of Alabama at Birmingham, Birmingham, Alabama 35294

Laurence A. Bradley, Division of Clinical Immunology and Rheumatology, Department of Medicine, University of Alabama at Birmingham, Birmingham, Alabama 35294

Janet M. Bronstein, Department of Health Care Organization and Policy, School of Public Health, University of Alabama at Birmingham, Birmingham, Alabama 35294

Kathleen C. Brown, Nursing Graduate Programs, School of Nursing, University of Alabama at Birmingham, Birmingham, Alabama 35294

Eli Capilouto, Department of Health Care Organization and Policy, School of Public Health, UAB Center for Health Promotion, University of Alabama at Birmingham, Birmingham, Alabama 35294

Stuart A. Capper, Department of Health Care Organization and Policy, School of Public Health, University of Alabama at Birmingham, Birmingham, Alabama 35294

Leslie F. Clark, Department of Health Behavior, School of Public Health, UAB Center for Health Promotion; University of Alabama at Birmingham, Birmingham, Alabama 35294

Brenda Cobb, School of Nursing, UAB Center for Health Promotion, University of Alabama at Birmingham, Birmingham, Alabama 35294

David Coombs, Department of Health Behavior, School of Public Health, UAB Center for Health Promotion, University of Alabama at Birmingham, Birmingham, Alabama 35294

Carol E. Cornell, Behavioral Medicine Unit, Division of Preventive Medicine, Department of Medicine, School of Medicine, UAB Center for Health Promotion, University of Alabama at Birmingham, Birmingham, Alabama 35294

Susan L. Davies, Department of Health Behavior, School of Public Health, UAB Center for Health Promotion, University of Alabama at Birmingham, Birmingham, Alabama 35294

Ralph J. DiClemente, Department of Behavioral Sciences and Health Education, Rollins School of Public Health, Emory University, and Emory/Atlanta Center for AIDS Research, Atlanta, Georgia 30322

Molly Engle, Department of Public Health, College of Health and Human Performance, Oregon State University, and Oregon State Extension Service, Corvallis, Oregon 97331

Philip R. Fine, Injury Control Research Center, University of Alabama at Birmingham, Birmingham, Alabama 35294

Larry Fish, Department of Health Behavior, School of Public Health, UAB Center for Health Promotion, University of Alabama at Birmingham, Birmingham, Alabama 35294

Eugene A. Gallagher, Department of Health Behavior, School of Public Health, UAB Center for Health Promotion, University of Alabama at Birmingham, Birmingham, Alabama 35294

Melissa M. Galvin, Department of Health Behavior, School of Public Health, University of Alabama at Birmingham, Birmingham, Alabama 35294

Marilyn M. Gardner, Department of Health Behavior, School of Public Health, University of Alabama at Birmingham, Birmingham, Alabama 35294

M. Janice Gilliland, Behavioral Medicine Unit, Division of Preventive Medicine, Department of Medicine, School of Medicine, Department of Health Behavior, School of Public Health, UAB Center for Health Promotion, University of Alabama at Birmingham, Birmingham, Alabama 35294

Diane M. Grimley, Department of Health Behavior, School of Public Health, UAB Center for Health Promotion, University of Alabama at Birmingham, Birmingham, Alabama 35294

Kathleen F. Harrington, Department of Health Behavior, School of Public Health, University of Alabama at Birmingham, Birmingham, Alabama 35294

Renée A. Harrison, Department of Epidemiology, School of Public Health, University of Alabama at Birmingham, Birmingham, Alabama 35294

James C. Hilyer, Division of Preventive Medicine, School of Medicine, University of Alabama at Birmingham, Birmingham, Alabama 35294

Wendy S. Horn, Injury Control Research Center, University of Alabama at Birmingham, Birmingham, Alabama 35294

Betty Keltner, School of Nursing, University of Alabama at Birmingham, Birmingham, Alabama 35294

Lorraine V. Klerman, Department of Maternal and Child Health, School of Public Health, UAB Center for Health Promotion, University of Alabama at Birmingham, Birmingham, Alabama 35294

Connie L. Kohler, Department of Health Behavior, School of Public Health, UAB Center for Health Promotion, University of Alabama at Birmingham, Birmingham, Alabama 35294

Polly P. Kratt, Behavioral Medicine Unit, Division of Preventive Medicine, Department of Medicine, School of Medicine, UAB Center for Health Promotion, University of Alabama at Birmingham, Birmingham, Alabama 35294

Laura Leviton, Department of Health Behavior, School of Public Health, UAB Center for Health Promotion, University of Alabama at Birmingham, Birmingham, Alabama 35294

Cora E. Lewis, Division of Preventive Medicine, School of Medicine, UAB Center for Health Promotion, University of Alabama at Birmingham, Birmingham, Alabama 35294

MaryAnn Littleton, Department of Health Behavior, School of Public Health, UAB Center for Health Promotion, University of Alabama at Birmingham, Birmingham, Alabama 35294

David M. Macrina, Department of Human Studies, School of Education, UAB Center for Health Promotion, University of Alabama at Birmingham, Birmingham, Alabama 35294

Walter Mason, Department of Epidemiology and International Health, School of Public Health, UAB Center for Health Promotion, University of Alabama at Birmingham, Birmingham, Alabama 35294

Vel S. McKleroy, Department of Health Behavior, School of Public Health, UAB Center for Health Promotion, University of Alabama at Birmingham, Birmingham, Alabama 35294

Jesse B. Milby, Behavioral Medicine Unit, Division of Preventive Medicine, Department of Medicine, School of Medicine, UAB Center for Health Promotion, University of Alabama at Birmingham, Birmingham, Alabama 35294

Katina Pappas-Deluca, Department of Health Behavior, School of Public Health, UAB Center for Health Promotion, University of Alabama at Birmingham, Birmingham, Alabama 35294

Mary Ann Pass, Department of Maternal and Child Health, School of Public Health, University of Alabama at Birmingham, Birmingham, Alabama 35294

Martha M. Phillips, UAB Civitan International Research Center, Department of Epidemiology, School of Public Health, UAB Center for Health Promotion, University of Alabama at Birmingham, Birmingham, Alabama 35294

James M. Raczynski, Behavioral Medicine Unit, Division of Preventive Medicine, Department of Medicine, School of Medicine, Department of Health Behavior, School of Public Health, UAB Center for Health Promotion, University of Alabama at Birmingham, Birmingham, Alabama 35294

Christopher Reinold, Department of Pediatrics, School of Medicine, University of Alabama at Birmingham, Birmingham, Alabama 35294

Kim D. Reynolds, Center for Behavioral Studies, AMC Cancer Research Center, Lakewood, Colorado 80214

Matthew D. Rousculp, Injury Control Research Center, University of Alabama at Birmingham, Birmingham, Alabama 35294

Bonnie K. Sanderson, Division of Cardiovascular Disease, School of Medicine, UAB Center for Health Promotion, University of Alabama at Birmingham, Birmingham, Alabama 35294

Joseph E. Schumacher, Behavioral Medicine Unit, Division of Preventive Medicine, Department of Medicine, School of Medicine, UAB Center for Health Promotion, University of Alabama at Birmingham, Birmingham, Alabama 35294

John L. Shuster, Jr., Department of Psychiatry, School of Medicine, University of Alabama at Birmingham, Birmingham, Alabama 35294

Delia E. Smith, Behavioral Medicine Unit, Division of Preventive Medicine, Department of Medicine, School of Medicine, UAB Center for Health Promotion, University of Alabama at Birmingham, Birmingham, Alabama 35294

Bonnie A. Spear, Department of Pediatrics, School of Medicine, University of Alabama at Birmingham, Birmingham, Alabama 35294

Katharine E. Stewart, Departments of Psychology and Medicine, UAB Center for AIDS Research and UAB Center for Health Promotion, University of Alabama at Birmingham, Birmingham, Alabama 35294

Herman A. Taylor, Jr., University of Mississippi Medical Center, Jackson, Mississippi 39216

Judith E. Taylor, Division of Health and Kinesiology, Mississippi University for Women, Columbus, Mississippi 39701

Andrea D. Tomasek, Injury Control Research Center, University of Alabama at Birmingham, Birmingham, Alabama 35294

Anne Turner-Henson, School of Nursing, UAB Center for Health Promotion, University of Alabama at Birmingham, Birmingham, Alabama 35294

Sten H. Vermund, Department of Epidemiology, School of Public Health, UAB Center for AIDS Research, University of Alabama at Birmingham, Birmingham, Alabama 35294

John W. Waterbor, Department of Epidemiology, School of Public Health, University of Alabama at Birmingham, Birmingham, Alabama 35294

Michael T. Weaver, Nursing Graduate Programs, School of Nursing, UAB Center for Health Promotion, University of Alabama at Birmingham, Birmingham, Alabama 35294

Suzan E. Winders, Behavioral Medicine Unit, Division of Preventive Medicine, Department of Medicine, School of Medicine, UAB Center for Health Promotion, University of Alabama at Birmingham, Birmingham, Alabama 35294

Gina M. Wingood, Department of Behavioral Sciences and Health Education, Rollins School of Public Health, Emory University and Emory/Atlanta Center for AIDS Research, Atlanta, Georgia 30322

Scott D. Winnail, Department of Human Studies, School of Education, University of Alabama at Birmingham, Birmingham, Alabama 35294

Preface

The idea for this volume developed when we were co-teaching our introductory, master's-level course in the Department of Health Behavior at the UAB School of Public Health, a core course for all masters of public health students in the school regardless of the department in which they enrolled or the focus of their studies. Hence, in the course we sought to provide both students in our department, as well as those who might not ever again take a health behavior course, with an overview that would both truly represent the field and substantially provide educational, research, and public health practice benefits. This was, and continues to be, a challenge with the diversity of students specializing in fields that include not only health behavior but also biostatistics, environmental health sciences, epidemiology, health care organization and policy, international health, and maternal and child health. The course that we taught attempted to provide the students with an overview of some of the important health promotion and disease prevention theories, methods, and policy issues, while reviewing applications of these theories and methods to promoting health and preventing disease through a variety of channels, for a variety of disease outcomes, and among a variety of populations. Since no one text provided this variety of readings, we depended on readings and guest lectures. It was from this beginning that the idea for this book emerged: a compendium that would truly represent the burgeoning activities in the field of health promotion and disease prevention.

Although we wanted this compendium to be useful as a text that overviewed the field, we also anticipated that it would provide a reference for researchers and practitioners actively working in the field of health promotion and disease prevention as well as those working in related areas. Thus, contributors have attempted to provide an overview of each area, while outlining the critical issues and directions in each area.

For us, working with our many contributors and colleagues over the many months that it took to assemble this volume was truly an interesting opportunity to reflect on where our field is and where it seems to be heading. While we came to the work on this book knowing that health promotion and disease prevention research and practice has far to go before it truly converges into a science, we complete this project with optimism for the directions we are headed and the progress that we are beginning to make.

J. M. R.
R. J. D.

Contents

IV. BEHAVIOR CHANGE FOR RISK REDUCTION

V. BEHAVIOR CHANGE FOR PREVENTING DISEASE AND DISABILITY OUTCOMES

PART I

Health Promotion and Disease Prevention
History and Areas of Importance

CHAPTER 1

The Importance of Health Promotion and Disease Prevention

Ralph J. DiClemente and James M. Raczynski

Introduction

Understanding human behavior is a daunting challenge. The noted mathematician Sir Isaac Newton once remarked that he could predict the motion of heavenly bodies but not the behavior of people. So, too, do we, who are dedicated to understanding human behavior, specifically as it affects the health of human populations, acknowledge the complexities inherent in our enterprise. Equally, if not more challenging, are our efforts to modify human behavior.

Despite these challenges, as discussed in the chapters of this book, significant progress is being made in understanding theoretical models to predict better the impact and outcome of specific methods and approaches; to endeavor to change risk factors to prevent disease and other behaviors to promote health; and to evaluate these endeavors in ways that will allow us to learn more about these efforts, as discussed in Section II. Progress is also being made in what may be considered as crosscutting areas of health promotion and disease prevention, such as those addressed in Section III: factors that influence symptom perception; health care seeking for routine and preventive care as well as signs and symptoms of illness that may, at least in some cases of acute health problems, dramatically influence the type of medical care possible and ultimately affect morbidity, mortality, and even the costs of care; and issues involving stress, coping, and the influence of social support.

The science of health promotion and disease prevention clearly has a long way to go to determine optimal methods of influencing people's health behaviors. Nonetheless, developments are being made to determine more effective theoretical

Ralph J. DiClemente • Department of Behavioral Sciences and Health Education, Rollins School of Public Health, Emory University, and Emory/Altanta Center for AIDS Research, Atlanta, Georgia 30322. *James M. Raczynski* • Behavioral Medicine Unit, Division of Preventive Medicine, Department of Medicine, School of Medicine, Department of Health Behavior, School of Public Health, UAB Center for Health Promotion, University of Alabama at Birmingham, Birmingham, Alabama 35294.

Handbook of Health Promotion and Disease Prevention, edited by Raczynski and DiClemente. Kluwer Academic/Plenum Publishers, New York, 1999.

models to understand risk behaviors and to modify these behaviors for risk reduction in areas such as smoking, obesity, physical activity, and substance use and abuse, as discussed in Section IV. The medical model approach has largely structured federal funding mechanisms in such a manner as to influence research to address risk factors related to particular disease outcomes; however, the crosscutting nature of risk factors for most of the chronic, and even many infectious diseases, argues for a continued strong focus on risk factors rather than solely focusing on disease outcomes. Nonetheless, differences in psychosocial outcomes and risk factors do emerge with particular diseases, arguing for not abandoning completely a medical model to examine different disease outcomes, as is addressed in Section V, and examining such prevention outcomes as cardiovascular diseases, cancer, intentional and unintentional injury, pulmonary disorders, pain and musculoskeletal disorders, and human immunodeficiency virus (HIV) infection.

In addition to making progress in developing theories and methods in areas of risk factors and disease outcomes, progress is also being made with respect to developing approaches and evaluation methodologies for particular settings and with particular populations. These include interventions delivered in settings such as those discussed in Section VI: schools, communities, health care settings, and work sites. Accommodations in theory and methods also are necessary with some populations with unique needs based on ethnicity, culture, and differences in population-specific health care problems and/or risk factors, as discussed in Section VII, for maternal and child health issues, adolescents, older populations, women, cultural and ethnic groups, and populations in developing countries.

Finally, as discussed in Section VIII, policy perspectives are important when considering intervention programs that involve health care organizations and health departments. Additionally, as managed care evolves and health promotion and disease prevention programs move along with all of medical care to be scrutinized based largely on cost-effectiveness, issues of cost evaluation have moved to the forefront in evaluating health promotion and disease prevention programs.

The Science of Health Promotion and Disease Prevention

Before proceeding with other chapters in this volume, a basic understanding of the science of health promotion and disease prevention is essential. This is a science that does not have an inveterate tradition. It is not comparable to the so-called "hard" sciences with respect to its genealogy. In actuality, the field of health promotion and disease prevention is not a unitary discipline but rather a newly emerging, multidisciplinary, and even interdisciplinary field of inquiry with a singular focus, namely, enhancing health and preventing disease. As a relatively fledgling field of inquiry, health promotion and disease prevention does not have as long a legacy of scientific theory, principles, and axioms to provide a foundation for informing research as most other sciences. Indeed, one measure of the multidisciplinary and interdisciplinary nature of health promotion and disease prevention is the degree with which other social and behavioral sciences, public health, medical, and other allied health disciplines participate and are engaged in the development of theories, research methodologies, and application techniques. The field is reflected in the wide diversity of disciplines that are represented among investigators and practitioners engaged in health promotion and disease prevention activities. Contributors to the field are often eclectic in practice, using varied conceptual models for understanding and modifying behavior, research methodologies (such as quantitative and qualitative approaches), and differing philosophical frameworks for contextualizing risk and protective behaviors associated with health promotion and disease prevention.

In one sense, the absence of a single discipline, with well-established principles and theories, may be seen as hindering the maturation of the field we call health promotion and disease prevention. The multifactorial nature of influences that affect health and the pheonomena of study, such as beliefs, attitudes, perceptions and their interactions, are complex and often difficult to isolate, operationalize, and quantify at a pace that would allow rapid convergence. The development of the field therefore cannot be characterized as smooth and linear, leading to rapid convergence. This is not to say, however, that other branches of scientific inquiry have not experienced a similar developmental trajectory. Indeed, the history of science is replete with examples of theories and principles that have been discarded or markedly modified based on new empirical data. This is the process of science.

In another way, however, the breadth of disciplines involved in health promotion and disease prevention, while certainly contributing to slow initial progress, may lead eventually to more rapid convergence of the science of health promotion and disease prevention. Understanding the complexity of human behavior clearly rivals that of any scientific endeavor and may even exceed the complexity of at least some. Changing individuals' behaviors is unquestionably a formidable challenge, influenced not just by one virus, gene, or physiological process, but through the complex, reciprocal determinism (Bandura, 1986) of individuals' physiological processes, cognitions, and emotional responses; his or her behavior; the environment; and interpersonal, social, economic, and psychological influences within a cultural context that is superimposed over traditions, values, and patterns of social organization. Such a complex process that must be addressed for behavior change is not likely to be understood in simplistic, unidimensional, or linear terms. Thus, the multidisciplinary and interdisciplinary nature of the field is critical to developing a coherent, integrated body of empirical data that acknowledges and accommodates the myriad genetic, physiological, intrapersonal, interpersonal, social system, and cultural forces that exert influence on whether individuals adopt and maintain health-promoting behaviors. These empirical data will enable development of theory and associated methods, particularly when the empirical data are guided by a starting theoretical framework. Thus, the broader initial diversity of disciplines, with the unique theoretical models and methodological approaches that they bring to the study of health promotion and disease prevention, have unquestionably led to great diversity or a wide opening of the "funnel" of activity in the field. Nonetheless, this great diversity may ultimately lead to more rapid progress toward a more focused science as the funnel of activity narrows.

Like all human endeavors, developing a truly effective technology for health promotion and disease prevention will require significant knowledge-based effort. The field to date can be characterized as showing promise. While certainly requiring a convergence of theory to guide and interpret data, significant methodological challenges also remain for the field of health promotion and disease prevention in order to generate an adequate knowledge base. These challenges are inherent in all field trial research and evaluation but may be particularly great in a field that attempts to address the complexity of modifying human behavior to overcome the myriad factors that work toward behavioral inertia. Fortunately, the standards for judging programmatic success are well developed. That is, to be successful, programs must demonstrate a reduction in the rates of risk behaviors associated with adverse health consequences and disease-related, morbidity and/or mortality outcomes. The same standards must be applied to evaluating all programmatic efforts.

In the end, success in advancing the field of health promotion and disease prevention requires the development of a significant knowledge base, built on and contributing to the development of theoretical underpinnings. Although often also encountered in aspects of chronic disease prevention, the field unfortunately is dominated by individuals and groups who believe strongly, almost blindly, in the value of health promotion and disease prevention, particularly in areas of rapid growth, such as HIV prevention. All too often, such activist approaches to prevention substitute adequate methodological knowledge and rigor with a determination to succeed. Unfortunately, such approaches seldom, if ever, achieve prevention goals. No matter how widespread, politically viable, or popular a program may be, demonstrable effectiveness in reducing risk behaviors and their adverse sequelae must remain the primary and sole criterion by which programs are judged. The science of health promotion and disease prevention must be able to meet the most rigorous methodological standards applied to any scientific area of inquiry.

Priorities should be directed away from programs in which success is based solely on marketing, persuasive philosophy, or anecdotal evidence and toward those that are based on solid empirical research, derived from rigorous, methodologically sound endeavors and demonstrable effectiveness. Approaches that have demonstrated promise should form the basis for refinements and experimentation, grounded in theoretical underpinnings, until a technology of prevention can be fully developed. In the end, empirically grounded theory and extensive field testing will result in the development of effective programs. The promise of a "quick fix" must be understood to be an illusion. The demand for ready solutions should be responded to with the development of technically sound solutions.

In a similar vein, Gochman (1997) notes,

> attempts to change individual health behaviors, either through individual therapeutic interventions or through larger-scale health promotion or health education programs, have been less than impressive. Many attempts are purely programmatic, hastily conceived, and lacking in theoretical rationale or empirical foundation. A major reason for this is the lack of basic knowledge about the target behaviors, about the contexts in which they occur, and about the factors that determine and stabilize them. (p. xiii)

Theoretically driven, methodologically sound, evidence-based research in health promotion and disease prevention programs when rigorously evaluated offers the greatest promise for contributing to our understanding of how best to modify individuals' risk behaviors. Greater specificity will be necessary to more effectively tailor interventions to target populations, taking into account their genetics, physiology, gender, sexual orientation, ethnicity, and developmental level, as well as the setting and social environment in which programs are implemented. For the field of health promotion and disease prevention to progress more rapidly, however, a comprehensive and coordinated infrastructure to conceptualize, stimulate, and support the continuum of social and behavioral intervention research necessary to impact the continuing and emerging health threats that confront the United States is still of critical importance.

The Focus of Health Promotion and Disease Prevention: The Swinging Pendulum

At the turn of the 20th century, the majority of morbidity and mortality resulted from infectious diseases. As medical science advanced during the early 20th century to develop effective treatments and even preventive vaccines for infectious diseases, public health emerged and epidemiology evolved to develop the methods of a scientific discipline to identify the sources of infectious disease for public health initiatives. As medical and public health approaches brought infectious diseases under better control in most industrialized countries and life spans increased, major sources of mortality shifted from infectious to chronic diseases, as well as, to at least some extent, other sources of mortality, such as intentional and unintentional injury.

It is somewhat ironic that, as we enter the next millennium, the pendulum has begun shifting back toward infectious diseases as a major source of morbidity and mortality. The rapid emergence of HIV as a devastating health threat for all age groups, coupled with the lack of an effective treatment, catapulted health promotion and disease prevention interventions into a critical role in stopping the spread of this new disease. The scientific development of chronic disease health promotion and disease prevention has evolved in a relatively systematic and programmatic manner with primarily academically based researchers developing the programs. In contrast, given the need to actively confront the growing threat of HIV, most HIV prevention programs had been historically developed without an adequate theoretical basis and without sufficient empirical information about the strategies that would be most effective in motivating individuals to adopt HIV-preventive behaviors. Often these behavioral interventions were developed without an understanding of the forces that maintain risk-taking behavior and, as important, without knowledge of the influences that promote the adoption and maintenance of HIV-preventive behaviors.

Despite evidence from chronic disease interventions that strictly education-based methods result in only limited behavior change, early HIV prevention interventions were primarily information based, disseminating information through public communication channels and outreach efforts. The assumption, of course, was that with a greater understanding of the behaviors associated with HIV transmission and infection, individuals would be more likely to adopt HIV-preventive behaviors. Despite the clear need to provide information to a public that knew little about HIV and had many misconceptions, the assumption that information alone would result in major health-protective behavior changes was ill-founded. There have been marked increases in the public's awareness of HIV/AIDS, but these increases have not resulted in corresponding changes in preventive behaviors. The relationship between acquisition of HIV/AIDS knowledge and subsequent adoption of preventive behaviors is often confusing, oversimplified, and at times contradictory. However, knowledge about HIV alone, or any health problem for that matter, is clearly not sufficient to promote the adoption and maintenance of preventive behaviors (DiClemente & Peterson, 1994).

The evolution of chronic disease health promotion and disease prevention programs can be characterized as slower than that for HIV, hence probably accounting for what may be characterized as more systematic development of programs for chronic disease prevention. Chronic disease risk factors have been identified by epidemiological methods over a period of the past 40 years; as data amass, our knowledge about genetic, physiological, and behavioral risk factors for chronic diseases continues to expand. With this slow expansion of our epidemiologic knowledge for chronic diseases, there was not the time-urgency that has been imposed on the health promotion and disease prevention community by the threat of the HIV epidemic of the past decade.

As the early rush to educate the public about HIV/AIDS abated, behavioral interventions for HIV prevention slowed in their evolution to parallel the more methodologically sound and theoretically based empirical approaches commonly seen in chronic disease prevention development. This also evolved as academically based HIV researchers began to be more active to balance the enthusiasm of community-based organizations devoted to implementing HIV prevention programs. Empirical data derived from longitudinal cohort studies identifying the determinants of safer sex behavior began emerging and have now been integrated into more recent prevention programs. For HIV interventions, a new generation of health promotion and disease prevention interventions that are theory driven emphasize motivational factors, provide skills training, and attempt to modify peer norms have been developed (Coates, 1990; DiClemente, 1997; Fisher & Fisher, 1992; Kelly & Murphy, 1992; Peterson & DiClemente, 1994). Recent reports suggest that the new generation of prevention interventions are more efficacious at promoting the adoption of HIV-preventive behaviors. These newer infectious disease programs will complement those that have evolved for chronic disease risk factors. While much remains ahead for the evolving field of health promotion and disease prevention, progress is being made in amassing incremental advancement of knowledge, building on previous research experiences, and integrating information into new, innovative, and more effective health promotion and disease prevention intervention programs. The goal is now to develop convergence of the field, combining what is learned about modifying risk factors to prevent both chronic and infectious diseases and promote health.

Conclusion

As discussed throughout this volume, individuals' willingness to tolerate, seek, and participate in risk behaviors represents the outcome of a multifactorial decision-making process in which many influences affect their eventual choices. Much more remains to be learned about factors determining the adoption and maintenance of risk and health-promoting behaviors. Future studies will need to define more precisely the interrelationship between determinants and their applicability for different populations and then define the theories and approaches that will be most effective in optimizing health promotion and disease prevention programs. While progress may be slowed somewhat by the diversity of disciplines that are essential in health promotion and disease prevention programs, the eventual convergence of the field from this broad diversity may lead to better theoretical models and more effective intervention approaches in the long term. It is imperative that we, as a society, begin to address the cost, both financially and in terms of damaged lives, that risk behaviors exact every year. Only by addressing this problem on the broadest of all possible levels will we meaningfully address the causes, antecedents, and adverse health outcomes associated with the risk behaviors. Without prompt redirection of our resources, commitment, and concern, we, as a nation, will face continued and perhaps even greater challenges to avoid behaviors that rob our population of the opportunity to be healthy, fulfilled, and productive individuals. In redirecting our resources, however, it is essential that this be done so as to ensure that adequate attention is being devoted to developing theoretically based, methodologically sound, and adequately evaluated programs; this approach will contribute not only to better infectious and chronic disease prevention programs but to advancements in the field of health promotion and disease prevention as well.

References

Bandura, A. (1986). *Social foundation of thought and action: A social cognitive theory.* Englewood Cliffs, NJ: Prentice-Hall.

Coates, T. J. (1990). Strategies for modifying sexual behavior for primary and secondary prevention of HIV disease. *Journal of Consulting and Clinical Psychology, 58,* 57–69.

D'Angelo, L., & DiClemente, R. J. (1996). Sexually transmitted diseases and human immunodeficiency virus infection among adolescents. In R. J. DiClemente, W. Hansen, & L. Ponton (Eds.), *Handbook of adolescent risk behavior* (pp. 333–368). New York: Plenum Press.

DiClemente, R. J. (1997). Looking forward: Future directions for prevention of HIV among adolescents. In L. Sherr (Ed.), *AIDS and adolescents* (pp. 189–199). Reading, Berkshire, UK: Harwood Academic.

DiClemente, R. J., & Peterson, J. (1994). Changing HIV/AIDS risk behaviors: The role of behavioral interventions. In R. J. DiClemente & J. Peterson (Eds.), *Preventing AIDS: Theories and methods of behavioral interventions* (pp. 1–4). New York: Plenum Press.

DiClemente, R. J., & Peterson, J. L. (in press). The importance of behavioral interventions in preventing HIV. In J. L. Peterson & R. J. DiClemente (Eds.), *Handbook of HIV prevention.* New York: Plenum Press.

Fisher, J. D., & Fisher, W. A. (1992). Changing AIDS risk behavior. *Psychological Bulletin, 111,* 455–474.

Gochman, D. S. (1997). *Handbook of health behavior research. I. Personal and social determinants.* New York: Plenum Press.

Kelly, J. A., & Murphy, D. A. (1992). Psychological interventions with AIDS and HIV: Prevention and treatment. *Journal of Consulting and Clinical Psychology, 60,* 476–485.

Peterson, J., & DiClemente, R. J. (1994). Lessons learned from behavioral interventions: Caveats, gaps and implications. In R. J. DiClemente & J. Peterson (Eds.), *Preventing AIDS: Theories and methods of behavioral interventions* (pp. 319–322). New York: Plenum Press.

CHAPTER 2

Historical and Conceptual Perspectives on Health Promotion

David M. Macrina

Health Promotion—Evolution of the Concept

The historical development of health promotion has paralleled to some degree the sweeping changes that have occurred in the evolution of public health. The nature of these developmental changes have been strongly influenced by the current basic belief systems relating to concepts of disease causation, prevention, and intervention. Furthermore, the changing nature of the definition of "health" as well has affected how health promotion is defined and operationalized. Many varied definitions of health have surfaced throughout the years. The depiction of health as not merely the absence of disease imparted a positive value that had significant quality of life implications.

What has occurred over time is a reconceptualization of the notion of health and subsequently that of health promotion. The definition of health as currently stated by the World Health Organization (WHO) is:

> the extent to which an individual or group is able, on the one hand, to realize aspirations and satisfy needs; and, on the other hand, to change or cope with the environment. Health is therefore seen as a resource for everyday life, not the object of living; it is a positive concept emphasizing social and personal resources, as well as physical capabilities. (Robertson & Minkler, 1994, p. 298)

It is significant to note that the implication of such a definition is that health promotion goes beyond disease prevention and risk reduction. Health promotion in its truest context has a much broader, enabling emphasis as distinct from the limited focus of disease prevention. The implicit ethical, social–economic, and political considerations inherent within those concepts helped to shape the operational context for answering basic questions such as what causes disease, how can disease be prevented, whose responsibility is prevention and health promotion, and what is the ethical between personal and social responsibility for disease prevention and health promotion?

David M. Macrina • Department of Human Studies, School of Education, UAB Center for Health Promotion, University of Alabama at Birmingham, Birmingham, Alabama 35294.

Handbook of Health Promotion and Disease Prevention, edited by Raczynski and DiClemente. Kluwer Academic/Plenum Publishers, New York, 1999.

Health Promotion—Historical Development

Developmentally, Ashton (1991) outlines four phases of development of public health that have implications for the concept of health promotion. The major characteristics of each phase have significantly contributed to our current understanding and approaches to health promotion. The initial phase of sanitary reform, which spanned the 1800s and early 1900s, brought wide-ranging and effective notions of individual and community hygiene to the notion of disease prevention and health protection. Subsequent advancements in the field of microbiology, extending into the 1930s, brought a second phase of public health progress characterized through an increased emphasis on child and family health, immunization, and the enhancement of protective services. This "preventive" phase underscored the early development of the concept of primary prevention. Interestingly, it is reported that most of the reduction in mortality from tuberculosis, bronchitis, pneumonia, influenza, and food- and waterborne disease had occurred before effective immunizations and treatments were available (Ashton, 1991).

The third phase of public health development, noted as the therapeutic phase, was highlighted by the increasing sophistication of antibiotic therapies and other technology-based interventions. The period from the 1930s until the mid-1970s brought an increasing enchantment and belief in the possibilities of technology as a means to not only disease prevention but health enhancement. The explosive growth of the medical care and pharmaceutical industry during this time reflected the willingness and trust of the public and governments in the potential of technology as the basis for health protection and promotion.

There were, however, epidemiological and economic signs that the promise of technology as a means to health enhancement was at best a double-edged sword. The social and economic burdens inherent within the technology-rooted health care system underscored that the cost-benefit and -effectiveness of many interventions were marginal. A health care system faced the issues that the economic cost of increased technological intervention was limited by virtue of the economic dynamics inherent in the delivery system and the limited potential of advanced therapies to prevent major causes of death and disability or necessarily enhance quality of life.

The fourth phase of public health development evolved from this realization and discontent. In the mid-1970s, voices of caution were increasingly heard noting the limited potential and accompanying hardships inherent in a health protection, care, and promotion system that was based on the delivery of increasingly sophisticated and expensive technological interventions to fewer and fewer numbers of people. Authors such as Illich (1974) noted that such efforts could not only be economically burdensome but questionable from a health outcome perspective in the best of circumstances and actually harmful in some.

The implications of such understanding are noted by Terris (1992) in his characterization of public health history as a series of "revolutions." His characterization of developments as revolutions highlights that in essence what had occurred was the construction of new paradigms to understand the etiology of health and disease. The paradox lies in the reality that the essence of the capabilities inherent in one paradigm potentially lessened the ability of society to respond to new and potentially more effective health paradigms. Thus, the knowledge, products, and benefits produced from the understanding of the germ theory of disease causation (first public health revolution) produced a series of potentially counterproductive by-products. Society's understanding of disease as caused by single organisms and of single-entity technology (such as by antibiotics) produced both a dependence on and expectation of this model as the means to understand both the causes of ill health and the potential sources of health improvement. The development of multicausal models of health and disease (second public health revolution) runs counter to the one cause–one solution model of early public health advancement. The historical vestige of the single-entity model of disease causation (and resultant single entity model of health promotion) is evident in society's search for the "magic" nutrient, medicine, exercise machine, vitamin, or health product that is the one answer to a healthy and productive life.

Health Promotion—Questions of Responsibility

The irony of the counterproductive relationship between the first and second public health revolutions noted above is further delineated in the debate between micro and macro orientation to health promotion (O'Rourke & Macrina, 1989). The micro orientation to health promotion as a function of individual responsibility acknowledges the ability of the individual to play a role in one's health protection and enhancement. Furthermore, this micro emphasis implies a responsibility of the individual to accept this role. The distinct possibility exists that the extent to which we envision health and health promotion as a function and responsibility of "self" underestimates the reality of health as a social function.

While there are numerous examples in the literature that stress the value of incorporating an individual-responsibility-oriented health promotion strategy, there is a growing concern regarding the need for caution in a wide variety of health problem areas, including lifestyle modification (Allegrante, 1986; Allegrante & Green, 1981; Becker, 1986), mental health promotion (Macrina & Tubbs, 1987), delimiting health protection (Ratcliffe & Wallack, 1986) and work site health promotion (Sloan, Gruman, & Allegrante, 1987).

Like the relationship between the first and second public health revolutions, the problems result not from the innate nature of the strategy (micro vs. macro), but rather the tendency to focus on one orientation to the exclusion of other possibilities. The reality that singular focus not only is limited in its effectiveness but potential counter productive remains a distinct possibility.

Health Promotion—Parallels of Iatrogenesis

The problem with singular approaches to health promotion is not necessarily that they do not make inroads into the causes of the problem, but rather that the short-term gains may have a long-term consequences. The concept of iatrogenesis as applied to medicine by Illich (1974) has implications for the practice of health promotion. Thus, the concept of individual responsibility, which originated as a means of improving health status, implies little or no responsibility on the part of collective society to share in the resolution of the situations that may be at the root of the health problems. Ironically, the micro focus of health promotion has been criticized in ways that parallel the criticisms of the technology focus of medicine (ORourke & Macrina, 1989). Like the focus on new technology as the "silver bullet" for medical problems (which is often criticized as being of limited value and at times counterproductive), the micro focus shares several characteristics. Both are looked at as being singular routes to solve health problems; both focus on "here-and-now" type changes, and both may have produced iatrogenic spinoffs. The strides that acute care and tertiary oriented technology have made indirectly deflect money, personnel, and other resources from primary prevention efforts. Likewise, the micro individual-oriented health promotion preoccupation that has dominated policy agendas may have lessened our desire, insight, and ability to pursue broader based interventions.

The concept of health promotion, while generally being touted for its laudable and idealistic goals, has also been criticized as a paradigm that has become an end unto itself. Becker (1986) called the individual behavior change and lifestyle focus of health promotion a form of "tyranny." In challenging the tyranny of health promotion, he chastised the development of the notion of health promotion that equated being sick with being guilty. He further suggested that substituting personal health goals for more important, humane societal goals is not necessarily in the best interest of the health of populations.

This new concept of health promotion also underscores health as a tool, whose value lies in its capability to facilitate one accomplishing one's goals rather than being a goal unto itself.

The Practice of Health Promotion

Health Promotion and the Marketplace

One of the unfortunate consequences of the concept of health as an end to be attained rather than a means to achieving ones goals has been the commercialization of health. The implication that "health" is a commodity that can be bought and sold has contributed to the marketplace and industry of health promotion. Society's trust in the technological ability of science to provide for the answers to the problems of disease have given rise to a similar trust in technology to provide the means to health. Health products in various forms ranging from nutrition supplements, exercise equipment (and of course the necessary clothing), health-measuring devices, and so on are a mammoth industry. The implication that "products" are necessary if one is to be really healthy has significantly expanded the health product marketplace. The health care industry has not neglected society's significant interest in health. Health promotion programs have evolved in workouts and medical care settings often as a corollary of facility marketing strategies. Many of these efforts are secondary prevention screening efforts via health fairs, mall displays, community newsletters, and presentations.

Health Promotion as Public Policy

Much of the recent evolution of the concept of health promotion has been influenced by several notable policy documents. There has been considerable discussion as to the policy implications of health promotion. The realization that the ever-increasing resource (technological and financial) expansion of health care did not necessarily translate into a corresponding elevation of health status of the population blossomed into a series of policy documents depicting a need for a change in direction in health promotion. In Canada, the Minister of Health and Welfare issued a report in 1974 (New Perspective) that emphasized the causal role of individual behavior in premature death and disability. It also outlined the resulting health and economic savings that a focus on individual responsibility related to lifestyle decisions could bring. Such a "health promotion" emphasis was reinforced by the Healthy People Report of the United States Surgeon General in 1980. While some criticized the reports as a national abdication of responsibility and a shift backward toward the notion of "blaming the victim," these reports have served as benchmarks in the modern era of health promotion. The Ottawa charter, Epp Report in Canada, the Healthy Cities project, and several other such documents have expanded the discussion on the variety of factors affecting health and quality of life as well as the variety of means to influence such outcomes. The Ottawa Charter has influenced the WHO in fostering the new approach to health promotion, namely, through building appropriate health public policy and strengthening community action (Raeburn & Beaglehole, 1989). The Ottawa Charter states that the "fundamental conditions and resources for health are peace, shelter, education, food, income, a stable ecosystem, sustainable resources, social justice and equity. Improvement in health (health promotion) requires a secure foundation in these basic prerequisites" (Terris, 1994, p. 5). Critical analysis of the "self"-orientation to health promotion has given rise to the popularization of the concepts of "empowerment" and "community participation" As noted by Robertson and Minkler (1994), the new health promotion movement includes features that expand beyond the limited notions of self and individual responsibility. These characteristics of the health promotion movement include: (1) broadening the definition of health and its determinants to include the social and economic context within which health, or more precisely, nonhealth, is produced; (2) going beyond the earlier emphasis on individual lifestyle strategies to achieve health through broader social and political strategies; (3) embracing the concept of empowerment—individual and collective—as a key health promoting strategy; and (4) advocating the participation of the community in identifying health problems and strategies for addressing those problems.

Health promotion has been defined as the process of enabling people to increase control over their health and to improve it. This process places emphasis on personal participation, supportive environments, and the shared responsibility of all sectors in improving individual and collective health. Health promotion puts health on the agenda of policymakers at all levels, it demands that health aspects be taken into account in shaping public policy, and it reminds those who shape it that they are responsible for the health consequences of their decisions.

Health promotion calls for efforts to create supportive environments; it urges a redelegation of responsibilities through the strengthening of community action; it emphasizes the importance of developing personal skills and enabling people to exercise more control over their health and their environment; and it calls for a reorientation of health services that need to be sensitive to the total needs of the individual as a whole person (Erben, 1991). Similarly, Lee and Paxman (1997) stress the need to incorporate the broader dimensions of health promotion as a part of "reinventing public health." This has significant implications for increasing the role of collaboration in health promotion among health professionals and community alike (Smille, 1992).

Philosophical Orientation and Practice

The development of health promotion as a guiding ideal has had significant impact on the ways in which the concept has been operationalized. Variation in perspective has produced differences in the manner in which health promotion programs are conceptualized, planned, operationalized, and evaluated. Nutbeam (1996) defines this variation as originating in how evidence is used to guide decision making in health promotion. He characterizes three basic models of health promotion practice, namely, planned, responsive, and reactive, differentiated by key operational differences and potential measures of success. The planned approach to health promotion relies on systematic assessment of need and research evidence leading to health-outcomes-focused decision making. The PRECEDE–PROCEED health education program planing model of Green and Kreuter (1991) probably best exemplifies a health promotion planning model conceptually based on an approach to health promotion practice that attempts to develop effective interventions based on need and to incorporate evaluation strategies that facilitate program effectiveness and integrity. The responsive orientation to health promotion practice places a priority similarly on need assessment, but increasingly emphasizes the role of the population in the identification of needs, determination on the appropriate response to this need, and measures by which success will be identified. The planned approach to community health developed by the Centers for Disease Control and Prevention (CDC) (1990) is firmly rooted in the concept of community participation in all phases of need identification, development of program intervention strategies, and criteria for determining success. The reactive model of health promotion is characterized as a attempt to develop answers for problems as they arise. Often this orientation is evident in programs swiftly developed in response to an urgent public health crises. In the school health education field, categorical programs such as those targeting illicit drug use, teen pregnancy, or sexually transmitted disease (STD) prevention are common examples. These programs are often short term and pragmatic in nature, politically driven and funded, and limited in terms of conceptual development and evaluation.

The changes in societal perspectives of the need for health promotion and the means by which to accomplish it are apparent in the microcosm of the history of school health. In the United States, early public health documents such as Shattuck's Report of the Sanitary Commission of Massachusetts in 1850 cited a need for the public to be educated about ways to protect and improve health (Shattuck, 1850). This early concept of health equated health promotion with the elemental factors of basic hygiene. As such, early school health promotion efforts evolved to teach students the need for washing their hands, appropriate personal sanitary practices, and basic food sanitation. The emphasis was on disease prevention based on then current understanding of the nature and causes of disease. Communicable diseases and their prevention were then the principle concern and were the essence of these early school and community health promotion efforts.

The Women's Christian Temperance Union was among the first organizations to promote public health education on the health risks inherent in certain individual behaviors. As early as the 1870s, this organization was a major proponent of public education on the dangers of alcohol, tobacco, and narcotics. These efforts were among the first organized attempts to educate the public on the relationship between individual behavior and the resulting consequences on personal health. It should be noted that these early health education and health promotion efforts reflected the notion of the day that the basis of health promotion was disease prevention. Little emphasis was made to promote health as a means to enhanced quality of life. It is understandable, given the living conditions of early settlers, that disease prevention would be a paramount concern.

The development in the early 1900s of voluntary health organizations such as the American Cancer Society, Tuberculosis Association, and Society for Mental Hygiene further promoted the notion that individual responsibility and actions could be taken to protect against and deal with disease. One of the first official collaborations between health and education professionals attempting to foster health promotion was the Joint Committee on Health Problems in Education, which originated in 1911. The committee was composed of representatives from the American Medical Association and the National Education Association and combined a concern for the future health and physical education needs of the school-age population. This landmark health promotion venture resulted in one of the first health promotion texts in 1924. The book, *Health Education: A Program for Public Schools and Teacher Training Institutions*, the present and future health concerns of society and what could be accomplished through individual health education and proper school and community health practices (Wood, 1924).

Reflecting the response of society to health concerns, the majority of school health promotion advancements have been typically crisis oriented. The ravages of a particular disease, an increase in the numbers of people involved in drug use, a rise in the number of injuries of a particular type, and similar such occurrences often prompted societal health and education promotion responses. Perceived health crises in communicable diseases such as STDs and AIDS, drug and tobacco use, or the alarming increase in youth violence have all given rise to health promotion efforts. These efforts often shared three characteristics: (1) they evolved as a result of a particular health issue and thus focused on that particular issue; (2) they were founded in the hopes that a sharing of information and personal life and decision-making skills might effectively limit the problem; and (3) they often had a short-term focus in the hopes of achieving results in a relatively short time span.

These characteristics reflect a fundamental health promotion belief that an informed individual will make a decision regarding their own health behavior that is in the best interests of their own health. Teach people about the dangers of smoking and they will not smoke. Teach people about the dangers of drugs and they will not use them. Teach people about the threat of AIDS and they will do what is necessary to protect themselves. Unfortunately, as research has confirmed, the relationship between information, education, and health-promoting behavior is not quite as direct as these categorical programs implied. The adage that "knowledge alone is not enough" is often acknowledged as a caution to health promotion program developers and policymakers. Other factors including personal motivation, values, skills, and resources contribute significantly to health behavior decision making and as such need to be addressed in health promotion interventions.

As noted by Nolte (1994), school and community health education reflecting a more comprehensive and developmental approach (as differentiated from the topic-oriented categorical approach) has given rise to health promotion initiatives such as the School Health Education study, the President's Committee on Health Education, the Michigan Model for health education, Seaside, State School Health Task Force, Growing Healthy, and Healthy Me.

Perhaps two of the most significant recent clarion calls for the need for health promotion among our young population that reflect this more comprehensive perspective are the report of the Carnegie Corporation's Task Force on Education of Young Adolescents and Code Blue, a report of the National Commission on the Role of the School and Community in Improving Adolescent Health.

Health Promotion: Future Crossroads

Health promotion has historically reflected the complex interaction of science, economics, politics, and individual decision making in formulating its agenda for future action. Like the domain of public health, health promotion will continue to reflect the tension in our society between collective and individual responsibility both as it relates to the causes of problems and to their solutions. Perhaps no single issue better represents this dynamic interaction in both a past and future tense than the relationship between tobacco and health. The complex interaction between science, business, politics, communities, and individuals epitomizes the diverse challenges to the future health promotion agenda.

Health promotion is a concept that implies activities across the life span in a variety of settings: home, school, community, and workplace. The significance of the comprehensive nature of health promotion lies in its goals of quality of life enhancement in addition to disease prevention. The progression of society's knowledge of the causes and cures for disease has ranged from microbial agents to ecological, genetic, and lifestyle risk factors. In response to these discoveries, the concept of health promotion has evolved from an initial emphasis on disease prevention through basic hygiene to a health enhancement perspective. This perspective, which emphasizes quality of life, recognizes the functional role that "being healthy" plays in our daily lives. In addition, it recognizes the spiritual role that mental, physical, social, and spiritual well-being play in our sense of purpose and fulfillment as humans.

This evolution of health promotion into both the dimensions of disease prevention and quality of life enhancement is not without its limitations and consequences. The quest for mortality reduction and increased longevity has produced a variety of dilemmas that will continue to confront the future of the health promotion field. Ethical dilemmas posed by genetic screening and manipulation are already on the horizon. The genetic manipulation issue beckons as the frontier of health promotion raises the hopes of health interventions that were unthinkable in previous years. The specter of eugenic interventions, while potentially helpful in terms of health status, bring society perilously close to an ethical abyss.

Furthermore, the issue of the individual's right to choose will continue to be at the heart of future health promotion debates. The right to knowingly expose oneself to risk factors will increasingly become an issue as the egalitarian desires of society confront the libertarian ethic of the individual. The debate concerning the future efficacy and relevance of health promotion may center around the manner in which the ethical perspectives of social justice versus market justice are resolved. The market justice perspective implies that persons are entitled to the rewards of that which they earn through their own efforts. The market justice philosophy stresses the significance of individual responsibility and lessens the opportunity for collective responsibility and obligation. This argument parallels the increasing focus on the role and responsibility of the individual in health promotion and protection. While the emphasis on individual responsibility may be a positive factor in fostering healthy behaviors, the paradoxical corollary of market justice is the lessening of society's sense of obligation for the common good. As stated by Beauchamp (1976), the market justice ethic is a powerful detriment, as it frees members of society from their sense of obligation and responsibility to foster the health of others. The implication of market justice perspective is that all behaviors are in essence the result of individual choice. Thus, the individual is responsible for the consequences of those choices, be they positive or negative. The sense of obligation to protect, through societal action such as regulation or legislation, or foster the provision of care by collective action is minimized and indeed discouraged as counterproductive. Within the market justice paradigm the individual is the beneficiary and primary determinant of both the contributors to health and disease as well as being responsible for earning the merits of protecting and preserving these benefits.

The perspective of social justice emphasizes the collective entitlement and obligation of members of society to foster individual and communal health. Within the paradigm of social justice the individual is best protected and provision of care fostered when actions for the common good are encouraged and actions harmful to the common good are discouraged or punished. Again, the current discussions of the actions of the tobacco industry in possibly knowingly bringing harm to persons who decided to use their products reflect the dilemma of the social versus market justice struggle. The extent to which these ethical paradigms are operationalized and resolved may determine the future extent to which the goals of public health and health promotion are realized. The issues inherent in both the right to individual choice and the obligation for the consequences of that choice continue to be at the core of public health action.

To some, the concept of health promotion represents the ultimate manifestation of humankind's progress and desires to live a longer, richer life. To others, health promotion may be viewed as that referred by Huxley as the "myth of progress" (Pickett & Hanlon, 1990). The argument that disease and selective premature mortality are nature's means of natural selection runs counter to the best long-term interests of our species. This argument is at best unsettling in its fatalism and questions the innate desire for self-betterment of humans. To what extent it is possible and advisable to tinker with life remains open to question, as it has throughout the history of health promotion. The striving of humans to lengthen the span and enrich the quality of life represents both the hope and folly of our species.

References

Allegrante, J. (1986). Potential uses and misuses of education in health promotion and disease prevention. *Eta Sigma Gamman, 3,* 2–8.

Allegrante, J., & Green, L. (1981). When health policy becomes victim blaming. *New England Journal of Medicine, 305,* 1528–1529.

Ashton, J. (1991). The healthy cities project: A challenge for health education. *Health Education Quarterly, 18(1),* 39–48.

Beauchamp, D. (1976). Public health as social justice. *Inquiry, XIII,* 3–14.

Becker, M. (1986). The tyranny of health promotion. *Public Health Review, 14,* 15–23.

Centers for Disease Control and Prevention. (1990). *Planned approach to community health: Guide for the local coordinators.* Atlanta: US Department of Health and Human Services.

Erben, R. (1991). Health challenges for the year 2000: Health promotion and AIDS. *Health Education Quarterly, 18(1),* 29–37.

Green, L., & Kreuter, M. (1991). *Health promotion planning: An educational and environmental approach.* Mountain View, CA: Mayfield.

Illich, I. (1974). Medical nemesis. *Lancet, 1,* 8–21.

Lee, P., & Paxman, D. (1997). Reinventing Public Health. *Annual Review of Public Health, 18,* 1–35.

Macrina, D., & Tubbs, L. (1987). Limitations of health education strategies in mental health promotion. *Health Education, 18,* 40–43.

Nolte, A. (1994). School health education: Highlights and milestones. In P. Cortese & K. Middleton (Eds.), *The comprehensive school health challenge-promoting health through education* (pp. 21–29). Santa Cruz, CA: ETR Associates.

Nutbeam, D. (1996). Improving the fit between research and practice in health promotion: Overcoming structural barriers. *Canadian Journal of Public Health, 87,* 18–23.

O'Rourke, T., & Macrina, D. (1989). Beyond victim blaming: Examining the micro–macro issue in health promotion. *Wellness Perspectives: Research, Theory and Practice, 6(1),* 7–16.

Pickett, G., & Hanlon, J. (1990). *Public health: Administration and practice.* St. Louis: Times Mirror Mosby.

Raeburn, J., & Beaglehole, R. (1989). Health promotion: Can it redress the health effects of social disadvantage? *Community Health Studies, 13(3),* 289–93.

Ratcliffe, J., & Wallach, L. (1986). Primary prevention in public health: An analysis of basic assumptions. *International Quarterly of Health Education, 6(3),* 215–237.

Robertson, A., & Minkler, M. (1994). New health promotion movement: A critical examination. *Health Education Quarterly, 21(3),* 295–312.

Shattuck, L. (1850). *Report of the Commission of Massachusetts.* Cambridge, MA: Harvard University Press.

Sloan, R., Gruman, J., & Allegrante, J. (1987). *Investing in employee health: A guide to effective health promotion in the workplace.* San Francisco: Josey & Bass.

Smille, C. (1992). Preparing health professionals for a collaborative health promotion role. *Canadian Journal of Public Health, 83(4),* 279–282.

Terris, M. (1992, Autumn). Concepts of health promotion: Dualities of public health theory. *Journal of Public Health Policy,* 267–275.

Terris, M. (1994). Determinants of health: A progressive political platform. *Journal of Public Health Policy, 15(1),* 5.

Wood T. D. (1924). *Health education: A program for public schools and teacher training institutions.* Joint Committee on Health Problems in Education of the National Education Association and the American Medical Association. New York: National Education Association.

PART II

Theoretical Models and Evaluation Methods in Health Promotion and Disease Prevention

Theoretical Approaches Guiding the Development and Implementation of Health Promotion Programs

Connie L. Kohler, Diane Grimley, and Kim Reynolds

Introduction

This chapter describes several theories and models that have been used to explain behavior and to design health promotion and disease prevention programs. Behavioral theories are explanations of what influences people to do the things they do. Behavioral theories generally identify the determinants of behavior, that is, those factors that are thought to be causally related to the behavior. Theories may also identify the mechanisms by which the determinants influence the behavior. Theories are used in several ways to guide the researcher in deciding what research questions are important to ask and to guide the development, implementation, and evaluation of health promotion programs. Theories guide health promotion research by providing propositions about what behavioral factors are related to a health problem and what factors are important to address in working on the problem. For example, smoking is a behavior causally related to many types of cancer. To address smoking and cancer as a public health problem, health researchers and practitioners may ask such questions as: Why do people smoke? What influences people to start smoking? What makes it hard to stop smoking? Why don't people quit in the face of so much information that it is dangerous? A theory can provide a starting place to look for answers to these questions.

In addition to looking for factors that influence a behavior, theory is used to develop programs to modify the behavior. For example, a theory that youth begin to smoke because of peer influence and the desire to rebel against parents could be tested by interviewing smoking and nonsmoking youth and comparing them to see if

Connie L. Kohler and Diane Grimley • Department of Health Behavior, School of Public Health, UAB Center for Health Promotion, University of Alabama at Birmingham, Birmingham, Alabama 35294. *Kim Reynolds* • Center for Behavioral Studies, AMC Cancer Research Center, Lakewood, Colorado 80214.

Handbook of Health Promotion and Disease Prevention, edited by Raczynski and DiClemente. Kluwer Academic/Plenum Publishers, New York, 1999.

the factors of peer influence and desire to rebel actually differentiate those who begin to smoke from those who do not. If the data support the theory, the theory can be used to develop smoking prevention programs that employ positive peer influences and constructive means of rebelling against parents. Other solutions to the problem of smoking may be based on different theories. For example, based on a theory that people do things that they have the most reasons for doing, a stop-smoking class may ask people to identify reasons for quitting that outweigh their reasons for smoking.

Finally, a theory can guide efforts to evaluate the solutions to health problems by helping answer such questions as: Did the intervention work as the theory predicted it would? Should the intervention be altered or do the results suggest that the theory is not appropriate for this application?

Development of Modern Behavioral Theories

Several theories have been developed to explain the factors that determine behavior and the mechanisms by which they do so. The behavioral theories reviewed in this chapter come from behavioral and social psychology. Early behavioral theory was based on the idea that actions are driven by external reinforcements which "stamp in" the behavior as a response to a particular stimulus. Such radical behaviorism has given way to more recent views theorizing that *external* factors (e.g., reinforcements) determine behavior to the extent that they are *internally* processed (e.g., thought about and desired) by the individual. For example, one cognitive–behavioral view is that external reinforcements, such as rewards, can cause certain behaviors when a person expects and values (cognitive processes) that reward. Thus, a supervisor's approval would be a determinant of an employee's behavior (e.g., arriving on the job 5 minutes early) only if the employee expects early arrival to elicit supervisor approval and supervisor approval is valued by the employee. Theories that employ this notion are often referred to as *expectancy value theories* (Bandura, 1997).

Expectancy value theories are those that explain behavior, at least in part, in terms of the *expected outcome* or consequences of the behavior (e.g., if I show up for work 5 minutes early, my supervisor will approve of me), and the *value* the individual puts on that consequence or outcome (e.g., I value my supervisor's approval). Thus, a particular behavior is more likely if the individual perceives it will lead to a valued outcome. Viewed in this way, learned behavior can be thought of as influenced by a combination of: (1) external social and environmental factors that provide the cues for and consequences of behavior, and (2) internal cognitive factors that influence a person's perceptions of the environment and their evaluation of what they perceive.

Overview

This chapter will cover four theories commonly applied to health behavior. The health belief model of Rosenstock and colleagues (Rosenstock, 1974), the theory of reasoned action developed by Ajzen and Fishbein (1980); social cognitive theory developed by Bandura (1986), and the transtheoretical model of change (Prochaska & DiClemente, 1983, 1984) explain why people behave as they do and suggest how people may go about changing their behavior. For each theory, the components are outlined, research applying the theory is reviewed, and suggestions are made for the use of the theory in health promotion and disease prevention.

The Theory of Reasoned Action

In the theory of reasoned action, developed by Ajzen and Fishbein (1980), a number of factors related to values and expectations explain behavior. Figure 1 shows the model that summarizes the theory of reasoned action. Analyzing Fig. 1 from right to left reveals that the immediate determinant of behavior is *intention*. A woman puts her young toddler into a safety seat in the backseat of the car as a result of a conscious intention to do so. Intention is a function of two other variables: attitude and subjective norm. The woman with a positive attitude toward putting her child into the safety seat is more likely to intend to do so. This positive attitude is viewed as a result of two additional factors: (1) the belief that the behavior (e.g., putting the child into the safety seat) results in a particular outcome (e.g., increased safety); and (2) the evaluation of that outcome (e.g., increased safety is viewed as a good thing). Thus, the attitude that determines intention is a function of expectations and values.

Intention is also a function of subjective norm. Subjective norm is defined as the person's subjective belief about what those people important to her or him think about the behavior. If the woman believes that the norm is positive (e.g., most people important to her think putting children into safety seats is a good thing to do), she is more likely to intend to do so. Like the attitude, the subjective norm has two cognitive determinants: (1) beliefs about what significant others think one should do; and (2) one's motivation to comply with those significant others. In the case of the woman and her toddler, she may feel that her husband feels strongly that safety seats are actually dangerous because they could trap children in burning or sinking cars; however, the mothers with whom she has social contact strongly believe in using safety seats at all times. If the woman is more motivated to comply with her husband, the subjective norm will be negative; if she is more motivated to comply with her group of friends, the subjective norm will be positive. Subjective norm is based on the perceived opinions of all people felt to be important and the strength of the woman's motivation to comply with each person's opinion.

All the variables in the model are also influenced by other factors as illustrated in the far left of Fig. 1. These are considered to be external to the model and to be mediated by the model factors to predict behavior. When applying the theory of reasoned action, it is necessary to define the model variables in terms of the specific target group and behavior. Ajzen and Fishbein (1980) have provided detailed strategies for doing so. They recommend that representatives of target groups for whom the theory will be used be employed to identify the likely beliefs, values, and attitudes of that group and to identify the people most commonly viewed as salient by that group. When these variables are specifically defined in this way, the authors provide a means of measuring their relative influence on intention. Thus, to predict the intention of young mothers to use child safety seats in the back of car, the most prevalent beliefs, values, and attitudes, as well as the most influential people, are first identified by interviewing women representative of the target audience. The next step is to construct a questionnaire that measures the degree to which individuals in the target audience hold the identified attitudes and normative beliefs and intend to use child safety seats. This questionnaire is then administered to the target audience and the resulting data are analyzed to determine the relative influence of the factors on the intention of the mothers to use child safety seats. The strength of the association of intention with actual safety seat use can also be determined.

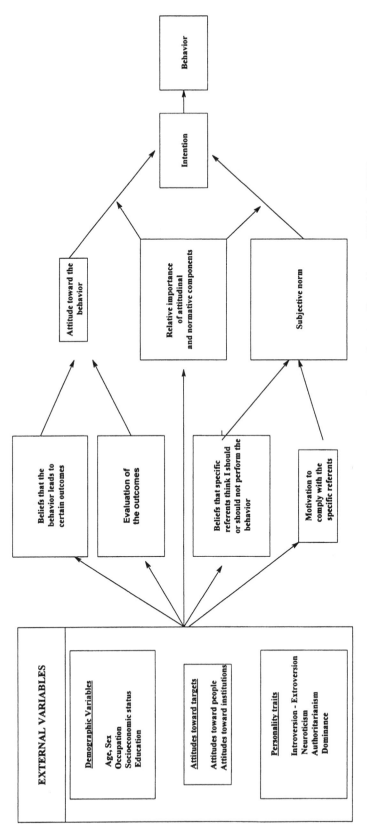

Figure 1. Relationships among the variables in the theory of reasoned action. From Ajzen and Fishbein (1980).

Health Behavior Research Using the Theory of Reasoned Action

The theory of reasoned action has been used as a tool for predicting certain health behaviors based on beliefs and values. The theory also has been applied to the development of health promotion interventions. The theory and its components have been shown to be weakly to moderately associated with such behaviors as contraception, condom use, physical activity, health screening, and provider behavior (Adler, Kegeles, Irwin, & Wibblesman, 1990; Baker, Morrison, Carter, & Verdon, 1996; Fisher, Fisher, & Rye, 1995; Ford & Norris, 1995; Blue, 1995; Taylor, Montano, & Koepsell, 1994; Millstein, 1996). Because the theory of reasoned action explicitly examines the role played by perceptions of norms, it has been viewed as a useful theory for adolescent behavior and for couple behavior.

Critique and Suggestions for Use

A major limitation of the theory is that it appears most appropriate for explaining behaviors that are entirely under a person's control, and this is not often the case for a number of health-related behaviors. Behaviors that are in response to an addiction, such as drug use or unprotected sex among drug users, may not be entirely intentional. Similarly, behaviors that have been practiced for a long time and have become more or less habitual, such as brushing and flossing teeth or taking birth control pills, may not be seen as a function of rational decision making that leads to intention each time the behavior is performed. Indeed, the theory of reasoned action may provide a reasonable explanation for the adoption of new practices that may later become routine, but the roles of attitude and subjective norm become overshadowed by the strength of past behavior in predicting habitual or routine health behaviors (Bentler & Speckert, 1979; Kohler, 1991).

The theory of planned behavior (Ajzen, 1988, 1991) is a later adaptation of the theory of reasoned action that adds a component: *perceived behavioral control*. Perceived behavioral control is thought to influence behavior both directly and indirectly through intention. Perceived behavioral control is a person's perception of how difficult a behavior is to perform. Just as attitude and subjective norm are influenced by specific categories of beliefs, perceived behavioral control is influenced by control beliefs and perceived power. Control beliefs are defined as beliefs about the resources for or impediments to doing the behavior. Perceived power is defined as the perceived effect of each resource or impediment on the difficulty of performance (Montano, Kasprzyk, & Taplin, 1996). Thus, a person who believes (1) that prayer is an available resource in quitting an addictive behavior and (2) that prayer can have a strong impact on making quitting less difficult should have higher perceived behavioral control over quitting. This higher perceived behavioral control should contribute to stronger intentions to quit and greater quitting success.

The theory of planned behavior has been used to identify factors that influence children's participation in vigorous activity (Craig, Goldberg, & Dietz, 1996), to predict intention to participate in physical activity and blood donation (Godin, Valois, & Lepage, 1993; Courneya & McAuley, 1995; Giles & Cairns, 1995), and to predict physician delivery of preventive services (Millstein, 1996).

Both the theory of planned behavior and the theory of reasoned action can be applied to developing health behavior interventions. In doing so, it is most useful to know the target audiences' response to assessments of the distal components of the model: behavioral belief and outcome evaluations, normative beliefs, and motivation to comply, and, in the theory of planned behavior, control beliefs and perceived power. Modifying these beliefs and values should lead to a change in attitudes and subjective norms and a resulting change in intention and behavior. For example, based on theory of reasoned action research on acquired immunodeficiency syndrome (AIDS) preventive behavior, Fisher *et al.* (1995) developed interventions to change attitudes, subjective norms, and intentions by focusing on the underlying beliefs and values that were empirically identified in the research. Similarly, Thuen and Rise (1994) used the theory of reasoned action to identify promising messages for persuasive communications to young adolescents regarding seat belt use. They found the "most promising messages" would be those that emphasize injury reduction and feelings of safety from seat belt use. The theory of planned behavior can also be applied to the development of interventions. When using this framework, attempts to modify beliefs and values are accompanied by attempts to modify people's perceptions of competence for performing the behavior, thus influencing perceived behavioral control.

The Health Belief Model

The health belief model (HBM) was originally developed by researchers in the public health service to explain the use of preventive health services (Rosenstock, 1974). Since that time, the model has been modified and used to explain a wide array of health-related behaviors (Bluestein and Rutledge, 1993; Gielen, Faden, O'Campo, Kass, &Anderson, 1994; Harrison, Mullen, & Green, 1992; Hyman, Baker, Ephraim, Moadel, & Philip, 1994; Janz & Becker, 1984; Lux & Petosa, 1994; Mirotznik, Feldman, & Stein, 1995; Schafer, Keith, & Schafer, 1995). In addition, the model has been used to design interventions targeting a range of behaviors and populations (Reynolds, West, & Aiken, 1990; Aiken, West, Woodward, Reno, & Reynolds, 1994). This section will review the components and empirical support for the model and will make suggestions for the use of the HBM in health promotion and disease prevention. Several reviews of the HBM have been published recently and should be consulted for a more in-depth analysis of the model (Sheeran & Abraham, 1996; Strecher & Rosenstock, 1997).

The main components of the HBM have remained intact since its inception in the 1950s (Rosenstock, 1974). These components include perceived severity of a disease threat, perceived susceptibility to the disease threat, perceived benefits of an advocated health action, perceived barriers to the completion of that action, and cues to action (Fig. 2). The component of perceived self-efficacy was added to the model some years later in recognition of the importance of this construct in the explanation of health behavior (Strecher & Rosenstock, 1997; Bandura, 1986, 1997; Rosenstock, Strecher, & Becker 1988). Various other factors that might influence behavior, such as socioeconomic status, gender, and environmental factors, are assumed to influence behavior by modifying the levels of one of the existing HBM components. In essence, the HBM components mediate the effects of these variables on behavior. For example, the level of education that a person has attained may influence his or her perception of susceptibility to a disease. A person of higher educational attainment may get health information from different sources than someone of lower educational attainment, influencing his or her

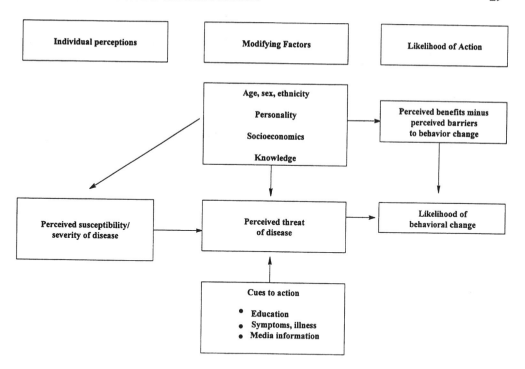

Figure 2. The health belief model. From Glanz, Marcus-Lewis, and Rimer (1997).

notions of the way in which the disease is spread and the likelihood of contracting the disease. Thus, the relationship between level of education and health behavior is mediated through the person's perception of susceptibility to disease.

The HBM Components

The HBM is defined as a single model with components that interact to explain health behavior. In order to illustrate the HBM in more detail, the components are presented separately in the following sections.

Perceived Susceptibility and Severity

The HBM postulates that increased perceived severity and increased perceived susceptibility combine to increase perceived threat from a disease. Higher perceived threat, in turn, increases the probability that a person will engage in an advocated health action. For example, the degree to which a middle-aged woman feels that heart disease is a threat to her will depend on her assessment of the likelihood that she can get heart disease (perceived susceptibility) and her perception of the consequences for her health and quality of life if she develops heart disease (perceived severity). If she feels that her personal susceptibility is high and that the consequences of heart disease are severe, she will believe that heart disease is a higher threat and will be more likely to take action than a woman who feels that she is not susceptible or that the consequences of heart disease are minimal.

Perceived Benefits and Barriers

The perceived benefits of the advocated health action also influence the likelihood that a person will take action. The higher the perceived benefits of a health action, including both positive health outcomes and positive social outcomes, the higher the likelihood that a person will take action. Perceived barriers are the costs associated with taking the advocated action. These can include monetary costs, but also include physical discomfort and social costs such as resistance from family members to taking a preventive action. The lower the perceived barriers to action, the more likely someone is to take action. The HBM also states that the perceived benefits of a health action and the perceived barriers to that action will combine. If the benefits outweigh the costs, the individual will be more likely to take action. If the barriers outweigh the benefits, the person is less likely to take action. Consider again the example of a woman who is considering action to prevent heart disease. She may be considering beginning an exercise program as a means of preventing heart disease. Before deciding to pursue an exercise program, she will first decide whether a regular program of exercise will reduce the threat posed by heart disease. She may consider whether a regular program of exercise will substantially reduce the probability that she will get heart disease and have a heart attack in the coming years. If she feels that this preventive effect is a benefit of exercise, she is more likely to take action. She may also consider other benefits of exercise including the advantage of helping to control her weight, the feeling of well-being that occurs when she exercises, and the possibility of meeting new friends while exercising. However, prior to exercising, the woman will also consider the costs of exercising, including the physical pain of beginning a new exercise regimen, the monetary costs of equipment or an exercise club membership, and the additional time needed to exercise regularly. If, in her mind, the benefits (e.g., reduced heart disease risk, increased fitness) outweigh the barriers (monetary cost, time commitment), she will be more likely to take action.

Perceived Self-Efficacy

Perceived self-efficacy acts in the HBM as a special case of a perceived barrier (Strecher & Rosenstock, 1997; Rosenstock *et al.*, 1988). If a person does not feel capable of taking a health action, this lack of perceived self-efficacy can serve as a barrier to action. In the earlier example, if the woman does not feel capable of beginning or maintaining an exercise program, this lack of perceived self-efficacy increases her perceived barriers and decreases the chance that she will start exercising.

Cues to Action

Cues to action occur to help trigger the health action. Cues to action can be external to the person, such as a news story about a health problem or the occurrence of a disease in a friend, or cues can be symptoms that a person feels from a disease, such as pain. For example, the woman who is considering starting an exercise program (because her perceived threat from heart disease is high and the benefits to exercise outweigh the barriers) may begin the exercise program only after hearing about a co-worker having a heart attack; that information cues her to act.

Health Behavior Research Using the HBM

Empirical support for the HBM has been received through numerous studies that have related the model components to an outcome measure, usually using correlational methods. In the majority of these studies, the separate components of the model have been examined rather than testing the full model and its posited interrelationships, although some attempts have been made to test different versions of the model as a whole (Chen & Land, 1986; Rundall & Wheeler, 1979). Two major reviews of the HBM have been published. Most recently, Harrison *et al.* (1992) conducted a meta-analysis on four of the major HBM constructs: susceptibility, severity, benefits, and barriers. Starting with 488 studies on adults, the authors applied various exclusion criteria and applied a meta-analysis methodology to 16 studies that examined the relationship of the four HBM constructs to a screening, risk reduction, or adherence outcome measures. The authors found that for all studies combined, each component had a significant relationship with the outcomes measured. The percentage of variance in the outcome measures accounted for by the HBM constructs ranged between 0.1 and 9%. The retrospective studies in the analysis produced stronger effects for benefits and costs compared to the prospective studies, while the prospective studies demonstrated a stronger effect for severity compared to the retrospective studies. In sum, this meta-analysis suggests that each of the four major HBM components of susceptibility, severity, benefits, and barriers are related to behavior, but that these relationships are modest, accounting for a very small percentage of variance in a wide range of outcomes.

An earlier review was completed in 1984 by Janz and Becker (1984) and computed significance ratios for HBM components of susceptibility, severity, benefits, and barriers in 46 studies of preventive behavior and sick role behavior, such as compliance with a therapeutic regimen. This review found substantial support for the HBM components, with associations found with various measures of health action in both prospective and retrospective studies. The perceived barriers component was found to have the strongest association with both preventive health behavior and sick-role behavior across the 46 studies reviewed, while perceived severity had the weakest associations. Perceived severity was more strongly associated with sick-role behavior than with preventive health behavior. Perceived susceptibility and perceived benefits were associated with both preventive health behavior and sick-role behavior; however, perceived susceptibility was a stronger contributor to preventive health behavior than to sick-role behavior, while perceived benefits was more strongly related to sick-role behavior than to preventive health behavior.

Critique and Suggestions for Use

The HBM provides a reasonable organization of several key psychosocial concepts that appear to influence health behavior. As such, the model can be used by health promotion and disease prevention specialists to organize their thinking to target these key influences on behavior. Intervention components can be developed that address these important determinants of health behavior. Below is a simple hypothetical example of how the HBM can be used for the design of a primary prevention intervention.

Primary prevention involves the actions taken to prevent chronic or infectious diseases before they occur (Simons-Morton, Greene, & Gottlieb, 1995). One example of primary prevention is the modification of eating behaviors, which can help prevent heart disease, cancer, and other diseases and reduce mortality in the United States (McGinnis & Foege, 1993). This example describes an intervention developed to reduce the amount of fat consumed by adults and to be delivered as part of an adult education class on diet and exercise. In developing the intervention, the first consideration is the way in which each of the components of the HBM relate to changes in dietary behavior. Perceived susceptibility and severity, related to the types of diseases that are influenced by poor diet, include heart disease and certain forms of cancer. To increase perceived susceptibility to these diseases, the intervention might include information on the relationship between fat consumption and heart disease and cancer. In addition, the consequences of these diseases should be described to help increase perceived severity. Next, the classes could include activities focusing on the benefits for decreased fat consumption, for example, the reduction of risk for heart disease and cancer, to improve one's appearance, and to increase feelings of good health. This should increase perceived benefits for reduced fat consumption.

A diverse set of barriers might exist for the modification of an individual's diet, including resistance from family members, reduced preference for foods made with less fat, increased monetary cost of purchasing foods with less fat, and the need to learn new food preparation skills. The intervention program must identify and directly address these factors to reduce the participants' perceived barriers for taking the steps necessary to reduce dietary fat intake. Intervention steps to reduce perceived barriers might include teaching participants to purchase lower-fat food items in a cost-effective way, teaching participants to prepare appetizing low-fat food items, and teaching participants to slowly introduce low-fat food items to the family to prevent resistance to dietary modifications. Many of these activities will also increase perceived self-efficacy to eat foods with less fat. If participants are taught to purchase and prepare low-fat foods, they will feel more strongly that they are able to modify their diets, thus increasing perceived self-efficacy and reducing perceived barriers. Finally, cues to action can be structured into the intervention in several ways. For example, follow-up postcards or newsletters can be sent to participants a few months after they leave the program, reminding them to eat less fat in their diet.

Although limited in scope to perceptual variables, the HBM can provide a useful framework for analyzing the psychosocial determinants of health behavior and for developing several components for use in interventions. Health promoters should consider the HBM as one of several models they might use when designing disease prevention interventions.

Social Cognitive Theory

A social cognitive theory of behavior has been developed extensively by Albert Bandura (1986, 1997). To understand Bandura's social cognitive theory (referred to in his earlier work as social learning theory), it is important to view *behavior* in the context of the *environmental* events and *personal* factors that influence it and are, in turn, influenced by the *behavior*. This phenomenon of the three elements (behavior, environment, and person) all influencing each other is known as *reciprocal determinism* and is often diagramed as in Fig. 3. For example, consider the behavior of lighting a ciga-

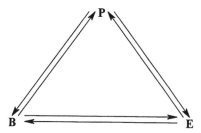

Figure 3. Reciprocal determinism in social cognitive theory. From Bandura (1986).

rette in the nonsmoking section of a restaurant. The behavior itself was probably in-fluenced by the person's thoughts about wanting to smoke and some environmental cues, such as the server removing the dinner plates from the table. However, the light-ing up behavior has an immediate influence on the environment in which other din-ers turn and glare at the smoker. This hostile environment influences the person's thought patterns, he realizes he is in a nonsmoking area, and initiates a nonsmoking behavior (i.e., puts out the cigarette).

Cognitive Capabilities within the Person

Given the framework of reciprocal determinism, social cognitive theory focuses on personal and environmental factors that influence behavior. Persons are seen as hav-ing a number of capabilities that enable them to learn and behave in complex ways:

1. *Symbolizing capability and forethought capability.* A person can use symbols to represent what is encountered in their world, and using this symbolizing ca-pability can think ahead (forethought) about what might happen in a given situation.
2. *Vicarious capability.* Because of symbolic capability, a person need not di-rectly experience something to learn about it; learning can occur vicariously by observing others' behavior and its consequences.
3. *Self-regulatory capability.* A person can set internal standards or goals and evaluate their own actions against these goals.
4. *Self-reflective capability.* A person can reflect on their own thoughts and be-haviors and adjust them if they appear invalid.

Determinants of Behavior

Similar to expectancy value theories, Bandura's social cognitive theory views the expected consequences or outcomes of a behavior (generally referred to as outcome expectations) as a major determinant of the behavior. For example, a person whose ex-pectation is that using a seat belt leads to the desired consequence of protection is more likely to buckle up than one whose expectation is that seat belts trap drivers in burn-ing cars. People learn these expectations primarily through four mechanisms:

1. Direct experience of the effects produced by their actions.
2. Vicarious experience of the effects produced by somebody else's actions.

3. Judgments voiced by others.
4. Inferred knowledge from what is already known.

Direct experience refers to learning expectations through directly experiencing outcomes produced by one's own actions. When people try a new behavior, they observe the effects of their action. If the action successfully leads to a desired outcome, the behavior will likely be performed again in the expectation that it will again result in the desired outcome. For example, an amateur musician picking out a tune on a piano may try F# in the hope that it is the next note in the song. If it sounds like expected, the person will continue to play F# at that point in the song. On the other hand, behaviors that do not lead to desired outcomes are discarded, for example, if F# sounds higher or flatter than expected, the person will not play it again at that point in the song. Enactive learning, that is, learning from direct experience, is more than a response conditioned by its desired consequences in the absence of any mental activity. Symbolizing capability and forethought play a large role. That is, the person thinks about (symbolizes) how the next note should sound and predicts that playing F# will produce the sound.

Vicarious learning refers to learning expectations from the outcomes produced by somebody else's actions. Vicarious learning is a type of observational learning and the ability of humans to use this type of information greatly accelerates human development by making trial-and-error learning unnecessary in many cases. Social learning is heavily influenced by observing the actions of others—often referred to as *models*—and the consequences they experience as a result of their actions. Because people can learn vicariously through mass media such as television and books, vicarious learning is a powerful influence on behavior. Television audiences, for example, observe the rewarding outcomes experienced from purchasing a particular car, drinking a certain soft drink, or using a certain cleaning product. On the other hand, behavior can be inhibited by vicarious learning if the modeled behavior is not rewarded. If a child in daycare sees that another child gets only a teacher's frown in response to using baby talk, the child is much less likely to try that behavior. The outcomes we expect from our behaviors are most often learned from either vicarious learning or direct experience.

Persuasory learning refers to learning expectations through judgments voiced by others. Not all knowledge is available to all humans through direct or vicarious experience. Knowledge of highly specialized information or of religious beliefs, for example, must often come from various experts in these fields. Although we may have learned from direct or vicarious experience that eating too many fatty foods can lead to obesity, we rely on the judgments of experts to tell us it can also lead to high cholesterol levels or cancer risk. In another domain, an expectation that committing certain sins will result in eternal damnation comes from the persuasive judgments of religious leaders.

Inferred knowledge refers to the fact that people can hold expectations about outcomes when they have not experienced, observed, or been told what to expect. This is so if they can derive knowledge from what they already know by using rules of inference. When the world consistently responds as expected to a given behavior, an individual may begin to infer rules about what types of things lead to what, generalizing the knowledge gained from direct, vicarious and persuasory learning. For example, a 2-year-old takes his brother's cookie and gets scolded. He then observes a fellow preschooler take another child's cookie and get scolded. From these experiences he may come to expect that taking cookies leads to scolding. Although he has not seen, experienced, or been told that taking candy leads to scolding, he may infer this knowledge from his experience with cookies.

Efficacy expectations are another determinant of behavior. A major component of social cognitive theory is the concept of efficacy expectations. Efficacy expectations differ from outcome expectations. Knowing that eating less than 1000 calories a day will result in weight loss does not mean the person desiring weight loss will perform in the desired way. The behavior of cutting calories depends on both the expected outcome of weight loss and the person's judgment that he or she is capable of cutting calories. This judgment of one's capability to behave in a way that attains desired outcomes is called *perceived self-efficacy*. Whatever outcome is expected from a given behavior (outcome expectation), if the person does not expect that the behavior can be performed efficaciously (efficacy expectation), it likely will not be tried. Thus, if a man who wishes to be slimmer feels incapable of cutting back on fried foods and desserts, he will not perform the behavior of cutting back, even though he may expect that it would lead to the desired outcome of slimness.

Perceived self-efficacy also influences people's thought patterns and emotional reactions as they anticipate behaving and as they behave in certain ways. A person who has poor self-efficacy for a behavior, such as public speaking, may dwell on a perceived lack of skill or other deficiency and potential problems may appear worse than they really are. This could lead to poor performance because the person is distracted from the task by negative feelings. In contrast, a person whose self-efficacy is strong will put their attention and effort into the demands of the situation.

People's beliefs about their own efficacy come from several sources. The most powerful source is direct experience. Direct successful experience leads to more positive perceptions of efficacy; direct failure experience leads to more negative perceptions of efficacy. If the magazine seller who starts out with little or no self-efficacy first encounters a couple of kind souls or avid readers who eagerly order subscriptions, self-efficacy may be boosted by the experience.

Another source of self-efficacy information is vicarious experience. Watching a model succeed at something can increase the observer's self-efficacy for doing the same thing, especially if the model and circumstances are seen as similar to those of the observer. Children have been known to imitate fairly risky behaviors seen on television because a young performer made it look easy. Many teenagers feel very efficacious about their driving skills long before ever getting behind the wheel of a car. This is, at least in part, a function of the thought, "If my parents can do that, I can do it."

A third source of efficacy information is verbal persuasion. Although verbally persuading someone that they have the skills to carry out a task is less effective than direct or vicarious experience with success, it can get people to put greater effort into the task (e.g., "Keep trying, I know you can do it"). This increases effort and persistence, leading to increased chances of success and potentially increased perceived self efficacy.

Finally, people interpret their physiological state as information about their own ability to do a behavior. That is, when a person is in a performance situation and feels symptoms such as increased heart rate or "butterflies," the feelings are often interpreted as signs of failure, thus lowering the person's perception of capability. As noted above, this can divert the person's attention from performing the behavior to the physical feelings, contributing to a resulting poor performance, which reinforces the perception of impaired efficacy to perform.

Perceived self-efficacy has been widely studied, and there are many examples of perceived self-efficacy mediating health behavior. Better perceived self-efficacy has been associated with smoking cessation, increased physical activity in chronic obstructive pulmonary disease (COPD) patients, self-control of pain, self-management of chronic disease, and consistent use of condoms (Condiotte & Lichtestein, 1981; Colleti, Supnick, & Payne, 1985; Strecher, DeVellis, Becker, & Rosenstock, 1986; Holman & Lorig, 1992; Wulfert & Wan, 1993). This association is easy to understand: if a person does not believe the health behavior can be mastered and adhered to, there is little likelihood that the necessary effort to succeed will be put forth. Efficacy beliefs theoretically affect several processes of behavior change: whether people consider changing health habits; whether they have the necessary motivation and endurance to succeed at the change; whether they regain control after relapse; and how well the change is maintained (Bandura, 1997).

Efficacy expectations are differentiated from outcome expectations. People may believe that a given behavior can produce a certain outcome, but fail to behave in that way because they question whether they can actually do that behavior. For example, many of us would expect to experience a thrill from standing atop Mount Everest, but few of us will ever attempt the climb. On the other hand, outcome expectations can rarely be separated from efficacy expectations in analyzing behavior. This is because expected outcomes depend to a great extent on a person's judgment of how well they will be able to perform in given situations. Thus, the outcome expectation for running in a 10-kilometer race may be quite different for a 60-year-old woman who has not trained and for a 20-year-old woman who has run races for several years. The older woman's expectation may be to finish the race; the younger woman's may be to win the race.

Perceived self-efficacy may determine choice of action, how much effort to expend, and how long to persevere at the activity in the face of obstacles or unpleasantness. As noted above, few people even choose the action of climbing Mount Everest. People with low self-efficacy for correctly solving math problems often put less than maximum effort into taking math tests. People who do not feel they can sell may be persuaded to go door to door to sell magazines but may not persevere after one or two refusals. People may want the firm muscles that come from a regular exercise regimen but may not stick to it long enough to see the results.

Health communications should focus on self-efficacy in addition to providing knowledge about how to behave in a healthy manner. Bandura states that the most effective health communications give people the belief that they can alter their health habits and emphasize that success requires perseverant effort (Bandura, 1986).

Incentives and motivators are a third type of determinant of behavior. In social cognitive theory, incentives and motivation to behave come from outcome expectations. Motivation is often viewed as an *antecedent* of behavior, that is, the motivation occurs prior to the behavior. However, the incentive or motivation to behave actually comes from outcomes that occurred when the behavior was previously enacted. For example, if the outcome of helping a "little old lady" across the street was a generous tip, the expectation of a tip is the incentive for helping more "little old ladies." Such outcomes create expectations of similar outcomes on future occasions: If the outcome was rewarding, it increases the likelihood of repeating the action; if the outcome was punishing, the likelihood of repeating the action is decreased. As noted earlier, expected outcomes are generally determined by past direct experience or by observed consequences experienced by others (vicarious learning). Outcomes that are valued become the incentive to behave in a particular manner. For example, a person may find that cutting back on caffeine for a day resulted in a better night's rest. Similarly, the person may learn of this outcome from observing a colleague appear more rested and inquiring about the cause of this change. Either way it is learned—directly or vicariously—the expected outcome of more rest (if rest is valued) becomes the incentive for decreasing caffeine consumption in the future.

Observed outcomes experienced by others (vicarious incentives) motivate behavior most readily in situations where new learning is occurring; maintaining already learned behavior occurs most readily with direct incentives. Thus, seeing a fellow student receive praise for speaking up in class may motivate the shy student to try this behavior, but if the praise continues to go to others and is not directly experienced by the shy student, the speaking-up behavior will not be maintained. Pairing vicarious with direct incentives is also motivating because it provides the basis for comparative judgment: If Joe receives more praise than Adam, Adam may try harder for praise because he sees, through Joe, that it is possible to get even more of what he likes.

Not all vicarious experience of outcomes is motivating, even if the outcome is highly valued. Vicarious motivation is most effective when the model is considered to be similar to oneself, the context in which the behavior is performed is relevant to the observer's environment, the observer does not have much direct experience with the behavior, and the behavior is not perceived as complex. For example, if a man who has been married for 20 years watches a soap opera in which a virile young actor experiences the outcome of warm affection from his partner for using condoms, he (the married man) will not find it all that motivating to use condoms himself. That is because the model (young) was not similar to him (middle-aged) and the context was not similar to his (20 years of marriage). On the other hand, if a female college student watches a soap opera in which a young woman learns one of her partners is HIV positive and exclaims, "Thank God I always use condoms!", the college student may indeed find the vicarious incentive of HIV protection to be motivating for condom use.

Vicarious outcomes affect motivation through two mechanisms: they create outcome expectations that can serve as negative or positive incentives for action, and they create efficacy expectations when the model succeeds or fails.

Social Cognitive Theory and Health Behavior Change

Social cognitive theory is often applied to the development of programs to promote health behavior change. Behavior change includes two processes: acquisition of knowledge about the new behavior and adoption of the new behavior (Bandura, 1986). Knowledge of health-promoting behavior is often conveyed through models. It is fairly commonplace to question a person who is looking or acting especially "healthy" about their secrets of success. Knowledge is necessary but insufficient to change behavior. For the adoption of the new healthy behavior several conditions are necessary: (1) motivational conditions, such as aversive experiences or promises of immediate, desirable rewards; (2) the means to change through self-regulation skills such as monitoring behavior, setting goals, and arranging incentives; (3) the self-belief in one's capability to put forth the needed effort; and (4) possession of prerequisite knowledge and skills ("behavioral capability") and resources. Change happens more readily when the individual perceives that there is utility in the new behavior, that it is not too complex for the individual's skills, that it can be tried out briefly for purposes of evaluation, and that it is compatible with social norms and values.

Bandura (1997) lists four major components to include when developing health promotion programs aimed at changing populations. The first is an informational component to increase knowledge of the health risks and benefits of given health behaviors, providing a reason to change. Risks and benefits that are close in time to the behavior and personalized are most motivating. The second component is aimed at providing the means to change and includes teaching social and self-regulation skills to use in initiating preventive action. The third component is meant to build efficacy necessary to persevere in using skills in difficult situations. The final component is a social support component to address factors in the environment that can support change.

Critique and Suggestions for Use

Because the social cognitive theory is very complex and includes the notion of a dynamic interaction among the person, the environment, and behavior, it is not possible to test the theory as a whole in a single study. It may be for this reason that researchers often choose other, simpler models to use in developing and testing health behavior interventions, often adding the construct of self-efficacy as a mediator between other model constructs and behavior. Indeed, the most widely tested component of this theory is the construct of perceived self-efficacy and the extent to which it influences behavior has been well documented. The concept of outcome expectations also has been included in a number of other behavioral theories, including those addressing health behavior, often under different labels, such as beliefs about outcomes (theory of reasoned action), pros and cons of behavior change (transtheoretical model of change), and perceived benefits from the health behavior. The construct of outcome expectations also has empirical support in health behavior literature. Incentive motivators also are well studied, perhaps more so outside the realm of health behavior, and studies of their role in motivating health behavior change are less prominent than studies of the other determinants (although perceived threat, as conceptualized in the health belief model, is a potential incentive). The components of social cognitive theory provide a useful framework for explaining and predicting health behaviors and for developing interventions to change behavior. For example, to differentiate between teenage girls who do and do not become sexually active, it may be useful to measure girls' self-efficacy to refuse sex from a well-liked boy. In developing an intervention to promote sexual abstinence, increasing girls' self-efficacy for refusal behavior may be an important objective to address. Social cognitive theory suggests several ways to address efficacy expectations and outcome expectations in interventions, such as training in small, incremental units to promote success and showing models successfully performing the behavior.

The Transtheoretical Model of Change

The transtheoretical model of change (TMC) (Prochaska & DiClemente, 1983, 1984, 1986), evolved from research with smoking cessation and psychotherapy and more recently has been applied to a broad range of health behaviors. The basic premise of the TMC is that behavior change is a *process*, not an event, and that individuals are at varying levels of motivational readiness for change. Individuals at different points on the continuum of change can benefit from different intervention strategies that are matched to their current level, or stage, of change. The TMC offers promise in the development of health promotion and disease prevention programs by providing a useful framework for determining who may respond to what types of treatment strategies and when.

The model includes four key constructs: (1) the stages of change; (2) the processes of change; (3) decisional balance (pros and cons of change); and (4) situational self-efficacy (confidence and temptation). The stages of change reflect motivational, social learning, and relapse theories, whereas the processes of change, decisional balance, and self-efficacy are constructs derived from a wide range of major psychosocial theories; it is in this sense that the model is *trans*theoretical (Prochaska, DiClemente, Velicer, & Rossi, 1993).

Stages of Change

A major limitation of efforts to impact populations at risk is the failure to take into account the readiness of individuals to change target behaviors. The majority of health promotion and disease prevention programs have been developed based on the implicit or explicit assumption that individuals are ready to change when, in fact, research has shown that only a small percentage of individuals at risk (20 to 30%) are adequately prepared to change their behavior (DiClemente *et al.*, 1991; Grimley, Prochaska, & Prochaska, 1997; Prochaska *et al.*, 1993). Such action-oriented programs are missing the majority of populations at greatest risk because these individuals are less likely to respond to public health messages or to sign up for health promotion programs (Prochaska *et al.*, 1993).

To address this limitation of action-oriented programs so as to impact a greater number of individuals at risk, the TMC offers an alternative conceptualization of the structure of change by defining behavior change as an incremental and dynamic process (Prochaska, DiClemente, & Norcross, 1992b). The basic premise of the TMC is that individuals pass through a series of five stages of change in their efforts to modify behaviors, of which "action" is only one: precontemplation, contemplation, preparation, action, and maintenance. Understanding the stages of change provides health educators and practitioners with information regarding when a particular shift in attitudes, intention, and behavior may occur.

Precontemplation (Not Ready for Change)

Precontemplation describes the stage in which a person is not considering change in the foreseeable future, usually defined as some time within the next 6 months. Individuals in the precontemplation stage may be uninformed or underinformed about the consequences of their behavior, demoralized about their ability to change, or simply resistant to change. In the precontemplation stage, individuals tend to underestimate the positive aspects of change and overestimate the negative aspects (i.e., pros and cons).

Contemplation (Thinking about Change)

Contemplation is the stage in which individuals are seriously thinking about change. They realize that their behavior may be a problem and they are better informed and more open to feedback about their behavior. In the contemplation stage, people are more aware of the advantages of making a health behavior change, but they still overestimate the disadvantages. In other words, individuals in the contemplation stage are ambivalent about change; part of them wants to change, and part does not. This indecision, in conjunction with a lack of commitment to change, is the most distinctive characteristic of the contemplation stage.

Preparation (Ready to Change)

Preparation is the stage that combines intention with a behavioral criterion. Individuals in the preparation stage are intending to take action in the near future, usually within the next 30 days, and have taken some behavioral steps toward modifying the specific behavior (e.g., using condoms "sometimes" or "almost always" for STD/HIV prevention). The balance between the costs and benefits of engaging in the new healthy behavior has tipped to the positive side, but individuals still may have some doubts about their ability to engage consistently in the new behavior. Decision making and commitment are the most distinctive characteristics of the preparation stage.

Action (Initiating Change)

Action is the stage in which a person is overtly engaged in the new behavior. To reach the action stage, strict criteria, which vary depending on the behavior, must be met. For example, with condom use, the action criterion is using a condom "every time" one engages in sexual intercourse; with smoking cessation, the action criterion is zero cigarettes smoked. The action stage usually lasts for 6 months with most behaviors. Originally with smoking cessation, this stage was separated into 0- to 3-month early action and a 3- to 6-month later action period. No differences were found between early and late action in terms of the frequency of use of change processes used to quit smoking. Therefore, the 0- to 6-month period has been used to define the action stage, which is the busiest period of change (Prochaska & DiClemente, 1983).

Maintenance (Continuing Change)

Maintenance is the stage reached after 6 months of sustained action. In the maintenance stage, people do not have to work as hard as they did in the action stage because temptation to engage in the unhealthy behavior is decreasing and confidence in engaging in the new healthy behavior is increasing. Stabilizing behavior change and avoiding relapse are the hallmarks of the maintenance stage. In other words, maintenance is a continuation, not an absence, of change (Prochaska et al., 1992b).

Progression through the stages of change is often not linear; many individuals backslide and recycle through earlier stages. Individuals may cycle through the stages several times before they succeed in their efforts to change. Within the TMC, relapse is viewed as a normal part of the change process as opposed to a failure. This notion of relapse supports the idea that change is difficult; it is unreasonable to expect people not to have some problems with acquiring the new habit and to experience some "slips" (Grimley et al., 1997).

The notion that behavior change occurs in a series of stages is not unique to the TMC. Precursors of this stage model can be found in the writings of Horn and Waingrow (1966), Cashdan (1973), and Egan (1975). What is unique to the TMC as compared with other models of behavior change is its focus on the process of change, as well as the outcome.

Processes of Change

What do individuals do to progress from one stage to the next? The second dimension of the TMC, the processes of change, provides information on *how* people change. The processes of change represent both covert and overt activities individuals use in order to alter their experiences or environments, or both, in order to affect behavior, cognitions, or relationships. The processes of change emerged from a comparative analysis of the leading systems of psychotherapy (Prochaska, 1979). This comparative analysis identified a finite number of change processes among these theories. Each process is a broad category encompassing multiple techniques, methods, and intervention strategies historically associated with disparate theoretical orientations (Prochaska, DiClemente, Velicer, & Rossi, 1992a).

Table 1 provides a brief description of the ten processes of change that have received the most theoretical and empirical support to date. Five of the processes of change are cognitive–affective and evaluative in nature and have been labeled "experiential" and include consciousness raising, dramatic relief, environmental reevaluation, self-reevaluation, and self-liberation. The remaining five processes are behavioral in nature and, therefore, labeled as such (i.e., "behavioral): helping relationships, stimulus control, counterconditioning, contingency management, and social liberation. A brief description of each of the ten processes of change, with some sample intervention strategies, are given.

Research based on the TMC has shown that individuals tend to emphasize certain processes at certain stages in their efforts to modify unhealthy behaviors or to acquire new healthy ones (Prochaska, Velicer, DiClemente, & Fava, 1988). With most behaviors, the experiential processes (such as consciousness raising and environmental reevaluation) are used most often by individuals in the earlier stages of change (i.e., precontemplation, contemplation, and preparation), whereas the behavioral processes (such as stimulus control) are used by people in the later stages of action and maintenance. The integration of the processes with the stages of change provides a useful guide for delivering interventions (see Fig. 4). Once an individual's current stage has been assessed, interventionists can facilitate the use of the appropriate processes to help individuals progress to the next stage and, ultimately, to action more quickly. Limited success in a behavior change program may be the result of not matching change processes and techniques to a person's actual stage of readiness for change. Such mismatches may result in little or no effect, or even negative effects. Figure 4 displays the integration of the processes with stages of change for many health behaviors.

Decisional Balance and Self-Efficacy

In addition to the stages and processes of change, the TMC incorporates other core constructs: *decisional balance* (Prochaska *et al.*, 1994; Velicer, Prochaska, DiClemente, & Brandenburg, 1985), based on the decision-making theory of Janis and Mann (1977), and self-efficacy, which Bandura (1977, 1982, 1986) considers to be the most important construct in social cognitive theory.

Table 1. Titles, Definitions, and Sample Intervention Strategies of the Processes of Change

Process	Definition: sample intervention strategies
Consciousness raising	Increasing information about the healthy behavior change and awareness of one's risks: media campaigns, feedback, confrontations
Dramatic relief	Experiencing and expressing emotions associated with engaging in unhealthy behaviors: role plays, psychodrama, personal testimonies
Self-reevaluation	Realizing how one thinks and feels about oneself (i.e., self-image) with regard to engaging in an unhealthy behavior and how one's self-image might change if the behavior were to be changed: values clarification, imagery, exposure to healthy role models
Environmental reevaluation	Assessing how one's behavior may negatively impact others in her or his personal–social environment, or affect the physical environment: empathy training, documentaries, couple–family system interventions
Self-liberation	Choosing and firmly committing to change: go "public" with one's decision to change, set a "quit," or "start" date, empowerment
Helping relationships	Having someone to talk to, share feelings with, and get feedback from regarding the healthy behavior change: increasing social support, rapport building, therapeutic alliances
Counterconditioning	Learning new healthy behaviors to substitute for old unhealthy ones: relaxation exercises, assertiveness training, increasing positive "self-talk"
Contingency management	Rewarding oneself or being rewarded by others for making a healthy change: contingency contracts, overt and covert reinforcements
Stimulus control	Avoiding people, places, or situations that might trigger unhealthy behavior and adding cues to trigger healthy behavior: avoidance techniques, restructuring one's environment (e.g., removing alcohol or fatty foods; carrying condoms, etc), posting reminders to engage in healthy behaviors (e.g., taking prescribed medications)
Social liberation	Realizing changes in social norms with regards to certain health behaviors: advocacy, public policy changes (e.g., smoke-free malls, restaurants, etc.)

Stages of Change --->

    Processes

Precontemplation	Contemplation	Preparation	Action	Maintenance
Consciousness raising				
Dramatic relief				
Environmental reevaluation				
	Self-reevaluation			
		Self-liberation		
			Contingency management	
			Helping relationships	
			Counterconditioning	
			Stimulus control	
			Social liberation	

Figure 4. Integration of the processes with the stages of change.

The construct of decisional balance represents the cognitive and motivational aspects individuals consider about changing their behavior. Simply stated, individuals tend to weigh the subjective benefits (pros) against the costs (cons) involved with modifying an unhealthy behavior or adopting a new healthy behavior. This concept is very similar to the concept of perceived benefits and barriers in the health belief model and to the concept of outcome expectations in the social cognitive theory described earlier. Research based on the TMC has shown that a positive decisional balance (i.e., pros outweigh cons) is a good predictor of successful change with a broad range of health behaviors.

The pattern of the pros and cons across the stages of change is revealing. The cons of changing always outweigh the pros for individuals in the precontemplation stage; the opposite is true for those in the action and maintenance stages, with the pros always outweighing the cons. The crossover in relative importance of the pros and cons always takes place *before* an individual takes action [i.e., during the contemplation or preparation stage, depending on the problem under study (Prochaska *et al.*, 1994]. Figure 5

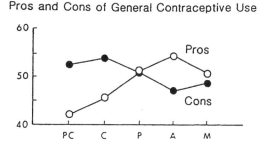

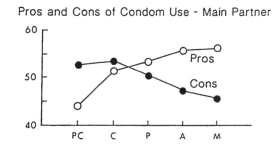

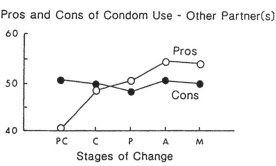

Figure 5. Pros and cons across the stages of change.

depicts representations of the pros and cons across the stages of condom use with main and other partner(s).

These findings with the pros and cons point out that the construct of decisional balance is relevant for understanding and predicting transition between the earlier stages of precontemplation, contemplation and preparation. During the later stages of action and maintenance, however, decisional balance is less important as a predictor of progress.

Within the framework of the TMC, the construct of self-efficacy represents an integration of the model of self-efficacy proposed by Bandura (1982, 1986) and the coping models of relapse and maintenance described by Shiffman (1986). Like the construct of decisional balance, self-efficacy has been integrated into the TMC as one of the critical constructs for assessing intermediate outcome and predicting future success (DiClemente, Prochaska, & Gilbertini, 1985; Velicer, DiClemente, Rossi & Prochaska, 1990).

The TMC has developed measures that operationalize self-efficacy in two ways: (1) confidence, which represents the level of confidence individuals have to engage in a particular behavior across specific situations; and (2) temptation, which represents individuals' reports of how tempted they would be not to engage in the target behavior in these same situations.

Across the stages of change, self-efficacy scores increase almost linearly from precontemplation to maintenance. More specifically, in the precontemplation stage, self-efficacy scores are the lowest; in the action and maintenance stages, self-efficacy scores are the highest. Figure 6 displays the representation of self-efficacy (confidence) across the five stages of change for condom use with main and other partners.

The Transtheoretical Model and Health Behavior

The TMC has been extensively applied to the measurement of a broad range of health behaviors such as smoking cessation, exercise, low-fat diet adoption, sun exposure, mammography screening, alcohol and other substance abuse, safer sex, physicians practicing preventive medicine (Prochaska *et al.*, 1994), condom and other contraceptive use (Galavotti *et al.*, 1995; Grimley *et al.*, 1996; Grimley, Riley, Bellis, & Prochaska, 1993; Grimley, Prochaska, Velicer, & Prochaska, 1995), adherence to prescribed medications (Johnson, Grimley, Bellis, Velicer, & Prochaska, 1996; Johnson, Grimley, & Prochaska, 1997), pharmacist readiness for rendering pharmaceutical care (Berger & Grimley, 1997), to name a few. However, many studies have been cross-sectional in nature, which is highly appropriate for measurement development and model testing, but is not useful in establishing causal effects. Although there are a number of ongoing intervention studies with results forthcoming, the effectiveness of the TMC has been demonstrated to date in published outcome studies only with smoking cessation, low-fat diets, and exercise.

Critique and Suggestions for Use

One of the major limitations of the TMC is that the stages of change construct is based on individual intention and behavior. For instance, the stages of change do not

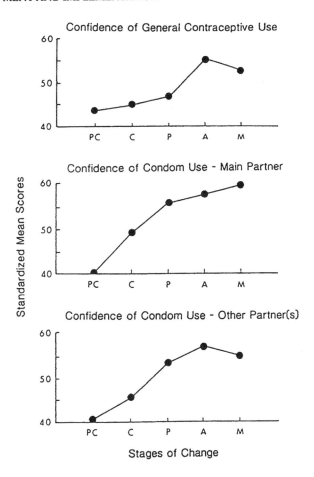

Figure 6. Self-efficacy across the stages of change.

take into account the dyadic nature of behaviors related to sex and condom use. The use of condoms and some other contraceptive methods is not always exclusively under one person's control, and this may influence the model's predictive ability (Galavotti *et al.*, 1995). Research is needed to clarify dyad, rather than individual, indicators of condom and other contraceptive use.

Many researchers and practitioners in the field are beginning to recognize that a "one-size-fits-all" intervention approach may not be appropriate for all individuals engaging in unhealthy behaviors. Change agents are shifting the focus of their efforts toward identifying the "best fit" between an individual's characteristics and intervention strategies. The transtheoretical model of change offers promise for this endeavor by matching behavioral interventions to where a person may be in the process of change. There also are other factors that could form the basis of an intervention that is matched to an individual, such as their perceived susceptibility, perceived self-efficacy, and knowledge about behavioral consequences. Such matching could be more effective and potentially cost-effective in changing unhealthy behaviors.

Summary

This chapter has outlined four theories that were developed to explain human behavior and have been used to explain why people do or do not engage in certain behaviors that lead to health-related outcomes. The theories have much in common: They share a focus on the perceptions of a person that influence his or her behavior, especially perceptions of the consequences of behavior, of what other people think about the behavior, and of their own ability to successfully perform the behavior. These theories have been tested and found useful in the context of explaining and changing health behavior. However, there is much more work to be done. Systematic, consistent use of the theories across a range of behaviors is necessary to advance the science of health behavior. Also, the theories must be applied to a range of populations, including population groups with different cultural perspectives and children. There are a number of theories that may be useful that were beyond the scope of this chapter and these, too, should be systematically and consistently applied to evaluate their usefulness. Finally, health behavior is an ideal context for developing new theories that build on what we already know but have greater explanatory power.

References

Adler, N. E., Kegeles, S. M., Irwin, C. E., & Wibbelsman, C. (1990). Adolescent contraceptive behavior: An assessment of decision processes. *The Journal of Pediatarics, 116,* 463–471.

Aiken, L. S., West, S. G., Woodward, C. K., Reno, R. R., & Reynolds, K. D. (1994). Increasing screening mammography in asymptomatic women: Evaluation of a second generation, theory-based program. *Health Psychology, 13,* 526–538.

Ajzen, I. (1988). *Attitudes, personality, and behavior.* Chicago: Dorsey Press.

Ajzen, I. (1991). The theory of planned behavior. *Organized Behavior and Human Decision Processes, 50,* 179–211.

Ajzen, I., & Fishbein, M. (1980). *Understanding attitudes and predicting social behavior.* Englewood Cliffs, NJ: Prentice-Hall.

Baker, S. A., Morrison, D. M., Carter, W. B., & Verdon, M. S. (1996). Using the theory of reasoned action (TRA) to understand the decision to use condoms in an STD clinic population. *Health Education Quarterly, 23,* 528–542.

Bandura, A. (1977). Self-efficacy: Toward a unifying theory of behavior change. *Psychological Review, 84,* 191–215.

Bandura, A. (1982). Self-efficacy mechanism in human agency. *American Psychologist, 37,* 122–147.

Bandura, A. (1986). *Social foundations of thought and action. A social cognitive theory.* Englewood Cliffs, NJ: Prentice Hall.

Bandura, A. (1997). *Self efficacy. The exercise of control.* New York: W. H. Freeman.

Bentler, P. M., & Speckert, G. (1979). Models of attitude–behavior relations. *Psychological Review, 86,* 452–464.

Berger, B., & Grimley, D. M. (1997). Pharmacists' readiness for rendering pharmaceutical care. *Journal of the American Pharmaceutical Association, 37,* 535–542.

Blue, C. L. (1995). The predictive capacity of the theory of reasoned action and the theory of planned behavior in exercise research: An integrated literature review. *Research in Nursing and Health, 18,* 105–121.

Bluestein, D., & Rutledge, C. M. (1993). Psychosocial determinants of late prenatal care: The health belief model. *Family Medicine, 25,* 269–272.

Cashdan, S. (1973). *Interactional psychotherapy: Stages and strategies in behavioral change.* New York: Grune & Stratton.

Chen, M. S., & Land., K. (1986). Testing the health belief model: LISREL analysis of alternative models of causal relationships between health beliefs and preventive dental behavior. *Social Psychology Quarterly, 49,* 45–60.

Colleti, G., Supnick, J. A., & Payne, T. J. (1985). The smoking self-efficacy quastionnaire (SSEQ): Preliminary scale development and validation. *Behavioral Assessment, 7,* 249–260.

Condiotte, M. M., & Lichtenstein, E. (1981). Self-efficacy and relapse in smoking cessation programs. *Journal of Consulting and Clinical Psychology, 49,* 648–658.

Courneya, K. S., & McAuley, E. (1995). Cognitive mediators of the social influence–exercise adherence relationship: A test of the theory of planned behavior. *Journal of Behavioral Medicine, 18,* 499– 515.

Craig, S., Goldberg, J., & Dietz, W. H. (1996). Psychosocial correlates of physical activity among fifth and eighth graders. *Preventive Medicine, 25,* 506–513.

DiClemente, C. C., Prochaska, J. O., & Gilbertini., M. (1985). Self-efficacy and the stages of self-change for smoking. *Cognitive Therapy and Research, 9,* 181–200.

DiClemente, C. C., Prochaska, J. O., Fairhurst, S. K., Velicer, W. F., Velasquez, M., & Rossi, J. S. (1991). The processes of smoking cessation: An analysis of precontemplation, contemplation and preparation stages of change. *Journal of Consulting and Clinical Psychology, 59,* 295–304.

Egan, G. (1975). *The skilled helper: A model for systematic helping and interpersonal relating.* Monterey, CA: Brookes/Cole.

Fisher, W. A., Fisher, J. D., & Rye, B. J. (1995). Understanding and promoting AIDS preventive behavior: Insights from the theory of reasoned action. *Health Psychology, 14,* 255–264.

Ford, K., & Norris, A. E. (1995). Factors related to condom use with casual partners among urban African-American and Hispanic males. *AIDS Education and Prevention, 7,* 494–503.

Galavotti, C., Cabral, R. J., Lansky, A., Grimley, D. M., Riley, G. E., & Prochaska, J. O. (1995). Validation of measures of condom and other contraceptive use among women at high risk for HIV infection and unintended pregnancy. *Health Psychology, 14,* 570–578.

Gielen, A. C., Faden, R. R., O'Campo, P., Kass, N., & Anderson, J. (1994). Women's protective sexual behaviors: A test of the health belief model. *AIDS Education and Prevention, 6,* 1–11.

Giles, M., & Cairns, E. (1995). Blood donation and Ajzen's theory of planned behaviour: An examination of perceived behavioural control. *British Journal of Social Psychology, 34(2),* 173–188.

Glanz, K., Marcus-Lewis, F., & Rimer, B. K. (1997). *Health behavior and health education: Theory, research, and practice.* San Francisco: Jossey-Bass.

Godin, G., Valois, P., & Lepage, L. (1993). The pattern of influence of perceived behavioral control upon exercising behavior: An application of Ajzen's theory of planned behavior. *Journal of Behavioral Medicine, 16,* 81–102.

Grimley, D. M., Riley, G. E., Bellis, J. M., & Prochasaka, J. O. (1993). Assessing the stages of change and decision-making for contraceptive use for the prevention of pregnancy, STDs, and HIV. *Health Education Quarterly, 20,* 455–470.

Grimley, D. M., Prochaska J. O., Velicer, W. F., & Prochaska, G. E. (1995). Contraceptive and condom use adoption and maintenance: A stage–paradigm approach. *Health Education Quarterly, 21,* 20–35.

Grimley, D. M., Prochaska, G. E., Velicer, W. F., Prochaska, J. O., Galavotti, C., Cabral, R. J., & Lansky, A. (1996). Cross-validation of measures assessing decisional balance and self-efficacy for condom use. *American Journal of Health Behavior, 20,* 406–416.

Grimley, D. M., Prochaska, G. E., & Prochaska, J. O. (1997). Application of the transtheoretical model to condom use. *Health Education and Research: Theory to Practice, 12,* 61–75.

Harrison, J. A., Mullen, P. A., & Green, L.W. (1992). A meta-analysis of studies of the health belief model with adults. *Health Education Research: Theory and Practice, 7,* 107–116.

Holman, H., & Lorig, K. (1992). Perceived self-efficacy in self-management of chronic disease. In R. Schwarzer (Ed.), *Self-efficacy: Thought control of action* (pp. 305–323). Washington, DC: Hemisphere.

Horn, D., & Waingrow, S. (1966). Some dimensions of a model for smoking behavior change. *American Journal of Public Health, 56,* 21–26.

Hyman, R. B., Baker, S., Ephraim, R., Moadel, A., & Philip, J. (1994). Health belief model variables as predictors of screening mammography utilization. *Journal of Behavioral Medicine, 17,* 391–406.

Janis, N. K., & Mann, L. (1977). *Decision making: A psychological analysis of conflict, choice and commitment.* New York: Free Press.

Janz, N. K., & Becker, M. H. (1984). The health belief model: A decade later. *Health Education Quarterly, 11,* 1–47.

Johnson, S. S., Grimley, D. M., Bellis, J. M., Velicer, W. F., & Prochaska, J. O. (1996). The transtheoretical model and compliance: A prediction study with oral medication use. Paper presented at the 4th International Congress of Behavior Medicine, Washington, DC.

Johnson, S. S., Grimley, D. M., & Prochaska, J. O. (1998). Prediction of adherence using the transtheoretical model: Implications for pharmacy care practice. *Journal of Social and Administrative Pharmacy, 15,* 135–148.

Kohler, C. L. (1991). *A test of a model to predict and explain contraceptive use.* Unpublished doctoral dissertation. The University of Alabama at Birmingham.

Lux, K. M., & Petosa, R. (1994). Using the health belief model to predict safer sex intentions of incarcerated youth. *Health Education Quarterly, 21,* 487–497.

McGinnis, J. M., & Foege, W.H. (1993). Actual causes of death in the United States. *Journal of the American Medical Association, 270,* 2207–2212.

Millstein, S. G. (1996). Utility of the theories of reasoned action and planned behavior for predicting physician behavior: A prospective analysis. *Health Psychology, 15,* 398–402.

Mirotznik, J., Feldman, L., & Stein, R. (1995). The health belief model and adherence with a community center-based, supervised coronary heart disease exercise program. *Journal of Community Health, 20,* 233–247.

Montano, D. E., Kasprzyk, D., & Taplin, S. H. (1996). The theory of reasoned action and the theory of planned behavior. In K. Glanz, F. M. Lewis, & B. K. Rimer (Eds.), *Health behavior and health education theory, research, and practice* (2nd ed., pp. 85–112). Second Edition. San Francisco: Jossey-Bass.

Prochaska, J. O. (1979). *Systems of psychotherapy: A transtheoretical analysis.* Pacific Grove, CA: Brookes/Cole.

Prochaska, J. O., & DiClemente, C. C. (1983). Stages and processes of self-change in smoking cessation: Toward an integrated model of change. *Journal of Consulting and Clinical Psychology, 51,* 390–395.

Prochaska, J. O., & DiClemente, C. C. (1984). *The transtheoretical approach: Crossing the traditional boundaries of therapy.* Homewood, IL: Dow Jones/Irwin.

Prochaska, J. O., & DiClemente, C. C. (1986). Toward a comprehensive model of change. In W. R. Miller and N. Heather (Eds.), *Treating addictive behaviors: Processes of change* (pp. 3–28). New York: Plenum Press.

Prochaska, J. O., Velicer, W. F., DiClemente, C. C., & Fava, J. (1988). Measuring processes of change: Applications to the cessation of smoking. *Journal of Consulting and Clinical Psychology, 56,* 520–528.

Prochaska, J. O., DiClemente, C. C., Velicer, W. F., & Rossi, J. S. (1992a). Criticism and concerns of the transtheoretical model in light of recent research. *British Journal of Addiction, 87,* 825–828.

Prochaska, J. O., DiClemente, C. C., & Norcross, J. C., (1992b). In search of how people change: Applications to addictive behaviors. *American Psychologist, 47,* 1102–1114.

Prochaska, J. O., DiClemente, C. C., Velicer, W. F., & Rossi, J. S. (1993). Standardized, individual, interactive, and personalized self-help programs for smoking cessation. *Health Psychology, 12,* 399–405.

Prochaska, J. O., Velicer, W. F., Rossi, J. S., Goldstein, M.G., Marcus, B. H., Rakowski, W., Fiore, C., Harlow, L. L., Redding, C. A., Rosenbloom, D., & Rossi, S. R. (1994). Stages of change and decisional balance for 12 problem behaviors. *Health Psychology, 13,* 39–46.

Reynolds, K. D., West, S. G., & Aiken, L. S. (1990). Increasing the use of mammography: A pilot program. *Health Education Quarterly, 17,* 429–441.

Rosenstock, I. M. (1974). Historical origins of the health belief model. *Health Education Monographs, 2,* 328–335.

Rosenstock, I. M., Strecher, V. J., & Becker, M. H. (1988). Social learning theory and the health belief model. *Health Education Quarterly, 15,* 175–183.

Rundall, T. G., & Wheeler, J. R. C. (1979). The effect of income on use of preventive care: An evaluation of alternative explanations. *Journal of Health and Social Behavior, 20,* 397–406.

Schafer, R. B., Keith, P. M., & Schafer, E. (1995). Predicting fat in diets of marital partners using the health belief model. *Journal of Behavioral Medicine, 18,* 419–433.

Sheeran, P., & Abraham, C. (1996). The health belief model. In M. Conner & P. Norman (Eds.), *Predicting health behaviour* (pp. 23–61). Buckingham, England: Open University Press.

Shiffman, S. (1986). A cluster analytic classification of smoking relapse episodes. *Addictive Behaviors, 11,* 295–307.

Simons-Morton, B. G., Greene, W. H., & Gottlieb, N. H. (1995). *Introduction to health education and health promotion.* Prospect Heights, IL: Waveland Press.

Strecher, V. J., & Rosenstock, I. M. (1997). The health belief model. In K. Glanz, F. Marcus-Lewis, & B. K. Rimer (Eds.), *Health behavior and health education: Theory, research, and practice* (pp. 41–59). San Francisco, CA: Jossey-Bass.

Strecher, V. J., DeVellis, B. M., Becker, M. H., & Rosenstock, I. M. (1986). The role of self-efficacy in achieving health behavior change. *Health Education Quarterly, 13,* 73–91.

Taylor, V. M., Montano, D. E., & Koespell, T. (1994). Use of screening mammography by general internists. *Cancer Detection and Prevention, 18,* 455–462.

Thuen, F., & Rise, J. (1994). Young adolescents' intention to use seat belts: The role of attitudinal and normative beliefs. *Health Education Research, 9,* 215–223.

Velicer, W. F., Prochaska, J. O., DiClemente, C. C., & Brandenburg, N. (1985). Decisional balance measure for assessing and predicting smoking status. *Journal of Personality and Social Psychology, 48,* 1279–1289.

Velicer, W. F., DiClemente, C. C., Rossi, J. S., & Prochaska, J. O. (1990). Relapse situations and self-efficacy: An integrated model. *Addictive Behaviors, 15,* 271–283.

Wulfert, E., & Wan, C. K. (1993). Condom use: A self-efficacy model. *Health Psychology, 12,* 346–353.

CHAPTER 4

Program Evaluation

Larry Fish and Laura Leviton

Introduction

The purpose of this chapter is to acquaint researchers with program evaluation as it applies to health promotion and disease prevention projects. Readers of this handbook are likely to become acquainted with evaluation in one or more contexts: They will read evaluation studies, they will purchase or commission evaluations, or they will evaluate programs that are planned or in progress. Each of these contexts has different requirements:

- The reader of evaluation studies should be sufficiently well-versed in research methods that he or she can critically appraise the appropriateness of evaluation given the program's stage of development. In addition, readers of evaluation reports should be acquainted with issues of research design, operationalization of treatments and measures, data collection procedures, and data analysis. To this end, we will (1) present information on evaluation stages and types, (2) briefly touch on major issues of methodology, and (3) present selected issues that are particularly important in health promotion program evaluation.
- The purchaser or client of an evaluation needs to know that many research questions may be appropriate, but only some of these questions can be answered, given logistics, resources available, and time constraints. The client must be able to appraise the evaluation critically. In addition, the client needs to be familiar with several issues presented in this chapter: the specification of goals and objectives, negotiations on an evaluation contract and budget, and ethical and professional issues for evaluators.
- The novice program evaluator is likely to have received at least some training in health promotion program techniques and theory-based applications to health promotion, as well as some exposure to traditional research methods,

Larry Fish and Laura Leviton • Department of Health Behavior, School of Public Health, UAB Center for Health Promotion, University of Alabama at Birmingham, Birmingham, Alabama 35294.

Handbook of Health Promotion and Disease Prevention, edited by Raczynski and DiClemente. Kluwer Academic/Plenum Publishers, New York, 1999.

measurement, and data analysis. In order to apply high-quality research methods, the new evaluator needs a careful orientation to the needs and dynamics of health promotion programs. The evaluator needs to understand and anticipate several issues that are discussed in this chapter: (1) how programs evolve; (2) how the evaluator can assist in the development of better goals and measurable objectives; (3) how to protect evaluation quality (and the evaluator's role) through contract and budget negotiations; and (4) how to maintain professional integrity.

Space does not permit a full discussion of these issues. Instead, we raise the issues here and refer the reader to the rich literature on the subject. Although a bibliography is presented for each point, it is worthwhile to introduce the reader to certain evaluation texts that are particularly important for further reading. We recommend two comprehensive texts that provide examples from many policy sectors: those by Rossi and Freeman (1993) and Wholey, Hatry and Newcomer (1994). The health promotion field frequently cites texts by Windsor, Baranowski, Clark, and Cutter (1984), Green and Lewis (1986), as well as the chapter on evaluation in Green and Kreuter's (1991) second edition of *Health Education Planning: An Educational and Environmental Approach,* one of the seminal texts in the field of health promotion. However, these health promotion-oriented texts provide only some of the information that is essential for the reader, client, or professional who conducts evaluation. Further, this chapter balances prescriptive and descriptive information about evaluation. On the one hand, the goal is to assure that readers know enough about mainstream evaluation viewpoints to make informed decisions in their roles as reader, client, or evaluator. However, we also want to portray the variety of legitimate viewpoints in evaluation.

The Evolution of Program Evaluation

Program evaluation evolved during the first half of the 1900s, along with a growing concern for scientific methods of assessment in business and education. It received its strongest impetus from the government-funded social programs that were implemented during and after the 1960s. At first, evaluation's goal was to determine whether social and educational programs were "working," and therefore whether they were worth the money spent on them. For this purpose, it was rarely distinguished from social research in any significant way. Beginning with Edward Suchman (1967), in the field of public health, writers on evaluation became more sensitive to the differences between evaluation and other applied research, and they described several goals and functions for their profession besides the assessment of whether something has "worked" (Shadish, Cook, & Leviton, 1991).

A Diversity of Viewpoints

There is a wide variety of viewpoints on the aims of evaluation and types of evaluation to be performed. As a field, evaluation has borrowed from social and behavioral research methodology, management, political science, and organizational behavior. It is employed in education, welfare studies, criminal justice, and urban development, as well as in health care and health promotion. Although there is some crossover, somewhat independent traditions of evaluation have evolved within these social service fields, notably in health care. Inevitably, there are differences among various authorities with respect to everything from terminology to ultimate purpose. While evaluators may differ in terminology and even in their ultimate purposes for evaluation, all serious evaluators subscribe to fundamental principles of scientific inquiry and ethical professional conduct. In practice, the purpose and particular approach to evaluation are often tailored to the problem at hand.

Because evaluation developed in several policy sectors simultaneously, different terminology developed to describe similar concepts. In the sections that follow, we present the equivalent terms for evaluation in health promotion and other fields, because readers should not confine their attention to evaluations of health promotion and because important evaluation techniques that are common in other policy sectors have yet to gain currency in health promotion.

One key differentiation can be seen in the definition of evaluation proposed by two leading evaluators. Alkin (1985) has defined* evaluation to be the "activity of systematically collecting, analyzing, and reporting information that can then be used to change attitudes or to improve the operation of a project or program" (pp. 11–12). Scriven (1991) described the "key sense" of evaluation very differently, as "the process of determining the **merit, worth** or **value** of something, or the product of that process" (p. 139). By Scriven's definition, Alkin's collection and analysis of information are not in themselves sufficient to make a study an evaluation. In practice, evaluations often require *both* information gathering and the determination of worth (Cronbach *et al.*, 1980). In fact, some of the major successes in evaluation have come about because the evaluator diagnosed a need, either for program improvement or for a determination of merit (e.g., Leviton & Boruch, 1983, 1984).

Some evaluation writers have developed explicit evaluation "models" that guide the practitioner, stepwise, through well-defined stages (Rossi & Freeman, 1993; Stake, 1967). Other writers have adopted expansive philosophical principles applicable to any evaluation (Scriven, 1967; Cronbach *et al.*, 1980). Some adhere fairly closely to the image of the evaluator as a provider of reliable and objective information (Alkin, 1985; Patton, 1982); others, though they may not disagree with this view, see the evaluator also as a mediator, participant, or teacher within the community of stakeholders, defined as all parties affected by the program or its evaluation (Cronbach *et al.*, 1980; Guba & Lincoln, 1981; Stake, 1975). In the face of diversity, we present a "distillation" of terms, concepts, and issues on which most evaluators would be likely to agree. Scriven (1967) has argued that evaluation is always fundamentally the same activity, whether we are evaluating "coffee machines or teaching machines" (p. 40). That may be so, but as with most issues in evaluation this view is controversial, and in this chapter we shall be concerned primarily with the evaluation of social interventions, with a special emphasis on the field of health promotion and disease prevention.

Viewpoints Most Evaluators Share

Is there a methodology of evaluation? In spite of differences in expert opinion concerning goals, philosophy, and specific research approaches, there does appear to be a core that can be termed evaluation methods. These methods emerged largely out of

---

*In reading what follows, the reader should bear in mind that no short definition ever does full justice to a theorist's beliefs.

the collective experience of evaluators and fall into two major categories: epistemology and the standards of evaluation practice. The interested reader can find more information on these points in Shadish *et al.* (1991) or Worthen and Sanders (1987) for overall theories of evaluation, Patton (1980) for a discussion of qualitative and quantitative methods, and the Joint Committee on Standards for Educational Evaluation (1994).

Evaluation methods are greatly preoccupied with epistemology, defined as how we establish that something is true or factual (e.g., Shadish *et al.*, 1991). While evaluators may differ about the relative merits of qualitative methods, quantitative methods, and specific standards of evidence, they do nevertheless agree that evaluation should be systematic and replicable and adhere to rules of social science. Those rules may vary across the disciplines that do evaluation (psychology, sociology, education), but rules do exist; evaluation is not a free-for-all. Evaluators may need to adhere to careful methods even more than laboratory scientists, because the evaluator's questions are more difficult to answer and the range of forces that can interfere with clear conclusions is so great. An evaluation that overcomes these problems can be ingenious; a mediocre evaluation is even more depressing than a mediocre laboratory experiment.

Standards of evaluation practice emerged from the hard experience of many practitioners. Some of the methods derived from this experience may fail to win the approval of all theorists, but most of these methods are geared to the problems that evaluators confront in the field. Methods belonging uniquely to evaluation will be outlined below. They include evaluability assessment, also known as exploratory evaluation (Wholey, 1994); logic models of programs and policies (Wholey, 1994); statistical models, termed state–stage models, that reflect the logic models (Lipsey, 1993); methods to elicit better evaluation questions (Patton, 1978; Cronbach *et al.*, 1980); and methods to generalize conclusions about programs, from initial sites to new exemplars elsewhere (Cronbach, 1982).

Readers with a serious interest in evaluation are strongly advised to use this chapter primarily as a guide to further reading. For the student or practitioner, the important task is to become familiar with the range of ideas that the major theorists have put forth so as to choose one's own approach intelligently.

Stages and Types of Evaluation

Determining whether a social program "worked" is often termed outcome evaluation. It is usually only one of several questions the evaluator needs to answer. In addition, there are questions that might be posed, both before and after an evaluation of outcome. Those that logically precede outcome evaluation are:

- Defining the evaluation's focus through several preevaluation activities: What questions need to be answered, and for whom?
- Implementation (also known as process): Was the program implemented as planned?
- Fine-tuning (also known as formative evaluation): How might the program be improved?

Those that might be posed after or in addition to outcome evaluation include:

- Mediating variables: Do we know why the program worked, and what factors must be present if it is to be successful?
- Comparison: Did the program work significantly better than alternative programs?
- Generalization: What kinds of intervention will work with what types of population, and in which settings?
- Efficiency: Are the benefits of the program worth its cost?

Addressing these questions systematically and in turn would constitute what Rossi and Freeman (1993) term a *comprehensive evaluation*. Comprehensive evaluations are often desirable since the evaluation questions appear in a logical series. However, comprehensive evaluations often are not feasible given the resources allocated to the enterprise (Cronbach *et al.*, 1980). It has been our observation that even the most prominent, most generously funded evaluations of health promotion and disease prevention usually cannot address all these questions at the same level of research quality. Since priorities often must be chosen, part of the art and science of evaluation practice has become choosing the more useful and important questions.

Ideally, the evaluator will be involved when a program commences and while it is in progress, as well as at the end when the final assessment is required. Consequently, there are several types of activity in which the evaluator may be engaged, and evaluation theorists have identified and labeled—not always consistently—several types of evaluation. Some of these types can stand alone, while others are more likely to be incorporated into more comprehensive studies. Like the verbs of classical Greek, most can be classified by time and aspect: certain types of evaluation are geared toward particular points in the time line of a project, while others are geared toward specific evaluation questions. There can be some overlap between the two groups, and with few exceptions (e.g., cost-effectiveness analysis), no stage or type of evaluation is tied to a particular methodology.

Preevaluation Activities

Certain activities are not evaluations as such. However, they are often prerequisites to asking the right evaluation question or to educating stakeholders about the implications of choosing an evaluation focus.

Needs Assessment

A full-scale evaluation is sometimes preceded by a needs assessment. Needs assessment is initiated when members or leaders of a community sense strongly that a problem must be addressed; the purpose of needs assessment is to define the problem and test assumptions about it. In the words of Rossi and Freeman (1993) it is a "systematic appraisal of the type, depth, and scope of a problem" (p. 56). Excellent models for needs assessment in the health promotion field can be found in Green and Kreuter (1991) and in the PATCH (planned approach to community health) model for community-based health promotion (Centers for Disease Control, 1985). Evaluators at this stage must be careful to distinguish needs from interests; and among needs themselves, evaluators must distinguish those that can be justified objectively from those that are merely perceived by the stakeholders. It is possible that the several stakeholder groups will perceive needs differently and part of what can be identified as evaluation practice involves accommodating these contending interests.

Program Design/Setting the Evaluation Question

Needs assessment as such may not be sufficient to inform stakeholders about the assumptions under which their program is operating. In fact, stakeholders often need to make those assumptions explicit. Public health differs from other policy sectors in that professionals are accustomed to setting measurable goals and objectives for their programs (e.g., Suchman, 1967; Peoples-Sheps et al., 1990). Nevertheless, goals and objectives can benefit from additional scrutiny over time. They may have proven infeasible; also, the assumptions under which they were created may have changed. Furthermore, different stakeholders may hold different expectations that need either to be resolved or made explicit as differences, and these need to be reflected in the goals.

In the preevaluation phase, a diplomatic evaluator may be able to turn a mediocre or even a "doomed" evaluation into an effective one by understanding stakeholder concerns. Some clients or stakeholders may be inherently supportive of a program or intervention, while others are hostile to it. Prior prejudices may stem from ideological beliefs that resist hard data: For example, persons who believe that sex education is morally wrong may remain unmoved by a positive report for a sex education program. In the preevaluation phase, the evaluator may have the opportunity to identify these special concerns and to negotiate a study that will be of value to as many stakeholders as possible.

Scriven (1973) has advocated "goal-free evaluation" to avoid buying into the assumptions of one or the other set of stakeholders. Although this approach is valuable to the field in its cautions against *cooptation* and its focus on unintended side effects, it is not widely used in the health sector.

Evaluability assessment offers some unique insights for program design (Wholey, 1994). This is an iterative method of arriving at better and more useful evaluation questions. Program stakeholders are first consulted about their goals, which are then compared to each other and to the program on paper. This information is shared and discussed until agreement on goals and objectives is reached. Sometimes agreement will not be reached; evaluation should then clearly specify which stakeholder goals are being addressed. Subsequently, the program design on paper is compared with program actuality; this information is again provided to stakeholders. Several outcomes of this process are possible, all of which can lead to program improvements. Sometimes, stakeholders can abandon infeasible goals. Sometimes, they will revise program design on the basis of the evaluability assessment. Finally, they may arrive at a more useful or relevant evaluation question. Clients of evaluation find this approach highly useful, both nationally and locally (Rog, 1985).

Logic models (Wholey, 1994) also represent an important technique to explicate the assumptions underlying programs. Logic models explicitly link problems to be addressed, activities to address them, and outcomes desired by stakeholders. This technique can be combined with the application of the PRECEDE–PROCEED model developed by Green and Kreuter (1991) for some extremely useful modifications to program design and improvement of evaluation questions.

An example combines the use of evaluability assessment and logic models to illustrate the importance of reviewing goals and objectives. A local project in Birmingham, AL, was developed in order to provide experiences in the arts to inner-city children. An evaluability assessment was conducted (Collins, Stephens, & Leviton, 1994). In the first stage, the evaluators were surprised when stakeholders expressed several other goals: They wanted to prevent drug abuse and teen pregnancy among children at risk, improve race relations in Birmingham, and develop a better image for the city nationally. The disparity of goals was brought to the attention of the stakeholders; they still wanted all five goals addressed. The evaluators agreed that they would eventually have to prioritize among these goals. They then moved to the second step of evaluability assessment, which was to scope out the reality of the program. They observed the program and conducted interviews with teachers, children, and others affected by the program. They discovered that high-risk children simply did not participate. Also the program activities were simply not compatible with the objectives of drug abuse prevention and preventing teen pregnancy. This information was provided to the stakeholders and led to a variety of program development activities.

The program developers and stakeholders in this example were intelligent people. Nevertheless, they needed coaching on focusing evaluation, because they were breaking new ground with a very attractive concept. This is common. Indeed, the same process occurs at the state and federal levels, for various reasons. Evaluability assessments are frequently cost-effective: For example, an evaluability assessment of the federally funded Follow Through Program was conducted for under $100,000; it proved very useful to stakeholders, while a $20 million evaluation of outcomes was never documented as being used at all (Leviton and Boruch, 1983).

Summative and Formative Evaluation

Summative and *formative* are two of the many terms that Scriven has contributed to the common vocabulary of evaluation. Formative evaluation is undertaken while the program is in progress; Scriven (1967) stated that the "role of formative evaluation is to discover deficiencies and successes in the intermediate versions of a new curriculum" (p. 51). Its chief purpose is to identify areas for change or improvement. One important function of the formative stage is to determine whether the treatment underway is in fact the same as the treatment envisioned. Most evaluators would agree that this stage is conducted primarily within the program agency and is not intended for broad circulation. Summative evaluation is conducted "*after* completion of the program . . . and *for* the benefit of some *external* audience or decision-maker . . ." (Scriven, 1991, p. 340). Summative evaluation summarizes the program's performance, often for outsiders, whether it be a summary of implementation ("200 people at risk were reached through the health fair"), outcomes ("hypertension in the group was reduced by 20%"), or comparison to alternative programs ("the community-oriented, peer-led intervention led to greater condom use than did the traditional health education intervention"). Many evaluators will use this term loosely to refer to the final evaluation report and recommendations.

Other Common Terms

Many evaluators (in particular, those in health promotion) use the term *process evaluation* with approximately the same meaning as formative evaluation: Fink (1993), for example, defined process evaluation to be "concerned with the extent to which planned activities are executed . . ." (p. 10) (see also Green and Kreuter, 1991, p. 228; Windsor *et al.*, 1984, p. 3). Other evaluators reserve this term for something beyond the narrow mandate of quality control. Patton (1980), for example, defined process evaluations to be those "aimed at elucidating and understanding the internal dynamics of program operations" (p. 60). Evaluators such as Patton would reserve the term *implementation evaluation* for the narrower description of program activities. Viewed this way, process evaluation can occur within either the formative or the summative stage. It is important for professionals in health promotion to realize that process and formative evaluation are not always the same; process information can be used either for formative or summative purposes.

The terms *outcome* and *impact* evaluation occur frequently and often with different meanings. Along with much of the field of health education, Green and Kreuter (1991) use "the term *impact* to refer to the immediate effect of a program or process and the term *outcome* to refer to the distant or ultimate effect" (p. 228). They note that this is "established use in biomedical and health services research" (p. 228), but health promotion is increasingly a multidisciplinary field, and not all of those who work in the field use this terminology.

Sometimes both terms are used to designate the final stage of evaluation, though with subtle differences between them. To many evaluators, *impact* refers to the extent to which the program has changed the behavior of the participants. An impact evaluation will certainly seek "changes in the desired direction" (Rossi and Freeman, 1993, p. 36); under some evaluators it will be sensitive to other, unanticipated changes as well. *Outcomes* is a related term often used to designate the broader range of changes or effects brought about by the program. If an antiviolence program has had a strong impact on the participants, one outcome may be fewer arrests in the community. Outcomes, like impacts, may sometimes be unplanned or unwanted.

Finally, Suchman (1967) developed terminology that is prevalent in the public health field, distinguishing among the achievement of: (1) immediate objectives, relating to those activities undertaken by program staff ("staff will recruit 1000 people into blood pressure screening"); (2) ultimate objectives, which are the ultimate aim of a program or project ("hypertension will be reduced by 20% in the target group"); and (3) intermediate objectives, also termed *bridging variables,* which are intermediate effects necessary to the achievement of ultimate objectives ("90% of program participants will adhere to taking their blood pressure medication"). Figure 1 attempts to clarify the correspondence of terminologies. It uses, as an illustration, abbreviated goals of a smoking cessation program for pregnant women.

As discussed further in Chapter 31, analyses of cost, cost-effectiveness, cost-utility, and cost-benefit are increasingly required in the evaluation of health promotion programs (Haddix, Teutsch, Shaffer, & Dunet, 1996; Russell, 1986). Many of these concepts can be closely linked to the use of a series of objectives (Suchman, 1967), to logic models (Wholey, 1994), and more recently to state–stage modeling as developed by Lipsey (1993). Cost-effectiveness examines the unit cost per unit achievement of a stated objective; the objective can be at any of the levels indicated above. Note, however, that in health promotion programs the achievement of intermediate or ultimate objectives is likely to cost more than the achievement of immediate objectives, because many health promotion programs have dropouts at each step.

Cost-benefit analysis examines the dollar benefits achieved by a health promotion program; the net of the direct and indirect costs of the program. (Some evaluation

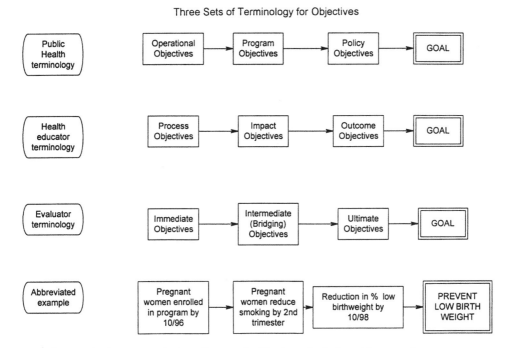

Figure 1. Evaluation terminology illustrated with a hypothetical smoking cessation program.

texts in health promotion still stress a cost-to-benefit ratio, but this approach is highly misleading and should not be used. Benefits net of program costs are a superior methodology.) It is generally not possible to reach agreement on a dollar value for benefits such as life, health, and functional status. Analyses have therefore focused on two alternatives: breakeven analysis, and cost-utility analysis. Breakeven analysis focuses on those benefits that can be monetarized and leaves aside those that cannot, to simply examine whether the program can cover its costs. For example, Leviton (1989) determined that work site health promotion programs focusing on seat belt use, hypertension control, and some smoking cessation programs could cover their cost under most conditions, even though benefits such as improved morale, attracting desirable employees, and increased work productivity could not be addressed. Cost-utility analysis focuses on people's subjective preferences about the quality of their lives, using the method of quality adjusted life years (Haddix *et al.*, 1996).

Elements of an Evaluation

Specification of Goals and Objectives

A social program must have well-defined goals; based on those goals, explicit and realistic objectives should be constructed. Objectives should be stated in "behavioral" terms, they should lend themselves to measurement even though they may not specify a target level of achievement, and they should provide specific time frames for accomplishment. Shortell and Richardson (1978) advise that a "clearly written objective must have *both* a single aim and a single end-product or result" (p. 26). By these criteria, the statement, "at least 70% of the participants will report having abstained from cigarettes for at least 6 weeks prior to final contact," though somewhat long, is a superior objective to "participants will quit smoking." (Specific numeric thresholds, like "at least 70%," may be avoided in objectives written for untested interventions.) Objectives must be measurable not only in theory but in practice; a common mistake is to specify objectives that even if achieved, cannot be measured with existing instruments or within the funding period of the evaluation.

Scriven (1967) has advised evaluators to be attentive to significant outcomes other than those specified by the formal objectives, and he has also maintained that the program goals themselves be subject to evaluation. As noted above, Scriven (1973) also recommends "goal-free evaluation," an often-misunderstood model in which the evaluator enters the field unaware of the formal goals and objectives, and measures all important outcomes. Whether the evaluator has any "business" questioning the objectives that he or she has been hired to study is still a controversial issue in evaluation.

Contract Negotiations and the Budget

In addition to the usual matters of budgets and deadlines, the negotiations between evaluator and client should anticipate and, if possible, address some important ethical and professional issues that may arise. The administrative decision-making process that evaluation is designed to serve is often political; money and careers will be at stake, group interests will have to be balanced, and there will be considerable room for error or abuse. The ethical problems that the program and the evaluator might encounter are often unpredictable, but many will fall into these broad categories:

- Harmful outcomes are observed or favorable outcomes are seen but not those anticipated in the objectives.
- Certain project staff members are uncooperative with the evaluation. Worse yet, they may conduct themselves incompetently, unethically, or illegally.
- Clients expect the evaluation to support a foregone conclusion, or publicly misrepresent the findings so it appears to do so; or they may withhold those findings from concerned audiences.

Clear and comprehensive negotiations between the evaluator and the client at the commencement of a project should be directed toward minimizing the possibility of such abuses. Evaluators have a stake in maintaining professional standards, and in particular should resist expectations that evaluation will "prove" that the program is worthwhile. Evaluation cannot prove worth solely through scientific methods. To maintain ethical standards, evaluators will find support in the professional guidelines issued by the Joint Committee on Standards for Educational Evaluation (1994).

Design, Measurement, and Analytic Method

The evaluator must formally establish the design of the study, the measurements to be made, and the methods by which these measurements will be analyzed. The design is, essentially, the "plan"; it specifies how subjects are to be selected, the treatment groups into which they will be placed and how they will be placed there, the measurements to be taken, and when they will be taken. The term *measurement* is used in the broad sense to include all observations taken on the subjects. Measurements will often be quantitative, that is, numeric, but they also may be verbal or anecdotal, especially in qualitative evaluations that employ anthropology's technique of ethnography or naturalistic designs. When resources permit, evaluators should "triangulate" on variables of interest by using different measurements. The rationale for this strategy is that virtually any kind of data has flaws; but if several flawed measures do not all share the same flaws, inferences are stronger (Cook & Campbell, 1979). For example, Baer, Holt, and Lichtenstein (1986) estimated personal smoking rates by asking their subjects how much they smoked and by taking carbon monoxide measures.

Measurements are made with instruments: in evaluation these instruments are often tests, surveys, questionnaires, and observation forms. In health promotion, they can also include standardized physiological measurements such as blood pressure, human immunodeficiency virus (HIV) and sexually transmitted disease (STD) tests, or skin fold measurement. An instrument must be reliable, that is, it must measure "something" (ability, attitude, etc.), and it must be valid, that is, it should measure what it is intended to measure and without consistent bias. (A math test consisting of "word problems" may not be valid; that is, it may measure reading ability better than it measures math skills, but it may nonetheless measure reading reliably.) Evaluators should be familiar with the theory of psychological measurement, including classical test theory (Lord & Novick, 1968; Crocker & Algina, 1986) and item response theory (Hambleton & Swaminathan, 1985).

The evaluator must specify the methods by which the data yielded by the measurements will be analyzed. For many evaluators this is the most difficult element of the study to specify in advance, at least when statistical methodology is required, and the evaluator may be tempted to list a "smorgasbord" of methods—correlation, regression, chi-square—in the hope of being correct somewhere. In fact, when the objectives, design, and measurements are specified well, the appropriate data analytic technique should "fall out" naturally.

Selection of measurements and analytic methods should be made at the same time, not in sequence, lest the evaluator end up with measurements that cannot be analyzed reliably by any existing method. Most statistical techniques place restrictions on the data that can be analyzed; the more sophisticated the technique, the more severe the restrictions usually are. It is not unusual for an evaluator to select a statistical method that is appropriate in principle for the measurements, only to discover later that the measurements have yielded data that fail to meet the method's restrictive assumptions. In this event there are often very few clean ways to "rescue" the analysis, and the evaluator will be forced to select the least adverse of unsatisfactory options. To guard against this problem, Cook, Leviton, and Shadish (1985) have argued for the development of "fallback options" for design, data collection, and analysis, so that if the preferred plan cannot be achieved, at least the project has some prospect of meaningful results. This strategy has been employed in evaluations of programs as diverse as the Peace Corps and school-based nutrition education.

Design, measurement, and analysis for quantitative evaluation are covered in many textbooks in the behavioral and social sciences, and there is widespread agreement on most issues. For qualitative evaluation, in contrast, few well-defined and universally accepted analytic methods exist; theoretical and practical issues are discussed extensively in Patton (1980).

The Final Report

The style of the final report and the scope of its circulation are subjects for negotiation at the commencement of the evaluation process. In most cases this report will begin with a relatively short "executive summary," in which the study design, the major findings, and the recommendations are summarized in nontechnical language. A full description of design, sampling, and methodology will appear in a full report or perhaps in a separate "technical report." In many settings the executive summary, not the full report, will have the wider circulation and the greater impact. Guidelines for effective report style can be found in Chapter 5 of Alkin (1985) and Chapter 8 of Fink (1993).

Special Issues in Evaluation

Technical Issues

Program evaluation grew out of the positivist scientific philosophy that dominated much of the 20th century. Positivism asserts that it is possible to find objective, scientific solutions to social problems. However, over the past few decades many evaluators have come to acknowledge (some more reluctantly than others) the special problems encountered when applying laboratory methods in difficult real-world settings. Some of those problems are discussed below.

Research Design

To determine whether a program "works" (whether this is in the context of outcome evaluation, comparisons, mediating variables, or efficiency), an evaluator compares two or more treatment groups: an experimental group of individuals who have been subject to the intervention under evaluation and at least one comparison group of individuals who have received an alternative intervention. (The latter is called a control group when its members have received no special treatment at all.) An evaluation is said to be internally valid when the outcomes can confidently be attributed to the treatment and to no other cause. Many factors threaten the internal validity of a study; part of the stimulating and challenging aspect of research design is to determine whether such factors could plausibly be said to operate in a given study. If no alternative explanations are plausible, the inference that a program caused an outcome is strengthened. Cook and Campbell (1979) list several threats to internal validity against which the evaluator must guard. Cronbach's (1982) response to Cook and Campbell also should be studied.

The ideal design for an internally valid evaluation is experimental, in which individuals are assigned randomly to the different groups. The purpose of random assignment is to maximize the likelihood that the groups do not differ on any relevant factor except the treatments they have received. Roughly put, random assignment "evens out" differences among the groups, so that at the end of the program differences between experimental and comparison groups can confidently be attributed to the program (i.e., the treatment).

In the development and testing of innovations for health promotion, randomized experiments are the standard for credible evidence of merit. When reading research on the development of these innovations, the reader needs to assess the degree to which the investigators achieved an unbiased, randomized experiment. If an experiment was not feasible for any reason, then readers should judge the plausibility of threats to internal validity that might have influenced the outcomes of evaluation, independent of any program treatment.

When local evaluators assess individual programs, however, the ideal of the randomized experiment is rarely achieved. People often cannot be assigned randomly to social programs; even when they can be, random assignment to alternative treatments may sometimes be politically infeasible or unethical where there are serious reservations about some of the alternatives. A frequently used strategy in health promotion overcomes both the ethical and political obstacles: the use of a *lagged-intervention group*, also termed a *wait-list control*. In this strategy, participants are randomly assigned to intervention (for example, to quit smoking) or to the lagged-intervention group. To combat political pressures, it should be noted that people regard lotteries as a fair method of allocating resources; and what is a lottery but random assignment (Wortman & Rabinowitz, 1979).

It is not possible, indeed not advisable, for health promotion professionals to rely on a chapter such as this for an in-depth discussion of all the alternative explanations and their operation in the context of prevention. However, acquaintence with these threats is vitally important both to critically appraise effectiveness of interventions and to conduct competent outcome studies. Numerous textbooks present tables of the different outcome evaluation designs and the threats to validity that routinely accompany those designs.

Though it will not usually be possible to account for every conceivable threat to validity in a particular design, the evaluator should study the data and all supporting documentation in search of explanations, other than intervention effect, which may account for the observed results. We illustrate this point with an example of a search for threats to internal validity that occur in context.

A study of 12 rural villages in Tanzania was conducted to determine whether improved care for STDs would prevent HIV infection (Grosskurth *et al.*, 1995). Infectious disease professionals have long suspected that STDs may facilitate the transmission of HIV; improved cures for STDs therefore might prevent HIV infection. Villages were affiliated with a regional health clinic. Villages were matched on geographic location and characteristics linked to HIV risk, and pairs were then randomly assigned to receive additional STD care, over and above what was previously available, or no additional care. The investigators were able to demonstrate significantly fewer new cases of HIV infection in the treatment villages at 2-year follow up, compared to controls.

We will illustrate the need to appraise internal validity with only one example: selection. One definition of selection is "identification of a comparison group not equivalent to the treatment group because of demographic, psychosocial, or behavioral characteristics" (Windsor *et al.*, 1984, p. 131). Because this study employed random assignment, we might dismiss selection as a possibility; after all, random assignment is supposed to "even out" such differences between treatment and control groups. However, the data dictate whether selection is a problem in any given evaluation study. Although villages were randomly assigned, three of the matched pairs showed higher HIV infections in control than in treatment villages at baseline. In the other three pairs, the trend was reversed but the differences were much smaller. The article simply does not speak to whether these differences between pairs were significant, and thus the possibility is raised that systematic differences between villages at the start of the study may have affected results later. With only 12 units being randomly assigned, it is possible that the study experienced bad-luck random assignment, such that a higher prevalence of HIV infection occurred in these three control villages; higher prevalence initially would be associated with greater change to HIV positive (seroconversion) later.

Note several things about these comments. First, we raise the possibility of selection as a threat to validity; we do not claim that selection is proven to be responsible for results. Second, the design reflects potential problems that are often seen in health promotion programs: random assignment of a fairly small number of units (people cannot be randomly assigned because they live within villages). Third, raising the specific possibility of selection (systematic differences between treatment and control villages at baseline) also presents specific opportunities to defend the conclusions. The investigators could easily defend their conclusions and make the threat less plausible, if they were able to demonstrate that the three control villages with higher initial rates of HIV infection were not solely responsible for differences between treatment and control groups at follow up.

Should the reader take away the message that this study is fatally flawed? By no means. Every evaluation study is vulnerable to some concerns such as these. Instead, the message is to understand exactly where and how individual studies may be vulnerable and to pose specific research questions, open to investigation, that can refute these plausible alternatives.

A study should be externally as well as internally valid. The concept of external validity includes the idea of generalization, though a precise definition is difficult to pin down. According to Campbell and Stanley (1963), "[e]xternal validity asks the question of generalizability: To what population, settings, treatment variables, and measurement variables can this effect be generalized" (p. 175); these authors observed that the question of external validity "is never completely answerable" (p. 175). Later, Cook and Campbell (1979) used the term external validity "to refer to the approximate validity with which conclusions are drawn about the generalizability of a causal relationship to and across populations of persons, settings, and times" (p. 39).

In "pure" behavioral research, generalizability to a particular population is assured, insofar as this is possible, by selecting subjects randomly from that population. In most program evaluations, random selection is neither possible nor appropriate, for the evaluator will be hired to study a particular implementation of a program, by clients who want to know how well their program worked in their institution. Naturally, cautious clients will want to know the range of conditions under which additional implementations of the program will produce results similar to those observed in the evaluation, but there is no easy method for making such inferences. It is important to understand that where they are achieved, internal and external validity result from the design of the study. The methods of statistical inference cannot be used to "prove" that one's findings are valid in either sense; on the contrary, these methods assume that the study was designed to be valid.

Cronbach's (1982) response to the theory of Campbell and Stanley cannot be presented here, but without doing full justice to Cronbach's analysis we present a few main ideas. Not only are the subjects of an evaluation a sample from a wider population, so are the measurement instruments and the varieties of program implementation. In a well-planned study, evaluators and clients will usually have in mind "populations" of individuals, instruments, and implementations to which they intend to generalize; for Cronbach, this is a question of internal validity. One may also be interested in generalizing to a population of individuals, instruments, or implementations different from the ones represented in the actual study; for Cronbach, this is the question of external validity.

Most writers acknowledge the practical problems with experimental design, but their responses to the problem differ in emphasis. Some (Guba & Lincoln, 1981; House, 1980) will tolerate, even advocate, a complete break with statistical research methodology; others will make this break only reluctantly, or will attempt to accommodate these real-world constraints in ways that still permit statistical inferences (Cook & Campbell, 1979; Cronbach et al., 1980; Cronbach, 1982).

Evaluators usually work perforce with quasi-experimental designs, in which the groups have not been formed by random assignment. In these designs, preexisting or latent differences between the experimental and comparison groups challenge the evaluator's demonstration of a true treatment effect. Methods for designing and interpreting reliable quasi-experimental studies can be found in Campbell and Stanley (1963) and Cook and Campbell (1979). Evaluators also should be familiar with the theory of regression–discontinuity designs (Trochim, 1984), which are relevant to programs (frequent in education) in which subjects are assigned to treatments according to their scores on well-defined numeric scales. Such designs have a great deal of potential, as yet unrealized, in health promotion. Regression–discontinuity designs were developed because programs had to be given to people based on their needs or merit. The astute reader will see that health-related treatments are frequently given to people on the basis of carefully defined needs; for example, hypertension control is only considered for people whose blood pressure readings are above 140/90; medication is only considered for truly elevated readings. The same applies to cholesterol reduction. Two other designs, more frequently used in health promotion, include interrupted time series and longitudinal panel studies of the same individuals across time (Cook & Campbell, 1979).

Evaluators should also be aware that even genuine treatment effects may wear off over time; for example, 80% of people who quit smoking can be expected to start again within the year (Pechacek, 1979). Sometimes, evaluations are not funded for a period of time long enough to detect such relapses; in such cases, evaluators and their clients must be careful not to overinterpret positive findings. For example, Sikkema et al. (1996) have noted that small-group interventions for HIV prevention in at-risk populations produce positive effects, but sometimes they decay over time. Under such circumstances, more sustained efforts, such as changes in community norms or relapse prevention strategies, may be needed.

Data Collection and Analysis

Closely related to the issue of research design is that of methodology: the kinds of data to be collected and the methods by which they are to be analyzed. There is an endless debate in evaluation between advocates of quantitative and qualitative methodology. Quantitative methodology is statistical and employs counts of predefined data. Qualitative methodologies are diverse and range from ethnography and participant observation, through carefully constructed case studies and focus groups, to detailed and highly structured content analyses of text, spoken words, or content of media. Qualitative "data" consist primarily of verbal observations and the data are not highly categorized or defined in advance of data collection. Instead, independent raters or judges often come to agreement on themes within the content and criteria for classifying instances of those themes. Although the methods vary greatly, for the most part they share the standard that independent investigators could replicate the data or come to similar conclusions. Most credible evaluators have accepted the premise that qualitative research is a full-fledged scientific methodology in its own right, not a "second-best" alternative to quantitative methods to be used when the latter are impractical or insufficient. Researchers who conduct health promotion studies in other cultures have long recognized that surveys and participant observation or in-depth interviews can often obtain radically different data; sometimes the survey data produce their own response biases.

Realistic evaluators must anticipate finding themselves in a double bind: Resource constraints (time and money) may prevent them from implementing high-quality experimental studies, while the constraints of an organizational culture that still regards statistical research as the norm will prevent them from employing innovative methodologies (e.g., ethnographic research). Since quantitative methodology is likely to be the standard for some time, evaluators must at least understand its limitations. For one thing, most methods of statistical inference have restrictive assumptions for data which usually cannot be satisfied in evaluation (see section titled "Research Design," above). Consequently, statistical methods may lack sufficient power to detect genuine treatment effects. (Put crudely, this means that even when a program "works," the statistics may say it did not.) Second, statistical inference is primarily intended for drawing conclusions about large, well-defined populations, and this will not always be the evaluator's task. The criteria of statistical significance are arbitrary, and the logic of the method is poorly understood by behavioral researchers and their audiences alike (Carver, 1978). Furthermore, in many evaluations the subjects being studied are, for all practical purposes, a population, not a sample, and so methods of statistical inference may be inappropriate, even meaningless. The use of statistical methods in settings for which they were not designed is obviously an ethical as well as a scientific issue.

Level of Analysis

A critical issue for data analysis in health promotion involves the unit of analysis. Frequently, we intervene with entire schools, classrooms, small groups, or communities. When this happens, both the larger unit (e.g., school) and the individuals within those units must be represented in the analysis. This principle is important enough (and in practice, violated enough) to be explained in some detail. Factors that affect behavior originate at the group* as well as at the individual level: Academic

*Here we are referring to natural or "real-world" groups like families, schools, and communities, not to the experimental and comparison groups that were defined above in the discussion of experimental research.

achievement, for example, will be affected by the characteristics of the student's family and school as well as by individual ability and motivation. The term *unit of analysis* refers to who or what is measured. Typically, program evaluators measure (*i.e.*, gather data on) individuals, but they often need to measure one or more units at the group level as well: These group-level units may include families, classrooms, schools, and so on. Group-level measures, that is, measurements taken when the group is the unit of analysis, may include averages of the member individuals, such as mean household income among the students in a school, as well as measures that can be taken only for a group-level unit, such as teacher–student ratio.

When designing a study, the evaluator must specify whether data will be collected and analysis conducted at the individual or group level. Whether individuals or groups are to serve as units of analysis is a question to be established when the evaluation is being planned and negotiated, and the decision will be based on theoretical factors (at what level do we expect to see results?) as well as practical ones (at which level are we able to collect data?). Among the theoretical factors that evaluators must consider in deciding among units of analysis is the fact that statistical relationships among the same kinds of measurement differ between group and individual levels. For example, in an oft-cited paper, Robinson (1950) observed that within the United States the relationship between literacy and national origin (United States vs. foreign) computed at the individual level was very different from that computed at the regional (census area) level, and naively interpreted, the group and individual level correlations led respectively to opposite conclusions. Cronbach, Deken, and Webb (1976) and House, Glass, McLean, and Walker (1978) cite examples of educational findings that vary with level of analysis and provide extensive discussion and criticism of issues in multilevel research. Once the unit of analysis has been chosen, therefore, evaluators and their clients must guard against making cross-level inferences (Burstein, 1980; Pedhazur, 1982, pp. 527–530); that is, drawing conclusions about individual behavior based on group-level findings, or vice versa.

Ideally, evaluations should include group- and individual-level measurements when both are theoretically justified, but separating group from individual effects has long been a major challenge in social research. (The methodological problems are discussed extensively in Burstein, 1980.) This challenge has been met effectively only recently, with the development of multilevel (alternatively, hierarchical) modeling methods that allow researchers to analyze effects at individual and group levels simultaneously (Bryk & Raudenbush, 1992; Goldstein, 1995).

Ethical and Political Issues

It is important to understand that evaluation is often part of a political process, a fact of life that some evaluators relish and others just learn to tolerate. All evaluators, however, will have to confront political and ethical issues that distinguish their profession from pure social research. In this section some of the more important of these issues are discussed.

Internal versus External Evaluation

Some evaluators are salaried members of the very organizations that run the programs to be evaluated; others are independent consultants or contractors. Though certain authorities may have strong opinions favoring one or the other group, there is no consensus on this question within the profession as a whole. Advantages and disadvantages of each should be readily apparent. "In-house" evaluators may benefit from intimate knowledge of the programs and their personnel, but they may be susceptible to criticism of personal bias by antagonistic stakeholders, especially if their conclusions are favorable, and they are certainly susceptible to such bias. Outside evaluators are less likely to be favorably biased, or so they may be presented to the audiences (there is something reassuring in the phrase "independent evaluator"). However, there are ethical pitfalls for independent evaluators as well. They may be less familiar with the goals, values, and culture of the organizations they study, so that their conclusions may not be fair. Although not biased toward the programs as such, they may succumb to the pressure of providing favorable reports in the hope of winning future contracts.

Stakeholders

Many public social programs will affect, if only indirectly, large numbers of persons in addition to those who actually have been targeted for the intervention. All community residents, for example, will have a "stake" in a program involving treatment for drug addicts in a local half-way house. Most evaluators acknowledge the existence of such stakeholder groups; they disagree, however, on the extent to which these groups should be involved in the evaluation, or on the evaluator's personal responsibility to respond to their interests. Some evaluators advocate a broad political process; others believe that their primary obligation is to the paying client. Whatever the evaluator's orientation, the identity of legitimate stakeholders and the extent to which they will be involved in the evaluation or given access to the results should be established during planning and contract negotiations.

Utilization

The evaluator's role in knowledge building is debatable; what is certain is that the evaluator will be obliged to meet short-term administrative demands. The evaluation must be conducted so as to have the greatest possible potential for impact on decisions. Some of the factors that will increase an evaluation's potential for impact are suggested by common sense and have been discussed above: advance negotiations between evaluator and client, identifying legitimate stakeholders, and an effective executive summary of the final report. Another important factor is timeliness: An evaluation should be completed in time to play its anticipated role in the decision-making process and certainly by the negotiated deadline. Experienced evaluators sometimes find it necessary to compromise with sound research procedure in order to produce a report by deadline and within the allotted resources.

Only the naive evaluator will expect every client who commissions an evaluation to be interested in scientific decision making. Some evaluations are commissioned only because the funding agencies required them; administrators and staff may be indifferent to the evaluation, perhaps even hostile. Evaluations may be commissioned by administrators whose minds are made up but who must appear "objective"; in these cases the evaluator may be under some pressure to produce the "desired" findings.

A finished evaluation may be misutilized: The evaluation will be quoted dishonestly or inaccurately to support conclusions much different from the ones the evaluator had actually recommended, or it will be withheld from legitimate stakeholders. (Sometimes the evaluator can anticipate corrective action: see the discussion of contract negotiations under the section titled "Elements of an Evaluation," above.) Often, especially in government programs, the evaluation will be only one of many factors employed by decision makers, and possibly not the one most heavily weighed. Research into the use of evaluation has become a full-fledged subspecialty, and evaluators should be familiar with the major publications, which include Alkin, Daillak, and White (1979), and Leviton and Hughes (1981). Alkin (1985, Chapter 5) discusses factors affecting evaluation use that can be anticipated from the beginning. Patton (1978) has specialized in evaluation methods designed to maximize the potential for use at the client level.

In the interest of pragmatism, the preceding discussion has focused on instrumental use of evaluation (Rich, 1977), in which decisions are based directly on evaluation findings. However, use may also be conceptual (Rich, 1977; Weiss, 1977); here, the evaluation is a source of insight, clarification, or enlightenment, even though it does not lead clients directly to their decisions. (An evaluation used conceptually usually competes with social and political factors for influence on decision makers.) Conceptual use may occur long after the evaluation is finished and in contexts neither the evaluator nor the client anticipated. Subtly different is what Leviton and Hughes (1981) called persuasive use, in which evaluation findings are used by an advocate of a program (or by an opponent) in "attempts to convince others to support a political position, or to defend such a position from attack" (p. 528). Among large-scale government programs involving diverse stakeholders and conflicting political interests, conceptual and persuasive uses of evaluation are more likely than instrumental use (when any use is made at all) and according to several experts are more appropriate (Weiss, 1988; Cronbach et al., 1980).

Evaluation as a Profession

Professional evaluators are employed routinely by public agencies at most levels of government. Standards for employment differ among the states, though a graduate degree will be required almost everywhere. At least one state (Louisiana) certifies evaluators hired to evaluate state programs. Under the leadership of Daniel Stufflebeam, the Joint Committee on Standards for Educational Evaluation (1994) published a comprehensive set of professional and scientific standards for evaluators to follow. Adherence to these standards is generally voluntary.

The largest professional organization for program evaluation is the American Evaluation Association, which holds annual conferences, publishes the journal *Evaluation Practice*, and accepts individual membership from professionals and students.

Evaluation as a profession holds many rewards, including variety (since many programs may be evaluated), challenges due to the logistical limitations on studies, and sometimes the realization that a program or funding agency has used one's input to improve or support a worthwhile program. Evaluation in all its complexity is a key skill for the health promotion professional.

References

Alkin, M. C. (1985). *A guide for evaluation decision makers.* Beverly Hills: Sage.

Alkin, M. C., Daillak, R. H., & White, P. (1979). *Using evaluations: Does evaluation make a difference?* Beverly Hills: Sage.

Baer, J.S., Holt, C. S., & Lichtenstein, E. (1986). Self-efficacy and smoking reexamined: Construct validity and clinical utility. *Journal of Consulting and Clinical Psychology, 54*(6), 846–852.

Bryk, A. S., & Raudenbush, S.W. (1992). *Hierarchical linear models: Applications and data analysis methods.* Newbury Park, CA: Sage.

Burstein, L. (1980). The analysis of multi-level data in educational research and evaluation. *Review of Research in Education, 8,* 158–233.

Campbell, D.T., & Stanley, J.C. (1963). *Experimental and quasi-experimental designs for research on teaching.* Chicago: Rand-McNally.

Carver, R. P. (1978). The case against statistical significance testing. *Harvard Educational Review, 48*(3), 378–399.

Centers for Disease Control. (1985). PATCH: *Planned approach to community health.* Atlanta: Author.

Collins, C., Stephens, B., & Leviton, L. (1994, November). *Evaluability assessment of an inner city arts program.* Paper presented at the meeting of the American Evaluation Association, Boston, MA.

Cook, T. D., & Campbell, D. T. (1979). *Quasi-experimentation: Design and analysis issues for field settings.* Boston: Houghton Mifflin.

Cook, T. D., Leviton, L. C., & Shadish, W. R. (1985). Evaluation research. In G. Lindzey & E. Aronson (Eds.), *The handbook of social psychology* (3rd ed., pp. 699–777). New York: Random House.

Crocker, L. M., & Algina, J. (1986). *Introduction to classical and modern test theory.* New York: Holt, Rinehart and Winston.

Cronbach, L. J. (1982). *Designing evaluations of educational and social programs.* San Francisco: Jossey-Bass.

Cronbach, L. J., Deken, J., & Webb, N. (1976). *Research on classrooms and schools: Formulation of questions, design and analysis.* Stanford: California Stanford Evaluation Consortium.

Cronbach, L. J., Ambron, S. R., Dornbusch, S. M., Hess, R. D., Hornik, R. C., Phillips, D. C., Walker, D. F., & Weiner, S. S. (1980). *Toward reform of program evaluation.* San Francisco: Jossey-Bass.

Fink, A. (1993). *Evaluation fundamentals: Guiding health programs, research, and policy.* Newbury Park, CA: Sage.

Goldstein, H. (1995). *Multilevel statistical models.* London: Edward Arnold.

Green, L. W., & Kreuter, M. W. (1991). *Health promotion planning: An educational and environmental approach.* Mountain View, CA: Mayfield.

Green, L. W. & Lewis, F. M. (1986). *Measurement and evaluation in health education and health promotion.* Palo Alto, CA: Mayfield.

Grosskurth, H., Mosha, F., Todd, J., Senkaro, K., Newell, J., Klokke, A., Changalucha, J., West, B., Maynard, P., Gavyole, A., et al. (1995). A community trial of the impact of improved sexually transmitted disease treatment on the HIV epidemic in rural Tanzania: 2. Baseline survey results. *AIDS, 9*(8), 927–934.

Guba, E. G., & Lincoln, Y. S. (1981). *Effective evaluation.* San Francisco: Jossey-Bass.

Haddix, A. C., Teutsch, S. M., Shaffer, P. A., & Dunet, D. O. (1996). *Prevention effectiveness: A guide to decision analysis and economic evaluation.* New York: Oxford University Press.

Hambleton, R. K., & Swaminathan, H. (1985). *Item response theory: Principles and applications.* Norwell, MA: Kluwer Academic Publishers.

House, E. R. (1980). *Evaluating with validity.* Beverly Hills: Sage.

House, E. R., Glass, G. V., McLean, L. D. & Walker, D. F. (1978). No simple answer: Critique of the follow through evaluation. *Harvard Educational Review, 48*(2), 128–160.

Joint Committee on Standards for Educational Evaluation. (1994). *The program evaluation standards* (2nd ed.). Thousand Oaks, CA: Sage.

Leviton, L. C. (1989). Can organizations benefit from worksite health promotion? *Health Services Research, 24*(2), 159–189.

Leviton, L. C., & Boruch, R. F. (1983). Contributions of evaluation to education programs and policy. *Evaluation Review, 7,* 563–598.

Leviton, L. C., & Boruch, R.F. (1984). Why the compensatory education evaluation was useful. *Journal of Policy Analysis and Management, 3,* 299–305.

Leviton, L.C., & Hughes, E. F. X. (1981). Research on the utilization of evaluation: A review and synthesis. *Evaluation Review, 5*(4), 525–548.

Lipsey, M. W. (1993). Theory as method: Small theories of treatments. *New Directions for Program Evaluation*, *57*, 5–38.

Lord, F. M., & Novick, M. R. (1968). *Statistical theories of mental test scores.* Reading, MS: Addison-Wesley.

Patton, M. Q. (1978). *Utilization-focused evaluation.* Beverly Hills, CA: Sage.

Patton, M. Q. (1980). *Qualitative evaluation methods.* Beverly Hills, CA: Sage.

Patton, M. Q. (1982). *Practical evaluation.* Beverly Hills, CA: Sage.

Pechacek, T. F. (1979). Modification of smoking behavior. In N. A. Krasnegor (Ed.), *The behavioral aspects of smoking* (pp. 127–188). NIDA Research Monograph 26, Washington, DC: DHEW. (ADM 79-882).

Pedhazur, E. J. (1982). *Multiple regression in behavioral research.* New York: Holt, Rinehart and Winston.

Peoples-Sheps, M. D., Byars, E., Rogers, M. M., & Finerty, E. J. (1990). *Using objects for program planning.* Chapel Hill, NC: University of North Carolina School of Public Health.

Rich, R. F. (1977). Uses of social science information by federal bureaucrats. In C. H. Weiss (Ed.), *Using social research in public policy making* (pp. 199–212). Lexington, MA: DC Heath.

Robinson, W. S. (1950). Ecological correlations and the behavior of individuals. *American Sociological Review*, *15*, 351–357.

Rog, D. J. (1985). *A methodological analysis of evaluability assessment.* Unpublished doctoral dissertation, Vanderbilt University.

Rossi, P. H., & Freeman, H. E. (1993). *Evaluation: A systematic approach.* Newbury Park, CA: Sage.

Russell, L. B. (1986). *Is prevention better than cure?* Washington, DC: Brookings Institute.

Scriven, M. (1967). The methodology of evaluation. In R. W. Tyler, R. M. Gagne, & M. Scriven (Eds.), *Perspectives of curriculum evaluation* (pp. 39–83). Chicago: Rand-McNally.

Scriven, M. (1973). Goal-free evaluation. In E. R. House (Ed.), *School evaluation: The politics and process* (pp. 319–328). Berkeley, CA: McCutchan.

Scriven, M. (1991). *Evaluation thesaurus* (4th ed.). Newbury Park, CA: Sage.

Shadish, W. R., Cook, T. D., & Leviton, L.C. (1991). *Foundations of program evaluation:Theorists and their theories.* Newbury Park, CA: Sage.

Shortell, S. M., & Richardson, W. C. (1978). *Health program evaluation.* St. Louis: C. V. Mosby.

Sikkema, K. J., Heckman, T. G., Kelly, J. A., Anderson, E. S., Winett, R. A., Solomon, L. J., Wagstaff, D. A., Roffman, R. A., Perry, M. J., Cargill, V., Crumble, D. A., Fuqua, R. W., Norman, A. D., & Mercer, M. B. (1996). HIV risk behaviors among women living in low-income, inner-city housing developments. *American Journal of Public Health*, *86*, 1123–1128.

Stake, R. E. (1967). The countenance of educational evaluation. *Teachers College Record*, *68*, 523–640.

Stake, R.E. (Ed.). (1975). *Evaluating the arts in education: A responsive approach.* Columbus, OH: Charles E. Merrill.

Suchman, E. A. (1967). *Evaluative research: Principles and practice in public service and social action programs.* New York: Russell Sage Foundation.

Trochim, W. M. K. (1984). *Research design for program evaluation: The regression discontinuity approach.* Beverly Hills: Sage.

Weiss, C. H. (1977). Research for policy's sake: The enlightenment function of social research. *Policy Analysis*, *3*(4), 531–545.

Weiss, C. H. (1988). Evaluation for decisions: Is anybody there? Does anybody care? *Evaluation Practice*, *9*(1), 5–19.

Wholey, J. S. (1994). Assessing the feasibility and likely usefulness of evaluation. In J. S. Wholey, H. P. Hatry, & K. E. Newcomer (Eds.), *Handbook of practical program evaluation* (pp. 15–39). San Francisco, CA: Jossey-Bass.

Wholey, J. S., Hatry, H. P., & Newcomer, K. E. (Eds.). (1994). *Handbook of practical program evaluation.* San Francisco, CA: Jossey-Bass.

Windsor, R. A., Baranowski, T., Clark, N., & Cutter, G. (1984). *Evaluation of health promotion and education programs.* Palo Alto, CA: Mayfield.

Worthen, B. R., & Sanders, J. R. (1987). *Educational evaluation: Alternative approaches and practical guidelines.* White Plains, NY: Longman

Wortman, C. B., & Rabinowitz, V. C. (1979). Random assignment: The fairest of them all. In L. Sechrest, S. G. West, M. A. Phillips, R. Redner, & W. Yeaton (Eds.), *Evaluation studies review annual* (vol. 4, pp. 177–184). Beverly Hills, CA: Sage.

PART *III*

General Cross-Cutting Issues

CHAPTER 5

Symptom Perception

Martha M. Phillips, Carol E. Cornell, James M. Raczynski,
and M. Janice Gilliland

Introduction

A physical symptom is a "perception, feeling, or even belief about the state of (one's) body" (Pennebaker, 1982, p. 1). Symptoms are often—but not always—based on a somatic change, "a departure from a personalized norm of physical functioning" (MacGregor & Fleming, 1996, p. 774) and represent information about the internal state of the individual (Pennebaker, 1982). The perception of symptoms plays an important role in many aspects of health maintenance, including detection of signals of illness, decisions to seek medical attention, completeness and accuracy of reporting of symptoms to health care providers, and adherence to medical regimens. It is readily recognized that early detection and appropriate attribution of symptoms for many medical conditions, such as heart attack, stroke, and breast and colon cancer, are desirable; the more rapidly patients perceive symptoms and seek treatment, the greater the chances of a positive outcome and reduced morbidity and mortality. The ability to detect subtle physical symptoms and to distinguish types of symptoms plays an equally important role following diagnosis of disease, as individuals use perceived symptoms to guide illness-regulation behaviors. Research shows that individuals with disorders such as hypertension, diabetes, and asthma use detection of symptoms to guide behaviors such as taking medication or monitoring blood pressure or blood glucose levels (e.g., Freund, Bennett-Johnson, Rosenbloom, Alexander, & Hansen, 1986; Meyer, Leventhal, & Gutmann, 1985). Other behaviors, such as taking time off from school or work, are also affected by symp-

Martha M. Phillips • UAB Civitan International Research Center, Department of Epidemiology, School of Public Health, UAB Center for Health Promotion, University of Alabama at Birmingham, Birmingham, Alabama 35294.   *Carol E. Cornell* • Behavioral Medicine Unit, Division of Preventive Medicine, Department of Medicine, School of Medicine, UAB Center for Health Promotion, University of Alabama at Birmingham, Birmingham, Alabama 35294.   *James M. Raczynski and M. Janice Gilliland* • Behavioral Medicine Unit, Division of Preventive Medicine, Department of Medicine, School of Medicine, Department of Health Behavior, School of Public Health, UAB Center for Health Promotion, University of Alabama at Birmingham, Birmingham, Alabama 35294.

Handbook of Health Promotion and Disease Prevention, edited by Raczynski and DiClemente.
Kluwer Academic/Plenum Publishers, New York, 1999.

tom perception and interpretation (e.g., Leiken, Firestone, & McGrath, 1988; Matteson & Ivancevich, 1982).

"Symptom perception" will be presented in this chapter as a sequence of events, a continuous process, beginning with the presentation of a sensory cue or somatic change through awareness, interpretation, attribution, and acknowledgment of the symptom. Increasingly, researchers conceptualize symptom perception as a natural psychological process through which individuals actively seek to (1) explain their physical state and (2) reduce uncertainty about factors or conditions that may cause them to feel as they do (MacGregor & Fleming, 1996). Each of the processes inherent in symptom perception is affected by a variety of physiological, psychological, and demographic variables. Theoretical models have been developed to explain relationships between symptom processes and influential variables. In addition, aspects of symptom perception affect the development of intervention programs.

Background

A change in somatic condition does not necessarily mean that a symptom will be perceived by an individual or will be perceived accurately. Moreover, perceived symptoms do not always correlate closely with underlying pathology (Barsky, Cleary, Barnett, Christiansen, & Ruskin, 1994). For example, in cardiac disease, a large proportion of arrhythmias are asymptomatic, and persons who report palpitations do not always evidence arrhythmias on examination. Similarly, arthritic pain cannot be predicted from the extent of joint involvement (Lichtenberg, Swensen, & Skehan, 1986), and symptom reports are not reliably associated with the size of peptic ulcers (Bodemar & Walan, 1978). When symptom clusters accompany a disorder, idiosyncratic symptom patterns may be associated with somatic condition variation within and among individuals. For example, hypertension and diabetes are two chronic diseases that appear to have idiosyncratic symptom constellations. Pennebaker et al. (1981) examined the relationships between self-reported symptoms and blood glucose levels in 30 insulin-dependent diabetics. Most patients had clusters of symptoms that covaried reliably with fluctuations in blood glucose level, but the specific symptoms comprising each cluster varied from person to person. Freund et al. (1986) reported similar findings in adolescents with insulin-dependent diabetes (IDDM). Both studies showed that some specific symptoms ("hungry," "shaky," "tired, weak, no energy") were more often associated with hypoglycemia, so certain symptoms may be experienced more frequently than others, even when symptom clusters are idiosyncratic.

Individuals appear to vary in the accuracy with which they perceive symptoms. Fritz and his colleagues (Fritz, Klein, & Overholser, 1990; Fritz, McQuaid, Spirito, & Klein, 1996) assessed the accuracy of symptom perception among asthmatic children, comparing subjective estimates of severity to spirometry measurements. A wide range of perceptual ability among the children was found, but no reliable predictors of accuracy could be identified. Similarly, Gonder-Frederick, Cox, Bobbitt, and Pennebaker (1986) tested the accuracy of blood glucose symptoms in 26 insulin-dependent diabetic patients by identifying symptoms related to low and high glucose levels in individual patients and then comparing symptom reports to actual glucose levels. Accuracy differed greatly within and across individual subjects, in part related to gender and stability of symptom–glucose relationships across time. This variability in accuracy of symptom perceptions may be related to a number of different factors.

Schemas, beliefs, and attributions have been related to the accuracy of symptom estimates. Hypertension and diabetes provide good examples. Most hypertensives believe they can tell when their blood pressure is elevated. Moreover, once these individuals are diagnosed and adopt beliefs regarding their hypertensive symptoms, they use these beliefs to guide further symptom perception and health behavior concerning their disorder. Pennebaker and Watson (1988) investigated differences between hypertensive, normotensive, and hypotensive university employees in terms of beliefs about blood pressure changes and accuracy of blood pressure reports. Subjects who held accurate beliefs about their symptom and mood–blood pressure correlations were more accurate in their blood pressure estimates, while inaccurate symptom beliefs were related to poor blood pressure estimation. Thus, correct beliefs appeared to enhance and false beliefs seemed to impede subjects' abilities to estimate their blood pressure accurately.

Pennebaker (1982) similarly reported that individuals with poorly controlled diabetes (and therefore extremely variable blood glucose) were relatively accurate in their hypotheses about which symptoms covaried with their blood glucose levels. With treatment, however, these patients' blood glucose levels moderated and the symptoms that covaried with blood glucose changed. Nevertheless, the patients' beliefs about their symptom–blood glucose levels did not change, resulting in initially accurate beliefs and symptom reports becoming inaccurate.

Pennebaker (1982) also notes that individuals may encode general changes in physiological status rather than absolute autonomic levels, so that greater autonomic lability provides more sensory information, which is therefore more readily encoded. This suggests that individuals may have increased ability to detect fluctuations in blood pressure, blood glucose, or heart rate, but may not necessarily be able to specify accurately the amount or even the direction of change. For example, Mandler and colleagues (Mandler & Kahn, 1960; Mandler, Mandler, & Uviller, 1958) found that greater autonomic variability increased the likelihood of symptom reporting, apparently by increasing the probability that internal changes would be detected. However, while autonomic lability increased attention to symptoms, accuracy of self-reports was not related to symptom score.

Theoretical Models

Researchers seeking to identify factors affecting symptom perception have drawn from a variety of theoretical orientations. Early theoretical models were founded in the medical and psychodynamic traditions. These models assumed that the existence of a disease or condition led to the existence of symptoms and signs, that unique symptom clusters were associated with particular illnesses, and that symptom reporting was directly related to disease state, that is, the more symptoms individuals reported, the sicker they were, up to a point. When patients presented such a number and variety of symptom complaints that they could not all be believed, they were assumed to have crossed the line from "normal" to psychopathological, to be manifesting underlying psychological disorders, such as hypochondriasis and conversion reaction (Costa & McCrae, 1985; Pennebaker, 1982).

Later models focused on how "normal" individuals evaluate and label their internal states. Research support for this approach comes from clinical–biofeedback and cognitive–social psychology traditions. The data show that individuals differ in their reporting of symptoms and their sensitivity to pain, so that more sensitive individuals are more likely to perceive symptoms and present medical complaints. However, other factors are also important, including early learning, external reinforcement or punishment for symptom reporting, health beliefs, demographic characteristics, high emotional distress, and general maladjustment (neuroticism). Costa and McCrae (1985) assert that "there are enduring and consistent individual differences in the perception, interpretation, and reporting of bodily symptoms" (p. 20) and that the relationships between symptom complaints and medical condition vary along a continuum from "persistent underreporting to frank hypochondriasis" (p. 20).

Studies on cognitive labeling and attribution theory are particularly relevant to a theoretical model of symptom perception. Research related to cognitive labeling and attribution theory indicates that individuals seek causal explanations for their own and other's behavior, and that a perceived change in internal state (even in the absence of actual physiological change) can activate the search for a label for that change (e.g., Ross, Rodin, & Zimbardo, 1969). This labeling process can lead to interpretation of a physical symptom as due to an emotional state or other internal sensations, such as hunger (Schachter, 1971; Schachter & Rodin, 1974), as well as to illness (e.g., Mechanic, 1972).

Like Pennebaker (1982) and Costa and McCrae (1985), Mechanic (e.g., 1972, 1980) observed that reported physical symptoms reflect a variety of environmental cues and person variables. He described how normal attribution processes work in the determination of symptoms and asserted that people tend to notice symptoms when they depart from ordinary experience. Mechanic (1972) based much of his discussion of how stress, emotion, symptoms, and external cues interact on Schachter and Singer's (1962) theory of emotion as a two-stage process requiring physiological arousal and labeling of the internal sensation. Mechanic asserted that variation in symptom perception and response is most likely to occur when symptoms are diffuse and ambiguous; since assessment of symptoms, conceptualization of possible causes, and decisions about whether to seek medical help occur most often during the early, unorganized phases of illness. External cues become important for symptom explanation when ambiguous symptoms occur concomitantly with emotional arousal and cannot be readily explained. Which cues are attended to and used for symptom explanation may depend on prior experience and on psychological, social, and/or cultural factors.

Recent theoretical models of symptom perception have recognized that "percepts, beliefs, and physiological state are highly interdependent" (Pennebaker & Epstein, 1983, p. 469). The self-regulatory model of illness behavior proposed by Leventhal and colleagues (Cameron, Leventhal, & Leventhal, 1993; Leventhal, 1970; Leventhal, Meyer, & Nerenz, 1980b) proposes that illness behavior can be conceptualized as a self-regulating process incorporating a number of influential factors and interactions. According to the model, changes in somatic activity initiate a process whereby individuals generate a *cognitive representation* of the illness. This representation of the illness is based, in part, on comparisons of the current somatic activity with memories of prior symptom experiences. In addition, symptom attributes, such as label (e.g., "pain"), duration, consequences and severity, possible causes, and expectations about controlling the symptom (Cameron *et al.*, 1993) are important. The representation is subsequently used to guide the selection and initiation of *coping responses*. As coping strategies are applied, an *appraisal process* ensues, during which individuals monitor symptoms and assess efficacy of coping strategies in achieving the goal of symptom elimination. The three activities are repeated in cycles, as individuals revise representations, generate and implement new coping responses, and evaluate the outcomes. In addition, the self-regulatory model includes, in parallel to the cognitive process, an emotional process, in which emotions (e.g., fear, anger, stress) are triggered by the recognition of the symptom and its cognitive representation. The emotional reactions modify the identification and selection of coping strategies and are modified themselves by the appraisal process.

Social cognitive theory, described in some detail in Chapter 3, can also contribute to the understanding of symptom perception processes. Social cognitive theory takes the position that individuals' behaviors are the result of complex, dynamic interactions between personal factors, environmental influences, and behavior (Bandura, 1986). Personal factors may include individuals' abilities to predict outcomes of behaviors, to learn by observing others, and to reflect and analyze experiences. In addition, individuals' expectations and beliefs about efficacy are likely to influence behavior. Environmental influences include characteristics of the situation, as well as information, feedback, reinforcement, and punishment received from others. In terms of symptom perception processes posed by the self-regulatory model, personal factors may influence the development and nature of the cognitive representation of the symptom, as well as the emotional reactions. External factors in the environment may also influence the emotional state and the illness representation. Beliefs about efficacy and other expectations may influence the development and implementation of coping strategies. Information and feedback from the environment, as well as reinforcement or punishment, will likely be incorporated into the appraisal process and used to modify the illness representation and coping efforts.

Variables Affecting Symptom Perception

Both self-regulatory and social cognitive theories highlight the contribution of a variety of factors to the processes of symptom perception. Key mediators within the processes may be physiological, psychological, cognitive, demographic, or environmental.

Physiological Mediators

Symptom Characteristics

Funch (1988) reported that the best predictors of symptom reporting were the characteristics of symptoms themselves. Symptoms can vary in a number of important ways that may affect perceptual processes. Specifically, symptoms vary in duration, intensity, magnitude, location, and clarity. Conceptually, symptoms that are intense (such as pain) or pervasive (i.e., affecting several areas of the body) are thought to be perceived more clearly. In a similar manner, symptoms associated with some areas of the body (e.g., severe pain in the chest or head) might be perceived differently than similar symptoms in other areas (e.g., in the leg or back). Further, vague symptoms (such as fatigue or edema) may be perceived less readily and explained differently than more specific symptoms. Research supports the importance of symptom characteristics in the perceptual process. Symptoms that are severe, unusual, or sudden are reported more often (Funch, 1988), and very painful symptoms are reported more readily than other symptoms (Safer, Tharps, Jackson, & Leventhal, 1979).

Physiological

A variety of physiological mechanisms may influence symptoms and symptom perceptions, such as the effects of referred types of pain; autonomic, neurohormonal, and other psychophysiological responses; and medical conditions, such as diabetes and surgeries that may affect nocioception. Referred types of pain are commonly found with a number of painful symptoms, such as back pain and angina, that is, ischemic pain associated with insufficient blood getting to the heart muscle through the coronary arteries. Back pain is often associated with sciatica as the sciatic nerve is irritated by the bulging of the disk in the back, and pain is felt down the sciatic nerve through the hip and back of the leg. The origin of the symptom is thus in the back, although the pain is felt in the hip and leg. With angina, symptoms are commonly found in the chest, but these symptoms are often not the only ones perceived, and chest symptoms may not be perceived at all by some patients with this type of heart pain; instead, pain may be perceived in the back, left arm, neck, jaw, or abdomen (Raczynski et al., 1994).

Autonomic, neurohormonal, and other psychophysiological mechanisms may also influence symptom perception. For example, while coronary artery disease is associated with ischemia, it is well documented that, among at least some patients, silent or asymptomatic ischemia occurs during both usual activities of living (Deanfield et al., 1983; Subramanian, 1986) and during mild laboratory stressors (Rozanski et al., 1988). At least some of the mechanisms associated with silent ischemia are thought to be physiological in nature (Kaufmann et al., 1998). Patients who evidence ischemia during mental stress have been observed to have heightened cardiovascular reactivity (Krantz et al., 1991; Specchia et al., 1984), and this heightened cardiovascular reactivity has been suggested as mediating ischemia (Specchia et al., 1984). These mechanisms may be related through homeostatic mechanisms that tend to regulate physiological functioning but also have cognitive influences, such as for the baroreflex. Neurohormonal influences also may be present. For instance, plasma noradrenaline has been associated with ischemia (De-Ping Lee, Kimura, & DeQuattro, 1989; Robertson, Bernard, & Robertson, 1983; Tamada, Ito, & Fukuzaki, 1985). Finally, endogenous opiods may also influence expression of ischemia as silent versus symptomatic (Cantor, Shapiro, Eyal, Gueron, & Danon, 1990; Sheps et al., 1987).

Medical conditions may also influence symptom perception. For instance, a well-documented effect of diabetes is damage to the peripheral nervous system that influences nocioception and may influence perception of symptoms from more central sources, such as the perception of angina (Nesto et al., 1988). Damage to the nervous system through trauma or even surgical procedure will also have effects on symptom perception.

Psychological and Emotional State–Trait Characteristics

A number of psychological and emotional characteristics, both transient (i.e., state characteristics) and more enduring (i.e., trait characteristics) have been associated with symptom perception.

Neuroticism

Costa and McCrae (1980, 1985) define neuroticism as a dimension of normal personality that encompasses traits such as self-consciousness, a vulnerability to stress, an inability to inhibit cravings, and a tendency to experience negative emotions such as anxiety, hostility, and depression. They note that several other constructs, including distress and low self-esteem, are closely related to neuroticism and often show similar relationships to symptom reporting. Costa and McCrae (1980, 1985, 1987) studied psycholgical factors and symptom reporting as part of the Baltimore Longitudinal Study of Aging (BLSA), in which initially healthy men and women returned at regular intervals for medical examinations and psychological testing. Costa and McCrae (1980) dichotomized a sample of 912 men into groups scoring high and low in neuroticism and found that neurotic individuals reported two to three times more symptoms than less neurotic individuals. These findings were later replicated in 806 "normals" by eliminating from analyses individuals with characteristics that might be classified as hypochondriacal (Costa & McCrae, 1985). The authors concluded that individuals who are not hypochondriacal but are high on neuroticism may report more somatic complaints because their personality leads them to different styles of noticing, interpreting, and reporting physical sensations.

The association of neuroticism with symptom reporting holds true for angina pectoris, the primary symptom of coronary heart disease (CHD), as well as for general, somatic symptoms. A number of prospective studies found that neuroticism predicted the development of angina pectoris and anginalike chest pain, while more objective measures of CHD were not predictive (Costa, 1981; Costa, Fleg, McCrae, & Lakatta, 1982; French-Belgian Collaborative Group, 1982; Medalie & Goldbourt, 1976; Medalie *et al.*, 1973; Ostfeld, Lebovitz, Shekelle, & Paul, 1964). Costa and McCrae (1985) examined how classical symptoms of chest pain related to CHD and to other patient characteristics in 72 patients referred for cardiac catheterization. Neither number nor severity of self-reported chest pain episodes was significantly related to documented arterial disease. The data also showed that CHD was not associated with mood descriptors, individual pain sensations, or other symptoms accompanying chest pain. In contrast, neuroticism was positively correlated with patient descriptions of their pain as "stabbing" and with several symptoms accompanying chest pain, including breathlessness, dizziness, and palpitations. Neuroticism was not uniquely related to CHD independent of chest pain. Thus, neuroticism appears to be an important factor in the diagnosis of angina pectoris, but not in the development of CHD.

Costa and McCrae (1985) similarly found that BLSA men who developed symptoms of angina without objective signs of cardiac disease were significantly higher in neuroticism than men who reported no chest pain despite electrocardiographic (ECG) evidence of ischemia. Subjects who remained CHD-free were no more or less neurotic than those who later developed CHD. These findings indicating a link between symptom reporting and neuroticism were replicated in 347 adult women also from the BLSA. As with the male subjects, no relationship was evident between mortality and neuroticism (Costa & McCrae, 1987). Costa and McCrae (1985) concluded that neuroticism influences individuals' perceptions of their health but not their objective health status. Thus, many symptoms that prompt patients to seek medical attention and influence physicians' initial diagnoses and referrals may have little relationship to the actual condition of patients' coronary arteries (Costa & McCrae, 1985). Costa and McCrae (1987) note that neurotic individuals' increased attention to internal sensations may in some cases be adaptive if it leads to detection of early signs of disease and subsequent medical attention.

Negative Affect

Negative affective states (e.g., generalized distress, anxiety, depressed affect) and general emotional arousal tend to heighten symptom experiences (Mechanic, 1972). Negative affect has been associated with increased health complaints (Cohen *et al.*, 1995; Watson & Pennebaker, 1989), and several studies have indicated that individuals with higher anxiety report more symptoms than less anxious individuals (e.g., Lipman, Rickels, Covi, Derogatis, & Uhlenhuth, 1969; Pennebaker, 1982). In a prospective study of older adults, E. Leventhal and colleagues (Leventhal, Hansell, Diefenbach, Leventhal, & Glass, 1996) found that negative affect overall, as well as anxious and depressed affect specifically, predicted somatic complaints. Relationships between affect and symptom reporting were more robust in this study using state, rather than trait, measures of negative affect. Neitzert, Davis, and Kennedy (1997) compared the relationship between neuroticism, depression, and somatic symptoms in a sample of 106 male and female university students. Results indicated that both neuroticism and depression were related to symptom reporting in this healthy sample. Depressed mood remained significant in predicting symptom reporting after controlling for the effects of neuroticism.

Studies of adult asthmatics have suggested that poor perceptual accuracy may be also related to anxiety (Fritz *et al.*, 1996). Early work indicated that adult asthmatics with anxious or dependent personality characteristics had higher thresholds for detecting change in pulmonary function (Hudgel & Kinsman, 1983). In addition, recent research has demonstrated that beliefs about mood influence symptom reporting (Goldman, Kraemer, & Salovey, 1996). Undergraduate students provided information about their beliefs concerning attention to mood, as well as self-reports of stress, illness, and symptoms. Students who were more attentive to their moods and made efforts to maintain a positive mood were less likely to report symptoms or illness. Goldman and colleagues concluded that individuals' general manner of appraising mood is an important mediator of stress and symptom reporting.

Personality Characteristics

Personality characteristics and behavioral styles, such as introversion and type A behavior, may also influence symptom perception. Attentiveness to internal state has been found to correlate positively with symptom reporting. Pennebaker (1982) notes that introspective individuals, sensitizers, high self-monitorers, and individuals high in both public and private self-consciousness are more attentive to internal states and report more symptoms than less internally focused individuals. Furthermore, merely directing individuals' attention to internal sensations increases reports of symptoms (Pennebaker & Skelton, 1981). Hansell and Mechanic (1985) found that introspectiveness was correlated with psychological distress and symptom reporting in college freshmen. Emotional sensitivity and time spent alone were also positively associated with symptom reporting. Cioffi (1991) postulates that because attention is directed inward, more somatic information is available to individuals possessing these types of characteristics.

Mechanic (1978, 1980) suggested that people have characteristic styles of symptom reporting which develop early in life. Mechanic (1979) investigated developmental predictors of psychological distress in young adults who were initially assessed 16 years earlier. He concluded that symptom reporting depends on learned patterns of sensitivity and internal monitoring that are formed by developmental experiences, psychological state, actual occurrence of physical illness, and general sense of well-being. Both Mechanic (1979) and Pennebaker, Burnam, Schaeffer, and Harper (1977) found that reporting of specific symptoms was not related to past experience with a symptom. Rather, it appears that a general pattern of internal monitoring and reporting is established in the course of development.

A number of studies have examined the perception of physical symptoms in type A individuals. The earliest studies reported that type As underreported the frequency and intensity of physical symptoms relative to type Bs (Carver, Coleman, & Glass, 1976; Greene, Moss, & Goldstein, 1974; Matthews & Brunson, 1979; Weidner & Matthews, 1978). Hart (1983) later found that type A male college students reported fewer and less intense physical symptoms than type Bs during a high-stress week of examinations. He suggested that type As and Bs may differ in how they label an internal state. Type As may resist defining symptoms as signals of illness in order to avoid the sick role, which collides with their need for control. The type A tendency to suppress symptoms that interfere with work or task performance has been observed in children as well as adults. Leikin et al. (1988) found that type A children reported fewer symptoms immediately postsurgery and at follow-up than type Bs. Type A children also missed fewer days of school following surgery than type Bs. Consistent with assertions that children develop patterns of internal awareness that persist across the course of development (e.g., Mechanic, 1979; Pennebaker et al., 1977), these data suggest that type As develop a style of symptom underreporting that begins early in life and persists across the life span.

Cognitive Variables

Symptom perception is related to cognitive factors that affect focus of attention on internal versus external stimuli and labeling of internal sensations. The amount and nature of available external information are important both in terms of providing a label for symptoms and in competing with internal sensory information.

Labeling

Studies of cognitive variables affecting symptom perception emphasize the importance of Schachter and Singer's (1962) theory of emotions. This theory proposes that an individual first detects an internal change or arousal, then surveys the environment for appropriate cues in order to develop labels for the internal sensation. The availability of an appropriate label is an important component of perceived symptoms (Pennebaker *et al.*, 1977). The label chosen with regard to a given symptom depends on mood and personality variables, cognitive factors, and external cues, as well as on physiological characteristics of the symptom. Physiological changes and symptoms are often associated with mood states (e.g., racing heart and sweating palms associated with anxiety, fatigue related to depression). In many cases, these symptoms of mood mimic symptoms of disease (e.g., heart disease), and individuals may attribute symptoms to a mood state rather than to disease.

Competition of Cues

Pennebaker (1980, 1982) asserts that awareness of internal state is a function of the ratio of internal to external information, and thus depends on the *relative* processing of internal versus external cues. He postulates that individuals' capacity to attend to stimuli is fixed. When the external environment produces relatively less stimulation, attention turns inward to somatic information (Pennebaker, 1980). Pennebaker and Lightner (1980) investigated this hypothesis in an exercise setting. Strategies to focus subjects' attention on external auditory stimuli attenuated perception of physical symptoms and fatigue. Conversely, forcing attention to subjects' own amplified breathing during exercise increased perceptions of fatigue and symptoms, even though physical work remained constant. Furthermore, increased external information resulted in lower jogging times, and thus differential physical work despite comparable reports of fatigue and symptoms.

Fillingim and Fine (1986) directed undergraduate students to focus internally (attending to breathing and heart rate) or externally (listening for a target word heard repeatedly over headphones) while running a mile in the laboratory. Participants reported significantly fewer symptoms in the external focusing condition than in either the internal focusing or a control condition. These studies suggest that as individuals become highly focused on an external task, the ability to attend to alternative (internal) information decreases.

Control

Perceived or actual control over symptoms or environmental events also plays an important role in symptom perception. High levels of control correlate negatively with symptom reporting. Conversely, actual or perceived loss or lack of control correlates positively with symptoms. Thus, persons with low self-esteem, individuals scoring high on external locus of control, subjects in laboratory situations manipulated to elicit perceived lack of environmental control, and those experiencing major life changes and actual loss of control report more symptoms (see Pennebaker, 1982).

Pennebaker *et al.* (1977) conducted two studies using undergraduate college students, varying the amount of control subjects had over an aversive stimulus. Lack of control led to increased symptom reporting, independent of whether subjects experienced success or failure in performing tasks. These authors hypothesized that lack of control led to increased negative affect or arousal, which, in turn, precipitated a search for labels for the internal arousal. A symptom checklist presumably provided such labels, resulting in increased symptom reporting. Other researchers have similarly found that unpredictable aversive events are linked with greater symptom re-porting than are more predictable and controllable ones (Weidner & Matthews, 1978).

Beliefs, Schemas, Attributions

Individuals' expectations and beliefs also impact awareness and interpretation of sensory information, particularly ambiguous sensations like those experienced in the early stages of many illnesses. Individuals often rely on environmental informa-tion in developing hypotheses and interpreting symptoms, and the search for symp-tom labels is typically guided by expectations and beliefs. Leventhal and colleagues (Baumann, Cameron, Zimmerman, & Leventhal, 1989; Leventhal, Nerenz, & Straus, 1980a) elaborated on the ways in which cognitive illness representations influence perception of symptoms, as well as subsequent illness coping processes and adher-ence to prescribed medical regimens.

Leventhal *et al.* (1980a) investigated the roles of direct perception and inference in patients with hypertension, a condition that is commonly assumed to be asympto-matic. Hypertensive subjects tended to believe they had symptoms associated with blood pressure elevations, despite information from their physicians about the asymptomatic nature of hypertension. These patients selectively monitored the spe-cific symptoms they *believed* to accompany increased blood pressure. The symptoms monitored were directly related to individuals' conception of what events "caused" or which sensations signaled high blood pressure. These authors concluded that ex-pectations about an illness and its symptoms affect awareness and interpretation of ambiguous sensory information.

The role of prior beliefs in making attributions for symptoms is highlighted by Baumann *et al.* (1989), who examined symptom reporting and illness representations in volunteer college students given false feedback regarding their blood pressure lev-els. Subjects given high blood pressure feedback reported symptoms consistent with high blood pressure; subjects used external cues to decide whether their ambiguous "blood pressure" symptoms were due to illness or stress, and symptom reporting was affected by subjects' prior beliefs regarding blood pressure lability and by external cues regarding their own daily stress levels. Subjects given high blood pressure feed-back reported that they tended to have their blood pressure rechecked in a few weeks, in contrast to the normal blood pressure feedback group, who planned to be rechecked in 3 to 6 months. Baumann *et al.* concluded that prior illness schemas and contextual cues consistent with these schemas influence inferences involved in symp-tom interpretation, and these inferences, in turn, affect coping plans.

Two studies conducted by Pennebaker and colleagues yielded similar results. Pennebaker and Skelton (1981) varied information given to college students about the effects of ultrasonic noise on skin temperature. Despite the fact that the noise produced no physiological change, subjects selectively attended to bodily sensations in the in-struction-induced direction of change (increased vs. decreased skin temperature) and did not utilize sensory information indicating a change in the opposite sensory direc-tion. Subjects given no particular hypothesis paid very little attention to skin temper-ature sensations at all. Anderson and Pennebaker (1980) had subjects place their finger on a piece of sandpaper attached to a vibrator. One group was told that the experience might be somewhat painful, while the other group was told that the experience would be pleasant. Study participants rated their experience as painful or pleasant totally consistent with the expectation they had been given at the outset; that is, no "painful" subjects rated the experience as pleasant and no "pleasant" participants rated the experience as painful. These studies demonstrate that providing individuals with an illness label will stimulate selective, belief-guided searching for label-consistent symptom information, and vice versa; symptoms will stimulate the search for a label.

The findings reviewed above help to explain how many patients become aware of illness symptoms, make attributions for their symptoms, and choose strategies to cope with these symptoms. Previously healthy individuals will interpret symptoms consistent with their prior experiences with acute illness. So, for example, individuals may take an antacid tablet in response to ambiguous chest pressure and discomfort. Once diagnosed with a disease, patients have specific illness schema within which to interpret even ambiguous sensations that might be illness related. However, research by Pennebaker (1982) suggests that even within a chronic disease schema, changes in beliefs about symptoms do not immediately coincide with physiological change and, if they do occur, will do so gradually over time.

Examples of the influence of belief can also be found in the occurrence of "medical students' disease." Woods, Natterson, and Silverman (1978) state that a majority of first-year medical students experience symptoms not unlike the ones they study. Pennebaker (1994) suggests that

> the students, who are undoubtedly under stress from sleep deprivation, exams, or other reasons, can detect a number of subtle bodily sensations that probably reflect heightened autonomic activity . . . their disease beliefs or schema direct the ways they attend to their bodies and interpret their symptoms. (p. 500)

Similarly, mass psychogenic illness occurs when large groups of people report similar physical symptoms that have no clear basis (Colligan, Pennebaker, & Murphy, 1982). The phenomenon usually occurs when one person reports symptoms (e.g., fainting, vomiting). This symptom report affects the beliefs of others, who subsequently experience similar symptoms. Such "outbreaks" often occur when people are under stress or engaged in boring occupations (Pennebaker, 1994).

Perceived Risk

An emerging body of literature is linking the perception of risk with symptom perception and reporting, particularly in the area of chemical exposures. MacGregor and Fleming (1996), in a review of the literature, note that risk can be categorized as "acceptable" or "unacceptable." Acceptability tended to be greater for risks perceived as voluntary, chronic, common, familiar, known to science, and controllable. Thus, symptoms that are perceived as putting individuals at greater risk, particularly when the risk is less acceptable, will draw more attention and may be labeled differently than other symptoms.

Demographic Variables

In large national studies of symptom prevalence and reporting, many completed by the National Center for Health Statistics (NCHS), findings indicate that most individuals (greater than 70%) acknowledge symptoms (NCHS, 1970), use aspirin at least occasionally (NCHS, 1979), or visit a physician (Woodwell, 1997). Over

69 million physician office visits were estimated to have occurred in 1995 (Woodwell, 1997), an average of 2.7 visits per person. Of these office visits, 55% were stimulated by symptom reports. Respiratory and musculoskeletal symptoms were the most commonly reported symptoms.

There are indications that symptom perception, reporting, and coping varies systematically with demographics (Kroenke & Price, 1993; Pennebaker, 1982). A number of studies indicate that females report more symptoms (Kroenke & Price, 1993; NCHS, 1970; Stenberg & Wall, 1995) and make more physician visits (Woodwell, 1997), as do older persons (Kroenke & Price, 1993; NCHS, 1970; Woodwell, 1997). Despite the increased number of physician visits by older persons, Prohaska, Leventhal, Leventhal, and Keller (1985) found that elderly persons were less likely to interpret chronic mild symptoms as illness warnings. Older individuals also reported greater frequencies of health-promoting activities (e.g., greater attention to diet, regular sleep and mild exercise, regular medical checkups) and health practices aimed at controlling stress and emotions (e.g., avoiding stress, staying active). Several factors may account for the increased symptom reporting of both women and older persons. Women and older persons may experience greater variability in somatic symptoms or their beliefs may be affected by social or cultural factors. In addition, the increased symptom frequency experienced by these groups may influence cognitive processes related to an increased somatic focus and perceptual and attributional processes.

Socioeconomic status has been found to be inversely related with symptom reporting (Funch, 1988; Kroenke & Price, 1993; NCHS, 1970; Woodwell, 1997), but the data relating educational attainment to symptom perception are more limited. Hannan, Anderson, Pincus, and Felson (1992) reviewed National Health and Nutrition Examination Survey I (NHANES I) data to examine the cross-sectional association between formal education and knee pain. They found univariate associations between osteoarthritis and lower educational levels. After adjustment for known risk factors (age, knee injury, race, obesity, occupation) and the presence of radiographic changes, reporting of knee pain remained significantly associated with lower educational attainment.

Environmental Influences

External events have long been associated with health. Early models focused on the external events themselves (Holmes & Rahe, 1967), whereas subsequent models emphasized individuals' cognitive appraisal of situational demands and their ability to meet those demands (DeLongis, Coyne, Dakof, Folkman, & Lazarus, 1982). For example, stress has been routinely reported to be related to symptom development and reporting among patients with irritable bowel syndrome (IBS) (Whitehead, 1992). Recent studies, however, have indicated that the existence of prior IBS symptoms may be a better predictor of subsequent symptom reporting by patients under stress than the existence of stress per se (Suls, Wan, & Blanchard, 1994) .

Cameron, Leventhal, and Leventhal (1995) tested the hypothesis that ongoing stress changes the attribution of symptoms to illness. In a longitudinal study of middle-aged and elderly persons, subjects were less likely to seek care for ambiguous symptoms if there was a concurrent life stressor, and such symptoms were more likely to be attributed to stress than to illness. Life stress did not affect interpretation of symptoms that were clearly related to disease. Moreover, stress management training, through cognitive behavior therapy (Blanchard *et al.*, 1992) and identification of coping strategies (Guthrie, Creed, Dawson, & Tomenson, 1991), has been shown to reduce the number of IBS symptoms reported by patients.

Relevance to Interventions

The perception of symptoms is important in many aspects of health maintenance, and early detection and appropriate attribution of symptoms is a key factor in efficacious treatment for many medical conditions. An understanding of the biopsychosocial determinants and processes of symptom perception and reporting informs the development of interventions in important ways. Interventions can be developed to provide health information, enhance coping strategies, and encourage appropriate health care seeking.

Enhancing the Accuracy of Symptom Perception and Attribution to Increase the Likelihood of Seeking Care

If individuals' ability to perceive symptoms and correctly determine the seriousness of symptoms is positively related to health knowledge, then interventions that increase knowledge about symptomatology and severity could help to stimulate appropriate health-care-seeking behavior. Studies of patients with asthma indicate that accuracy of symptom perception is important for effective self-management, particularly among children with asthma (Fritz, Yeung, & Teitel, 1994): "Self-management by child or adolescent asthma patients leads to timely treatment . . . [and] can reduce the side effects of medications that may be associated with improper or excessive treatment" (p. 423). Information and training programs for patients and caregivers can also be effective in increasing accuracy in perception of respiratory symptoms (Stout *et al.*, 1992).

Studies of health knowledge and symptom perception provide important information for the development of health-care-seeking interventions. For example, Smith and Kane (1970) completed a survey in rural Kentucky and found that health knowledge was positively correlated with recognition of symptoms as severe and requiring medical attention. Personal experience with chronic illness in the immediate family was *not* associated with either increased health knowledge or severity perception, suggesting that persons gain relevant information from other sources. Survey data such as these can be invaluable in guiding the development and dissemination of intervention activities and materials.

It should be noted, however, that materials used to inform the public about health matters must be developed and evaluated with caution. MacGregor, Slovic, and Morgan (1994) report on an evaluation of materials developed to inform the public about the potential risk associated with electromagnetic fields. A brochure was carefully designed to present a balanced presentation of scientific evidence and uncertainty about the sources and health effects associated with electromagnetic fields. The results of the evaluation indicated that persons who read the brochure were sensitized to a broad range of possible symptoms, despite specific statements in the brochure about the lack of evidence for a causal relationship. The investigators speculated that readers used the brochure's information to create their own intuitive models to explain a range of potential consequences, despite information to the contrary.

Developing More Effective Coping Strategies by Addressing Factors Mediating
Symptom Perception and Attribution

Distraction and imagery are often a part of pain management programs designed to help patients cope more effectively with chronic pain (Worthington & Shumate, 1981), as well as the pain and discomfort associated with experiences such as childbirth (Leventhal, Leventhal, Shacham, & Easterling, 1989) and chemotherapy (Love, Nerenz, & Leventhal, 1983). Both distraction via imagery and focusing on concrete aspects of the physical sensation have been found to be effective in helping individuals cope with discomfort (Cioffi, 1991). As noted earlier, cognitive behavioral stress management training also has been shown to ameliorate the discomfort associated with these types of conditions and reduce the number of symptoms reported by patients (Blanchard *et al.*, 1992; Guthrie *et al.*, 1991).

Adherence to exercise protocols can be very important in maintaining healthy lifestyles as well as recovering from myocardial infarction, stroke, and injuries. The use of external competing cues (e.g., listening to audiotapes, running on a cross-country trail) has been shown to be effective in reducing symptom reports and increasing exercise tolerance (Fillingim & Fine, 1986; Pennebaker & Lightner, 1980). In addition, increasing individuals' perceived self-efficacy may positively affect exercise tolerance and performance. Studies of treadmill activity and cardiac patients have indicated that patients' expectations of their abilities to tolerate exertion is more predictive of performance than measured cardiac capacity (Ewart, Taylor, Reese, & Debusk, 1983).

Encouraging Appropriate Health-Care-Seeking Behavior

In addition to focusing on strategies for promoting more accurate symptom perception, comprehensive interventions also need to address health-care-seeking behaviors. Leventhal (1975) proposed that self-treating behavior and health care seeking arise from individuals' beliefs and inferences about their physical states rather than from their actual physiological conditions. Meyer *et al.* (1985) examined this proposal in patients with hypertension. Hypertensive patients who perceived that their medical treatments affected symptoms they believed to accompany elevated blood pressure were more adherent to mediation regimens and were more likely to have their blood pressure under control. Health-care-seeking behaviors and interventions are the focus of the next chapter.

Summary and Conclusions

To summarize many of the factors affecting symptom perception, Pennebaker (1982) offers a description of the high symptom reporter as young, often female, from a small town with a lower socioeconomic background who is self-conscious, anxious, has low self-esteem, and aspires (but may not succeed) to control her environment. When she perceives changes in her physical condition, she actively searches the environment (both internal and external, current and historical) for labels for the sensations. She makes attributions concerning the causes and consequences of the symptom(s) and applies coping strategies, both behavioral and emotional, to effect change in her perceived symptoms. Reappraisal of her physical condition follows, which may lead her to revise her coping strategies or to seek care. Taken together, the literature suggests that (1) symptom processes involve complex interactions between physiological and psychological variables and (2) the amount of interindividual and intraindividual variation is significant and important. Understanding the components and nature of these interactions and variation can help researchers and practitioners develop more effective and cost-efficient interventions to improve perceptual accuracy, change beliefs and attributions, enhance appropriate health-care-seeking behaviors, and limit inappropriate use of health care.

References

Anderson, D., & Pennebaker, J. W. (1980). Pain and pleasure: Alternative interpretations of identical stimulation. *European Journal of Social Psychology, 10,* 207–212.

Bandura, A. (1986). *Social foundations of thought and action.* Englewood Cliffs, NJ: Prentice-Hall.

Barsky, A. J., Cleary, P., Barnett, M. C., Christiansen, C. L., & Ruskin, J. N. (1994). The accuracy of symptom reporting by patients complaining of palpitations. *American Journal of Medicine, 97,* 214–221.

Baumann, L. J., Cameron, L. D., Zimmerman, R. S., & Leventhal, H. (1989). Illness representationas and matching labels with symptoms. *Health Psychology, 8,* 449–469.

Blanchard, E. B., Schwarz, S. P., Suls, J. M., Gerardi, M. A., Scharff, L., Greene, B., Taylor, A. E., Berreman, C., & Malamood, H. S. (1992). Two controlled evaluations of a multicomponent psychological treatment of irritable bowel syndrome. *Behavior Research & Therapy, 2,* 175–189.

Bodemar, G., & Walan, A. (1978). Maintenance treatment of recurrent peptic ulcer by cimetidine. *Lancet, 1,* 403–407.

Cameron, L., Leventhal, E. A., & Leventhal, H. (1993). Symptom representations and affect as determinants of care seeking in a community-dwelling, adult sample population. *Health Psychology, 12*(3), 171–179.

Cameron, L., Leventhal, E. A., & Leventhal, H. (1995). Seeking medical care in response to symptoms and life stress. *Psychosomatic Medicine, 57*(1), 37–47.

Cantor, A., Shapiro, Y., Eyal, A., Gueron, M., & Danon, A. (1990). Asymptomatic or mildly symptomatic effort-induced myocardial ischemia: Plasma β-endorphins and effect of naloxone. *Israeli Journal of Medical Science, 26,* 67–71.

Carver, C. S,. Coleman, A. E., & Glass, D. C. (1976). The coronary-prone behavior pattern and the suppression of fatigue on a treadmill test. *Journal of Personality and Social Psychology, 3,* 460–466.

Cioffi, D. (1991). Beyond attentional strategies: A cognitive–perceptual model of somatic interpretation. *Psychological Bulletin, 109*(1), 25–41

Cohen, S., Doyle, W. J., Skoner, D. P., Fireman, P., Gwaltney, J. M., & Newson, J. T. (1995). State and trait negative affect as predictors of objective and subjective symptoms of respiratory viral infections. *Journal of Personality and Social Psychology, 68,* 159–169.

Colligan, M., Pennebaker, J. W., & Murphy, L. (1982). *Mass psychogenic illness: a social psychological analysis.* Hillsdale, NJ: Erlbaum.

Costa, P. T. (1981). Neuroticism as a factor in the diagnosis of angina pectoris. *Behavioral Medicine Update, 3,* 18–20.

Costa, P. T., & McCrae, R. R. (1980). Somatic complaints in males as a function of age and neuroticism: A longitudinal analysis. *Journal of Behavioral Medicine, 3,* 245–257.

Costa, P. T., & McCrae, R. R. (1985). Hypochondriasis, neuroticism, and aging. *American Psychologist, 40,* 19–28.

Costa, P. T., & McCrae, R. R. (1987). Neuroticism, somatic complaints, and disease: Is the bark worse than the bite? *Journal of Personality, 55,* 301–316.

Costa, P. T., Fleg, J. L., McCrae, R. R., & Lakatta, G. (1982). Neuroticism, coronary artery disease, and chest pain complaints: Cross-sectional and longitudinal studies. *Experimental Aging Research, 8,* 37–44.

Deanfield, J. E., Maseri, A., Selwyn, A. P., Ribeiro, P., Chierchia, S., Krikler, S., & Morgan, M. (1983). Myocardial ischemia during daily life in patients with stable angina: Its relation to symptoms and heart rate changes. *Lancet, 2,* 753–758.

DeLongis, A., Coyne, J. C., Dakof, F., Folkman, S., & Lazarus, R. S. (1982). Relationship of daily hassles, uplifts, and major life events to health status. *Health Psychology, 1,* 119–136.

De-Ping Lee, D., Kimura, S., & DeQuattro, V. (1989, February). Noradrenergic activity and silent ischaemia in hypertensive patients with stable angina: Effect of Metoprolol. *Lancet, 1*, 403–406.

Ewart, C., Taylor, C., Reese, L., & Debusk, R. (1983). Effects of early postmyocardial infarction exercise testing on self-perception and subsequent physical activity. *American Journal of Cardiology, 51*, 1076–1080.

Fillingim, R. B., & Fine, M. A. (1986). The effects of internal versus external information processing on symptom perception in an exercise setting. *Health Psychology, 5*(2), 115–23.

French–Belgian Collaborative Group. (1982). Ischemic heart disease and psychological patterns: Prevalence and incidence studies in Belgium and France. *Advances in Cardiology, 29*, 25–31.

Freund, A., Bennett-Johnson, S., Rosenbloom, A., Alexander, B., & Hansen, C. A. (1986). Subjective symptoms, blood glucose estimation, and blood glucose concentrations in adolescents with diabetes. *Diabetes Care, 9*(3), 236–243.

Fritz, G. K., Klein, R. B., & Overholser, J. C. (1990). Accuracy of symptom perception in childhood asthma. *Journal of Developmental & Behavioral Pediatrics, 11*(2), 69–72.

Fritz, G. K., McQuaid, E. L., Spirito, A., & Klein, R. B. (1996). Symptom perception in pediatric asthma: Relationship to functional morbidity and psychological factors. *Journal of American Academy of Child and Adolescent Psychiatry, 35*(8), 1033–41.

Fritz, G. K., Yeung, A., & Teitel, M. S. (1994). Symptom perception and self-management in childhood asthma. *Current Opinion in Pediatrics, 6*, 423–427.

Funch, D. P. (1988). Predictors and consequences of symptom reporting behaviors in colorectal cancer patients. *Medical Care, 26*(10), 1000–1008.

Goldman, S. L., Kraemer, D.T., & Salovey, P. (1996). Beliefs about mood moderate the relationship of stress to illness and symptom reporting. *Journal of Psychosomatic Research, 41*(2), 115–128.

Gonder-Frederick, L. A., Cox, D. J., Bobbitt, S. A., & Pennebaker, J. W. (1986). Blood glucose symptoms beliefs of diabetic patients: Accuracy and implications. *Health Psychology, 5*(4), 327–341.

Greene, W. A., Moss, A. J., & Goldstein, S. (1974). Delay, denial, and death in coronary heart disease. In R. S. Eliot (Ed.), *Stress and the heart*. New York: Futura.

Guthrie, E., Creed, F., Dawson, D., & Tomenson, B. (1991). A controlled trial of psychological treatment for the irritable bowel syndrome. *Gastroenterology, 100*, 450–457.

Hannan, M. T., Anderson, J. J., Pincus, T., & Felson, D. T. (1992). Educational attainment and osteoarthritis: Differential associations with radiographic changes and symptom reporting. *Journal of Clinical Epidemiology, 45*(2), 139–47.

Hansell, S., & Mechanic, D. (1985). Introspectiveness and adolescent symptom reporting. *Journal of Human Stress, 11*(4), 165–76.

Hart, K. E. (1983). Physical symptom reporting and health perception among type A and B college males. *Journal of Human Stress, 9*(4), 17–22.

Holmes, T. H., & Rahe, R. H. (1967). The social readjustment rating scale. *Journal of Psychosomatic Research, 11*, 213–218.

Hudgel, D., & Kinsman, R. (1983). Interactions among behavioral style, ventilatory drive, and load recognition. *American Reviews of Respiratory Diseases, 128*, 246–248.

Kaufmann, P.G., McMahon, R.P., Becker, L. C., Bertolet, B., Bonsall, R., Chaitman, B., Cohen, J. D., Foreman, S., Goldberg, A. D., Freedland, K., Ketterer, M. W., Krantz, D. S., Pepine, C. J., Raczynski, J. M., Stone, P. H., Taylor, H., Knatterud, G. L., Sheps, D. S., for the PIMI Investigators. (1998). The Psychophysiological Investigations of Myocardial Ischemia (PIMI) Study: Objective, method, and variability of measures. *Psychosomatic Medicine, 60*, 52–55.

Krantz, D. S., Helmers, K. F., Bairey, C. N., Nebel, L. E., Hedges, S. M., & Rozanski, A. (1991). Cardiovascular reactivity and mental stress-induced myocardial ischemia in patients with coronary artery disease. *Psychomatic Medicine, 82*, 1296–1304.

Kroenke, K., & Price, R. K. (1993). Symptoms in the community: Prevalence, classification, and psychiatric comorbidity. *Archives of Internal Medicine, 153*, 2474–2480.

Leiken, L., Firestone, P., & McGrath, P. (1988). Physical symptom reporting in type A and type B children. *Journal of Consulting and Clinical Psychology, 56*, 721–726.

Leventhal, E. A., Leventhal, H., Shacham, S., & Easterling, D. V. (1989). Active coping reduces reports of pain from childbirth. *Journal of Consulting and Clinical Psychology, 57*, 365–371.

Leventhal, E. A., Hansell, S., Diefenbach, M., Leventhal, H., & Glass, D. (1996). Negative affect and self-report of physical symptoms: Two longitudinal studies of older adults. *Health Psychology, 15*(3), 193–199.

Leventhal, H. (1970). Findings and theory in the study of fear communications. *Advances in Experimental Social Psychology, 5*, 119–186.

Leventhal, H. (1975). The consequences of depersonalization during illness and treatment. In J. Howard & A. Strauss (Eds.), *Humanizing health care* (pp. 119–161). New York: Wiley.

Leventhal, H., Nerenz, D., & Straus, A. (1980a). Self-regulation and the mechanisms for symptoms appraisal. In D. Mechanic (Ed.), *Psychosocial epidemiology* (pp. 58–86). New York: Neal Watson.

Leventhal, H., Meyer, D., & Nerenz, D. (1980b). The common sense representation of illness danger. In S. Rachman (Ed.), *Contributions to medical psychology* (vol. 2, pp. 7–30). New York: Pergamon Press.

Lichtenberg, P. A., Swensen, C.H., & Skehan, M. W. (1986). Further investigation of the role of personality, lifestyle, and arthritic severity in predicting pain. *Journal of Psychosomatic Research, 30,* 327–337.

Lipman, R., Rickels, K., Covi, L., Derogatis, L., & Uhlenhuth, E. (1969). Factors of symptom distress. *Archives of General Psychiatry, 21,* 328–338.

Love, R., Nerenz, D., & Leventhal, H. (1983). Anticipatory nausea with cancer chemotherapy: Development through two mechanisms. *Proceedings of the American Society for Clinical Oncology, 2,* 62.

MacGregor, D. G., & Fleming, R. (1996). Risk perception and symptom reporting. *Risk Analysis, 16*(6), 773–783.

MacGregor, D. G., Slovic, P., & Morgan, M. G. (1994). Perception of risks form electromagnetic fields: A psychometric evaluation of a risk-communication approach. *Risk Analysis, 14,* 815–828.

Mandler, G., & Kahn, M. (1960). Discrimination of changes in heart rate: Two unsuccessful attempts. *Journal of the Experimental Analysis of Behavior, 3,* 21–25.

Mandler, G., Mandler, J. M., & Uviller, E. T. (1958). Autonomic feedback: The perception of autonomic activity. *Journal of Abnormal and Social Psychology, 56,* 367–373.

Matteson, M. T., & Ivancevich, J. M. (1982). Type A and B behavior patterns and self-reported health symptoms and stress: Examining individual and organizational fit. *Journal of Occupational Medicine, 24*(8), 585–589.

Matthews, K. A., & Brunson, B. I. (1979). Allocation of attention and the type A coronary-prone behavior pattern. *Journal of Personality and Social Psychology, 37,* 2081–2090.

Mechanic, D. (1972). Social psychologic factors affecting the presentation of bodily complaints. *New England Journal of Medicine, 286,* 1132–1139.

Mechanic, D. (1978). Effects of psychological distress on perceptions of physical health and use of medical and psychiatric facilities. *Journal of Human Stress, 4,* 26–32.

Mechanic, D. (1979). Correlates of psychological distress among young adults: A theoretical hypothesis and results from a 16-year follow-up study. *Archives of General Psychiatry, 36,* 1233–1239.

Mechanic, D. (1980). The experience and reporting of common physical complaints. *Journal of Health and Social Behavior, 21,* 146–155.

Medalie, J. H., & Goldbourt, U. (1976). Angina pectoris among 10,000 men. *American Journal of Medicine, 60,* 910–921.

Medalie, J. H., Snyder, M., Groen, J. J., Neufeld, H. N., Goldbourt, U., & Riss, E. (1973). Angina pectoris among 10,000 men: 5-year incidence and univariate analysis. *American Journal of Medicine, 55,* 583–594.

Meyer, D., Leventhal, H., & Gutmann, M. (1985). Common sense models of illness: The example of hypertension. *Health Psychology, 4,* 115–135.

National Center for Health Statistics (NCHS). (1970). *Selected symptoms of psychological distress.* Series 11, Number 37. Washington, DC: US Government Printing Office.

National Center for Health Statistics (NCHS). (1979). *Acute conditions: Incidence and associated disability, United States, July 1977–June 1978.* Series 10, Number 132. Washington, DC: US Government Printing Office.

Neitzert, C. S., Davis, C., & Kennedy, S. H. (1997). Personality factors related to the prevalence of somatic symptoms and medical complaints in a healthy student population. *British Journal of Medical Psychology, 79*(1), 93–101.

Nesto, R. W., Phillips, R. T., Kett, K. G., Hill, T., Perper, E., Yung E., & Leland, O. S., Jr. (1988). Angina and exertional myocardial ischemia in diabetic and nondiabetic patients: Assessment by exercise thallium scintigraphy. *Annals of Internal Medicine, 108,* 170–175.

Ostfeld, A. M., Lebovitz, B. Z. , Shekelle, R. B., & Paul, O. (1964). A prospective study of the relationship between personality and coronary heart disease. *Journal of Chronic Disease, 17,* 265–276.

Pennebaker, J. W. (1980). Perceptual and environmental determinants of coughing. *Basic and Applied Social Psychology, 1,* 83–91.

Pennebaker, J. W. (1982). *The psychology of physical symptoms.* New York: Springer-Verlag.

Pennebaker, J. W. (1994). Psychological bases of symptom reporting: Perceptual and emotional aspects of chemical sensitivity. *Toxicology and Industrial Health, 10*(4/5), 497–511.

Pennebaker, J. W., & Epstein, D. (1983). Implicit psychophysiology: Effects of common beliefs and idiosyncratic physiological responses on symptom reporting. *Journal of Personality, 51*(3), 468–496.

Pennebaker, J. W., & Lightner, J. (1980). Competition of internal and external information in an exercise setting. *Journal of Personality and Social Psychology, 41*, 213–223.

Pennebaker, J. W., & Skelton, J. A. (1981). Selective monitoring of physical sensations. *Journal of Personality and Social Psychology, 41*, 213–223.

Pennebaker, J. W., & Watson, D. (1988). Blood pressure estimation and beliefs among normotensive and hypertensive. *Health Psychology, 7*, 309–328.

Pennebaker, J. W., Burnam, M. A., Schaeffer, M. A., & Harper, D. C. (1977). Lack of control as a determinant of perceived physical symptoms. *Journal of Personality and Social Psychology, 35*(3), 167–174.

Pennebaker, J. W., Cox, D. J., Gonder-Frederick, L., Wunsch, M. G., Evans, W. S., & Pohl, S. (1981). Physical symptoms related to blood glucose in insulin-dependent diabetics. *Psychosomatic Medicine, 43*, 489–500.

Prohaska, T. R., Leventhal, E. A., Leventhal, H., & Keller, M. L. (1985). Health practices and illness cognition in young, middle aged, and elderly adults. *Journal of Gerontology, 40*(5), 569–578.

Raczynski, J.M., Taylor, H., Rappaport, N., Cutter, G., Hardin, M., & Oberman, A. (1994). Diagnoses, acute symptoms and attributions for symptoms among black and white inpatients admitted for coronary heart disease: Findings of the Birmingham–BHS project. *American Journal of Public Health, 84*(6), 951–995

Robertson, R. M., Bernard, Y., & Robertson, D. (1983). Arterial and coronary sinus catecholamines in the course of spontaneous coronary artery spasm. *American Heart Journal, 105*, 901–906.

Ross, L., Rodin, J., & Zimbardo, P. (1969). Toward an attribution therapy: The reduction of fear through induced cognitive–emotional attribution. *Journal of Personality and Social Psychology, 12*, 279–288.

Rozanski, A., Bairey, C. N., Krantz, D. S., Friedman, J., Resser, K. J., Morell, M., Hilton-Chalfen, S., Hestrin, L., Bietendorf, J., & Berman, D. S. (1988). Mental stress and the induction of silent ischemia in patients with coronary artery disease. *New England Journal of Medicine, 318*, 1005–1021.

Safer, M. A., Tharps, Q. J., Jackson, T. C., & Leventhal, H. (1979). Determinants of three stages of delay in seeking care at a medical clinic. *Medical Care, 17*(1), 11–29.

Schachter, S. (1971). *Emotion, obesity and crime.* New York: Academic Press.

Schachter, S., & Rodin, J. (1974). *Obese humans and rats.* Hillsdale, NJ: Erlbaum.

Schachter, S., & Singer, J. E. (1962). Cognitive, social, and physiological determinants of emotional state. *Psychological Review, 69*, 379–399.

Sheps, D. S., Adams, K. F., Hinderliter, A., Price, C., Bissette, J., Orlando, G., Margolis, B., & Koch, G. (1987). Endorphins are related to pain perception in coronary artery disease. *American Journal of Cardiology, 59*, 523–527.

Smith, L., & Kane, R. (1970). Health knowledge and symptom perception: A study of a rural Kentucky county. *Social Science and Medicine, 4*(5), 557–567.

Specchia, G., de Servi, S., Farcone, C., Gravazzi, A., Angoli, L., Bramucci, E., Ardissino, D., & Mussini, A. (1984). Mental arithmetic stress testing in patients with coronary artery disease. *American Heart Journal, 108*, 56–63.

Stenberg, B., & Wall, S. (1995). Why do women report "sick building symptoms" more often than men? *Social Science and Medicine, 40*(4), 491–502.

Stout, C., Kotses, H., & Creer, T. L. (1993). Improving recognition of respiratory sensations in healthy adults. *Biofeedback and Self-Regulation, 18*, 79–92.

Subramanian, V. B. (1986). Clinical and research applications of ambulatory Holter ST-segment and heart rate monitoring. *American Journal of Cardiology, 58*, 11B–20B.

Suls, J., Wan, C. K., & Blanchard, E. B. (1994). A multilevel data analytic approach for evaluation of relationships between daily life stressors: The case of irritable bowel syndrome. *Health Psychology, 13*, 103–113.

Tamada, K., Ito, Y., & Fukuzaki, H. (1985). Autonomic hyperactivity in patients with vasospastic angina. *Japanese Heart Journal, 26*, 715–726.

Watson, D., & Pennebaker, J. W. (1989). Health complaints, stress, and distress: Exploring the central role of negative effectivity. *Psychological Review, 96*(2), 234–254.

Weidner, G., & Matthews, K. A. (1978). Reported physical symptoms elicited by unpredictable events and the type A coronary-prone behavior pattern. *Journal of Personality and Social Psychology, 36*, 1213–1220.

Whitehead, W. E. (1992). Assessing the effects of stress on physical symptoms. *Health Psychology, 13*(2), 99–102.

Woods, S., Natterson, J., & Silverman, J. (1978). Medical students' disease: Hypochondriasis in medical education. *Journal of Medical Education, 41,* 785–790.
Woodwell, D. A. (1997). *National Ambulatory Medical Care Survey: 1995 summary. Advance data from vital and
health statistics;* No 286. Hyattsville, MD: National Center for Health Statistics.
Worthington, E., & Shumate, M. (1981). Imagery and verbal counseling methods in stress inoculation training for pain control. *Journal of Counseling Psychology, 28,* 1–6.

CHAPTER *6*

Health-Care-Seeking Behaviors

M. Janice Gilliland, Martha M. Phillips, James M. Raczynski, Delia E. Smith, Carol E. Cornell, and Vera Bittner

Introduction

Health-care-seeking behavior is that action taken by an individual in response to a stimulus (such as the perception of a symptom) that he or she decides is indicative of a condition needing evaluation by a health professional. This behavior is influenced by personal, physical, and psychological characteristics and by sociocultural and environmental factors. Structural barriers or facilitators can also hinder or abet the decision to seek care. Health-care-seeking behavior is closely related to symptom perception (Chapter 5) in that symptoms are often the stimulus or cue that initiates action by individuals. More urgent, unambiguous symptoms tend to encourage rapid care seeking (Alonzo, 1986; Ell *et al.*, 1994; Hartford, Herlitz, Karlson, & Risenfors, 1990); but even so, people often delay for days, weeks, or even months with symptoms of acute myocardial infarction (AMI), stroke, or cancer. Symptoms and symptom perceptions may contribute to delay or avoidance of care seeking because of psychological responses such as fear, anxiety, or denial (Bosl *et al.*, 1981; Hackett & Cassem, 1969; Millar & Millar, 1996).

Care-seeking behaviors affect both individuals and society in terms of health care costs, quality of life issues, and morbidity and mortality. Excessive or inappropriate care seeking may add to the costs of health care, but it is less likely than delayed care seeking to have health repercussions for individual patients. Delay in

M. Janice Gilliland, James M. Raczynski • Behavioral Medicine Unit, Division of Preventive Medicine, Department of Medicine, School of Medicine, Department of Health Behavior, School of Public Health, UAB Center for Health Promotion, University of Alabama at Birmingham, Birmingham, Alabama 35294. *Martha M. Phillips* • UAB Civitan International Research Center, Department of Epidemiology, School of Public Health, UAB Center for Health Promotion, University of Alabama at Birmingham, Birmingham, Alabama 35294. *Delia E. Smith and Carol E. Cornell* • Behavioral Medicine Unit, Division of Preventive Medicine, Department of Medicine, School of Medicine, UAB Center for Health Promotion, University of Alabama at Birmingham, Birmingham, Alabama 35294. *Vera Bittner* • Division of Cardiovascular Disease, School of Medicine, UAB Center for Health Promotion, University of Alabama at Birmingham, Birmingham, Alabama 35294.

Handbook of Health Promotion and Disease Prevention, edited by Raczynski and DiClemente. Kluwer Academic/Plenum Publishers, New York, 1999.

seeking medical care for acute symptoms or those symptoms suggestive of a life-threatening illness episode may have serious consequences both for the patient and for the health care system. For example, Weissman, Stern, Fielding, and Epstein (1991) found that patients who reported delays in seeking medical care prior to hospitalization for all types of medical conditions had longer hospital stays than did patients who sought more timely treatment. Longer hospital stays are associated with higher hospital costs, in part because of greater disease severity and complexity at presentation (Asenjo et al., 1994; Rosko & Carpenter, 1994). Inappropriate delay in care seeking is often associated with a poorer treatment outcome. Conversely, early treatment for AMI has been associated with a reduction in mortality (GISSI, 1986; Grines & DeMaria, 1990; ISIS-2 Collaborative Group, 1988). The natural course of the disease may affect the delay in seeking treatment and health outcomes. For example, delayed care seeking for breast and other cancers does not necessarily lead to poorer outcomes after controlling for other factors (Vernon, Tilley, Neale, & Steinfeldt, 1985), although increased mortality is associated with later stage at diagnosis for some cancers (Facione, 1993), suggesting that time of presentation to the health care system does play a role in many cancer outcomes.

Health care seeking involves a series of stages or phases, beginning with the patient becoming aware of a need and ending with medical assessment and treatment, if warranted. Delay can occur at any stage, including delay in patient care seeking and delay in treatment once contact is made with the health care system. While structural–environmental issues may play a role in treatment delay (e.g., access to care, poor emergency medical service, physician-instituted delays in diagnosis or treatment), the largest component of delay for acute problems occurs before the patient contacts the health care system (Hartford et al., 1990; Schroeder, Lamb & Hu, 1978; Wielgosz & Nolan, 1991). Although patient delay accounts for a longer period than health care system delays, the efficacy of programs for reducing treatment-seeking delay may be less easy and more challenging to demonstrate than for delays associated with evaluation and treatment components. For example, the National Heart, Lung, and Blood Institute's National Heart Attack Alert Program (NHAAP), after carefully reviewing the literature on delays associated with seeking and obtaining treatment for AMI, acknowledged that empirical support was lacking for methods to reduce patient delay, and initial delay-reducing efforts by the NHAAP were directed toward assessment, diagnosis, and treatment in the emergency department (ED) (Dracup et al., 1997). Nonetheless, issues concerning patient delay present the greatest challenges and the potentially greatest benefits for reducing overall delay. Hence, the focus of this chapter will be on why people delay seeking care, particularly for life-threatening conditions such as AMI and cancer, concentrating on those factors that are attributes of the individual or group and those that are more or less under personal control.

To understand why people delay seeking care in potentially life-threatening situations, it is important to understand the theoretical models that have been used to structure research in this area. Theory-based research into factors underlying decision making for care seeking can direct the development of more effective interventions to change health-care-seeking behaviors. The models commonly used to understand or predict care-seeking behaviors will be discussed briefly, with emphasis placed on studies that support or refute the models. See Chapter 3 for a more complete explication of the theories addressed here.

Theoretical Models

Researchers have employed several different theoretical models to predict and explain delay in care seeking. Factors of primary interest in studies of disease detection and delayed treatment have been behaviors, beliefs, and barriers that facilitate or hinder utilization. Conceptual models developed to address psychosocial factors associated with preventive, health-enhancing, or health-seeking behaviors include: the Health Belief Model (Becker, 1974; Rosenstock, 1966), Social Cognitive Theory (Bandura, 1986), Self-Regulatory Theory (Leventhal, 1970; Leventhal, Meyer, & Nerenz, 1980), and the Theory of Care Seeking (Lauver, 1992, 1994), among others.

The Health Belief Model (HBM) suggests that participation in early detection or care-seeking behaviors is influenced by: (1) perceived susceptibility; (2) perceived severity; (3) potential benefits; (4) barriers; and (5) cues to action that initiate the behavior (Becker, 1974; Rosenstock, 1966). The HBM has been used extensively for research on cancer behaviors. Application of the HBM to preventive and care-seeking behaviors has produced equivocal results. Although the model often has accurately predicted these behaviors (Champion, 1994; King, 1984), other studies have reported no relationships between the model constructs and preventive or care-seeking behaviors for cancer (Champion, 1985; Kash, Holland, Halper, & Miller, 1992; Trotta, 1980). Constructs of the HBM have demonstrated predictive value in explaining variation found in knowledge, attitudes about breast cancer, and changes in mammography usage in some (Saint-Germain & Longman, 1993; Stein, Fox, Murata, & Morisky, 1992) but not all studies (Aiken, West, Woodward, & Reno, 1994; Reynolds, West, & Aiken, 1990). Perceived barriers to mammography screening are consistently associated with poorer adherence (Aiken *et al.*, 1994; Baumann, Brown, Fontana, & Cameron, 1993; Burack & Liang, 1989; Kurtz, Given, Given, & Kurtz, 1993). Barriers may be most salient in the prediction of ongoing, regular screening behavior rather than in explaining which women have ever had a mammogram (Rimer, Trock, Engstrom, Lerman, & King, 1991). Perceived susceptibility has also been shown to be a strong predictor of breast cancer surveillance behavior in several studies (Aiken *et al.*, 1994; Champion, 1991; Fajardo, Saint-Germain, Meakem, Rose, & Hillman, 1992; Lerman, Rimer, Trock, Balshem, & Engstrom, 1990; Massey, 1986). Although some studies have found that women with higher perceived susceptibility were not more likely to engage in screening mammography (Aiken *et al.*, 1994; Burack & Liang, 1989), both studies found that mammography was predicted by cues to action. Stein *et al.* (1992) reported that perceived susceptibility use was a strong predictor of future intentions to have a mammogram, while cues to action predicted previous mammography (Stein *et al.*, 1992). Kash and colleagues (1992) have suggested that the HBM may predict risk-reducing behaviors, but may fail to predict health surveillance behaviors that produce anxiety and avoidance.

Social Cognitive Theory (Bandura, 1986) suggests that behavior is determined by reciprocal interactions among environmental events, behavior, and personal characteristics. The likelihood that individuals will initiate and maintain health-enhancing behaviors is influenced by social and environmental cues as well as by reinforcement contingencies. Furthermore, the effects of cues and contingencies are mediated by cognitive processes associated with outcome expectations and self-efficacy. Perceptions of self-efficacy influence the type of anticipatory scenarios that individuals construct. If an individual believes that he or she would be ineffective in initiating or maintaining the behavior, that individual is hypothesized to be less likely to engage in the behavior. Some studies have provided evidence that outcome expectations and self-efficacy are associated with seeking mammography (Calnan, 1984) and cervical cancer screening (Kegeles, 1969; Kegeles, Kirscht, & Haefner, 1965).

Self-Regulatory Theory (Leventhal, 1970; Leventhal *et al.*, 1980) proposes that illness and care-seeking behaviors can be understood as a self-regulating process in that individuals perceive symptoms and elaborate on them to create a cognitive representation and an emotional response to the symptom event. The cognitive representation and the emotional response then guide individuals in selecting and initiating coping responses, as well as reevaluating and making changes in these responses as necessary. The model proposes three main stages that are triggered with the threat of illness. Stage 1, *problem representation,* is composed of the individual use of a set of attributes to identify or specify the problems and actions to be taken. Coping responses are then generated in the *action plan* stage, and in the third stage, *appraisal process,* individuals use personal sets of rules to determine if the responses generated in the action stage have been effective. These stages may cycle repeatedly as individuals generate new hypotheses regarding the illness, and initiate and evaluate the responses and consequences. The theory also posits that emotional responses such as fear or anger coincide with the cognitive processes that develop in response to symptoms. The success or failure of responses can influence health care seeking.

The concepts of Social Cognitive Theory and Self-regulatory Theory are interrelated and have been used in a combined model to conceptualize the intervention for the Heart Attack REACT (Rapid Early Action for Coronary Treatment) project (Simons-Morton *et al.*, 1998). The Heart Attack REACT project is a multicenter community intervention study to reduce delay time for symptoms of AMI. See Chapter 12 for a more detailed discussion of the intervention.

Finally, Lauver (1992, 1994) has proposed the Theory of Care Seeking, based on an earlier general theory of behavior proposed by Triandis (1982). The theory proposes that care seeking can be explained by psychosocial and facilitator variables. Four psychosocial variables are proposed: *affect*—feelings about care seeking; *utility*—beliefs about perceived worth of care seeking; *habits*—usual patterns of care seeking; and *norms*—personal and societal opinions about the behavior. Facilitators are measured by their presence or absence, for example, whether individuals have an identified health care provider. According to the theory, demographic and clinical factors and personality characteristics affect behavior indirectly only by influencing psychosocial and facilitator variables (Lauver, 1992, 1994; Lauver, Nabholz, Scott, & Tak, 1997). Lauver (1994) studied care seeking for symptoms of breast cancer and found that promptness of care seeking was associated with habit and with an interaction between anxiety (affect) and having a source of health care (facilitation). Utility was associated with delayed care seeking. Race was not associated with care-seeking behavior, as predicted by the model. In a study of adherence to mammography screening (Lauver *et al.*, 1997), intention to have a mammogram was associated with utility beliefs, whereas anxiety interacted with barriers to influence screening practices. These results were similar to those from the earlier study on breast cancer (Lauver, 1994). The theory was contradicted in that age, family history of breast cancer, and belief in personal risk were associated with adherence to screening after controlling for psychosocial and facilitator variables.

Background

Although multiple factors have been shown to influence health-care-seeking behavior, patient delay for acute symptoms, such as those associated with an AMI, has generally been found to be the longest single component in delay to treatment (Alonzo, 1980; Andersen & Cacioppo, 1995; Bett, Aroney, & Thompson, 1993; Ell *et al.*, 1994; Safer, Tharps, Jackson, & Leventhal, 1979). Not unexpectedly, the natural course of the disease affects the magnitude of effect related to patient delay. In studies of care seeking for acute events such as AMI, delay is usually reported in terms of hours or even minutes. With the advent of reperfusion therapies, optimal time to treatment for AMI is within 1 hour of symptom onset [Fibrinolytic Therapy Trialists (FTT) Collaborative Group, 1994], with some benefits still accruing after 6 hours (AIMS Trial Study Group, 1990; GISSI, 1986, 1987; Grines & Demaria, 1990; Linderer *et al.*, 1993) to as long as 12 hours (ACC/AHA Committee on Management of Acute Myocardial Infarction, 1996; EMERAS Collaborative Group, 1993; LATE Study Group, 1993). In contrast, undue delay is defined in time spans of weeks or even months for most carcinomas. Facione (1993) quotes Pack and Gallo (1938) as defining undue delay in cancer-seeking treatment as 3 months or more elapsing between the individual's perception of symptoms and physician contact.

Phases of Delay in Care-Seeking Behavior

Delay in seeking treatment has been considered as either a single overall period or segmented into as few as 2 to as many as 11 phases (Gillum, Feinleib, Margolis, Fabsitz, & Brasch, 1976; Maynard *et al.*, 1991; Moss, Wynar, & Goldstein, 1969; Safer *et al.*, 1979; Schroeder *et al.*, 1978; Simon, Feinleib, & Thompson, 1972; Weissman *et al.*, 1991). Factors that influence care seeking in one phase may not be relevant in another. In a useful categorization of delay, Alonzo (1986) classified delay in care seeking for AMI symptoms into: (1) the prodromal phase: initial health deviation to acute symptom onset; (2) the definition period of self-evaluation: acute symptom onset to seeking lay consultation; (3) the lay consultation phase: the period from seeking lay advice to medical consultation or hospital transport; (4) the medical consultation phase: the beginning of medical consultation to initiation of hospital travel; (5) the travel phase; and (6) the hospital procedural phase: arrival at the emergency department to treatment initiation. Dracup *et al.* (1995) modified Alonzo's categories to include only three phases: the patient–bystander recognition and action phase, which begins when the patient or bystander becomes aware of symptoms and continues through to initiating transport to the hospital; the prehospital action phase is the interval following initiation of travel to the hospital to actual arrival, and the hospital action phase encompasses the period of time between hospital arrival and definitive treatment. Care seeking for cancer has been divided into similar phases, albeit with longer time frames. Andersen and Cacioppo (1995) list four stages—appraisal, illness, behavioral, and scheduling delay—and suggest that each phase is governed by different sets of decisional and appraisal processes. This agrees with other research indicating that delay can occur at any or all of these phases, but different factors exert influence at different stages (Crawford, McGraw, Smith, McKinlay, & Pinson, 1994). Some cardiovascular researchers have divided delay into similar stages of appraisal, illness, and utilization delay (Safer *et al.*, 1979). However defined, most delay occurs in the stage or stages prior to contact with the health care system, particularly during the decision or appraisal phases (Alonzo, 1980; Andersen & Cacioppo, 1995; Bett *et al.*, 1993; Ell *et al.*, 1994, 1995; Safer *et al.*, 1979; Weissman *et al.*, 1991).

Sources of Delay in Care-Seeking Behavior

Studies investigating patients' stated reasons for delay for AMI symptoms have found among the most frequently cited reasons: (1) thinking that the problem would go away or was not serious; (2) lack of time or conflicts with other priorities; (3) failure to perceive the symptoms as being cardiac related; (4) advice of family or friends; (5) difficulties in getting appointments; and (6) concern about treatment cost (Hartford, Karlson, Sjörn, Holmberg, & Herlitz, 1993; Meischke, Ho, Eisenberg, Schaeffer, & Larsen, 1995; Schmidt & Borsch, 1990; Weissman *et al.*, 1991). Similar reasons have been found to explain delays in seeking treatment for symptoms of cancer, with the addition of delay being related to a belief that a cure is unlikely and fear of surgery, debilitating treatments, or death (Facione, 1993; Mor, Masterson-Allen, Goldberg, Guadagnoli, & Wool, 1990).

Previous studies have described a host of factors as contributing to patient delays in seeking medical care for symptoms of possible cancer or cardiac origin. These include: (1) characteristics of the patient, such as age, gender, ethnicity and culture, socioeconomic status (SES) and education, and prior medical history; (2) psychological and cognitive factors, including personality and emotional factors, as well as patient beliefs, attributions, and expectations; (3) characteristics of symptoms, including their nature and severity; (4) environmental and behavioral factors, such as the situation, time, and setting in which the symptoms occur, as well as self-treatment behaviors; and (5) the health care system contacted after making the decision to seek treatment. As noted above, the following discussion will concentrate on those factors that are amenable to change or can help to target high-risk populations for delay-reducing interventions. The literature reviewed is summarized in Table 1.

Patient Characteristics

A number of patient characteristics have been investigated to illuminate reasons for delay in seeking treatment. These characteristics have included age, gender, ethnicity and culture, SES and education, and prior medical history. While many of these characteristics are nonmodifiable, they can be highly relevant in terms of selecting high-risk groups for targeting delay-reduction intervention efforts.

Age

Studies on the relationship of age to care seeking have shown inconsistent results. Leventhal and Prochaska (1986) found that older people are more likely to postpone seeking care, often minimizing or denying symptoms. In contrast, in a study of care seeking for several different symptoms, Berkanovic, Telesky, and Reeder (1981) report that older people are more likely to seek care and that the number of chronic conditions is positively related to care seeking. However, the study was limited in that the variables examined were highly interrelated. Some studies have found no ef-

Table 1. Risk Factors Associated with Patient Delay in Care Seeking[a]

Risk factor	No. Studies +/0/— for delay[b]	Comments
Patient characteristics		
Age		
AMI studies	8/10/1	The effect of age on AMI delay is unclear, but age does not appear
Cancer studies	1/5/0	to affect delay for care seeking for cancer symptoms. Methodological problems with sample size differences and age groups may account for some variation for both AMI and cancer.
Gender		
AMI studies	4/12/0	For AMI, 4 studies show females delay longer, 12 show no gender
Cancer studies	0/1/0	effect; 2 other studies show a greater but nonstatistically
Other studies	0/1/0	significant (n.s.) delay for women.
Ethnicity–culture		
AMI studies	7/4/0	Most studies show minorities delay longer for AMI and cancer
Cancer studies	6/2/0	symptoms and screening. Minorities delay longer in seeking care for cancer symptoms and are less likely to follow recommended screening guidelines. Many studies have serious methodological problems in that few control for SES factors in analysis.
SES characteristics		
SES–income	9/6/0	Some SES measures appear to be associated with delayed care
Educ.–Occup.	0/9/1	seeking, but comparisons across studies are risky because of the number of factors lumped under the term and differing operational definitions of SES-related constructs. Few studies control for confounding factors.
Medical history		
CHD	18/0/1	There is strong evidence that a history of CHD is associated with increased delay, although generalizing across the various types of CVD may not be possible. Again, methodological problems may influence the results.
Diabetes	5/0/0	The evidence supports a positive relationship between diabetes and longer delay for AMI.
Other	2/0/1	The evidence is slight for an association between delay and hypertension and fibrocystic breast disease.
Psychological characteristics		
Type A	1/3/0	Type A personality does not appear to influence delay.
Denial	6/2/0	Most studies show longer delay associated with denial; however, methodological problems limit interpretation.
Somatic awareness	2/0/0	Lower perceptions of physical sensations increases delay time
Fear	2/0/1	Fear may delay care seeking for cancer symptoms but apparently not for AMI.
Anxiety	3/2/2	Anxiety may increase delay for cancer care seeking, screening or time to detection, although the evidence is contradictory. Anxiety has not been reported as a factor in care seeking for AMI.
Fatalism	2/0/0	Fatalism is reported to cause delays in care seeking among African Americans.
Other	2/0/0	Locus of control, obsessiveness, phobia, and social support have all been positively associated with care-seeking behavior.

(continued)

Table 1. (Continued)

Risk factor	No. Studies +/0/— for delay[b]	Comments
Patient beliefs, attributions, and expectations		
Beliefs	2/2/8	Patient beliefs regarding seriousness increase delay in care seeking for cancer symptoms, but probably reduces delay for AMI.
Risk Perceptions	0/2/4	Increased perception of risk is associated with improved adherence to cancer screening.
Self-treatment	4/0/0	Self-treatment for AMI symptoms is associated with longer delay. There has been little research on self-treatment and care seeking for cancer symptoms.
Symptom characteristics	7/6/9	Most studies report that delay is associated with mild symptoms or a gradual onset, while severity is associated with shorter delay to treatment seeking. However, one study found longer delay associated with symptom severity.
Environment		
Setting	2/1/0	Being at home may increase delay time.
Social environment	5/1/5	This category includes several different social environments, and some studies report both increased or reduced delay associated with different variables. Being with strangers appears to reduce delay time, while being with family may increase it.
Timing	5/4/2	Night or weekend onset may increase delay. Some studies found this applied only to fatal AMIs; one study found shorter delay time with late night physician contact and, presumably, late night onset, and one study reported shorter delays on weekends for survivors only.
Health care system		
Phy.–staff contact	3/0/0	Contacting one's physician or physician's office appears to increase delay.
EMS	0/0/5	Use of EMS reduces delay.

[a] Numbers in table are not exhaustive, but show only those studies cited in the text.
[b] +, increased delay; 0, no or nonsignificant relationship; —, reduced delay.

fect on delay in care seeking for symptoms of AMI by age (Doehrman, 1977; Erhardt, Sjögren, Sawe, & Theorell, 1974; Gilchrist, 1973; Matthews, Siegel, Kuller, Thompson, & Varat, 1983; Ottesen *et al.*, 1996; Simon *et al.*, 1972; Wielgosz, Nolan, Earp, Biro, & Wielgosz, 1988). Other investigators have reported significant positive associations between age and delay for AMI (Dracup & Moser, 1997; GISSI, 1995; Maynard *et al.*, 1989; Moss *et al.*, 1969; Rawles & Haites, 1988; Schmidt & Borsch, 1990; Turi *et al.*, 1986), but the differences are not always statistically significant (Moss & Goldstein, 1970). Dracup and Moser (1991), in their excellent review of delay associated with symptoms of AMI, propose that these inconsistencies may be due to methodological differences, including differences in sample size and in the number of individual phases of delay that was examined.

Age has been associated with delay among British women with breast cancer (Nichols, Waters, Fraser, Wheeler, & Ingham, 1981), but the results may be limited by the small number of older women in the sample. As with reports on AMI and delay, most studies have not found a significant difference in cancer care seeking by age of the patient (Dent *et al.*, 1990; Elwood & Moorhead, 1980; Samet, Hunt, Lerchen, & Goodwin, 1988; Saunders, 1989). Facione (1993) suggests the earlier studies on delayed care seeking and breast cancer may reflect women's beliefs regarding the effectiveness of cancer treatment at the time these studies were conducted, whereas more recent studies may reflect positive changes in beliefs about cancer treatments and the potential for a cure. She postulates that these changes may have shortened delay patterns among more recent cohorts of women. This conjecture, if true, may apply to changes in attitudes about treatment for other forms of cancer as well. However, older women also are less likely to follow recommended screening guidelines for early cancer detection. Younger women are more likely to have had mammograms and Pap smears (Calle, Flanders, Thun, & Martin, 1993; Harris *et al.*, 1991) than older women. If age is indeed a risk factor for delayed care seeking, it may be that older persons are more likely to have chronic diseases and to attribute symptoms to these conditions (Leventhal & Prochaska, 1986). However, Mor *et al.* (1990) found that comorbidity did not increase patient delay in seeking care for three types of cancer.

Gender

Studies have also yielded inconsistent findings regarding the influence of gender on delay in treatment seeking. Women seek health care overall more frequently than men (Briscoe, 1987; Chien & Schneiderman, 1975; Waldron, 1983), and at least one study has found that women are more likely than men to encourage their spouses and others to seek care (Norcross, Ramirez, & Palinkas, 1996). Women have been shown to delay significantly longer than men in seeking treatment for AMI symptoms (Cunningham *et al.*, 1989; Ell *et al*, 1994; Turi *et al.*, 1986) for at least some phases of delay (Alonzo, 1986).

However, not all studies have found clear gender differences in treatment seeking. Some investigators found trends for longer delay times for women compared to men, but not statistically significant differences (Clark, Bellam, Shah, & Feldman, 1992; Moss *et al.*, 1969). Other studies reported no gender differences (Doehrman, 1977; Erhardt *et al.*, 1974, Gilchrist, 1973; Hackett & Cassem, 1969; Matthews *et al.*, 1983; Maynard *et al.*, 1989; Moss & Goldstein, 1970; Schroeder *et al.*, 1978; Simon *et al.*, 1972; Wielgosz *et al.*, 1988). Furthermore, no significant differences have been reported between men and women in care-seeking behavior for types of cancer common to both sexes (Marshall & Funch, 1986) or for low back pain (Carey *et al.*, 1996).

Ethnicity and Culture

Differences among ethnic groups in care-seeking behaviors have been reported (Raczynski *et al.*, 1994). Several studies on delay in treatment seeking for symptoms of a possible AMI suggest that nonwhites delay longer than whites (Clark *et al.*, 1992; Cooper *et al.*, 1986; Lee, 1997; Raczynski *et al.*, 1994). This delay appears to be due primarily to the time patients take to make the decision to seek treatment following symptom onset (Alonzo, 1986; Clark *et al.*, 1992). Weissman *et al.* (1991) reported that blacks delayed longer than whites in general and were more likely to judge the problem as not being serious, which was in itself a significant cause of care-seeking delay.

However, as with gender and age, findings have been somewhat inconsistent. For example, in a study of a low-SES population, Crawford *et al.* (1994) found little difference in African-American and white care-seeking patterns after controlling for SES and access to care, although average delay time was shorter for African-American women. Ell *et al.* (1994) report that African-American patients had care-seeking patterns for symptoms of AMI that were similar to those for white populations, but also noted some differences that were specific to African Americans, including issues related to SES, access to care, and gender. Further, in a second study, Ell and colleagues (1995) reported that SES, as determined by type of hospital (public vs. private), exerted a greater influence on care-seeking behavior than did race. Turi *et al.* (1986) found no significant difference in the average delay times between whites and nonwhites, but did note a trend for nonwhites to arrive later. It may be that racial differences in delay are affected by symptom perception and attribution, which appear to vary between African Americans and whites (Raczynski *et al.*, 1994).

At least one study has shown that African-American women are more likely than white women to delay seeking care for symptoms of breast cancer after controlling for SES (Richardson, Langholz, Bernstein, Burciaga, & Ross, 1992). African-American women tend to have a later stage breast cancer at diagnosis compared to white, non-Hispanic women (Saunders, 1989), perhaps because of their delayed care seeking (Richardson *et al.*, 1992) and lower rates of mammography screening (Pearlman *et al.*, 1996; Weinberg, Cooper, Lane, & Kripalani, 1997). Hispanic women also are less likely than white women to have had a recent mammogram, but are still almost twice as likely to have had one as African-American women (46.4% vs. 28.6%) (Weinberg *et al.*, 1997). White men have higher rates of screening for prostate or colon cancer compared to African-American men (Cowen, Kattan, & Miles, 1996). Other research has indicated that African Americans and Hispanics are less likely to follow up on lesions that may be indicative of skin cancer (Friedman *et al.*, 1994). In contrast, Vernon *et al.* (1985) found a nonsignificant effect on delay in seeking care for breast cancer symptoms and concluded that ethnicity does not affect delay; however, they did report some "ethnic specific patterns of association between stage of disease and length of delay . . . which showed that the pattern for Hispanics and whites differed noticeably from that for blacks" (p. 1569). Lauver (1994) also reported that race had no direct influence on care-seeking behavior for women with symptoms or actual breast cancer in a sample composed of socioeconomically disadvantaged patients.

The conflicting results from studies on race–ethnicity and delay may be explained at least partially by socioeconomic differences among ethnic groups. Facione (1993) has pointed out that few studies have controlled for differences in SES and access to health care when examining the effects of race on care-seeking delay. In one of the few studies of delay in breast cancer patients to address both SES and race, Richardson and colleagues (1992) reported an interaction between SES and race–ethnicity and what the researchers called "long duration of symptoms." The authors concluded that, after adjusting for socioeconomic factors, upper-SES white and Hispanic women appeared to have similar time to treatment seeking, while African-American women were at higher risk for extended delays.

It has been suggested that the longer delays observed in nonwhite patients, if real, may stem from cultural factors that have produced an increased tolerance for symptoms, combined with a tendency to engage in more self-treatment and to delay seeking medical treatment until an illness becomes serious (Harrison & Harrison, 1971). This may be especially true for Southern African Americans (Bailey, 1987). Moreover, there is some evidence to suggest that African Americans are more likely than whites to believe in the effectiveness of alternative treatments for serious illnesses (Loehrer *et al.*, 1991). Culturally mediated beliefs about disease and disease risk may explain some ethnic–racial differences in delay. Chavez, Hubbell, McMullin, Martinez, and Mishra (1995) report that among Hispanic women there is a "Latina model" of breast cancer causation that holds that the disease is caused by trauma to the breast or "bad behaviors." These beliefs likely affect care-seeking behavior in that Hispanic women with no risk factors, according to the accepted Latina model, may delay longer following onset of symptoms because they believe they are not at risk or fear being thought of as having engaged in socially unacceptable behaviors.

SES

Many studies examining socioeconomic factors have not found a significant effect of this variable on delay in treatment seeking for AMI. For example, in a sample of Canadian patients, Wielgosz *et al.* (1988) found no significant differences in decision time for sociodemographic variables or for urban versus rural areas. Gilchrist (1973) similarly found no delay differences due to social class in a sample of British patients. A number of studies with US cardiac patients have yielded similar results (e.g., Doehrman, 1977; Hackett & Cassem, 1969; Matthews *et al.*, 1983; Simon *et al.*, 1972). Other studies, however, have found SES to be significantly associated with delay in treatment seeking. Schmidt and Borsch (1990) studied a group of patients drawn from a largely rural population and found that low-income was an independent predictor of increased delay for symptoms of AMI. In a large multicenter study in Washington State, Dracup and Moser (1997) reported that delay for symptoms of AMI was associated with lower income. In a study of low- and middle-SES African Americans seeking care for symptoms of AMI, Ell and colleagues (1994) found a significant difference by SES. Haywood *et al.* (1993) also compared low- and middle-SES AMI patients and reported that low-SES patients were significantly more likely to use modes of transport, such as public transportation, that have a built-in delay.

Research on care seeking related to insurance lends further support to the importance of SES. Yarzebski, Goldberg, Gore, and Alpert (1994) reported that type of insurance (publicly subsidized vs. private insurance) was associated with increased delay for symptoms of AMI. Love (1991) found that indigent patients had later stage cancer at initial diagnosis than did patients with medical insurance, perhaps because disadvantaged persons wait longer than more advantaged persons before seeking medical care (Howard, 1982). Care seeking for other conditions, such as low back pain, also has been associated with income and insurance status (Carey *et al.*, 1996). Weissman *et al.* (1991) found higher probabilities of delay in patients who were uninsured and/or had lower SES.

The majority of studies have found no relationship between delay time and level of education (Dent *et al.*, 1990; Doehrman, 1977; Mor *et al.*, 1990; Moss & Goldstein, 1970; Moss *et al.*, 1969; Turi *et al.*, 1986; Wielgosz *et al.*, 1988) or occupation

(Simon *et al.*, 1972). One study has reported decreased delay times for care seeking for symptoms of AMI among less educated patients (Matthews *et al.*, 1983). Loehrer (1991) reported an inverse association between level of education and knowledge and beliefs regarding cancer-related care-seeking behaviors, with lower education levels being correlated with misconceptions about appropriate behaviors.

Medical History

Prior medical history has been associated with care-seeking behavior. Having a medical history of coronary heart disease (including previous myocardial infarction, coronary artery disease, or congestive heart failure), prodromal symptoms, and/or previous angina episodes does not necessarily prompt patients to respond more quickly to symptoms, and in fact may increase delay time (Clark *et al.*, 1992; Erhardt *et al.*, 1974; Goldstein, Moss, & Greene, 1972; Hackett & Cassem, 1969; Hofgren *et al.*, 1988; Kenyon, Ketterer, Gheorghiade, & Goldstein, 1991; Leitch, Birbara, Freedman, Wilcox, & Harris, 1989; Maynard *et al.*, 1989; Moss & Goldstein, 1970; Moss *et al.*, 1969; Ottesen *et al.*, 1996; Rawles, Metcalfe, Shirreffs, Jennings, & Kenmure, 1990; Rawles & Haites, 1988; Schroeder *et al.*, 1978; Simon *et al.*, 1972; Turi *et al.*, 1986; Wielgosz *et al.*, 1988). One study has reported a "borderline" association between prior AMI and decreased prehospital delay (Schmidt & Borsch, 1990), although exclusion of patients with "painless AMI" may have biased the sample. Erhardt and colleagues (1974) similarly found shorter delay among prior cardiac inpatients.

Research indicates that patients with a prior history of other medical conditions also wait longer before seeking treatment for AMI symptoms than patients without such prior histories. For example, patients with diabetes have increased delay times in several studies (Dracup & Moser, 1997; GISSI, 1995; Ottesen *et al.*, 1996; Schmidt & Borsch, 1990; Yarzebski *et al.*, 1994). Although an early report found shorter delay times for people with hypertension (Moss & Goldstein, 1970), methodological problems limit interpretations (Schroeder *et al.*, 1978). Schmidt and Borsch (1990) found a significant relationship between hypertension and delay in univariate analysis, but the relationship was not statistically significant in the multivariate analysis. Women with fibrocystic breast disease apparently are more likely to delay seeking treatment for breast cancer than women without such a history (Gould-Martin, Paganini-Hill, Casagrande, Mack, & Ross, 1982; Lierman, 1988), probably because they and their physicians are more likely to attribute a lump to the existing benign condition.

Psychological, Cognitive, and Behavioral Factors

Both psychological factors, such as personality type, affective response characteristics and coping strategies, and cognitive factors, including patient beliefs, attributions, and expectations, have been linked to delay in care-seeking behavior. These factors are more amenable to change through individual and group interventions, and thus become important aspects on which to intervene to reduce patient delay.

Psychological Factors

Some personality and emotional factors have been implicated in increased delay for care seeking. Individuals scoring high in some aspects of type A behavior have been reported to take somewhat longer to decide to seek treatment following symptom onset (Sjögren *et al.*, 1979). Matthews *et al.* (1983) found a positive but nonsignificant correlation between global type A behavior and decision time. This is consistent with the findings of both Wielgosz *et al.* (1988) and Kenyon *et al.* (1991) in suggesting that global type A behavior does not significantly affect decision time.

Some authors have suggested that patient denial plays a significant role in increasing delay for care seeking (e.g., Bleeker *et al.*, 1995; Gentry, 1978; Gentry & Haney, 1975; Hackett & Cassem, 1969; Worden & Weisman, 1975; Zervas, Augustine, & Friechione, 1993). Other studies have reported no significant influence of denial on delay (Goldstein *et al.*, 1972; Wielgosz *et al.*, 1988). Given the diverse ways in which denial has been defined and measured, conclusions about the role of denial are premature. Moreover, denial is likely to be confounded by individual differences in perception of physical symptoms. For example, AMI patients with decreased awareness of somatic sensations and emotions have longer delays between symptom onset and hospital arrival compared with those with greater awareness (Kenyon *et al.*, 1991). A conceptually similar construct, deficient psychological awareness (alexithymia), has been significantly associated with delay (Theisen *et al.*, 1995). Overall, denial has not been adequately defined and operationalized over comparable studies to allow a determination of its effect, if any, on prehospital delay.

Various affective responses have been found to affect care seeking. Fear causes delay in treatment seeking for breast cancer (Magarey, Todd, & Blizard, 1977; Mor *et al.*, 1990), but may result in a shorter time to treatment among AMI patients (Schwarz, Schobererger, Rieder, & Kunze, 1994). Anxiety has been reported to increase response time to detection of disease (Millar & Millar, 1996), although one study found it has no effect on adoption of regular mammography screening (Siegler, Feaganes, & Rimer, 1995). Anxiety has been found to be a significant predictor for intention to seek care for breast cancer symptoms (Lauver & Chang, 1991), but increased cancer anxiety may, in fact, decrease regular clinical examinations (Kash *et al.*, 1992) and adherence to repeat mammography (Lauver *et al.*, 1997; Lerman *et al.*, 1990). Not all studies have found anxiety to increase delay time for cancer care seeking (Keinan, Carmil, & Rieck, 1991). Fatalism has been associated with increased delay in care seeking among African-American women (Conrad, Brown, & Conrad, 1996; Powe, 1994). Theisen and colleagues (1995) hypothesize that believing in chance or fate may inhibit care-seeking behavior.

Other psychological characteristics have been associated with increased delay in care seeking. For example, after controlling for gender, race, marital status, education, and income, Theisen *et al.* (1995) found a positive relationship between delay in AMI patients and external locus of control. In a study that controlled for age and severity (Johnson, Gunning, & Lewis, 1996), men who sought care for heartburn exhibited higher levels of obsessiveness, phobia, and somatization than those who did not obtain treatment. Overall, the evidence suggests that psychological factors clearly affect care-seeking behaviors, but methodological problems, particularly in operational definition of constructs, often limit interpretation and generalizability of these studies.

Patient Beliefs, Attributions, Perceptions, and Expectations

Patient beliefs, attributions, perceptions and expectations regarding their symptoms have been found to affect delay times. Several authors have reported that AMI patients who believed that their symptoms were cardiac in nature (Burnett, Blumenthal, Mark, Leimberger, & Caliz, 1995; Gilchrist, 1973; Hackett & Cassem, 1969; Kenyon *et al.*, 1991; Moss *et al.*, 1969) and that coronary heart disease was preventable (Clark *et al.*, 1992) had shorter delays. Perceived inability to control the symptoms also reduced delay time, and perceived seriousness of the situation was the strongest predictor of short prehospital delay in a study of AMI patients (Burnett *et al.*, 1995). Such differences, however, are not statistically significant in all studies (Erhardt *et al.*, 1974; Moss *et al*, 1969). Other studies have reported no decrease in decision time associated with patients' belief that symptoms were cardiac in origin (Moss & Goldstein, 1970; Simon *et al.*, 1972). Similarly, patients' beliefs about cancer appear to contribute to delay in care seeking. Seffrin, Wilson, and Black (1991), in a review of American Cancer Society research on individuals' perceptions about cancer, found a common perception of cancer as a death sentence. The authors suggest that people delay care seeking because they dread having their worst fears confirmed. Similar cancer-related beliefs have been reported in a range of populations. Thirty-five percent of Appalachian women said that they would not want to know or were not sure they would want to know if they had cancer (Sortet & Banks, 1997). Underwood (1992) found that African-American men who perceived themselves as more helpless in controlling their health were significantly less likely to engage in early cancer detection and other risk reduction behaviors. The study was limited by the use of a small, nonrandom sample; nevertheless, it does suggest that perceptions may play an important role in determining care-seeking behaviors for cancer symptoms among this segment of the population.

Evidence from screening detection studies suggests that how people perceive personal risk may be a factor in delay for care seeking. Greater perceived risk has been associated with having a recent clinical breast examination (Rimer, Schildkraut, Lerman, Lin, & Audrain, 1996; Vernon, Vogel, Halabi, & Bondy, 1993), although not with increased screening for colon cancer (Helzlsouer, Ford, Hayward, Midzenski, & Perry, 1994). However, no association was found between degree of perceived risk and failure to undergo mammography or other cancer screening (Helzlsouer *et al.*, 1994). Risk perception may vary by nationality or ethnicity, which may help explain some racial differences in delay. Fontaine and Smith (1995) found a lower perceived cancer risk among British adults compared with Americans. Other studies have shown that African-American women tend to perceive themselves to be at increased risk for breast cancer (Royak-Schaler *et al.*, 1995; Vernon *et al.*, 1993), and perceived risk has been reported to be positively associated with screening rates (Royak-Schaler *et al.*, 1995). Still, African-American women have lower rates of mammography use (Pearlman *et al.*, 1996; Weinberg *et al.*, 1997). According to Lerman, Audrain, & Croyle (1994), perceived risk has been positively associated with interest in DNA testing for breast cancer. However, women with extremely high perceived risk for breast cancer report increased anxiety, and anxiety has been associated with delay in treatment seeking (Manheimer, 1993).

Expectations may also influence care-seeking behavior. Lauver and Angerame (1993) interviewed 40 women with no history of breast cancer about their expectations regarding care seeking for the disease. Perceived advantages to early care seeking were a reduction in worry, taking care of a medical problem, and increasing one's chances of living. Almost half of all participants identified no disadvantages of seeking care for symptoms of breast cancer, and almost two-thirds saw no advantages to delaying. Nonetheless, a substantial percentage of women did note some liabilities associated with care seeking and saw some advantages in adopting a "wait-and-see" attitude.

Raczynski and colleagues (1994), in study of black and white patients diagnosed with coronary heart disease, found some racial differences in attribution of symptoms. About half of white patients attributed their symptoms to heart problems, compared with only about one-third of black patients. In multiple logistic regression analysis, race was significantly and independently associated with attribution of symptoms to cardiac origins. Attributing symptoms to cardiac origins has been associated with shorter delays in seeking care (Schmidt & Borsch, 1990).

Self-treatment Behavior

Attempting to self-treat symptoms can significantly influence care-seeking delay. Wielgosz et al. (1988) reported that predictors of decision time included engagement in self-treatment strategies, such as resting and taking medication. Significant correlations have been found between delayed hospital arrival time and engaging in particular self-treatment activities for AMI, including taking prescribed and over-the-counter medications (Hofgren et al., 1988; Simon et al., 1972; Turi et al., 1986). Turi and colleagues (1986) reported increased time to hospital arrival for patients who took beta-blockers and nitroglycerin, with arrival time increasing directly with the amount of nitroglycerin taken per day in the 3 weeks prior to hospital arrival. Alonzo (1986) found that self-treatment variables, including resting, reducing activity level, and taking prescription and nonprescription medications, were significant predictors of a longer self-evaluation phase.

Little research has been conducted on self-treatment for cancer (Facione, 1993). Some women have been reported to pull on their nipples to try and correct inversion, or to remove brassiere padding (Lierman, 1988). Facione (1993) cites unpublished research (Dodd et al., n.d.) reporting that attempts at self-treatment prior to care seeking have included applying antibiotic ointments, washing the breast to remove secretions, changing brassieres to relieve pain, rubbing roughened areas of skin, or applying heat to painful or reddened areas. It remains to be determined how much these self-care practices contribute to patient delay in seeking treatment.

Symptom Characteristics

There is evidence that characteristics of the symptoms themselves may play a role in care seeking. Key characteristics include specificity, consistency, familiarity, rapidity of onset, and intensity or severity. Persons who experience symptoms that are typically associated with a specific disease are less likely to delay seeking treatment than individuals who have symptoms that are more generalized or ambiguous. For example, symptoms of chest and arm pain are associated with shorter delay time than other symptoms of AMI (Schmidt & Borsch, 1990). Similarly, women with breast lumps seek diagnosis and treatment more rapidly then women who have symptoms other than a lump (MacArthur & Smith, 1981). However, increased delay has also been found in colon cancer patients who present with rectal bleeding or a change in bowel habits (Mor et al., 1990). Delay time may vary by cancer site (Samet et al., 1988), probably as a result of symptom presentation or a lack of symptom specificity. Still, not all studies reporting an association between symptom specificity and delay find differences that are statistically significant (Kenyon *et al.*, 1991; Moss *et al.*, 1969), and some studies report no effect of symptom characteristics on delay (Erhardt *et al.*, 1974; Mor *et al.*, 1990).

Previous experience with cardiac-related symptoms influences time to presentation for AMI treatment. Patients having a myocardial infarction who had similar symptoms in the past (either as infarction or as acute angina) had shorter delays than patients who had not previously experienced these symptoms (Wielgosz *et al.*, 1988). In addition, a pattern of intermittent symptoms produces longer delays than continuous symptoms (Ell *et al.*, 1994). Schmidt and Borscht (1990) found that individuals who had initial symptoms that were low in intensity tended to delay longer and that slow symptom progression was the strongest independent predictor of increased delay. Alonzo (1986) found that, in the prodromal stage, symptoms that were relatively mild, manageable, and ambiguous allowed patients to normalize these sensations and continue to self-treat, but that when patients moved into the acute illness stage, sudden symptom onset reduced the length of the self-evaluation phase compared to symptoms that evolved more gradually. Wielgosz *et al.* (1988) reported that feeling invulnerable to reinfarction and having increased pain or illness in the month prior to reinfarction were significant predictors of increased delay for AMI symptoms. Gradual onset has been associated with increased delay in care seeking for other diseases as well (Cunningham-Burley, Allbutt, Barraway, Lee, & Russell, 1996).

Surprisingly, symptom severity has not been found consistently to affect delay time. Two studies (Hofgren *et al.*, 1988; Maynard *et al.*, 1989) found no association between symptom severity and delay, and one study reported that patients with more severe symptoms actually delayed longer (Hackett & Cassem, 1969). The GISSI (1995) study found that mild to moderate pain increased delay time. In contrast, some studies (Kenyon *et al.*, 1991; Sjögren *et al.*, 1979) have reported shorter delays in patients with more severe symptoms, and degree of incapacity has been inversely related to delay (Ell *et al.*, 1994). Rawles *et al.* (1990) found an inverse association between pain score and delay time. Gilchrist (1973) found that patients with the shortest delay times reported that they sought treatment due to the nature or severity of their pain. Taken together, these findings suggest the existence of a severity threshold below which there is increased likelihood of delay and above which there is a greater sense of urgency and less delay in seeking treatment.

Environmental Factors

Many factors relating to the environment are thought to influence health-care-seeking behavior. These factors include the setting and time of symptom presentation and the social environment within which symptoms occur. Understanding these factors can help inform the choice of content and target group for delay-reduction intervention efforts.

Setting

Data related to the setting or location of the patient at onset of symptoms are somewhat limited but clear in terms of the relationship between setting and care seeking delays. Alonzo (1986) found that individuals who were at home or who decided to travel to a home setting after AMI symptom onset had an increased self-evaluation phase that was primarily due to having greater opportunity to self-treat and monitor symptoms. Furthermore, having a spouse at home who was available for assistance and consultation increased the lay evaluation phase. Other authors have similarly observed longer delays in patients who were at home at the time of symptom onset (Erhardt et al., 1974; Turi et al., 1986). In contrast, Schmidt and Borsch (1990) found that setting did not effect hospital arrival time.

Social Environment

Studies of the effects of social factors on delay for AMI have shown that their impact depends on the phase of the prehospital period, the presence of other people, and whom the patient informs about the symptoms. Onset of AMI symptoms in the presence of friends or other nonfamily bystanders may reduce prehospital delay (GISSI, 1995), although not every study has reported this association (Moss et al., 1969). A majority of people with AMI symptoms consult with someone prior to deciding to seek treatment (Hackett & Cassem, 1969). Alonzo (1986) found that patients who informed others of their symptoms during the prodromal phase were more likely to consult a physician than patients who did not discuss their symptoms. Similarly, other researchers (Doehrman, 1977; Safer et al., 1979; Wielgosz et al., 1988) found that attempting to cope with acute pain without informing others of symptoms was associated with a longer delay.

Informing other people at symptom onset does not always reduce delay in care seeking. Apprising a spouse is likely to increase delay (Alonzo, 1986; Hackett & Cassem, 1969), while telling nonfamily others reduces it (Hackett & Cassem, 1969). Alonzo (1986) reported that patients who first informed a spouse or other family member of their symptoms (especially males who informed wives) experienced an increased lay evaluation phase when compared with patients who first informed nonfamily members, and suggests that the longer delay time may be influenced by the patient's desire to continue to self-treat and monitor symptoms and by the willingness of family members to go along with the patient's wishes. This, however, seems to contradict studies that show a shorter delay when the patient makes the decision to seek care (Hackett & Cassem, 1969; Moss et al., 1969). Being assisted in the care-seeking decision by family members, especially a spouse, may result in a longer prehospital delay (Hackett & Cassem, 1969), but at least one study has reported that married persons have shorter delays to treatment for AMI compared with nonmarried persons (Burnett et al., 1995). Nonetheless, delay may be shortest when the decision to seek treatment is made by the patient, rather than by family, friends, co-workers, or strangers (Hackett & Cassem, 1969; Moss et al., 1969).

Time of Symptom Onset

Night onset or being asleep at time of onset has been found to increase delay (GISSI, 1995). Wielgosz et al. (1988) found nighttime onset (12 to 8 AM) significant only for fatal AMIs. Individuals who seek treatment for AMI symptoms on weekends or during the day may engage in a longer decision time compared to symptom onset on a weekday or at night (Moss et al., 1969; Moss & Goldstein, 1970), or may be more reluctant to disturb their physicians (Gilchrist, 1973). Alonzo (1986) found that individuals who contacted their physicians between 12:00 and 6:00 AM had shorter medical evaluation phases than those who called their physicians during normal office hours.

Several authors have reported finding no significant relationships between time variables and delay, or between weekend versus weekday symptom onset and delay (Erhardt *et al.*, 1974; Schmidt & Borsch, 1990; Simon *et al.*, 1972). In a sample of Canadian patients, Wielgosz *et al.* (1988) found no difference in treatment delay time between weekdays and weekends for nonsurvivors of AMI, but survivors did have a shorter delay on weekends. The authors also reported longer delays for nonsurvivors between midnight and 8:00 AM, but virtually no differences in delay due to time of day for survivors.

Health Care System Contacts

There is some evidence that the component of the health care system initially contacted by patients can influence time to treatment. Studies have reported that patients with symptoms of an AMI who initially contacted their physicians rather than calling the emergency medical service or going to a hospital emergency department had longer delays due to physician intervention. Only about one-third (Alonzo, 1986) to one half (Schroeder *et al.*, 1978) of patients with AMI symptoms who initially contacted physicians were instructed to seek emergency care. Still, physicians were more likely to advise patients to seek emergency care than were nonphysician medical personnel (Simon *et al.*, 1972). The type of symptom reported may also influence physician recommendations for treatment. Physicians delay longer in referring to specialists women who have symptoms of breast cancer other than a lump (MacArthur & Smith, 1981). Interestingly, once the women were referred to a hospital, those with symptoms other than a lump got treated more quickly than women with breast lumps (MacArthur & Smith, 1981). Atypical symptoms for AMI may lead to providers recommending other than emergency treatment, also.

Several authors have found that AMI patients who traveled to the hospital by ambulance or other emergency rescue service had shorter delay times than patients who traveled by car (Clark *et al.*, 1992; Doehrman, 1977; Moss *et al.*, 1969; Simon et al, 1972; Wielgosz *et al.*, 1988). Doehrman (1977) found that transportation by ambulance was due to a shorter decision time, which, in turn, was associated with the perceived seriousness of symptoms. Moss *et al.* (1969) similarly noted shorter decision and unaccounted-for time in patients who traveled to the hospital by ambulance.

Summary: Putting It Together

As reviewed in this chapter, a number of factors have been demonstrated to affect health-care-seeking behavior, and inconsistencies are evident in the direction of the relationships found for many of these factors. In Table 1, we have provided a summary of the literature concerning factors that affect health care seeking. Among patient characteristics, inconsistent associations emerge for age and gender, although there is some evidence that women delay longer for AMI symptoms. Minorities and people from low-income, low-SES, and low-education groups may delay longer than their counterparts, although these factors are commonly not differentiated in analyses; since these groups tend to overlap, interpretation of these data is difficult. There is strong evidence that a history of coronary heart disease is associated with increased delay, although generalizing across the various types of cardiovascular disease may not be possible. A positive relationship also emerges between diabetes and longer delay for AMI.

Studies of psychological characteristics show few and generally weak associations with delay, with the exception of denial, but differing measures and operational definitions of the concept severely limit interpretation. Vagueness of symptoms associated with reduced perceptions of physical sensations increases delay time; similarly, mild symptoms or symptoms that are gradual in onset are associated with greater delay and, conversely, severe symptoms are associated with shorter delay. Fear and anxiety appear to be associated with increased delay in care seeking for cancer symptoms, but not for AMI. Patient beliefs regarding seriousness of the symptoms being experienced may increase delay in health care seeking for cancer, but reduces delay for AMI symptoms. The environment appears to affect delay: being at home increases delay; being with strangers reduces delay; and nighttime or weekend onset may increase delay. Health-care-seeking actions also may significantly affect eventual receipt of care in emergency situations: contacting a personal physician or office appears to increase delay, while using EMS reduces delay.

Interventions

Many interventions have been undertaken to educate individuals or communities on the health consequences of delayed care seeking. The American Cancer Society has been prominent in education for cancer signs and symptoms. Most large-scale intervention programs for cancer have focused on early detection by increasing screening for breast, cervical, prostate, skin, testicular, colorectal, and other cancers. These programs often have focused on high-risk or hard-to-reach populations such as minorities (Suarez, Lloyd, Weiss, Rainbolt, & Pulley, 1994; Yancey & Walden 1994), older women (Rimer, 1993; Mayer *et al.*, 1992), poor or underserved women (Harper, 1993), or some combination of these (Mandelblatt *et al.*, 1993; Saint-Germain & Longman, 1993). Use of screening, particularly for breast cancer, has increased steadily as a result. According to data from the National Health Interview Surveys, mammography use among women over age 40 years almost doubled between the 1987 and 1990 (Breen & Kessler, 1994). Although there is some dispute as to whether screening for cancer decreases mortality or merely increases the time between diagnosis and death (Cole & Morrison, 1980; US Preventive Services Task Force, 1996), it is generally agreed that screening can detect some cancers at an earlier stage, resulting in prolonged life, or even a cure, that might have been impossible had the diagnosis been delayed. Since cancer is the second most common cause of death in this country, even small percentage increases in mean survival time or cure rates can be significant in terms of numbers of persons affected.

Several interventions to reduce delay in care seeking for symptoms of AMI have been undertaken, both in the United States and in other countries. Outside this country, programs have demonstrated median delay decreases with a 6-month educational program (Rustige, Burczyk, Schiele, Werner, & Senges, 1990); an increased proportion of patients presenting at the emergency department within 2 hours of symptom onset with an 8-week campaign (Mitic & Perkins, 1984); an increase in coronary care unit patients admitted between 1 and 4 hours of symptom onset (O'Rourke,

Thompson, & Ballantyne, 1989); and increased community awareness, decreased median delay, increased numbers of patients presenting within 6 hours of symptom onset, and a 9% increase in use of thrombolysis (Blohm *et al.*, 1992; Herlitz *et al.*, 1991). In the United States, results of trials to reduce treatment-seeking delay for AMI have produced successes (Eppler, Eisenberg, Schaffer, Meischke, & Larson, 1994), although not consistently. No changes were found in either patient response or emergency department visits in an Illinois campaign (Moses *et al.*, 1991). Another campaign over a 7-week period revealed awareness of the campaign but no changes in delay or in the percent of patients transported by emergency medical services (Ho, Eisenberg, Litwin, Schaeffer, & Damon, 1989).

Several studies have shown that many people are not aware of risk factors for cancer and AMI and the need to seek care quickly for certain signs and symptoms. Interventions should concentrate on increasing people's knowledge of risk factors and the importance of screening for early screen-detectable cancers and AMI risk factors. Knowledge may not be sufficient to change behaviors, but it is more powerful than ignorance.

Summary and Conclusions

Much research has been conducted on the problem of health-care-seeking delay, but the evidence is far from conclusive as to which factors are most important in reducing delay or increasing early response. Socioeconomic, demographic, environmental, systemic, cultural, and psychological factors have all been implicated. Many studies have been atheoretical, making it difficult to reconcile study results with potentially explanatory models. Theoretical models may need to be further refined or developed to explore the myriad layers of the issues surrounding care-seeking behaviors. Methodological issues likely account for some portion of the inconsistency in study results. Differences in operational definitions of variables often do not allow cross-study comparisons, and thus limit the generalizability of findings. Also, uncontrolled confounding among variables in many studies may be the cause of some of the inconsistencies in research in this area. Much work remains to be done on separating out the effects of race–ethnicity, education, income, and access to care, among other issues. Interactions among these factors will be explored in the next phases of research.

References

ACC/AHA Committee on Management of Acute Myocardial Infarction. (1996). Guidelines for the management of patients with acute myocardial infarction. A report of the American College of Cardiology/American Heart Association Task Force on Practice Guidelines. *Journal of the American College of Cardiology, 28*(5), 1328–1428.

Aiken, L. S., West, S. G., Woodward, C. K., & Reno, R. R. (1994). Health beliefs and compliance with mammography screening recommendations in asymptomatic females. *Health Psychology, 13*, 122–129.

AIMS Trial Study Group. (1990). Long-term effects of intravenous anistreplase in acute myocardial infarction: Final report of the AIMS Study. *Lancet, 2*, 427–431.

Alonzo, A. A. (1980). Acute illness behavior: A conceptual exploration and specification. *Social Science and Medicine, 14A*(6), 515–526.

Alonzo, A. A. (1986). The impact of the family and lay others on care-seeking during life-threatening episodes of suspected coronary artery disease. *Social Science and Medicine, 22*(12), 1297–1311.

Andersen, B. L., & Cacioppo, J. T. (1995). Delay in seeking a cancer diagnosis: Delay stages and psychophysiological comparison processes. *British Journal of Social Psychology, 34*(1), 33–52.

Asenjo, M. A., Bare, L., Bayas, J. M., Prat, A., Lledo, R., Grau, J., & Sulleras, L. (1994). Relationship between severity, costs, and claims of hospitalized patients using the Severity of Illness Index. *European Journal of Epidemiology, 10*(5), 625–632.

Bailey, E. J. (1987). Sociocultural factors and health care-seeking behavior among black Americans. *Journal of the National Medical Association, 79*(4), 389–392.

Bandura, A. (1986). *Social foundations of thought and action: A social cognitive theory.* Englewood Cliffs, NJ: Prentice-Hall.

Baumann, L. J., Brown, R. L., Fontana, S. A., & Cameron, L. (1993). Testing a model of mammography intention. *Journal of Applied Social Psychology, 23,* 1733–1756.

Becker, M. H. (Ed.). (1974). The health belief model and personal health behavior. *Health Education Monograph, 2,* 409–419.

Berkanovic, E., Telesky, C., & Reeder, S. (1981). Structural and social psychological factors in the decision to seek medical care for symptoms. *Medical Care, XIX*(7), 693–709.

Bett, N., Aroney, G., & Thompson, P. (1993). Delays preceding admission to hospital and treatment with thrombolytic agents of patients with possible heart attack. *Australian and New Zealand Journal of Medicine, 23,* 157–161.

Bleeker, J. K., Lamers, L. M., Leenders, I. M., Kruyssen, D. C., Simoons, M. L., Trijsburg, R. W., & Erdman, R. A. (1995). Psychological and knowledge factors related to delay of help-seeking by patients with acute myocardial infarction. *Psychotherapy and Psychosomatics, 63,* 151–158.

Blohm, M., Herlitz, J., Hartford, M., Karlson, B. W., Risenfors, M., Luepker, R. V., Sjolin, M., & Holmberg, S. (1992). Consequences of a media campaign focusing on delay in acute myocardial infarction. *American Journal of Cardiology, 69,* 411–413.

Bosl, G. J., Vogelzang, N. J., Goldman, A., Fraley, E. E., Lange, P. A., Lewitt, S. H., & Kennedy, B. J. (1981). Impact of delay in diagnosis on clinical stage of testicular cancer. *Lancet, 2,* 970–972.

Breen, N., & Kessler, L. (1994). Changes in the use of screening mammography: Evidence from the 1987 and 1990 National Health Interview Surveys. *American Journal of Public Health, 84*(1), 62–67.

Briscoe, M. E. (1987). Why do people go to the doctor? Sex differences in the correlates of GP consultation. *Social Science and Medicine, 25*(5), 507–513.

Burak, R. C., & Liang, J. (1989). The acceptance and completion of mammography by older black women. *American Journal of Public Health, 79,* 721–726.

Burnett, R. E., Blumenthal, J. A., Mark, D. B., Leimberger, J. D., & Caliz, R. M. (1995). Distinguishing between early and late responders to symptoms of acute myocardial infarction. *American Journal of Cardiology, 75*(15), 1019–1022.

Calle, E. E., Flanders, W. D., Thun, M. J., & Martin, L. M. (1993). Demographic predictors of mammography and Pap smear screening in U.S. women. *American Journal of Public Health, 83,* 53–60.

Calnan, M. W. (1984). The health belief model and participation in programmes for the early detection of breast cancer: A comparative analysis. *Social Science and Medicine, 19,* 823–830.

Carey, T. S, Evans, A. T., Hadler, N. M., Lieberman, G., Kalsbeek, W. D., Jackman, A. M., Fryer, J. G., & McNutt, R. A. (1996). Acute severe low back pain. A population-based study of prevalence and care-seeking. *Spine, 21*(3), 339–344.

Champion, V. L. (1985). Use of the health belief model in determining frequency of breast self-examination. *Research in Nursing and Health, 8,* 373–379.

Champion, V. L. (1991). The relationship of selected variables to breast cancer detection behaviors in women 35 and older. *Oncology Nursing Forum, 18,* 733–739.

Champion, V. L. (1994). Strategies to increase mammography utilization. *Medical Care, 32,* 118–129.

Chavez, L. R., Hubbell, F. A., McMullin, J. M., Martinez, R. G., & Mishra, S. I. (1995). Understanding knowledge and attitudes about breast cancer. A cultural analysis. *Archives of Family Medicine, 4*(2), 145–152.

Chien, A., & Schneiderman, L. J. (1975). A comparison of health care utilization by husbands and wives. *Journal of Community Health, 1*(2), 118–126.

Clark, L. T., Bellam, S. V., Shah, A. H., & Feldman, J. G. (1992). Analysis of prehospital delay among inner-city patients with symptoms of myocardial infarction: Implications for therapeutic intervention. *Journal of the American Medical Association, 84*(11), 931–937.

Cole, P., & Morrison, A. S. (1980). Basic issues in population screening for cancer. *Journal of the National Cancer Institute, 64*(5), 1263–1272.

Conrad, M. E., Brown, P., & Conrad, M. G. (1996). Fatalism and breast cancer in black women. *Annals of Internal Medicine, 125*(11), 941–942.

Cooper, R. S., Simmons, B., Castaner, A., Prasad, R., Franklin, C., & Ferlinz, J. (1986). Survival rates and prehospital delay during MI among black persons. *American Journal of Cardiology, 57*, 208–211.

Cowen, M. E., Kattan, M. W., & Miles, B. J. (1996). A national survey of attitudes regarding participation in prostate cancer testing. *Cancer, 78*(9), 1952–1957.

Crawford, S. L., McGraw, S. A., Smith, K. W., McKinlay, J. B., & Pinson, J. E. (1994). Do blacks and whites differ in their use of health care for symptoms of coronary heart disease. *American Journal of Public Health, 84*, 957–964.

Cunningham, M. A., Lee, T. H., Cook, E. F., Brand, D. A., Rouan, G. W., Weisberg, M. C., & Goldman, L. (1989). The effect of gender on the probability of myocardial infarction among emergency department patients with acute chest pain: A report from the Multicenter Chest Pain Study Group. *Journal of General Internal Medicine, 4*, 392–398.

Cunningham-Burley, S., Allbutt, H., Barraway, W. M., Lee, A. J., & Russell, E. B. (1996). Perceptions of urinary symptoms and health-care-seeking behavior amongst men aged 40–79 years. *British Journal of General Practice, 46*(407), 349–352.

Dent, O. F., Goulston, K. J., Tennant, C. C., Langeluddecke, P., Mart, A., Chapuis, P. H., Ward, M., & Bokey, E. L. (1990). Rectal bleeding. Patient delay in presentation. *Diseases of the Colon and Rectum, 33*(10), 851–857.

Dodd, M. J., Lovejoy, N., Stetz, K., Larsen, P., Linsey, A. M., Musci, E., Lewis, B., Hauck, W., Paul, S., & Holzemer, W. (n.d.). Self-care interventions to decrease chemotherapy morbidity. Funded NIH National Cancer Institute R01 CA 48312.

Doehrman, S. R. (1977). Psychosocial aspects of recovery from coronary heart disease: A review. *Social Science and Medicine, 11*, 199–218.

Dracup, K., & Moser, D. K. (1991). Treatment-seeking behavior among those with symptoms and signs of acute myocardial infarction. In J. H. Lanosa, M. J. Hogan, & E. R. Posseman (Eds.), *Proceedings of the NHLBI symposium on rapid identification and treatment of acute myocardial infarction* (pp. 25–45). Washington, DC: National Heart, Lung, and Blood Institute.

Dracup, K., & Moser, D. K. (1997). Beyond sociodemographics: Factors influencing the decision to seek treatment for symptoms of acute myocardial infarction. *Heart and Lung, 26*(4), 253–262.

Dracup, K., Moser, D. K., Eisenberg, M., Meischke, H., Alonzo, A. A., & Braslow, A. (1995). Causes of delay in seeking treatment for heart attack symptoms. *Social Science and Medicine, 40*(3), 379–392.

Dracup, K., Alonzo, A. A., Atkins, J. M., Bennett, N. M., Braslow, A., Clark, L. T., Eisenberg, M., Ferdinand, K. C., Frye, R., Green, L., Hill, M. N., Kennedy, J. W., Kline-Rogers, E., Moser, D. K., Ornato, J. P., Pitt, B., Scot, J. D., Selker, H. P., Silva, S. J., Thies, W., Weaver, W. D., Wenger, N. K., & White, S. K. (1997). The physician's role in minimizing prehospital delay in patients at high risk for acute myocardial infarction: Recommendations from the National Heart Attack Alert Program. *Annals of Internal Medicine, 126*, 645–651.

Ell, K. S., Haywood, L. J., Sobel, E., deGuzman, M, Blumfield, D., & Ning, J-P. (1994, June). Acute chest pain in African Americans: Factors in the delay in seeking emergency care. *American Journal of Public Health, 84*(6), 965–970.

Ell, K., Haywood, L. J., deGuzman, M., Sobel, E., Norris, S., Blumfield, D., Ning, J. P., & Butts, E. (1995). Differential perceptions, behaviors, and motivations among African Americans, Latinos, and whites suspected of heart attacks in two hospital populations. *Journal of the Association for Academic Minority Physicians, 6*(2), 60–69.

Elwood, J. M., & Moorhead, W. P. (1980). Delay in diagnosis & long-term survival in breast cancer. *British Medical Journal, 280*, 1291–1294.

Eppler, E., Eisenberg, M. S., Schaffer, S., Meischke, H., & Larson, M. P. (1994). 911 and emergency department use for chest pain—Results of a media campaign. *Annals of Emergency Medicine, 24*, 202–208.

Erhardt, L. R., Sjögren, A., Sawe, U., & Theorell, T. (1974). Prehospital phase of patients admitted to a coronary care unit. *Acta Medica Scandinavia, 196*, 41–46.

Estudio Multicentrico Estreptoquinasa Reublicas de America del Sur (EMERAS) Collaborative Group. (1993). Randomized trial of late thrombolysis in patients with suspected acute myocardial infarction. *Lancet, 2*, 767–772.

Facione, N.C. (1993). Delay versus help seeking for breast cancer symptoms: A critical review of the literature on patient and provider delay. *Social Science and Medicine, 36*(12), 1521–1534.

Fajardo, L. L., Saint-Germain, M., Meakem III, T. J., Rose, C., & Hillman, B. J. (1992). Factors influencing women to undergo screening mammography. *Radiology, 184*, 59–63.

Fibrinolytic Therapy Trialists (FTT) Collaborative Group. (1994). Indications for fibrinolytic therapy in suspected acute myocardial infarction: Collaborative overview of early mortality and major morbidity results from all randomized trials of more than 1000 patients. *Lancet, 1,* 311–322.

Fontaine, K. R., & Smith, S. (1995). Optimistic bias in cancer risk perception: A cross-national study. *Psychological Reports, 77*(1), 143–46.

Friedman, L. C., Bruce, S., Weinberg, A. D., Cooper, H. P., Yen, A. H., & Hill, M. (1994). Early detection of skin cancer: Racial/ethnic differences in behaviors and attitudes. *Journal of Cancer Education, 9*(2), 105–110.

Gentry, W. D. (1978). Prehospital behavior after a heart attack. *Psychiatry Annals, 8,* 516–520.

Gentry, W. D., & Haney, T. (1975). Emotional and behavioral reaction to acute myocardial infarction. *Heart and Lung, 4,* 738–745.

Gilchrist, I. C. (1973). Patient delay before treatment of myocardial infarction. *British Medical Journal, 1,* 535–537.

Gillum, R. F., Feinleib, M., Margolis, J. R., Fabsitz, R. R., & Brasch, R. C. (1976). Delay in the prehospital phase of acute myocardial infarction: Lack of influence on incidence of sudden death. *Archives of Internal Medicine, 136,* 649–654.

Goldstein, S., Moss, A. J., & Greene, W. (1972). Sudden death in acute myocardial infarction. *Archives of Internal Medicine, 129,* 720–724.

Gould-Martin, K., Paganini-Hill, A., Casagrande, C., Mack, T., & Ross, R. K. (1982). Behavioral and biological determinants of surgical stage of breast cancer. *Preventive Medicine, 11*(4), 429–440.

Grines, C. L., & DeMaria, A. N. (1990). Optimal utilization of thrombolytic therapy for acute myocardial infarction: Concepts and controversies. *Journal of the American College of Cardiology, 16,* 223–231.

Gruppo Italiano per lo Studio della Steptochinasi nell'Infarto miocardico (GISSI). (1986). Effectiveness of intravenous thrombolytic treatment in acute myocardial infarction. *Lancet, 1,* 397–401.

Gruppo Italiano per lo Studio della Streptochinasi nell'Infarto Miocardico (GISSI). (1987). Long-term effects of intravenous thrombolysis in acute myocardial infarction: Final report of the GISSI Study. *Lancet, 2,* 871–874.

Gruppo Italiano per lo Studio della Steptochinasi nell'Infarto miocardico (GISSI). (1995). Epidemiology of avoidable delay in the care of patients with acute myocardial infarction in Italy. *Archives of Internal Medicine, 155,* 1481–1488.

Hackett, T. P., & Cassem, N. H. (1969). Factors contributing to delay in responding to the signs and symptoms of acute myocardial infarction. *American Journal of Cardiology, 24,* 651–658.

Harper, A. P. (1993). Mammography utilization in the poor and medically underserved. *Cancer, 9*(Suppl 4), 1479–1482.

Harris, R. P., Fletcher, S. W., Gonzalez, J. J., Lannin, D. R., Degnan, D., Ear, J. A., & Clark, R. (1991). Mammography and age: Are we targeting the wrong women? A community survey of women and physicians. *Cancer, 67,* 2010–2014.

Harrison, I., & Harrison, D. (1971). The black family experience and health behavior. In C. Crawford (Ed.), *Health and the family: A medical–sociological analysis* (pp. 175–199). New York: Macmillan.

Hartford, M., Herlitz, J., Karlson, B. W., & Risenfors, M. (1990). Components of delay time in suspected acute myocardial infarction with particular emphasis on patient delay. *Journal of Internal Medicine, 228,* 519–523.

Hartford, M., Karlson, B. W., Sjörn, M., Holmberg, S., & Herlitz, J. (1993). Symptoms, thoughts, and environmental factors in suspected acute myocardial infraction. *Heart and Lung, 22,* 64–70.

Haywood, L. J., Ell, K., DeGuman, M, Norris, S., Blumfield, D., & Sobel, E. (1993). Chest pain admissions: Characteristics of black, latino, and white patients in low- and mid-socioeconomic strata. *Journal of the National Medical Association, 85*(10), 749–757.

Helzlsouer, K. J., Ford, D. E., Hayward, R. S. A., Midzenski, M., & Perry, H. (1994). Perceived risk of cancer and practice of cancer prevention behaviors among employees in an oncology center. *Preventive Medicine, 23,* 302–308.

Herlitz, J., Hartford, M., Karlson, B. V., Risenfors, M., Blohm, M., Luepker, R. V., Wennerblom, B., & Holmberg, S. (1991). Effect of a media campaign to reduce delay times for acute myocardial infarction on the burden of chest pain patients in the emergency department. *Cardiology, 79,* 127–134.

Ho, M. T., Eisenberg, M. S., Litwin, P. E., Schaeffer, S. M., & Damon, S. K. (1989). Delay between onset of chest pain and seeking medical care: The effect of public education. *Annals of Emergency Medicine, 18,* 727–731.

Hofgren, K., Bondestam, E., Johansson, G., Jern, S., Herlitz, J., & Holmberg, S. (1988). Initial pain course and delay to hospital admission in relation to myocardial infarct size. *Heart and Lung, 17,* 274–280.

Howard, J. (1982). An approach to the secondary prevention of cancer. In D. L. Parron, R. Solomon, & C. D. Jenkins (Eds.), *Behavior, health risks, and social disadvantage* (pp. 51–61). Washington, DC: National Academy Press.

ISIS-2 Collaborative Group. (1988). Randomized trial of intravenous streptokinase, oral aspirin, both, or neither among 17,187 cases of suspected acute myocardial infarction: ISIS-2. *Lancet, 2,* 349–360.

Johnson, B. T., Gunning, J., & Lewis, S. A. (1996). Health care seeking by heartburn sufferers is associated with psychosocial factors. *American Journal of Gastroenterology, 91,* (12), 2500–2504.

Kash, K. M., Holland, J. C., Halper, M. S., & Miller, D. G. (1992). Psychological distress and surveillance behaviors of women with a family history of breast cancer. *Journal of the National Cancer Institute, 84,* 24–30.

Kegeles, S. S. (1969). Communications problems of experimental research in the ghetto. *Medicine Care, 7,* 395–405.

Kegeles, S. S., Kirscht, J. P., Haefner, D. P., & Rosenstock, I. M. (1965). Survey of beliefs about cancer detection and taking the Papanicolaou test. *Public Health Reports, 80,* 815–823.

Keinan, G., Carmil, D., & Rieck, M. (1991). Predicting women's delay in seeking medical care after discovery of a lump in the breast: The role of personality and behavior patterns. *Behavioral Medicine, 17,* 177–183.

Kenyon, L. W., Ketterer, M. W., Gheorghiade, M., & Goldstein, S. (1991). Psychological factors related to prehospital delay during acute myocardial infarction. *Circulation, 84,* 1969–1976.

King, J. B. (1984). Illness attributions and the health belief model. *Health Education Quarterly, 10,* 287–312.

Kurtz, M. E., Given, B., Given, C. W., & Kurtz, J. C. (1993). Relationships of barriers and facilitators to breast self-examination, mammography, and clinical breast examination in a worksite population. *Cancer Nursing, 16,* 251–259.

Late Assessment of Thombolytic Efficacy (LATE) Study Group. (1993). Late assessment of thrombolytic efficacy (LATE) study with alteplase 6–24 hours after onset of acute myocardial infarction. *Lancet, 342,* 759–766.

Lauver, D. (1992). Psychosocial variables, race, and intention to seek care for breast cancer symptoms. *Nursing Research, 41,* 236–241.

Lauver, D. (1994). Care-seeking behavior with breast cancer symptoms in Caucasian and African-American women. *Research in Nursing and Health, 17,* 421–431.

Lauver, D., & Angerame, M. (1993). Identifying women's expectations about care seeking for a breast cancer symptom. *Oncology Nursing Forum, 20,* 519–525.

Lauver, D., & Chang, A. (1991). Testing theoretical explanations of intentions to seek care for a breast cancer symptom. *Journal of Applied Social Psychology, 21,* 1440–1458.

Lauver, D., Nabholz, S., Scott, K., & Tak, Y. (1997). Testing theoretical explanations of mammography use. *Nursing Research, 46*(1), 32–39.

Lee, H. O. (1997). Typical and atypical clinical signs and symptoms of myocardial infarction and delayed seeking of professional care among blacks. *American Journal of Critical Care, 6*(1), 7–13.

Leitch, J. W., Birbara, T., Freedman, B., Wilcox, I., & Harris, P. J. (1989). Factors influencing the time from onset of chest paint to arrival at hospital. *Medical Journal of Australia, 150,* 6–8.

Lerman, C., Rimer, B., Trock, B., Balshem, A., & Engstrom, P. R. (1990). Factors associated with repeat adherence to breast cancer screening. *Preventive Medicine, 19,* 279–290.

Lerman, C., Audrain, J., & Croyle, R. T. (1994). DNA-testing for heritable breast cancer risks: Lessons from traditional genetic counseling. *Annals of Behavioral Medicine, 16*(4), 327–333.

Leventhal, E. A., & Prochaska, T. (1986). Age, symptom interpretation, and health behavior. *Journal of the American Geriatric Society, 34,* 185–191.

Leventhal, H. (1970). Findings and theory in the study of fear communications. *Advances in Experimental Social Psychology, 5,* 119–186.

Leventhal, H., Meyer, D., & Nerenz, D. (1980). The common-sense representation of illness danger. In S. Rachman (Ed.), *Medical psychology* (pp. 517–554). New York: John Wiley.

Lierman, L. M. (1988). Discovery of breast changes. Women's responses and nursing implications. *Cancer Nursing, 11,* 352–361.

Linderer, T., Schroder, R., Arntz, R., Heineking, M. L., Wunderlich, W., Kohl, K., Forycki, F., Henzgen, R., & Wagner, J. (1993). Prehospital thrombolysis: Beneficial effects of very early treatment on infarct size and left ventricular function. *Journal of the American College of Cardiology, 22,* 1304–1310.

Loehrer, P. J., Greger, H. A., Weinberger, M., Musick, B., Miller, M., Nichols, C., Bryan, J., Higgs, D., & Brock, D. (1991). Knowledge and beliefs about cancer in a socioeconomically disadvantaged population. *Cancer, 68,* 1665–1671.

Love, N. (1991). Why patients delay seeking care for cancer symptoms. What you can do about it. *Postgraduate Medicine, 89*(4), 151–152, 155–158.

MacArthur, C., & Smith, A. (1981). Delay in breast cancer and the nature of presenting symptoms. *Lancet, 1,* 601–603.

Magarey, C. J., Todd, P. B., & Blizard, P. J. (1977). Psychosocial factors influencing delay and breast self-examination in women with symptoms of breast cancer. *Social Science and Medicine, 11,* 229–232.

Mandelblatt, J., Traxler, M., Lakin, P., Kanetsky, P., Thomas, L., Chauhan, P., Matseoane, S., Ramsey, E., & the Harlem Study Group. (1993). Breast and cervical cancer screening of poor, elderly, black women: Clinical results and implications. *American Journal of Preventive Medicine, 9,* 133–138.

Manheimer, J. (1993). Medical risk, perceived risk, and body anxiety in women attending a high-risk breast surveillance clinic. *Dissertation Abstracts International [B], 54*(1), 502.

Marshall, J. R., & Funch, D. P. (1986). Gender and illness behavior among colorectal cancer patients. *Women and Health, 11*(3–4), 67–82.

Massey, V. (1986). Perceived susceptibility to breast cancer and the practice of breast self-examination. *Nursing Research, 35,* 183–185.

Matthews, K. A., Siegel, J. M., Kuller, L. H., Thompson, M., & Varat, M. (1983). Determinants of decisions to seek medical treatment by patients with acute myocardial infarction symptoms. *Journal of Personality and Social Psychology, 44*(6), 1144–1156.

Mayer, J. A., Slymen, D. J., Drew, J. A., Wright, B. L., Elder, J. P., & Williams, S. J. (1992). Breast and cervical cancer screening in older women: The San Diego Medicare Preventive Health Project. *Preventive Medicine, 21,* 395–404.

Maynard, C., Althouse, R., Olsufka, M., Ritchie, J. L., Davis K. B., & Kennedy J. W. (1989). Early versus late hospital arrival for acute myocardial infarction in the Western Washington Thrombolytic Therapy Trials. *American Journal of Cardiology, 63,* 1296–1300.

Maynard, C., Litwin, P. E., Martin, J. S., Cerqueira, M., Kudenchuk, P. J., Ho, M. T., Kennedy, J. W., Cobb, L. A., Schaeffer, S. M., & Hallstrom, A. P. (1991). Characteristics of black patients admitted to coronary care units in metropolitan Seattle: Results from the Myocardial Infarction Triage and Intervention Registry (MITI). *American Journal of Cardiology, 67,* 18–23.

Meischke, H., Ho, M. T., Eisenberg, M. S., Schaeffer, S. M., & Larsen, M. P. (1995). Reasons patients with chest pain delay or do not call 911. *Annals of Emergency Medicine, 25*(2), 193–197.

Millar, M. G., & Millar, K. (1996). The effects of anxiety on response times to disease detection and health promotion behaviors. *Journal of Behavioral Medicine, 19*(4), 401–413.

Mitic, W. R., & Perkins, J. (1984). The effect of a media campaign on heart attack delay and decision times. *Canadian Journal of Public Health, 75,* 414–418.

Mor, V., Masterson-Allen, S, Goldberg, R., Guadagnoli, E., & Wool, M. S. (1990). Prediagnostic symptom recognition and help seeking among cancer patients. *Journal of Community Health, 15*(4), 253–266.

Moses, H. W., Engelking, N., Taylor, G. J., Prabhakar, C., Vallala, M., Colliver, J. A., Silberman, H., & Schneider, J. A. (1991). Effect of a two-year public education campaign on reducing response time of patients with symptoms of acute myocardial infarction. *American Journal of Cardiology, 68,* 249–251.

Moss, A. J., & Goldstein, S. (1970). The prehospital phase of acute myocardial infarction. *Circulation, 41,* 737–742.

Moss, A. J., Wynar, B., & Goldstein, S. (1969). Delay in hospitalization during the acute coronary period. *American Journal of Cardiology, 24,* 659–665.

Nichols, S., Waters, W. E., Fraser, J. D., Wheeler, M. J., & Ingham, S. K. (1981). Delay in the presentation of breast symptoms for consultant investigation. *Community Medicine, 3,* 217–225.

Norcross, W. A., Ramirez, C., & Palinkas, L. A. (1996). The influence of women on the health care-seeking behavior of men. *The Journal of Family Practice, 43*(5), 475–480.

O'Rourke, M. F., Thompson, P. L., & Ballantyne, K. (1989). Community aspects of coronary thrombolysis: Public education and cost effectiveness. In D. G. Julian, W. Kubler, R. M. Norris, H. J. Swan, D. Collen, & M. Verstraete (Eds.), *Thrombolysis in cardiovascular disease* (pp. 309–324). New York: Marcel Dekker.

Ottesen, M. M., Køber, L., Jørgensen, S., & Torp-Pedersen, C., on behalf of the TRACE Study Group. (1996). Determinants of delay between symptoms and hospital admission in 5978 patients with acute myocardial infarction. *European Heart Journal, 17,* 429–437.

Pack, G. T., & Gallo, J. S. (1938). The culpability for delay in the treatment of cancer. *American Journal of Cancer, 33,* 443.

Pearlman, D. N., Rakowski, W., Ehrich, B., & Clark, M. A. (1996). Breast cancer screening practices among black, Hispanic, and white women: reassessing differences. *American Journal of Preventive Medicine, 12*(5), 327–337.

Powe, B. D. (1994). Perceptions of cancer fatalism among African Americans: The influence of education, income, and cancer knowledge. *Journal of National Black Nurses Association, 7*(2), 41–48.

Raczynski, J. M., Taylor, H., Rappaport, N., Cutter, G., Hardin, M., & Oberman, A. (1994). Diagnoses, acute symptoms and attributions for symptoms among black and white inpatients admitted for coronary heart disease: Findings of the Birmingham–BHS project. *American Journal of Public Health, 84,* 951–956.

Rawles, J. M., & Haites, N. E. (1988). Patient and general practitioner delays in acute myocardial infarction. *British Medical Journal, 296,* 882–884.

Rawles, J. M., Metcalfe, M. J., Shirreffs, C., Jennings, K., & Kenmure, A. C. F. (1990). Association of patient delay with symptoms, cardiac enzymes, and outcome in acute myocardial infarction. *European Heart Journal, 11,* 643–648.

Reynolds, K., West, S., & Aiken, L. S. (1990). Increasing the use of mammography: A pilot program. *Health Education Quarterly, 17*(4), 429–441.

Richardson, J. L., Langholz, B., Bernstein, L., Burciaga, C., & Ross, R. K. (1992). Stage and delay in breast cancer diagnosis by race, socioeconomic status, age and year. *British Journal of Cancer, 65,* 922–926.

Rimer, B. (1993). Improving the use of cancer screening for older women. *Cancer, 72*(Suppl 3), 1085–1087.

Rimer, B. K., Trock, B., Engstrom, P. F., Lerman, C., & King, E. (1991). Why do some women get regular mammograms? *American Journal of Preventive Medicine, 7,* 69–74.

Rimer, B. K., Schildkraut, J. M., Lerman, C., Lin, T. H., & Audrain, J. (1996). Participation in a women's breast cancer risk counseling trial. Who participates? Who declines? High-Risk Breast Cancer Consortium. *Cancer, 77*(11), 2348–2335.

Rosenstock, I. M. (1966). Why people use health services. *Milbank Memorial Fund Quarterly, 44,* 94–127.

Rosko, M. D., & Carpenter, C. E. (1994). The impact of intra-DRG severity of illness on hospital profitability: Implications for payment reform. *Journal of Health Politics, Policy and Law, 19*(4), 729–751.

Royak-Schaler, R., DeVellis, B. McE., Sorenson, J. R., Wilson, K. R., Lannin, D. R., & Emerson, J. A. (1995). Breast cancer in African-American families. *Annals of the New York Academy of Sciences, 768,* 281–285.

Rustige, J. M., Burczyk, U., Schiele, R., Werner, A., & Senges, J. (1990). Media campaign on delay times in suspected myocardial infarction—The Ludwigshafen Community Project [Abstract]. *European Heart Journal, 11*(Suppl), 171.

Safer, M. A., Tharps, Q. J., Jackson, T. C., & Leventhal, H. (1979). Determinants of three stages of delay in seeking care at a medical clinic. *Medical Care, 17*(1), 11–29.

Saint-Germain, M. A., & Longman, A. J. (1993). Breast cancer screening among older Hispanic women: knowledge, attitudes, and practices. *Health Education Quarterly, 20*(4), 539–553.

Samet, J. M., Hunt, W. C., Lerchen, M. L., & Goodwin, J. S. (1988). Delay in seeking care for cancer symptoms: A population-based study of elderly New Mexicans. *Journal of the National Cancer Institute, 80,* 432–438.

Saunders, I. D. (1989). Differences in the timeliness of diagnosis, breast and cervical cancer, San Francisco 1974–85. *American Journal of Public Health, 79*(1), 69–70.

Schmidt, S. B., & Borsch, M. A. (1990). The prehospital phase of acute myocardial infarction in the era of thrombolysis. *American Journal of Cardiology, 65,* 1411–1415.

Schroeder, J. S., Lamb, I. H., & Hu, M. (1978). The prehospital course of patients with chest pain: Analysis of the prodromal, symptomatic, decision-making, transportation and emergency room periods. *American Journal of Medicine, 64,* 742–748.

Schwarz, B., Schobererger, R., Rieder, A., & Kunze, M. (1994). Factors delaying treatment of acute myocardial infarction. *European Heart Journal, 15,* 1595–1598.

Seffrin, J. R., Wilson, J. L., & Black, B. L. (1991). Patient perceptions. *Cancer, 67,* 1783–1787.

Siegler, I. C., Feaganes, J. R., & Rimer, B. K. (1995). Predictors of adoption of mammography in women under age 50. *Health Psychology, 14*(3), 274–278.

Simon, A. B., Feinleib, M., & Thompson, H. K. (1972). Components of delay in the pre-hospital phase of acute myocardial infarction. *American Journal of Cardiology, 30,* 476–481.

Simons-Morton, D. G., Goff, D. C., Osganian, S., Goldberg, R. J., Raczynski, J. M., Finnegan, J. R., Zapka, J., Eisenberg, M. S., Proschan, M. A., Feldman, H. A., Hedges, J. R., & Luepker, R. V. (1998). Rapid early action for coronary treatment: Rationale, design, and baseline characteristics. *Academic Emergency Medicine, 5,* 726–738.

Sjögren, A., Erhardt, L. R., & Theorell, T. (1979). Circumstances around the onset of a myocardial infarction. *Acta Medica Scandinavia, 205,* 287–292.

Sortet, J. P., & Banks, S. R. (1997). Health beliefs of rural Appalachian women and the practice of breast self-examination. *Cancer Nursing, 20(4)*, 321–235.

Stein, J. A., Fox, S. A., Murata, P. J., & Morisky, D. E. (1992). Mammography usage and the health belief model. *Health Education Quarterly, 19(4)*, 447–462.

Suarez, L., Lloyd, L., Weiss, N., Rainbolt, T., & Pulley, L. (1994). Effect of social networks on cancer-screening behavior of older Mexican-American women. *Journal of the National Cancer Institute, 86*, 775–779.

Theisen, M. E., MacNeill, S. E., Lumley, M. A., Ketterer, M. W., Goldberg, A. D., & Barzak, S. (1995). Psychosocial factors related to unrecognized acute myocardial infarction. *American Journal of Cardiology, 75(17)*, 1211–1213.

Triandis, H. (1982). A model of choice in marketing. In L. McAlister (Ed.), *Choice models for buyer behavior* (pp. 147–162). Greenwich, CT: JAI Press.

Trotta, P. (1980). Breast self-examination: Factors influencing compliance. *Oncology Nursing Forum, 7*, 13–17.

Turi, Z. G., Stone, P. H., Muller, J. E., Parker, C., Rude, R. E., Raabe, D. E., Jaffe, A. S., Hartwell, T. D., Robertson, T. L., & Braunwalk, E., the Milis Study Group. (1986). Implications for acute intervention related to time of hospital arrival in acute myocardial infarction. *American Journal of Cardiology, 58*, 203–209.

Underwood, S. (1992). Cancer risk reduction and early detection behaviors among black men: Focus on learned helplessness. *Journal of Community Health Nursing, 9*, 21–31.

US Preventive Services Task Force. (1996). *Guide to clinical preventive services*. Baltimore: Williams & Wilkins.

Vernon, S. W., Tilley, B. C., Neale, A. V., & Steinfeldt, L. (1985). Ethnicity, survival, and delay in seeking treatment for symptoms of breast cancer. *Cancer, 55*, 1563–1571.

Vernon, S. W., Vogel, V. G., Halabi, S., & Bondy, M. L. (1993). Factors associated with perceived risk of breast cancer among women attending a screening program. *Breast Cancer Research and Treatment, 28(2)*, 137–144.

Waldron, I. (1983). Sex differences in illness incidence, prognosis and mortality: Issues and evidence. *Social Science and Medicine, 17(16)*, 1107–1123.

Weinberg, A. D., Cooper, H. P., Lane, M., & Kripalani, S. (1997). Screening behaviors and long-term compliance with mammography guidelines in a breast cancer screening program. *American Journal of Preventive Medicine, 13(1)*, 29–35.

Weissman, J.S., Stern, R., Fielding, S. L., & Epstein, A. M. (1991). Delayed access to health care: Risk factors, reasons, and consequences. *Annals of Internal Medicine, 114(4)*, 325–331.

Wielgosz, A. T., & Nolan, R. P. (1991). Understanding delay in response to symptoms of acute myocardial infarction: A compelling agenda. *Circulation, 84(5)*, 2193–2195.

Wielgosz, A. T., Nolan, R. P., Earp, J. A., Biro, E., & Wielgosz, M. B. (1988). Reasons for patients' delay in response to symptoms of acute myocardial infarction. *Canadian Medical Association Journal, 139(9)*, 853–857.

Worden, J. W., & Weisman, A. D. (1975). Psychosocial components of lagtime in cancer diagnosis. *Journal of Psychosomatic Research, 19*, 69–79.

Yancey, A. K., & Walden, L. (1994). Stimulating cancer screening among Latinas and African-American women. *Journal of Cancer Education, 9(1)*, 46–52.

Yarzebski, J., Goldberg, R. J., Gore, J. M., & Alpert, J. S. (1994). Temporal trends and factors associated with extent of delay to hospital arrival in patients with acute myocardial infarction: The Worcester Heart Attack Study. *American Heart Journal, 128*, 255–263.

Zervas, I. M., Augustine, A., & Friechione, G. L. (1993). Patient delay in cancer. A view from the crisis model. *General Hospital Psychiatry, 15(1)*, 9–11.

CHAPTER *7*

Stress, Coping, Social Support, and Illness

Leslie F. Clark, Leslie Aaron, MaryAnn Littleton,
Katina Pappas-Deluca, Jason B. Avery, and Vel S. McKleroy

Introduction

Social and behavioral scientists have a great deal to offer to public and private sector efforts directed toward health promotion and disease prevention. This chapter focuses on stress, coping, and social support. Research questions in these domains revolve around the interconnections among individuals' emotions, motivation, goals, cognitions, and social relationships. The utility of such research lies in establishing behavioral predictors of individuals' likelihood of becoming ill and the ease of their recovery from illness (Clark, 1994). A second contribution lies in the abilities of these fields to inform and guide health promotion and disease prevention intervention.

The work in this chapter is largely guided by the biopsychosocial model of health and illness in which there is an interchange among social, psychological, and biological levels of human functioning as they contribute to health and illness. The chapter will cover stress, coping, and social support separately. For each topic, the chapter will discuss research on sociodemographic findings, health risks, and amelioration or exacerbation of medical conditions. Finally, we discuss interventions that have been designed to reduce stress and enhance coping and social support in particular illness domains.

Leslie F. Clark, Leslie Aaron, MaryAnn Littleton, Katina Pappas-Deluca, Jason B. Avery, and Vel S. McKleroy • Department of Health Behavior, School of Public Health, UAB Center for Health Promotion, University of Alabama at Birmingham, Birmingham, Alabama 35294.

Handbook of Health Promotion and Disease Prevention, edited by Raczynski and DiClemente. Kluwer Academic/Plenum Publishers, New York, 1999.

Stress

Conceptualization and Measurement of Stress

The term *stress* is frequently used interchangeably to denote either a stressful event or the experience of psychological distress. However, it is helpful to maintain a distinction between the event itself (the stressor) and the person's reaction to the event (psychological distress) (Lobel, 1994). This distinction is made in Table 1, which lists some common self-report measures of stressful events and psychological distress. Some of the instruments in Table 1 include a separate assessment of the person's appraisal of the event as distressing (e.g., Perceived Stress Scale), while others do not (e.g., Social Readjustment Rating Scale).

Modified measures of stressful events have been developed to apply to specific populations. For example, the Gay Affect and Life Events Scale (GALES) assesses both the degree of life change and level of emotional distress associated with life events in homosexual men (Rosser & Ross, 1989). Assessment techniques for stress include self-report or observational coding in natural and laboratory settings.

Stress and Demographic Characteristics

There is growing recognition that individual characteristics traditionally defined as demographic variables (e.g., gender, socioeconomic status, ethnicity) are associated with a greater vulnerability to stress and its health-related consequences. Inclusion of women in health outcome studies introduces the necessity of considering factors that might interact with stress to produce disease specifically in women. For example, the multiple roles in which many women function as mother, wife, and employee may increase stress and perhaps produce adverse effects on health and well-being (Barnett, 1993). Yet, this expectation has not received support from studies examining the role of women in the workforce. They found that women who work

Table 1. Stress and Psychological Distress Constructs and Instruments

Construct	Appraisal of event	Instrument
Major life events	No	Social Readjustment Rating Scale (Holmes & Rahe, 1967)
		Psychiatric Epidemiology Research Interview Life Events Scale (Dohrenwend *et al.*, 1978)
	Yes	Perceived Stress Scale (Cohen, Kamarck, & Mermelstein, 1983)
		Life Experiences Survey (Sarason, Sarason, & Shearin, 1986)
Daily life stressors	Yes	Hassles Scale (DeLongis *et al.*, 1982)
	No	Survey of Recent Life Experiences (Kohn & MacDonald, 1992)
Psychological distress	N/A	Speilberg State–Trait Anxiety Scale (Speilberg *et al..* 1983)
		Center for Epidemiologic Studies Depression Scale (Radloff, 1977)
		Beck Depression Inventory (Beck *et al.*, 1961)

outside the home show overall better physical and psychological health than women who do not work outside the home (Thoits, 1983; Verbruggee, 1983). These findings have been explained by the concept of "identity-relevant stressors." This position proposes that only those negative events that threaten a valued and meaningful role in an individual's social functioning will exert an adverse influence on health and well-being (Thoits, 1991). This theory would predict then that those women who highly value their work role, perhaps to the exclusion of other life domains, might be at greater risk for development of work-stress-induced illness.

Socioeconomic status (SES) also has been linked to an increased vulnerability to the effects of stress. Persons with low SES, as indexed by income, educational level, and occupation, encounter more negative events and may be more susceptible to adverse effects because they may have fewer social and psychological resources to cope with these events (Adler et al., 1994; McLeod & Kessler, 1990). It has been shown that individuals with low education particularly may attempt to cope in stressful circumstances by using a variety of unhealthy behaviors such as cigarette smoking, excessive use of alcohol, or poor eating and exercise habits (Seeman, Seeman, & Budros, 1988). Evidence also exists that links SES (i.e., educational level) and stress directly to health consequences. Both stressful events and educational level have been shown to independently predict mortality over a 3-year period among male survivors of myocardial infarction (Ruberman, Weinblatt, & Goldberg, 1984). However, when stressful events were rated as high, education no longer accounted for mortality, suggesting a close interdependence between stress and educational level.

Finally, ethnicity itself consistently relates to health outcomes, although it often has been subsumed under the rubric of SES. Repeated empirical studies show, however, that ethnic differences in health status persist after SES indicators have been taken into account, emphasizing the unique effects of ethnicity on health (Williams & Collins, 1995). For example, African Americans have greater blood pressure elevations than whites in response to laboratory stressors, suggesting that cardiovascular reactivity to stress is differentially associated with race. Cardiovascular reactivity, in turn, is believed to account in part for the relation between stress and development of hypertension and heart disease (Light, Obrist, Andrew, Jones, & Strogatz, 1987; Tofler et al., 1990).

Stress and Health Risks

An individual's perception or appraisal of a situation as stressful may be accompanied by emotional distress, which is believed to produce a chain of physiological changes in the body. These acute changes consist primarily of suppression of immune system functioning in response to pathogens and the release of a variety of pituitary and adrenal hormones in the brain (Rose, 1984). Moreover, there is a bidirectional relationship between the body's hormonal and immunologic response systems. Although much is still unknown, this relationship generally provides an explanation as to the specific pathways by which stress leads to the development of infections and tumors in both humans and animals (Stein & Miller, 1993).

Few studies have linked stress directly to the development of chronic disease (e.g., breast cancer: Chen et al., 1995). In a series of investigations, Schneiderman et al. (1993) demonstrated that stressful events act to produce specific dysfunctional immune and endocrine reactions in human immunodeficiency virus type 1 (HIV-1) seropositive versus HIV-1 seronegative gay men. These aberrant physiological reactions are hypothesized to increase the probability of acquiring opportunistic infections in HIV-1 seropositive patients.

Comparatively stronger evidence exists implicating the role of stress in the development of acute illnesses. For example, DeLongis, Folkman, and Lazarus (1988) prospectively examined daily hassles among married couples and found a significant relationship between daily stress and the occurrence of concurrent health problems such as flu, sore throat, headaches, and backaches. Overall, however, associations between stress and infection have been modest (see Cohen & Williamson, 1991, for a review).

The influence of individual differences in stress reactivity has been proposed as a way to account for these modest effects (e.g., cardiovascular reactivity to a stressor). A prospective study of cardiovascular reactivity showed that children who display high cardiovascular reactivity were more likely to develop respiratory illness during periods of high environmental stress compared to children with low cardiovascular reactivity (Boyce *et al.*, 1995). Other studies have shown similar effects in adult populations (Kiecolt-Glaser, Duran, Speicher, Trask, & Glaser, 1991; Miller, Markides, Chiriboga, & Ray, 1995). These studies demonstrate the important role that individual differences can play in creating illness episodes during stress.

Stress may affect health directly as well as indirectly through unhealthy self-care practices. Generally, individuals under stress are more likely to engage in poor health behaviors (e.g., smoking, excessive alcohol consumption) and are less compliant with medical recommendations (Caldwell *et al.*, 1983). In a Canadian national survey, community-based elderly residents who reported a greater number of negative stressful life events were more likely to smoke and be at an increased risk for respiratory problems (Maxwell & Hirdes, 1993). Similarly, pregnant women who experience a greater number of negative life events were more likely to abuse drugs or alcohol (Bresnahan, Zuckerman, & Cabral, 1992). These studies suggest that negative health behaviors often are correlates of stress, which can in turn adversely affect health status.

Finally, one study suggests circumstances in which distress, evidenced as concern over one's symptoms, can be beneficial to health care practices. Lauver and Chang (1991) investigated psychosocial, demographic, habit, and facilitating (e.g., health insurance) factors influencing women's intentions to seek care promptly for breast cancer symptoms. Women's anxiety in response to finding a suspicious lump in the breast predicted the intention to seek care for cancer screening independently of facilitating conditions. The authors concluded that clinicians can increase the intention to seek care by promoting a moderate amount of concern along with clear instructions for routine follow-up to women who exhibit symptoms of early breast cancer.

Stress and the Amelioration or Exacerbation of Medical Conditions

Individuals who suffer from chronic illness may be especially vulnerable to stress in exacerbating a preexisting condition. For example, rheumatoid arthritis (RA) patients with more active disease show increased reactivity between daily stressful events and next-day joint pain (Affleck, Tennen, Urrows, & Higgins, 1994). Stressful interpersonal conflicts also have been related to increases in the immune-stimulating hormones prolactin and estradiol and higher clinician ratings of disease activity for rheumatoid arthritis patients (Zautra, Burleson, Matt, Roth, & Burrows, 1994).

Stress may also interfere with treatment of high blood pressure and make it more difficult to manage by diminishing the effectiveness of antihypertensive medications. Brody (1980) found that patients who scored in the highest quartile on a measure of psychological distress received more antihypertensive medications but had smaller reductions in blood pressure than those who scored lower on psychological distress. However, it is unclear from the study methodology if these effects are due to direct mediation of stress on blood pressure or whether patients experiencing more distress were simply less compliant with the medication regimen. Indeed, multiple maladaptive health behaviors may occur in association with distress to put individuals with various chronic medical conditions at even greater risk for exacerbation of their illness. For example, patients with diabetes mellitus who experienced high levels of psychological distress used more alcohol and cigarettes and monitored their blood glucose level less often, thus placing themselves at higher risk for severe hypoglycemia (Spangler, Konen, & McGann, 1993).

Perhaps some of the most definitive studies that demonstrate the relationship between stress and illness are those that link stress to mortality. For example, Denollet, Sys, and Brutsaert (1995) reported that among the best predictors of subsequent mortality following myocardial infarction in a sample of men with coronary artery disease were life stress and depression.

The combined results from these studies suggest that psychosocial interventions may be beneficial in modifying the effects of stress within target populations to prevent acute illness or ameliorate chronic illness. However, prior to the development of an intervention, it is necessary to further elucidate the specific physiological and behavioral pathways by which stress produces adverse effects for particular diseases. Identification of the moderators of these pathways can then be used to devise interventions that seek to modify the effects of stress on illness. Thus, the remainder of this chapter will review two important moderators of the relationship between stress and illness: coping and social support.

Coping

Conceptualization and Measurement of Coping

Coping is conceptualized as an individual's ongoing efforts to manage specific external and internal demands that are appraised as taxing or exceeding personal resources (Folkman & Lazarus, 1988b). Contemporary theories view coping as a continuous process that changes through time and within the context of a changing stressful event. The "coping as a process" view underscores the importance of the interaction between a person and his or her environment. This interaction determines the person's appraisals or perceptions, efforts, and outcomes. Individuals draw on coping resources such as social support from friends, families, and institutions, as well as personal resources such as beliefs, abilities, and dispositions, in order to cope with a stressful event.

Coping efforts have been divided into two broad functions: problem-focused or emotion-focused. In any stressful encounter, coping includes efforts to control or change the emotional and/or problem-solving aspects of situations (Folkman & Lazarus, 1988b). Also, coping efforts have been classified as either approach or avoidance strategies; that is, whether efforts to manage stress include approach or avoidance of the stress-inducing aspects of a situation (Moos, 1992).

Coping research comprises the measurement of the various efforts (e.g., problem focused–emotional focused), strategies (e.g., avoidance–approach), and personal resources (e.g., beliefs, dispositions) found to influence adaptational outcomes. Table 2 summarizes these major constructs. Personal resource constructs are still being investigated in terms of whether or not they are valid and reliable measures. For example, "hardiness," "dispositional optimism," and "sense of coherence" have received criticism with regard to their similarity with each other and to other constructs such as negative affectivity (Jennings & Staggers, 1994; Sullivan, 1993).

Ways of Coping Questionnaire

Perhaps the most widely used instrument in the research on coping efforts is the Ways of Coping Questionnaire. In general, studies employing this instrument have found eight distinct efforts (three emotion focused, four problem focused and seeking support effort) that individuals use to deal with a stressful event (e.g., self-controlling, positive reappraisal, escape–avoidance, planful problem solving). This research shows that individuals often use both emotion- and problem-focused efforts in any one situation. Moreover, research has not substantiated in a generalizable manner that one effort is superior to another. In any coping situation, the utility of any coping effort or strategy is dependent on many factors: the type of stressor experienced, availability of personal and social resources, and which outcome modality is being measured (Lazarus, 1993a).

Coping and Demographic Characteristics

A variety of sociodemographic variables including gender, SES, and age are associated with coping differences among individuals. Coping research has mirrored stereotypical gender differences that women are more emotionally expressive and use passive coping strategies, while men tend to control emotions and engage in more problem-solving efforts (Thoits, 1995). Some of the differences found between women and men in their problem-solving efforts may be attributable to perceived control in a role-relevant domain (Thoits, 1995). Evidence shows that when work, health, and family-related stress are held constant, men and women show similar coping patterns (Lazarus, 1993a).

In general, low-SES populations in general are exposed more often to a greater degree of stressors and may lack the resources (financial and otherwise) to enact successful coping strategies compared to middle- or high-SES individuals (Adler et al., 1994; James, 1994). Research on age does not conclusively show that there are wide disparities in coping efforts in the young versus old (Costa & McCrae, 1993). However, there are differences in the kinds of stressors experienced as one ages as well as how stressors are appraised, which influences coping efforts (Feifel & Strack, 1989). Also, personality variables that influence coping efforts, such as negative affectivity, have been shown to become more predominate as one ages (Costa & Mc-Crae, 1993).

Table 2. Coping Constructs and Instruments

Construct	Definition	Instrument
Coping efforts	Ongoing efforts in thought and action to manage specific demands appraised as taxing or overwhelming (e.g., emotion- and problem-focused efforts, and/or avoidance and approach efforts) (Folkman & Lazarus,1988).	Ways of Coping Questionnaire (Folkman & Lazarus,1988) Coping Responses Inventory (Moos, 1992) Medical Coping Modes Questionnaire and Life Situations Inventory (Feifel *et al.*, 1987; Feifel & Strack,1989) Multidimensional Coping Inventory (Carver *et al.*, 1989) Coping Inventory for Stressful Situations (Endler & Parker, 1991)
Dispositional optimism	A general expectancy for positive outcomes, especially in difficult and ambiguous situations (Scheier & Carver, 1985)	Life Orientation Test (Scheier & Carver, 1985)
Pessimistic explanatory style	Habitually explaining bad events in a fatalistic manner using stable and internal explanations (Peterson & Villanova, 1988)	Expanded Attributional Style Questionnaire, (Peterson & Villanova, 1988)
Sense of coherence	Pervasive, enduring confidence about the outcome including comprehensibility, manageability, and meaningfulness (Antonovsky, 1993)	Sense of Coherence Scale (Antonovsky, 1993)
Hardiness	Three components: control, commitment and challenge (Kobasa, 1979)	Hardiness Scale (Kobasa, 1979) Health-related Hardiness Scale (Pollack, 1986)
Negative affectivity	Chronic negative emotions, low self-esteem, excess worry and complaining (Watson & Clark, 1984)	Hopkins Symptom Checklist (Watson & Pennebaker,1989)
Type A	Aggressive, competitive style with a sense of time urgency (Rosenman *et al.*, 1964)	Structure Interview (Rosenman *et al.*, 1974) Jenkins Activity Survey (Jenkins *et al.*, 1979) Bortner Scale (Bortner, 1969) Framingham Type A Scale (Haynes, Levine, & Scotch, 1978)
John Henryism	Active coping including efficacious mental–physical vigor, commitment to hard work, and single-minded determination to succeed (James *et al.*, 1983)	John Henryism Scale for Active Coping (James *et al.*, 1983)
Monitor–blunter processing styles	Seeking out threat-relevant information (monitoring) versus avoiding threat-relevant information (blunting) (Miller, 1987)	The Miller Behavioral Style Scale (Miller, 1987)
Locus of control	Generalized belief that circumstances are under own or others control (Rotter, 1966)	Locus of Control Scale (Rotter, 1966) Health Locus of Control (Wallston *et al.*, 1978)
Self-efficacy	Perception of ability to enact the necessary actions to obtain a specific outcome (Bandura, 1977)	Situational Confidence Questionnaire for Alcohol Relapse (Soloman & Annis, 1990)

Coping and Health Risks

Positive Coping Influences

The hardiness construct is defined in terms of individuals who are less likely to report illness due to stressful events. Psychologically, hardy individuals show high levels of perceived control, commitment to succeed, and a propensity to see stressful life events as challenges (Kobasa, 1979). Cross-sectional studies have confirmed that hardiness is associated with decreases in smoking, drinking, and reckless behaviors. Problem-focused and support-seeking coping efforts have been shown to mediate the relationship between the hardiness construct and health risks (Williams, Wiebe, & Smith, 1992) .

People who in general expect positive outcomes (i.e., optimists) are more likely to engage in active coping efforts, be better psychologically adjusted, and report less physical illness (Aspinwall & Taylor, 1997). Optimists also are more likely to practice health-enhancing behaviors than pessimists (Robbins, Spence, & Clark, 1991).

Studies of control and coping cite the importance of a match between the controllability of a situation and coping efforts employed in order to create adaptational outcomes (Folkman, 1984). In a study of residents living on Three Mile Island during the nuclear plant disaster, people who engaged in the use of problem-focused coping to deal with the chronic, uncontrollable aspects of the accident experienced more psychological symptoms than those who turned their efforts toward managing emotional aspects (Collins, Baum, & Singer, 1983). Also, belief in one's ability to cope with stressors (self-efficacy beliefs) have been shown to affect health outcomes. A study of self-efficacy beliefs and ability to cope with labor pain showed that confidence in the ability to control pain was related to reports of less labor pain obtained within 48 hours of delivery (Crowe & von Baeyer, 1989).

In a meta-analysis of avoidance and approach coping strategies, it was reported that avoidance strategies such as denial, distraction, repression, and suppression were more beneficial when dealing with acute short-term stressors, such as noise, pain, blood donation, and some uncomfortable medical diagnostic procedures than approach (attention-focused) strategies. In contrast, approach strategies that involved focusing one's attention on the stressor were superior to avoidance strategies for chronic stressors, especially if the attention is focused on sensory information rather than the emotional aspects of the situation (Suls & Fletcher, 1985).

Research on the ways people process information either by seeking or avoiding threat-relevant cues (monitor–blunter types) emphasizes costs and benefits for both strategies. Miller, Brody, and Summerton (1988) found that high monitors came to physicians with less severe medical problems than blunters but they reported the same amount of distress and dysfunction and requested more tests, information, and counseling. However, Davey, Tallis, and Hodgsen (1993) found blunters were less likely to respond to illness cues and therefore reported more symptoms related to opportunistic infections than monitors.

Negative Coping Influences

The association between pessimistic explanatory style and illness suggests that individuals who explain negative life events in terms of internal, stable, and global causes are less likely to take steps to combat illness than those with a more optimistic explanatory style (Lin & Peterson, 1990). Individuals with a pervading negative mood (i.e., negative affectivity) are more likely to experience alcoholism, depression, and suicidal behavior.

Type A behavior pattern (TABP) is known to be a risk factor for cardiovascular heart disease among white male populations (Rosenman, 1993). Competitive drive, impatience, and potential for hostility appear to be the most important predictive coronary-prone type A behaviors (Rosenman, 1993). Another behavioral pattern, known as John Henryism, has been shown to measure different characteristics than TABP (Weinrich, Weinrich, Keil, Gazes, & Potter, 1988). John Henryism is a coping strategy characterizing individuals as hard-working and using vigorous efforts to overcome obstacles. John Henryism has been implicated in studies of low SES African Americans to explain the higher prevalence of hypertension among African Americans (James, 1994). Although John Henryism is not yet a generalizable concept, study results have supported the theory that high-job-status blacks and white women also may be more susceptible to stress-related illness due to the use of active coping strategies measured by the John Henry Scale (Light *et al.*, 1995).

Coping and Amelioration or Exacerbation of Medical Conditions

Recovery from cardiac bypass surgery among optimists has been found to be associated with several positive outcomes including more activity immediately following postsurgical period, faster normalization of lives after discharge, and reports of less angina pain at 5-year follow-up when compared to pessimists (Scheier *et al.*, 1989). A study of adjustment to early breast cancer showed that pessimism about one's life increases a woman's risk for adverse psychological reactions to the diagnosis of and treatment for breast cancer (Carver *et al.*, 1993; Pozo *et al.*, 1990).

Hardy insulin-dependent diabetic patients have been shown to have increased psychosocial adaptation to chronic illness (Pollack, 1986). Hardy individuals with acquired immunodeficiency syndrome (AIDS) were more likely to have engaged in spiritual activities (prayer and meditation), exercised more often, and used special diets more often than nonhardy individuals with AIDS (Carson, 1993).

Studies of avoidance strategies, such as denial, have shown both positive and negative effects on chronic disease outcomes. For example, myocardial patients with high denial spent fewer days in the hospital; but at year-one follow-up, the high-denial group displayed poorer adaptation to disease, were less adherent, and required more days of rehospitalization (Levine *et al.*, 1987).

Perceptions of control have been found to improve adjustment to breast cancer (Taylor, Lichtman, & Wood, 1984), myocardial infarction (Michela, 1986), coronary bypass surgery (Mahler & Kulik, 1990), and AIDS (Taylor, Helgeson, & Reed, 1991). Feelings of personal control over symptoms, disease, medical care, or other aspects of life have been shown to increase health outcomes and relieve distress even when prognosis is not good (Taylor *et al.*, 1991).

In a study of control and depression among both HIV-positive and HIV-negative gay males, having symptoms of HIV disease explained only a small percentage of the variance in depressive mood. Instead, control-related coping efforts such as planful problem solving, seeking advice–information, and reappraising the situation in a positive light mediate the relationship between stress and depressive mood among HIV-infected gay males (Folkman, Chesney, Pollack, & Coates, 1993).

Social Support

Conceptualization and Measurement of Social Support

Social support may be conceptualized broadly as a social transaction between two or more individuals where either the "recipient" or the "donor" perceives the exchange to be supportive. Social support has been conceptualized in a variety of ways, including the presence or absence of a confidante or intimate partner, the nature of their social connections (e.g., size and density of an individual's social network), and the degree to which a person is integrated in society. Measures of social support have also varied according to conceptualization and study design. Table 3 provides an outline of some of the conceptualizations of social support and some of its more well-known measures.

Social support is perhaps best understood as a meta-construct, consisting of various subconstructs (Vaux, 1988; Wortman, 1984). Some of the more persistent and empirically observed subconstructs include: (1) emotional support, or the demonstrations of love, caring, esteem, sympathy, and group belonging; (2) instrumental support, or actions, materials, goods, or services provided to an individual; (3) informational support, such as advice, personal feedback and information that might make an individual's life circumstances easier; and (4) appraisal support, or information from others relevant to self-evaluation, or an individual's ability to interpret their situation (Cobb, 1976; House, 1981; Thoits, 1986; Dunkel-Schetter, Folkman, & Lazarus, 1987).

Social support and its subconstructs have been defined as support an individual actually receives. This is known as available, actual, or received support and may be related to any of the four subconstructs outlined above. Research on an individual's perception that support is available if it is needed, or perceived support, has also been studied. Studies show that perceived support is a stronger predictor of health outcomes than reported received support (Sarason, Sarason, & Shearin, 1986).

The effect of social support on health outcomes has largely been conceptualized as main effect of support and support producing a stress-buffering effect. These two positions address whether social support improves health outcomes independent of other stressors, or whether it interacts to increase (or decrease) susceptibility to poor health outcomes only in the presence of increased stress (Cohen, 1991).

The main effect hypothesis suggests that social support is beneficial to an individual's health and well-being overall. The protective quality of social support is hypothesized to function in many ways (Cohen, 1991). First, social support may facilitate health-promoting behaviors in an individual, encouraging them to take better care of themselves either by providing them with information regarding how to lead healthier lives or by applying social pressures on them to engage in health promoting behaviors. Individuals with adequate social support may be more likely to engage in health promoting behaviors and less likely to develop some health problems. Second, social support may cause positive changes in an individual's psychological states, such as affect, control, and self-esteem, which in turn influence their neuroendocrine response. Third, social support, particularly instrumental support, may prevent disease by providing material aid, such as food, clothing, and housing. Finally, social support may influence health by providing warnings and information that help persons avoid stress (Cohen, 1991).

Table 3. Social Support Constructs and Instruments

Construct	Definition	Instrument
Type		
Tangible social support	The instrumental, practical social support that one receives (Cohen & Willis, 1985)	The Interpersonal Subscale Evaluation List (ISEL) (Cohen & Willis, 1985) The Social Support Inventory of People with AIDS (SSIPWA), (Friedland, *et al.*, Renwick, & McColl, 1996) "Close Persons" Questionnaire (Rael 1995) The Social Support Receipt Scale (Dunkel-Schetter *et al.*, 1987)
Appraisal social support	The informational social support that one receives (Cohen & Willis, 1985)	The Interpersonal Subscale Evaluation List (ISEL) (Cohen and Willis, 1985) The Social Support Inventory of People with AIDS (SSIPWA), (Friedland *et al.*, 1996) The Social Support Receipt Scale (Dunkel-Schetter *et al.*, 1987)
Belonging social support	Support that gives a sense of identification and belonging (Cohen & Willis, 1985)	The Interpersonal Subscale Evaluation List (ISEL) (Cohen & Willis, 1985)
Self-esteem social support	Support that increases–decreases self-esteem and self-worth (Cohen & Willis, 1985)	The Interpersonal Subscale Evaluation List (ISEL) (Cohen & Willis, 1985)
Emotional social support	Warmth and nurturance provided by others, reassurance that the person is a valuable individual who is cared for by others (Dunkel-Schetter, Folkman, & Lazarus, 1987)	The Social Support Inventory of People with AIDS (SSIPWA) (Friedland *et al.*, 1996) "Close Persons" Questionnaire (Rael *et al.*, 1995) The Social Support Receipt Scale (Dunkel-Schetter *et al.*, 1987)
Global social support	Six components: attachment, social integration, reassurance of worth, guidance, reliable alliance, and opportunity for nuturance. These are assessed within social provisions in the individual's network (Cutrona & Russel, 1987)	Social Provisions Scale (Cutrona & Russel, 1987)
Domain-specific social support	Six components: attachment, social integration, reassurance of worth, guidance, reliable alliance, and opportunity for nurturance. These are assessed within specific social domains (e.g., friends, romantic partner, faculty advisor) (Davis, Morris, & Kraus, 1987)	Social Provisions Checklist (Davis *et al.*, 1987)
Available social support	Measures perceived availability of social support (Sarason *et al.*, 1987)	Social Support Questionnaire Satisfaction Scale (Sarason *et al.*, 1987) Perceived Available Social Support Scale (Pierce, Sarason, & Sarason, 1991)
Spiritual support	Social support felt by a relationship with a God, or participation in a religion (Maton, 1989)	Spiritual Support Scale (Maton, 1989)

(continued)

Table 3. (Continued)

Construct	Definition	Instrument
Source		
Partner social support	Three components: partner, partner interest, partner satisfaction (Locke & Wallace, 1959)	Partner Social Support Scale (Locke & Wallace, 1959)
Friend social support	Social support provided by friends (Procidano & Heller, 1983)	Parent Support and Friend Support Scales (Procidano & Heller, 1983)
		The Social Support Scale for Children (People in My Life) (Harter, 1975)
		The Social Support Appraisals Scale (Dubow & Ullman, 1989)
		The Social Support Receipt Scale (Dunkel-Schetter et al., 1987)
		Perceived Available Social Support Scale (Pierce et al., 1991)
		The Social Support Scale (Belle, 1982)
Parent–family social support	Social support provided by parents and family (Procidano & Heller, 1983)	Parent Support and Friend Support Scales (Procidano & Heller, 1983)
		The Social Support Scale for Children (People in My Life) (Harter, 1975)
		The Social Support Appraisals Scale (Dubow & Ullman, 1989)
		The Social Support Receipt Scale (Dunkel-Schetter et al., 1987)
		Perceived Available Social Support Scale (Pierce et al., 1991)
		The Social Support Scale (Belle, 1982)
Neighbor social support	Social support provided by those who live in close proximity.	
Teacher–classmate social support	Social support provided by teachers and classmates (Procidano & Heller, 1983)	Parent Support and Friend Support Scales (Procidano & Heller, 1983)
		The Social Support Appraisals Scale (Dubow & Ullman, 1989)
		The Social Support Receipt Scale (Dunkel-Schetter et al., 1987)
Network		
Degree of social support	Network size, the number of individuals providing child rearing assistance, the density of the network, and the average number of interactions with individuals outside the home (Wahler & Dumas, 1984)	Community Interaction Checklist (CIC) (Wahler & Dumas, 1984)
		Social Support Questionnaire (Sarason et al., 1983)
Social interaction	Four aspects: material and emotional exchange, quantitative and morphological features of the overall network, characteristics of a network member, and environmental influence (Cohen, Terisi, & Holmes, 1985)	Network Analysis Profile (Cohen et al., 1985)
Social satisfaction	Degree of satisfaction with social support received (Sarason, Levine, Basham, & Sarason, 1983)	Social Support Questionnaire (Sarason et al., 1983)
Communication competence	Degree to which one can derive support from communication within a network (Wienmann, 1977)	Communication Competence Scale (Wienmann, 1977)

Rather than contributing directly to health outcomes, the stress-buffering hypothesis suggests that social support buffers the effect of stress on an individual, positively influencing their health and well-being. Whereas stressors put one at risk for disease, individuals who perceive themselves to have sufficient social support may be protected from the negative effects from stress and therefore may be less likely to develop health problems related to stress (Wortman, 1984). Social support also may be reconceptualized as coping assistance in that it may provide information on how threatening an event actually is, thus (1) aiding in an individual's coping process, (2) discouraging maladaptive coping styles or (3) leading to the disengagement of a stress-triggered biological process (Cohen, 1991; Cohen & Willis, 1985).

Similarities between social support and coping may be observed between problem-focused coping and instrumental support, emotion-focused coping and emotional support, and perception-focused coping and informational support (Thoits, 1986). Social support and coping may interact to buffer the effects of stress. A person's coping response is facilitated by their (perceived) social support. This may occur by supportive others assisting the person to (1) change the situation, (2) the meaning of the situation, or (3) the individual's emotional reaction to the situation (Thoits, 1986).

Social Support and Demographic Characteristics

The amounts of support available and its effects may vary according to individual demographic characteristics such as sex, age, and ethnicity (Dunkel-Schetter *et al.*, 1987; see also Maton, Teti, Corns, & Vieira-Baker, 1996). More specifically, according to Turner and Marino (1994), women experience substantially higher levels of social support than do men; married individuals report more support than their nonmarried counterparts; higher occupational prestige level (used to estimate SES) is associated with higher levels of social support; and age revealed a convex relationship with the lowest levels of support found among 18 to 25-year-olds, and the highest levels were observed between 35 and 45 years of age. According to Lieberman (1982), the key factors that distinguish those who do and do not seek help are age and race. Seeking social support declines with age and is more prevalent among whites than blacks. In general, help seekers are characterized as young, white, educated, middle-class, and female.

Social Support and Health Risks

According to Berkman (1995), no other risk factor has gained attention as quickly as social support. Most of the early conclusions regarding social support and health outcomes were based on correlational data collected at a single time point, establishing a negative relationship between various forms of social support and a variety of individual health outcomes such as low birth weight, death, arthritis, tuberculosis, depression, and substance abuse (Wortman, 1984; Rook, 1984; Cobb, 1976).

Other studies, combining prospective data collection and quasi-experimental conditions, revealed similar findings. One of the more well-known prospective studies, the Alameda County, California, study revealed that healthy individuals with better social integration lived longer than their less socially integrated counterparts (Berkman & Syme, 1979). These findings have been supported in other prospective community health studies (House, Robbins, & Metzner, 1982; Blazer, 1982). Cohen and Willis (1985) found that high social support in the presence of high stress predicted long-term maintenance among ex-smokers and was most important during quitting and early maintenance stages. In addition, studies on social support and pregnancy outcome have consistently observed a relationship between high social support and fewer pregnancy complications (Sosa, Kennell, Klaus, Robertson, & Urrutia, 1980; Nuckolls, Cassel, & Kaplan, 1972).

Social Support and Amelioration or Exacerbation of Medical Conditions

Social support also affects the morbidity and mortality of individuals who are already ill. Higher levels of social support are associated with a reduction in the amount of medication required, accelerated recovery, and improved compliance with prescribed medical regimens (Cobb, 1976). High social support has been demonstrated to have a positive effect on recovery from cancer (Wortman, 1984). Low social support has been associated with increased mortality risk for individuals who have had a myocardial infarction (Ruberman et al., 1984; Williams et al., 1992).

It is uncertain whether or not a less favorable prognosis deters social support, or whether those with low social support have less favorable prognoses. For example, individuals with greater psychological symptoms may have greater needs for support, and therefore may perceive less support to be available. Regardless, the relationship between high social support and improved health outcomes of chronic illness is evident.

While it has been overwhelmingly observed that higher levels of social support produce positive outcomes, some evidence has emerged documenting negative consequences of well-intentioned support (Wortman, 1984). This primarily occurs when the type of support offered (e.g., emotional, informational, instrumental, appraisal) is not matched to the needs of the individual.

Treatment Interventions

Intervention strategies designed to alter the relationship between stress and illness employ a variety of approaches including behavioral strategies that directly reduce physiological arousal to stress (e.g., exercise, biofeedback, relaxation training), cognitive-based strategies that augment one's coping repertoire (e.g., cognitive therapy), or altering the person's environment by increasing social support. This section will briefly present representative intervention techniques, along with relevant empirical evidence, within each of these treatment strategy domains.

Stress-Based Interventions

One stress management technique shown to be effective in managing acute and chronic illness by reducing physiological arousal is biofeedback-assisted therapy. In this type of treatment intervention, the patient learns how to monitor and control some aspect of their physiological reaction to stress (e.g., heart rate). As with many stress management programs, biofeedback is combined with some form of relaxation training. This treatment combination has been shown to prevent the development of heart disease in high-risk individuals (Patel, Marmot, & Terry, 1981). An 8–week work site treatment program found that workers who received biofeedback and relaxation training displayed a significantly greater reduction in systolic and diastolic blood pressure than a control group who received health education material and standard medical treatment only. More importantly, these group differences persisted at 4 years follow-up and more subjects in the control versus the treatment group reported having angina and treatment for hypertension. Bradley *et al.* (1987) applied biofeedback and relaxation to patients with rheumatoid arthritis and found that it produced significant reductions in pain and disease activity indices, relative to attention–placebo and no adjunct treatment control conditions. Finally, another study applied this treatment combination to patients who were HIV positive but asymptomatic and found an overall significant improvement in emotional and health status posttreatment (i.e., significant increase in T-cell count, a measure of immune system functioning) (Taylor, 1995). These effects did not persist at 1–month follow-up, however, perhaps due to the reported poor compliance in self-practice of the techniques by the study patients. The latter results highlight the importance of patient motivation in the successful application of stress management interventions as well as the need to make the treatment effects generalizable to the patient's everyday life.

Another type of intervention, stress inoculation training (SIT), combines a range of techniques in an effort to provide successful response alternatives to future episodes of stress (Meichenbaum, 1993). Using the SIT paradigm, the individual is first taught to recognize the transactional nature between stress and illness symptoms as manifested in their daily life. Next, specific coping strategies are taught that reduce the effects of stress on the individual's symptoms. These strategies might be cognitive, behavioral, or environmentally based. Finally, after sufficient rehearsal in therapy, the individual is encouraged to use and integrate the strategies *in vivo*, that is, in their everyday experience. This gradual approach of teaching and implementing techniques is intended to "inoculate" the individual against the adverse effects of future stressful life episodes and has been successfully applied to a wide variety of patient populations (see Meichenbaum, 1993, for review).

Coping Interventions

Cognitive effectiveness training (CET) was developed from research demonstrating the importance of the match between a situation's amenability to change and the coping efforts utilized. CET incorporates cognitive–behavioral stress management techniques with added components that teach individuals to identify whether stressors are controllable or not and then encourages the selection of problem-focused efforts in changeable situations and emotion-focused efforts in less changeable situations. Preliminary findings with CET demonstrate that HIV-infected homosexual men receiving CET show greater increases in coping efficacy and less perceived stress and burnout than those in control conditions (Chesney, Folkman, & Chambers, 1996).

A self-efficacy enhanced self-management intervention was developed for patients with arthritis following results from earlier interventions that found that individuals who improved were those who had a positive outlook and felt a greater sense of control. The incorporation of new behaviors to relieve pain, or greater disease knowledge, was not strongly associated with improved health status. However, an individual's self-efficacy belief or confidence in their ability to control or change arthritis symptoms predicted enhanced health status. Subsequent interventions including more self-efficacy-related components showed significant improvements in symptoms and were cost-effectiveness (Lorig & Holman, 1993).

Within the health care field, information on patient and family coping styles has been found useful for teaching nurses better ways to care for patients and their families (Martin, 1995). Also, psychoeducational interventions that improve communication between hospital staff and patients and increase control for patients during and after major and minor surgical procedures have proven effective in reducing psychological distress and length of hospital stays (Devine, 1992). In addition, therapeutic touch, a hands-on healing technique used by nurses, has been found to be beneficial in helping patients cope with pain and stress during hospitalization (Heidt, 1981, 1991; Kramer, 1990; Meehan, 1991). The use of therapeutic touch within the medical setting is paralleled by the growing trend in society toward the use of complementary therapies, such as massage, as stress relieving, coping aids (Eisenberg *et al.*, 1993).

Social Support Interventions

Both individual- and community-level interventions have been designed to improve social support. Interventions may have a primary prevention focus, with social support attempting to influence health behavior change for healthier lifestyles to avoid illness and distress, or a secondary prevention emphasis, which may aim to avoid negative consequences of low social support on individuals already ill. These applications are consistent with well-known behavior change theories that include a role for social support on both an individual and societal or community level (Bandura, 1982).

According to Berkman (1995), interventions on social support may be more effective if they focus on increasing or improving existing, informal social support resources for individuals. However, support groups, or formalized systems of social support, have grown in popularity over the past decade. Many interventions involving social support also have centered on social support as a mechanism of coping. In particular, coping effectiveness training (Folkman *et al.*, 1993) has incorporated social support training as an important component. In this context, social support is not conceptualized as perceived support, but rather as coping assistance with appraisal. Using appraisal coping and social support encourages individuals to seek a match between their needs and their support resources. This approach attempts to avoid problems associated with inappropriate support discussed earlier.

Summary and Future Directions

In the past 25 years, an enormous amount of research has provided evidence for a link between stress and illness in a variety of general populations and specific patient populations. This chapter began with a review of the many ways in which stress can impact health behavior practices as well as the development and exacerbation of disease. We also have described some of the evidence showing interventions that can alter the impact that stress has on an individual's physical and emotional status.

Further progress in our understanding of the relationship between stress and health depends on clarification of several areas. For example, very little attention has been given to determining the health-related consequences of acute versus chronic stress(ors). These differences may require different intervention designs. A need also exists to further elucidate the unique relationships that occur between individuals' environmental, physiological, and psychological states that result in adverse health effects.

Coping efforts, strategies, and personal resources hold much potential for influencing health practices and increasing positive health outcomes within the public and private health arenas. Lazarus and Folkman's research findings suggest that coping is a powerful mediator of an individual's emotional state throughout a stressful event (Folkman & Lazarus, 1988a). The cognitive–motivation–relational theory of emotion proposed by Lazaurus, (1993b) posits that analysis of the changing emotional outcomes during a stressful event will provide richer information into the utility of coping efforts. Thoits (1995) found that individuals who are flexible in their choice of coping efforts show better adaptation. This suggests the need for developing indexes to assess the versatility or flexibility of coping responses and subsequent health outcomes.

Already, personal growth gained through confronting a stressor has been cited as an important new addition to coping theory, as many people experience improved coping abilities as a function of successfully dealing with stressors. Resiliency, wisdom, tolerance, and increased empathy are a few qualities that have been found to develop through coping with stressful encounters (Moos, 1992). Recent research on meaning of illness as a separate construct has shown important consequences for patients dealing with chronic illness (Lipowski, 1985; Fife, 1995). Finally, religious, spiritual, and financial coping resources also are being researched as important determinants of coping outcomes (Thoits, 1995; Carson, 1993; Mickley, Carson, & Soeken, 1995).

In an age where emphasis is being placed on preventive medicine and where we are experiencing a shift toward managed care strategies for health care delivery, psychosocial interventions that utilize coping research findings have an important role to play in disease prevention and in improving quality of life. In addition, the influence of social support on utilization of health care facilities and health care costs has been explored. Researchers have discovered that low social support may encourage high medical care utilization rates. Specifically, older individuals experiencing psychological distress and low social support may seek medical care for physical symptoms more often than individuals with high social support (Pilisuk, Boylan, & Acredolo, 1987; Counte & Glandon, 1991). These data suggest that interventions aimed at increasing social support may be a cost-saving mechanism for managed care. The necessity for studying transactions between person and environment continue to underscore the importance of integrating knowledge of stress, coping, and social support in efforts to understand the holistic experience of the person's health, illness, and well-being.

References

Adler, N. E., Boyce, T., Chesney, M. A., Cohen, S., Folkman, S., Kahn R. L., & Syme S. L. (1994). Socioeconomic status and health. The challenge of the gradient. *American Psychologist, 49,* 15–24.

Affleck, G., Tennen, H., Urrows, S., & Higgins, P. (1994). Person and contextual features of daily stress reactivity: Individual differences in relations of undesirable daily events with mood disturbance and chronic pain intensity. *Journal of Personality and Social Psychology, 66,* 329–340.

Antonvsky, A. (1993). The structure and properties of the sense of coherence scale. *Social Science Medicine, 36,* 725–733.

Aspinwall, L. G., & Taylor, S. E. (1997). A stitch in time: Self-regulation and proactive coping. *Psychological Bulletin, 112*, 417–436.

Bandura, A. (1977). Self-efficacy: Toward a unifying theory of behavioral change. *Psychological Review, 84*, 191–215.

Bandura, A. (1982). Self-efficacy mechanism in human agency. *American Psychologist, 37*, 122–147.

Barnett, R. C. (1993). Multiple roles, gender, and psychological distress. In L. Goldberger & S. Breznitz (Eds.), *Handbook of stress: Theoretical and clinical aspects* (2nd ed., pp. 427–445). New York: Free Press.

Beck, A. T., Ward, C. H., Mendelson, M., Mock, J., & Erbaugh, J. (1961). An inventory for measuring depression. *Archives of General Psychiatry, 56*, 53–63.

Belle, D. (1982). Social ties and social support. In D. Belle (Ed.), *Lives in stress: Women and depression* (pp. 133–144). Thousand Oaks, CA: Sage.

Berkman, L.F. (1995). The role of social relations in health promotion. *Psychosomatic Medicine, 57*, 245–254.

Berkman, L. F., & Syme, S. L. (1979). Social networks, host resistance, and mortality: A nine-year follow-up study of Alameda County residents. *American Journal of Epidemiology, 109*, 186–204.

Blazer, D. G. (1982). Social support and mortality in an elderly community population. *American Journal of Epidemiology, 115*, 684–694.

Bortner, R. W. (1969). A short rating scale as a potential measure of pattern A behavior. *Journal of Chronic Diseases, 22*, 87–91.

Boyce, W. T., Chesney, M., Alkon, A., Tschann, J. M., Adams, S., Chesterman, B., Cohen, F., Kaiser, P., Folkman, S., & Wara, D. (1995). Psychobiologic reactivity to stress and childhood respiratory illnesses: Results of two prospective studies. *Psychosomatic Medicine, 57*, 411–422.

Bradley, L. A., Young, L. D., Anderson, K. O., Turner, R. A., Agudelo, C. A., McDaniel, L. K., Pisko, E. J., Semble, E. L., & Morgan, T. M. (1987). Effects of psychological therapy on pain or behavior of rheumatoid arthritis patients: Treatment outcome and six month follow-up. *Arthritis and Rheumatism, 30*, 1105–1114.

Bresnahan, K., Zuckerman, B., & Cabral, H. (1992). Psychosocial correlates of drug and heavy alcohol use among pregnant women at risk for drug use. *Obstetrics and Gynecology, 80*, 976–980.

Brody, D. S. (1980). Psychological distress and hypertension control. *Journal of Human Stress, 6*, 2–6.

Caldwell, J. R., Theisen, V., Kaunisto, C. A., Reddy, P. J., Smythe, P. S., & Smith, D. W. (1983). Psychosocial factors influence control of moderate and severe hypertension. *Social Science and Medicine, 17*, 773–782.

Carson, V. B. (1993). Prayer, meditation, exercise, and special diets: behaviors of the hardy person with HIV/AIDS. *Journal of American Nursing and AIDS Care, 4*, 18–28.

Carver, C., Scheier, M., & Weintaub, J. (1989). Assessing coping strategies: A theoretically based approach. *Journal of Personality and Social Psychology, 15*, 267–283.

Carver, C. S., Pozo, C., Harris, S. D., Noriega, V., Scheier, M. F., Robinson, D. S., Ketcham, A. S., Moffat, F. L., Jr., & Clark, K. C. (1993). How coping mediates the effect of optimism on distress: A study of women with early stage breast cancer. *Journal of Personality and Social Psychology, 65*, 375– 390.

Chen, C. C., David, A. S., Nunnerley, H., Michell, M., Dawson, J. L., Berry, H., Dobbs, J., & Fahy, T. (1995). Adverse life events and breast cancer: Case-control study. *British Medical Journal, 311*, 1527–1530.

Chesney, M., Folkman, S., & Chambers, D. (1996). Coping effectiveness training for men living with HIV: Preliminary findings. *International Journal of STD and AIDS*.

Clark, L. F. (1994). Social cognition and health psychology. In R. S. Wyer & T. K. Srull (Eds.), *Handbook of social cognition* (vol. 2, pp. 239–288). Hillsdale, NJ: Erlbaum.

Cobb, S. (1976). Social support as a moderator of stress. *Psychosomatic Medicine, 38*, 10–14.

Cohen, C., Terisi, J., & Holmes, D. (1985). Social networks, stress, and physical health: A longitudinal study of an inner-city elderly population. *Journal of Gerentology, 40*, 478–486.

Cohen, S. (1991). Social supports and physical health: Symptoms, health behaviors, and infectious disease. In E. M. Cummings, A. L. Greene, & K. H. Karraker (Eds.), *Life span developmental psychology: Perspectives on stress and coping* (pp. 213–234). Hillsdale, NJ: Erlbaum.

Cohen, S., & Williamson, G. M. (1991). Stress and infectious disease in humans. *Psychological Bulletin, 109*, 5–24.

Cohen, S., & Willis, T.A. (1985). Stress, social support and the buffering hypothesis. *Psychological Bulletin, 5*, 310–357.

Cohen S., Karmack, T., & Mermelstein, R. (1983). A global measure of perceived stress. *Journal of Health and Social Behavior, 24*, 385–396.

Collins, D. L., Baum, A., & Singer, J. E. (1983). Coping with chronic stress at Three Mile Island: Psychological and biochemical evidence. *Health Psychology, 2*, 149–166.

Costa, P. T., & McCrae, R. R. (1993). Psychological stress and coping in old age. In L. Goldberger & S. Breznitz (Eds.), *Handbook of stress, theoretical and clinical aspects*, (2nd ed., pp. 403–412). New York: Free Press.

Counte, M. A., & Glandon, G. L. (1991). A panel study of life stress, social support, and the health services utilization of older persons. *Medical Care, 29,* 348–361.

Crowe, K., & Von Baeyer, C. (1989). Predictors of a positive childbirth experience. *Birth, 16,* 59–63.

Cutrona, C. E., & Russel, D. (1987). The provisions of social relationships and adaptation to stress. *Advances in Personal Relationships, 1,* 37–87.

Davey, G. C., Tallis, F., & Hodgsen, S. (1993). The relationship between information-seeking and information-avoiding coping styles and the reporting of psychological and physical symptoms. *Journal of Psychosomatic Research, 37,* 334–344.

DeLongis, A., Coyne, J. C., Dakof, G., Folkman, S., & Lazarus, R. S. (1982). Relationship of daily hassles, uplifts, and major life events to health status. *Health Psychology, 1,* 119–136.

DeLongis, A., Folkman, S., & Lazarus, R. S. (1988). The impact of daily stress on health and mood: Psychological and social resources as mediators. *Journal of Personality and SocialPsychology, 54,* 486–495.

Denollet, J., Sys, S. U., & Brutsaert, D. L. (1995). Personality and mortality after myocardial infarction. *Psychosomatic Medicine, 57,* 582–591.

Devine, E. C. (1992). Effects of psychoeducational care for adult surgical patients: A meta-analysis of 191 studies. *Patient Education Counselor, 19,* 129–142.

Dohrenwend, B. S., Krasnoff, A. R., Askenasy, A. R., & Dohrenwend, B. P. (1978). Exemplification of a method for scaling life events: The PERI Life Events Scale. *Journal of Health and Social Behavior, 19,* 205–229.

Dubow, E. F., & Ullman, D. G. (1989). Assessing social support in elementary school children: The survey of children's social support. *Journal of Clinical Child Psychology, 18,* 52–64.

Dunkel-Schetter, C., Folkman, S., & Lazarus, R. (1987). Correlates of social receipt. *Journal of Personality and Social Psychology, 53,* 71–80.

Eisenberg, D. M., Kessler, R. C., Foster, C., Norlock, F. E., Calkins, D. R., & Delbanco, T. L. (1993). Unconventional medicine in the United States: Prevalence, costs, and patterns of use. *New England Journal of Medicine, 328,* 246–252.

Endler, N. S., & Parker, J. D. (1991). *Coping inventory for stressful situations manual.* Toronto: Multi-Health Systems.

Feifel, H., & Strack, S. (1989). Coping with conflict situations: Middle-aged and elderly men. *Psychology and Aging, 4,* 26–33.

Feifel, H., Strack, S., & Nagy, V. T. (1987). Degree of life threat and differential use of coping modes. *Journal of Psychosomatic Medicine, 31,* 91–99.

Fife, B. L. (1995). The measurement of meaning in illness. *Social Science and Medicine, 40,* 1021–1028.

Folkman, S. (1984). Personal control and stress and coping processes: A theoretical analysis. *Journal of Personality and Social Psychology, 46,* 839–852.

Folkman, S., & Lazarus, R. S. (1988a). The relationship between coping and emotion: Implication for theory and research. *Social Science and Medicine, 26,* 309–317.

Folkman, S., & Lazarus, R.S. (1988b). *Manual for the ways of coping questionnaire.* Palo Alto, CA: Consulting Psychologist.

Folkman S., Chesney, M., Pollack, L., & Coates, T. (1993). Stress, control, coping and depressive mood in human immunodefieciency virus-positive and -negative gay men in San Francisco. *Journal of Nervous and Mental Disease, 181,* 409–416.

Friedland, J., Renwick, R., & McColl, M. (1996). Coping and social support as determinants of quality of life in HIV/AIDS. *AIDS Care, 8,* 15–31.

Harter, S. (1975). *Manual for the social support scale for children.* Denver, CO: University of Denver.

Haynes, S. G., Levine, S., & Scotch, N. (1978). The relationship of psychosocial factors to coronary heart disease in the Framingham Study: I. Methods and risk factors. *American Journal of Epidemiology, 107,* 362–381.

Heidt, P. (1981). Effect of therapeutic touch on anxiety level of hospitalized patients. *Nursing Research, 30,* 33–37.

Heidt, P. (1991). Helping patients to rest: Clinical studies in therapeutic touch. *Holistic Nursing Practice, 5,* 57–66.

Holmes, T. H., & Rahe, R. H. (1967). The social readjustment scale. *The Journal of Psychometric Research, 11,* 213–218.

House, J. S. (1981). *Work, stress and social support*. Reading, MA: Addison Wesley.

House, J. S., Robbins, C., & Metzner, H. L. (1982). The association of social relationships and activities with morality: Prospective evidence from the Tecumseh community health survey. *American Journal of Epidemiology, 116*, 123–140.

James, S. A. (1994). John Henryism and the health of African Americans. *Culture , Medicine, and Psychiatry, 18*, 163–82.

James, S. A., Hartnett, S., & Kalsbeek, W. D. (1983). John Henryism and blood differences among black men. *Journal of Behavioral Medicine, 6*, 259–278.

Jenkins, C .D., Zyanski, S. J., & Rosenman, R. H. (1979). *The Jenkins activity survey*. New York: Psychological Corporation.

Jennings, B. M., & Staggers, N. (1994). A critical analysis of hardiness. *Nursing Research, 43*, 274–281.

Kiecolt-Glaser, J. K., Dura, J. R., Speicher, C. E., Trask, J., & Glaser, R. (1991). Spousal caregivers of dementia victims: Longitudinal changes in immunity and health. *Psychosomatic Medicine, 53*, 345–362.

Kohn, P. M., & MacDonald, J. E. (1992). The survey of recent life experiences: A decontaminated hassles scale for adults. *Journal of Behavioral Medicine, 15*, 221–236.

Kobasa, S. C. (1979). Stressful life events, personality and health: An inquiry into hardiness. *Journal of Personality and Social Psychology, 37*, 1–11.

Kramer, N. A. (1990). Comparison of therapeutic touch and casual touch in stress reduction of hospitalized children. *Pediatric Nursing, 16*, 483–485.

Lauver, D., & Chang, A. (1991). Testing theoretical explanations of intention to seek care for a breast cancer symptom. *Journal of Applied Social Psychology, 21*, 1440–1458.

Lazarus, R. S. (1993a). Coping theory and research: Past, present, and future. *Psychosomatic Medicine, 55*, 234–247.

Lazarus, R. S. (1993b). From psychological stress to the emotions: A history of changing outlooks. *Annual Review of Psychology, 44*, 1–21.

Levine, J., Warrenburg, S., Kerns, R., Schwartz, G., Delaney, R., Fontana, A., Gradman, A., Smith, S., Allen, S., & Cascione, R. (1987). The role of denial in recovery from coronary heart disease. *Psychosomatic Medicine, 49*, 109–117.

Lieberman, M. A. (1982). The effects of social supports on responses to stress. In L. Goldberger & S. Breznitz (Eds.), *Handbook of stress* (pp. 764–782). New York: Free Press.

Light, K., Obrist, P., Andrew, S., Jones, S., & Strogatz, D. (1987). Effects of race and marginally elevated blood pressure on responses to stress. *Hypertension, 10*, 555–563.

Light, K. C., Brownley, K. A., Turner, J. R., Hinderliter, A. L., Girdler, S. S., Sherwood, A., & Anderson, N. B. (1995). Job status and high-effort coping infleunce work blood pressure in women and blacks. *Hypertension, 25*, 554–559.

Lin, E. H., & Peterson, C. (1990). Pessimistic explanatory style and response to illness. *Behavioral Research Therapy, 28*, 243–248.

Lipowski, Z. (1985). Physical illness, the individual and the coping process. *International Journal of Psychiatry in Medicine, 1*, 91–102.

Lobel, M. (1994). Conceptualizations, measurement, and effects of prenatal maternal stress on birth outcomes. *Journal of Behavioral Medicine, 17*, 225–272.

Locke, H., & Wallace, K. (1959). Short marital adjustment and prediction tests: Their reliability and validity. *Marriage and Family Living, 21*, 251–255.

Lorig, K., & Holman, H. (1993). Arthritis self-management studies, a 12 year review. *Health Education Quaterly, 20*, 17–28.

Mahler, H. M., & Kulik, J. A. (1990). Preferences for health care involvement, perceived control and surgical recovery: A prospective study. *Social Science Medicine, 31*, 743–751.

Martin, S. D. (1995). Coping with chronic illness. *Home Health Care Nurse, 13*, 50–54.

Maton, K. I. (1989). The stress-buffering role of social support: Cross-sectional and prospective investigations. *Journal for Scientific Study of Religion, 28*, 310–323.

Maton, K. I., Teti, D. M., Corns, K. M., & Vieira-Baker, C. C. (1996). Cultural specificity of support sources, correlates and contexts: Three studies of African American and Caucasian youth. *American Journal of Community Psychology, 24*, 551–562.

Maxwell, C. J., & Hirdes, J. P. (1993). The prevalence of smoking and implications for quality of life among the community-based elderly. *American Journal of Preventive Medicine, 9*, 338–345.

McLeod, J. D., & Kessler, R. C. (1990). Socioeconomic status differences in vulnerability to undesirable life events. *Journal of Health and Social Behavior, 31*, 162–172.

Meehan, T. C. (1991). Therapeutic touch and postoperative pain: A Rogerian research study. *Nursing Science Quarterly, 6,* 69–78.

Meichenbaum, D. (1993). Stress inoculation training: A 20-year update. In D. Meichenbaum (Ed.), *Handbook of stress management* (pp. 373–406). New York: Guilford Press.

Michela, J. (1986). Interpersonal and individual impacts of a husband's heart attacks. In A. Baum & J. Singer (Eds.), *Handbook of psychology and health: vol. 5. Stress and coping* (pp. 255–301). Hillsdale, NJ: Erlbaum.

Mickley, J. R., Carson, V., & Soeken, K. L. (1995). Religion and adult mental health: State of the science in nursing. *Issues in Mental Health Nursing, 16,* 345–360.

Miller, S. M. (1981). Predictability and human stress: Toward a clarification of evidence and theory. In L. Berkowitz (Ed.), *Advances in experimental social psychology* (Vol. 14, pp. 203–256). New York: Academic Press.

Miller, S. M. (1987). Monitoring and blunting: Validation of a questionnaire to assess styles of information-seeking under threat. *Journal of Personality, 57,* 345–353.

Miller, S. M., Brody, D. S., & Summerton, J. (1988). Styles of coping with threat: Implications for health. *Journal of Personality and Social Psychology, 54,* 142–148.

Miller, T. Q., Markides, K. S., Chiriboga, D. A., & Ray, L. A. (1995). A test of the psychosocial vulnerability and health behavior models of hostility: Results from an 11-year follow-up study of Mexican Americans. *Psychosomatic Medicine, 57,* 572–581.

Moos, R. (1992). *Coping responses inventory manual.* Palo Alto, CA: Center for Health Care Evaluation, Department of Veteran Affairs and Stanford University Medical Centers.

Nuckolls, K. B., Cassel, J., & Kaplan, B. H. (1972). Physhological assets, life crises, and prognosis of pregnancy. *American Journal of Epidemiology, 95,* 431–441.

Patel, C., Marmot, M. G., & Terry, D. J. (1981). Controlled trial of biofeedback-aided behavioral methods in reducing mild hypertension. *British Medical Journal, 282,* 2005–2008.

Peterson, C., & Villanova, P. (1988). An expanded attributional style questionnaire. *Journal of Abnormal Psychology, 97,* 87–89.

Pierce, G., Sarason, I., & Sarason, B. (1991). General and relationship-based perceptions of social support: Are two constructs better than one? *Journal of Personality and Social Psychology, 61,* 1028–1039.

Pilisuk, M., Boylan, R., & Acredolo, C. (1987). Social support, life stress, and subsequent medical care utilization. *Health Psychology, 6,* 273–288.

Pollack, S. E. (1986). Human responses to chronic illness: Physiologic and psychosocial adaptation. *Nursing Research, 35,* 90–95.

Pozo, C., Carver, C. S., Noriega, V., Harris, S. D., Robinson, D. S., Ketcham, A. S., Legaspi, A., Moffat, F. L, Jr., & Clark, K. C. (1990). Effects of mastectomy versus lumpectomy on emotional adjustment to breast cancer: A prospective study of the first year postsurgery. *Journal of Oncology, 10,* 1292–1298.

Procidano, M. E., & Heller, K. (1983). Measures of perceived social support from friends and from family: Three validation studies. *American Journal of Community Psychology, 11,* 1–24.

Radloff, L. S. (1977). The CES-D scale: A self-report depression scale for research in the general population. *Applied Psychological Measurement, 1,* 385–401.

Rael, E. G. S., Stansfield, S. A., Shipley, M., Head, J., Feeney, A., & Marmot, M. (1995). Sickness absence in the Whitehall 2 study, London: The role of social support and material problems. *Journal of Epidemiology and Community Health, 49,* 474–481.

Robbins, A. S., Spence, J. T., & Clark, H. (1991). Psychological determinants of health and preformance: The tangled web of desirable and undesirable characteristics. *Journal of Personality and Social Psychology, 61,* 755–765.

Rook, K. S. (1984). The negative side of social interaction: Impact on psychological well-being. *Psychiatric Clinics of North America, 46,* 1097–1108.

Rose, R. M. (1984). Endocrine responses to stressful psychological events. *Psychiatric Clinics of North America, 3,* 251–276.

Rosenman, R. H. (1993). Relationship of the type A behavior pattern with coronary heart disease. In L. Goldberger & S. Breznitz (Eds.), *Handbook of stress, theoretical and clinical aspects,* (2nd ed., pp. 449–476). New York: Free Press.

Rosser, B. S., & Ross, M. W. (1989). A gay life events scale (GALES) for homosexual men. *Journal of Gay and Lesbian Psychotherapy, 1,* 87–101.

Rotter, J. B. (1966). Generalized expectancies for internal versus external control of reinforcement. *Psychological Monographs, 80,* (609).

Ruberman, W., Weinblatt, E., & Goldberg, J. D. (1984). Psychosocial influences on mortality after myocardial infarction. *New England Journal of Medicine, 311,* 552–559.

Sarason, I., Levine, H., Basham, R., & Sarason, B. (1983). Assessing social support: The social support questionnaire. *Journal of Personality and Social Psychology, 49,* 127–139.

Sarason, B. R., Sarason, I. G., & Shearin, E. N. (1986). Assessing the impact of life changes: Development of experiences survey. *Journal of Consulting and Clinical Psychology, 46,* 932–946.

Scheier, M. F., & Carver, C. S. (1985). Optimism, coping and health: Assessment and implications of generalized outcome expectancies. *Health Psychology, 4,* 219–247.

Scheier, M. F., Matthews, K. A., Owens, J. F., Magovern, G. J., Sr., Lefebvre, R. C., Abbott, R. A., & Carver, C. S. (1989). Dispositional optimism and recovery from coronary artery bypass surgery: The beneficial effects on physical and psychological well-being. *Journal of Personality and Social Psychology, 57,* 1024–1040.

Schneiderman, N., Antoni, M. H., Fletcher, M. A., Ironson, N. K., Kumar, M., & LaPerriere, A. (1993). Stress, endocrine responses, immunity and HIV-1 spectrum disease. In H. Friedman *et al.* (Eds.), *Drugs of abuse, immunity, and AIDS* (pp. 225–233). New York: Plenum Press.

Seeman, M., Seeman, A. Z., & Budros, A. (1988). Powerlessness, work, and community: A longitudinal study of alienation and alcohol use. *Journal of Health and Social Behavior, 29,* 185–198.

Solomon, K. E., & Annis, H. M. (1990). Outcome and efficacy expectancy in the prediction of postdrinking behavior. *British Journal of Addiction, 85,* 659–665.

Sosa, R., Kennell, J., Klaus, M., Robertson, S., & Urrutia, J. (1980). The effect of a supportive companion on perinatal problems, length of labor, and mother–infant interaction. *New England Journal of Medicine, 303,* 596–600.

Spangler, J. G., Konen, J. C., & McGann, K. P. (1993). Prevalence and predictors of problem drinking among primary care diabetic patients. *Journal of Family Practice, 37,* 370–375.

Spielberger, C. D. (1983). *Manual for the state–trait anxiety inventory.* Palo Alto, CA: Consulting Psychologists Press.

Stein, M., & Miller, A. H. (1993). Stress, the immune system, and health and illness. In L. Goldberger, and S. Breznitz (Eds.), *Handbook of stress: Theoretical and clinical aspects* (2nd ed., pp. 127–141). New York: Free Press.

Sullivan, G. C. (1993). Towards clarification of convergent concepts: Sense of coherence, will to meaning, locus of control, learned helplessness and hardiness. *Journal of Advanced Nursing, 18,* 1172–1778.

Suls, J., & Fletcher, B. (1985). The relative efficacy of avoidant and nonavoidant coping strategies: A meta-analysis. *Health Psychology, 4,* 249–288.

Taylor, S. E. (1995). *Health psychology.* New York: McGraw-Hill.

Taylor, S. E., Helgeson, V. S., & Reed, G. M. (1991). Self-generated feelings of control and adjustment to physical illness. *Journal of Social Issues, 47,* 91–109.

Taylor, S. E., Lichtman, R. R., & Wood, J. V. (1984). Attributions, beliefs about control, and adjustment to breast cancer. *Journal of Personality and Social Psychology, 46,* 489–502.

Thoits, P. A. (1986). Social support as coping assistance. *Journal of Consulting and Clinical Psychology, 54,* 416–423.

Thoits, P. A. (1991). On merging identity theory and stress research. *Social Psychology Quarterly, 54,* 101–112.

Thoits, P. A. (1995). Stress, coping, and social support processes: Where are we? What next? *Journal of Health and Social Behavior: Extra Issue,* 53–79.

Tofler, G. H., Stone, P. H., Maclure, M., Edelman, E., Davis, V. G., Robertson, T., Antman, E. M., & Muller, J. E. (1990). Analysis of possible triggers of acute myocardial infarction (The MILIS Study). *The American Journal of Cardiology, 66,* 22–27.

Turner, R. J., & Marino, F. (1994). Social support and social structure: A descriptive epidemiology. *Journal of Health and Social Behavior, 35,* 193–212.

Vaux, A. (1988). *Social support: Theory, research, and intervention.* New York: Praeger.

Verbruggee, L. M. (1983). Multiple roles and the physical health of women and men. *Journal of Health and Social Behavior, 24,* 16–30.

Wahler, R. G., & Dumas, J. E. (1984). Changing the observational coding styles of insular and noninsular mothers: A step towards maintenance of parent training effects. In R. F. Dangel & R. A. Polster (Eds.), *Parent training* (pp. 379–416). New York: Guilford Press.

Wallston, K. A., Wallston, B. S., & DeVellis, R. (1978). Development of the multidimensional health locus of control (MHLC) scale. *Health Education Monographs, 6,* 161–170.

Watson, D., & Clark, L. A. (1984). Negative affectivity: The disposition to experience aversive emotional states. *Psychological Bulletin, 96,* 234–254.

Watson, D., & Pennebaker, J. W. (1989). Health complaints, stress and distress: Exploring the central role of negative affectivity. *Psychological Review, 96,* 233–253.

Weinrich, S. P., Weinrich, M. C., Keil, J. E., Gazes, P. C., & Potter, E. (1988). The John Henryism and Framingham type A scales: Measurement properties in elderly blacks and whites. *American Journal of Epidemiology, 128,* 165–178.

Wienmann, J. M. (1977). Explication and a test of a model of communicative competence. *Human Communication Research, 3,* 195–213.

Williams, D. R., & Collins, C. (1995). Socioeconomic and racial differences in health. *Annual Review of Sociology, 21,* 349–386.

Williams, P. G., Wiebe, D. J., & Smith, T. W. (1992). Coping processes as mediators of the relationship between hardiness and health. *Journal of Behavioral Medicine, 15,* 237–255.

Wortman, C. (1984). Social support and the cancer patient. *Cancer, 53,* 2339–2362.

Zautra, A. J., Burleson, M. H., Matt, K. S., Roth, S., & Burrows, L. (1994). Interpersonal stress, depression, and disease activity in rheumatoid arthritis and osteoarthritis patients. *Health Psychology, 13,* 139–148.

PART *IV*

Behavior Change for Risk Reduction

CHAPTER 8

Tobacco Use Prevention and Cessation

Suzan E. Winders, Connie L. Kohler, Diane M. Grimley, and Eugene A. Gallagher

Introduction

Cigarette smoking is one of the country's most important public health problems (US DHHS, 1990). Approximately 400,000 US citizens die yearly from tobacco-related diseases, including cardiovascular disease, cancer, and obstructive lung disease (CDC, 1993). Tobacco is also responsible for increased disability from a variety of causes including chronic obstructive lung disease (Renwick & Connelly, 1996; Higgens *et al.*, 1993), cerebrovascular accidents (Shinton & Beevers, 1989), myocardial infarction (Seeman, Mendes de Leon, Berkman, & Ostfeld, 1993; Chun, Dobson, & Heller, 1993), amputations secondary to peripheral vascular disease (Eneroth & Persson, 1993), and blindness due to macular degeneration (Seddon, Willett, Speizer, & Hankinson, 1996). Collectively, Americans spend approximately $50 billion annually in medical costs related to the negative health consequences of tobacco addiction (CDC, 1994c). Moreover, the cost of lost productivity and earnings due to disability is estimated at $47 billion per year (Herdman, Hewitt & Laschober, 1993).

Despite the widely publicized health risks and financial costs associated with cigarette smoking, approximately one quarter of the adult population—about 50 million people—are regular smokers (CDC, 1994b). Furthermore, the number of new smokers has not decreased appreciably over the last decade. Despite continuing efforts of public health officials, approximately 3000 teenagers start smoking each day (Giovino *et al.*, 1995).

Suzan E. Winders • Behavioral Medicine Unit, Division of Preventive Medicine, Department of Medicine, School of Medicine, UAB Center for Health Promotion, University of Alabama at Birmingham, Birmingham, Alabama 35294.   *Connie L. Kohler, Diane M. Grimley, and Eugene A. Gallagher* • Department of Health Behavior, School of Public Health, UAB Center for Health Promotion, University of Alabama at Birmingham, Birmingham, Alabama 35294.

Handbook of Health Promotion and Disease Prevention, edited by Raczynski and DiClemente. Kluwer Academic/Plenum Publishers, New York, 1999.

Epidemiology

Cigarette Consumption Since 1900

The US Department of Agriculture (USDA) has tracked adult (persons age 18 and over) per capita consumption of manufactured cigarettes since 1900. According to the USDA, total per capita yearly consumption rose from 54 cigarettes per person per year in 1900 to 4345 cigarettes per person per year in 1963; since the release of the first Surgeon General's report in 1964 (US PHS, 1964), cigarette consumption has declined steadily; current levels 2493 cigarettes per person are roughly equivalent to those that occurred in 1942 (Giovino et al., 1994).

Cigarette Smoking Since 1965

In 1965, the Centers for Disease Control (CDC) began collecting data on adult tobacco use through the National Health Interview Survey (NHIS) (Giovino et al., 1994; CDC, 1994a,b). Data were stratified by sex, race (black, white, other), and education. Overall sample sizes have ranged from 10,342 in 1980 to 86,332 in 1966. Data have been adjusted for nonresponse and weighted to provide national estimates. According to their estimates, overall prevalence rates have declined steadily since the release of the first Surgeon General's report in 1964. Specifically, in 1965, an estimated 42% of US adults were current smokers (Giovino et al., 1994). In 1993, the prevalence of smoking among adults was 26% overall (CDC, 1994b).

Smoking Prevalence by Sex

Overall prevalence of smoking by men and women is presented in Fig. 1. As can be seen in Fig. 1, cigarette smoking has declined steadily since 1965 among both groups— from 52% in 1965 to 28% in 1993 among men and from 34% to 22% during the same period among women. As can also be seen from Fig. 1, the prevalence of cigarette smoking has always been greater among men compared to women. However, the gender gap has narrowed considerably in recent years. The "converging of the sexes" is generally attributed to gender differences in initiation and cessation trends (Giovino et al., 1995). Specifically, although males and female adolescents are currently about equally likely to smoke, the prevalence of daily cigarette smoking was consistently higher among girls compared to boys during the late 1970s and 1980s (Giovino et al., 1994). Second, although cessation rates have increased among both men and women, the prevalence of quitting since 1965 has been higher among men compared to women. For example, in 1991, 51.5% of male smokers had quit compared to 44.7% of female smokers (Giovino et al., 1994).

Smoking Prevalence by Race–Ethnic Group

The NHIS categorized race as black, white, or other from 1965 to 1978. In 1979, a Hispanic and non-Hispanic race category was added (Giovino et al., 1994). And finally, in 1991, the race category was expanded to include American Indians/Alaska Natives and Asian/Pacific Islanders (CDC, 1994a,b). In 1993, the prevalence of cigarette smoking among adults was highest for American Indians and Alaska Natives (39%), intermediate for blacks (26%) and whites (25%), and lowest for Hispanics (20%) and Asian

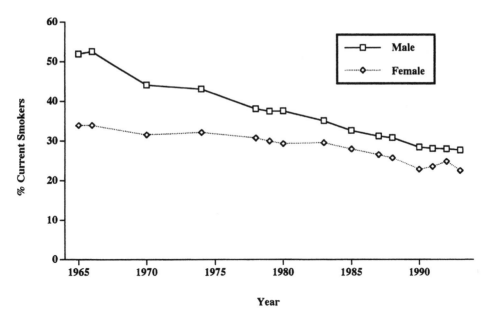

Figure 1. Trends in cigarette smoking by sex among adults 18 and over—United States, 1963–1993. *Source:* 1965–1993 National Health Interview Surveys (Giovino *et al.,* 1994; CDC, 1994b).

Americans/Pacific Islanders (18%) (CDC, 1994b). Until recently the prevalence of smoking has been higher comparing African Americans to their European-descended counterparts (Giovino *et al.,* 1994; CDC, 1994a,b) (see Fig. 2). Blacks are less likely than whites to have ever smoked (Giovino *et al.,* 1994), but are less likely to quit smoking (Giovino *et al.,* 1994; CDC 1994b). Thus, historically higher rates of smoking among African Americans appear to be related to a lower rate of cessation among this group. However, the prevalence of cigarette smoking among black adolescents has declined sharply since the 1970s, while the prevalence among white adolescents has remained relatively constant (US DHHS, 1994; Giovino *et al.,* 1994; CDC, 1994b). If this trend continues, smoking among whites will soon exceed the rates of blacks.

Smoking Prevalence by Education

The overall smoking prevalence rates by education is presented in Fig. 3. As can be seen in Fig. 3, the prevalence of smoking has decreased among all education groups. However, over time, the prevalence has declined most rapidly among persons with the most education. Lower smoking cessation rates among this group appear to be related to lower rates of initiation (Giovino *et al.,* 1995) and higher rates of cessation (Giovino *et al.,* 1994; CDC, 1994a).

Smoking Prevalence by Age

Smoking prevalence by age is presented in Fig. 4. As can be seen from Fig. 4, from 1965 to 1991, the prevalence of smoking has decreased among all age groups. The rate of decline has been greatest among younger (aged 18 to 44 years) persons (whose rates declined between 22 and 20.8%). Smoking prevalence is lowest among

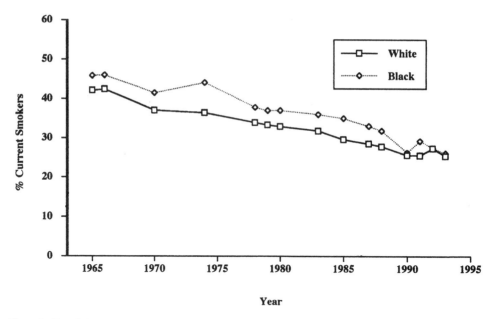

Figure 2. Trends in cigarette smoking by black and white race among adults 18 and over—United States, 1963–1993. *Source:* 1965–1993 National Health Interview Surveys (Giovino *et al.,* 1994; CDC, 1994b).

older individuals. This difference appears to be due to a higher rate of cessation among this group and the higher rates of mortality among older smokers compared to age-matched nonsmoking counterparts (Giovino *et al.,* 1995).

Associated Demographic Factors

In a recent review of trends in cigarette smoking (Giovino *et al.,* 1995), the following factors were found to be positively associated with higher prevalences of cigarette smoking: (1) living below the poverty line; (2) having a blue-collar job; (3) being an active duty military personnel; and (4) living in the southern United States. The lowest prevalence of smoking and greatest decline in smoking prevalence in the United States has occurred among physicians (Giovino *et al.,* 1995).

Health Behavior Models and Intervention Development

Tobacco use can be divided into three stages: acquisition, maintenance, and cessation. These stages can be further subdivided into various substages including thinking about trying tobacco, trying tobacco, experimenting with cigarettes, and so on. Several decades of research suggest that the factors that contribute to smoking behavior vary depending on what stage an individual is in. Therefore, current state-of-the-art interventions are generally stage-specific.

A wide variety of biological, psychological, and sociocultural factors contribute to the onset and maintenance of smoking behavior. It is generally assumed that smoking initiation and maintenance result from the interplay of these determinants. From

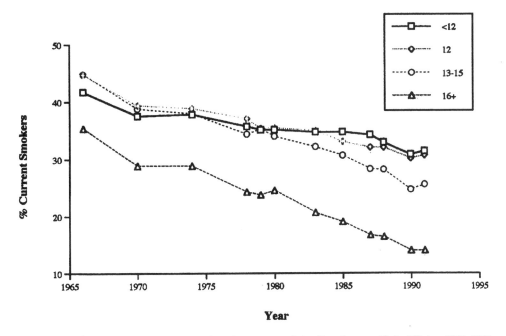

Figure 3. Trends in cigarette smoking by education among adults 18 and over—United States, 1966–1991. *Source:* 1965–1991 National Interview Surveys (Giovino *et al.*, 1994).

the preceding discussion, it is clear that tobacco use is a complex phenomenon that cannot be predicted from a simple formula. For this reason, theoretical models have been used to develop theories about the interrelationships among the determinants of smoking at each stage.

Tobacco control strategies can be divided into primary and secondary prevention interventions. Primary prevention interventions attempt to prevent individuals from becoming addicted. The vast majority of smokers start smoking in adolescence. Thus, primary prevention interventions tend to be school-based interventions targeting young children and adolescents. Applying a similar logic to the process of cessation, the majority of people who wish to quit smoking are adults. Thus, with few exceptions, secondary prevention interventions have targeted adults.

Early primary and secondary interventions relied more on common sense than empirically validated theories. As accumulating evidence called into question the efficacy of the early interventions, researchers began to incorporate concepts from newly developed theories about behavior and behavior change into their interventions. Thus, current approaches to prevent smoking onset and promote smoking cessation incorporate concepts from a variety of behavioral theories including the health belief model (Glanz, Lewis, & Rimer, 1997), theory of reasoned action (Glanz, Lewis, & Rimer, 1997), social cognitive theory (Bandura, 1982, 1986), and transtheoretical model (DiClemente, 1986; Prochaska & DiClemente, 1993; Prochaska *et al.*, 1992). Not surprisingly, decades of tobacco control research clearly demonstrates the superiority of theory-based smoking prevention interventions over nontheoretical interventions.

The purpose of this chapter is to review the psychosocial approaches to primary and secondary tobacco control that have been developed since the release of the first

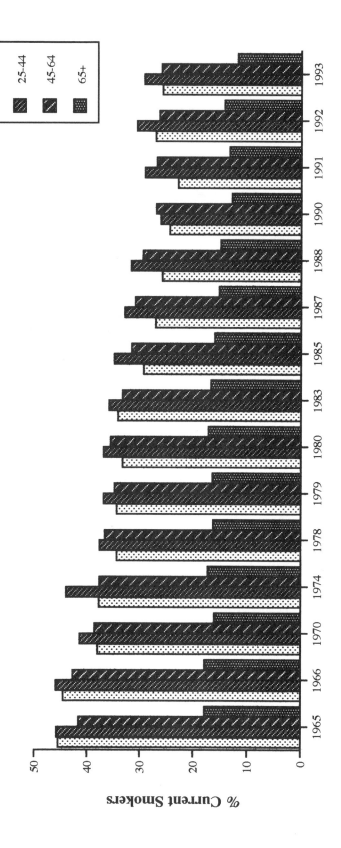

Figure 4. Trends in cigarette smoking by age among adults 18 and over—United States, 1963–1991. *Source:* 1965–1993 National Interview Surveys (Giovini *et al.*, 1994; CDC, 1994b).

Surgeon General's report in 1964. First, we will review the literature describing primary prevention approaches used with youth. Second, we will present the literature on interventions developed to promote cessation among adults. In reviewing the intervention literature, we will take a historical approach, emphasizing the influence of various models over time on the development of these interventions.

Primary Prevention

Preventing Youth Initiation

The majority of smokers report that they began smoking prior to graduation from high school. Therefore, most primary prevention efforts have centered on preventing children and adolescents from starting to smoke in the first place. Despite widespread knowledge among youth about the consequences of smoking (Crawford, Winders, & Kohler, 1996), approximately 3000 of them begin smoking each day (US DHHS, 1994). Based on current trends, it is estimated that 50% of these will go on to smoke for at least 16 to 20 years (Pierce & Gilpin, 1996) and 750 of them will eventually die from a tobacco-induced illness (Dawson & Henderson, 1987).

Stages of Smoking Initiation

Smoking acquisition among children and adolescents is thought to progress through five stages: preparation, trying, experimentation, regular use, and addiction (Flay, D'Avernas, Best, Kersell, & Ryan, 1983; Flay, 1993; Leventhal & Cleary, 1980; US DHHS, 1994). During the preparation phase, individuals form attitudes and beliefs about tobacco. During the second stage, individuals "try" smoking (i.e., smoke one to three cigarettes) to see if they like it. During the last phase prior to the adoption of regular smoking, smoking frequency increases in an unstable manner while the "experimenter" learns to smoke in new situations. During the regular smoking phase, the adolescent smokes on a regular basis (at least weekly). Addicted adolescents are physically dependent on nicotine as manifest by nicotine tolerance and the appearance of withdrawal symptoms (McNeill, West, Jarvis, Jackson, & Bryant, 1986). Smoking acquisition occurs over a period of from 1 to 3 years, prior to the onset of regular smoking (Leventhal, Fleming, & Glynn, 1988). Approximately 50% of all who experiment with cigarettes go on to become regular smokers within 1 year (McNeill, 1990).

Predictors of Initiation

The development of effective programs to prevent childhood smoking depends on the identification of reliable risk factors for adolescent smoking. Fortunately, a large number of longitudinal investigations since 1980 have examined a variety of predictors of smoking onset in children. Conrad, Flay, and Hill (1992) reviewed 27 longitudinal studies examining factors associated with the onset of smoking. Predictably, their review suggested that socioeconomic status was a strong predictor of smoking onset, with 76% of studies that used some measure of this variable showing a strong relationship between disadvantaged circumstances and smoking initiation.

Social bonding, particularly peer and school bonding, also emerged as a consistent predictor, with 60% of studies showing a relationship between this variable and smoking initiation. Social learning, especially from peers and older sibling, was also important, predicting smoking onset in 72% of studies. As expected, individual characteristics, especially rebelliousness and/or risk taking, and negative self-esteem were predictors of smoking initiation in multiple studies, while high self-efficacy to refuse offers to smoke was a strong predictor of abstinence in many studies. A number of other variables including locus of control, tolerence of deviance, alienation, curiosity, intelligence, constructiveness, personal efficacy, short time orientation, social helplessness, independence, and distress–stress have been examined, but too few data are available to draw firm conclusions. Affective beliefs were predictive of smoking in multiple studies, but negative attitudes and beliefs about smoking were only modest predictors of smoking onset. In contrast, intention to smoke was a powerful predictor, predicting use in 89% of studies that looked at it. Alcohol and other substance use were also predictive in multiple studies.

Early Prevention Interventions

Early approaches were based on the assumption that widespread dissemination of information about the health consequences associated with cigarette smoking would discourage nonsmoking adolescents from adopting the habit. Thus, the early approaches focused on educating school-aged youth about the short- and long-term health effects of smoking. Unfortunately, several decades of research examining the impact of various teaching approaches suggests that although educational programs can increase knowledge and favorably alter attitudes, they have little impact on actual smoking behavior (Thompson, 1978; Goodstadt, 1978; US DHHS, 1979). The reason for the failure of these approaches is thought to be twofold (Flay, 1993): (1) information is rarely sufficient to alter behavior (Flay et al., 1983; Leventhal & Cleary, 1980); and (2) information about long-term health consequences are not salient to youth, who focus on the present.

Early research suggested that children who smoked often had low self-esteem, were poor achievers, and had trouble making decisions. This led to the development of "affective" approaches (Flay, 1993). Programs based on the affective approach focused on self-esteem enhancement, values clarification, and decision making, but did not address tobacco or drug use per se (Durell & Bukoski, 1984; Goodstadt, 1978). Unfortunately, although these programs may have increased self-esteem, instilled values, and enhanced decision making, they had little impact on tobacco use (Hansen, Johnson, Flay, Graham, & Sobel, 1988; Tobler, 1986).

Current Prevention Interventions

Discovery of the various risk factors associated with smoking onset described above suggested that the process of becoming a smoker was complex. Various models from social psychology were used to generate hypotheses about the interrelation of these variables to account for smoking iniation and led to the development of a variety of classroom-based, psychosocial approaches to smoking prevention (Flay, 1993). The first intervention of this type (Evans, 1976) relied heavily on the social inoculation aspect of McGuire's (1969) persuasive communication model. The program was based on the belief that if adolescents were warned or inoculated against family, peer, and media pressure, they would be able to resist actual pressure. Subsequent interventions by Evans and his colleagues (Evans *et al.*, 1978, 1981) incorporated additional constructs from persuasive communication model (McGuire, 1969) and drew heavily on Bandura's (1977) social learning theory. Other approaches that have been used include Jessor and Jessor's (1977) multideterminant conceptual structure of problem behavior (Sherman *et al.*, 1982), attribution theory (Jones *et al.*, 1971), commitment theory (Kiesler, 1971), and Beck's (1976) cognitive–behavioral approach (Gilchrist, Schinke, & Blythe, 1979; Schinke & Blythe, 1981).

As summarized by Flay (1993), current psychosocial interventions typically include: (1) information on the consequences of tobacco use, with an emphasis on the short-term health and social consequences; (2) information on the prevalence of smoking among peers; (3) discussion of social influence from peers, family, and the media on tobacco use and ways to resist these influences; (4) modeling to show these influences and ways to cope with them; (5) role-playing and explicit learning and practice of behavioral skills; and (6) making a public commitment not to use tobacco (Flay, 1993). Some also include general self-esteem enhancement and social skills development (Botvin & Wills, 1985).

A comprehensive review of over 50 studies examining various psychosocial approaches conducted between 1976 and 1985 (Flay, 1985) suggested that these approaches could be effective at delaying the onset of smoking initiation; however, this conclusion could only be tentatively made due to a variety of methodological flaws (Flay, 1985). Reviews of recent, methodologically sound studies (Best, Thompson, Santin, Smith, & Brown, 1988; Tobler, 1986; Rundall & Bruvold, 1988; Rooney, 1992; Bruvold, 1992) all report a decreased prevalence of smoking among students exposed to the social influence programs compared to students in equivalent comparison groups or randomly assigned control groups. The difference between treated and nontreated groups ranges from 25 to 60% and lasts from 1 to 4 years (US DHHS, 1994). The following treatment components appear to enhance the effects of these programs: sustained treatment (e.g. several "booster sessions" over several years), incorporation of complementary communitywide and/or mass-media components, and presenting the antismoking intervention in the context of a more comprehensive school health education program.

Secondary Prevention

Secondary prevention refers to the prevention of morbidity related to smoking and encompasses a range of activities referred to as smoking control strategies (US DHHS, 1991). Smoking control strategies are implemented across a number of different social sectors and target both individual smokers and the environment where smoking occurs. Using a variety of social sectors, such as the political, occupational, educational, communications, and health care sectors, provides a synergistic effect to reach more smokers (US DHHS, 1991). This section will focus primarily on the health education and behavior efforts designed to encourage and help individual smokers to quit.

Over a quarter century of research has been devoted to determining the most effective methods to get smokers to want to quit, feel ready to quit, actually quit, and remain abstinent. Most smokers report they want to quit; when polled, about 70% of smokers say they would like to quit (CDC, 1994b). However, a smaller proportion actually feel ready to quit. When the transtheoretical model of change (Prochaska & DiClemente, 1983) is applied to populations of smokers, only about 20% intend to quit in the next month, with the majority of smokers desiring to quit falling into the "contemplation" category, which includes smokers who intend to quit in the next 6 months but not in the next month (Prochaska, 1994). About 50% of people who have ever smoked have actually quit and remained smoke free, while most quitters relapse on their first, second, and even third attempt. Each of these points in the quitting process has been the subject of behavioral research.

Smoking cessation is often broadly characterized as either "on one's own" or through a formal program. Most quitters report doing so on their own, but even among these, many have had help in one form or another. For example, a person who quits without a formal program may have actually attended one during a previous attempt and learned certain techniques that were helpful later in the successful attempt. Thus, although it appears that the majority of quitters quit on their own, there is a need for formal cessation programs that offer well-researched techniques to help smokers overcome the physical and psychological addiction to tobacco. The following paragraphs outline the process of quitting, which applies to all quitters whether or not a formal cessation program is used. Later in this chapter, a variety of cessation strategies will be reviewed.

Motivation—When Smokers Decide They Want to Stop Smoking

According to behavioral theory, a major determinant of health behavior is the expected outcome of the particular behavior (Bandura, 1986). For smokers, this means that they perceive the consequences of continuing to smoke to be more important or valuable than the consequences of quitting. For example, a valuable outcome of smoking for the newly initiated is often linked to an enhanced self-image: if I smoke, I will be seen as more like the people I wish to be like. For the smoker addicted to nicotine, a valuable outcome from smoking may be avoidance of withdrawal symptoms. For smokers, these outcomes are more highly valued at that time than outcomes associated with abstaining from smoking.

Using the same theoretical perspective, a person becomes motivated to stop smoking when the perceived outcomes of quitting begin to be more valued than those of continued smoking. For example, the young smoker may find that his athletic performance is compromised by continued smoking and this may become more important to his self-image than being a member of the smoking group. The addicted smoker may develop chronic bronchitis or another illness, and the importance of recovering his or her health may be great enough to get him or her past withdrawal. In fact, the majority of smokers who quit say they do so for health reasons (Duncan, Cummings, Hudes, Zahnel, & Coates, 1992).

Viewed in terms of the transtheoretical model of change, precontemplators—smokers who are not thinking about quitting within the next 6 months—can be given information to raise their consciousness about the negative consequences of smoking and the positive consequences of quitting. Motivational interventions for smokers have focused on shifting perceptions about the benefits of smoking versus the benefits of quitting. A technique known as motivational interviewing has been evaluated in several studies (Miller & Rollnick, 1991). Counselors using this technique enable smokers to identify personally relevant benefits of smoking along with personally relevant reasons for quitting. With subtle guidance smokers can shift their own perceptions and begin to value the reasons for quitting over the reasons for continuing to smoke (Miller & Rollnick, 1991). This is in contrast to methods that are based on the assumption that everyone should stop smoking now and is in keeping with the concept of decisional balance in the transtheoretical model of change (see Predictors of Cessation, below).

Another technique to motivate smokers has been to provide them with feedback regarding the damage they are doing to themselves, particularly their lungs. Pictures of emphysemic or cancerous lungs were once commonly used as a technique to convince smokers to quit. Such "scare tactics" have not proved to be highly motivating and it appears that personalizing this sort of message may be a more effective motivational technique. Some have suggested that providing smokers with results of lung function tests that estimate their "lung age" is a technique for motivating smokers (Morris & Temple, 1985). From a transtheoretical model of change perspective, this technique serves as both a consciousness-raising process and a dramatic relief process.

Preparation—Getting Ready to Quit

While people who are motivated to quit smoking are more "ready" to quit than those who express no interest in quitting, desiring to quit is not necessarily synonymous with being ready to quit soon. In terms of the transtheoretical model of change, these people may be in the contemplation stage—seriously thinking about quitting in the next 6 months—and must move into the preparation stage—planning to quit in the next 30 days. A major issue in preparation is building percieved self-efficacy to change a habit and to overcome problems related to nicotine addiction (Baer & Lichtenstein, 1988). The Confidence Questionnaire is a fairly typical example of an instrument that asks smokers to quantify their level of confidence to avoid smoking in response to a number of different smoking cues, such as social gatherings with alcohol, or after a meal, or in high-stress settings (Baer, Holt, & Lichtenstein, 1986). A common preparation intervention technique is to use small behavioral steps to increase the smoker's self-efficacy to quit altogether. For example, a smoker may delay the first cigarette of the day for a certain amount of time. As the smoker experiences success, the amount of time can be increased to build the smoker's self-efficacy that they can tolerate cravings for an increasing time period. Another efficacy-building exercise is to cut out altogether a certain "routine" cigarette, such as the one smoked while talking on the phone. Again, a success with this small step builds confidence toward larger steps.

Other preparation activities include (1) self-monitoring: keeping a record of smoking urges, the circumstances surrounding the urge, and whether or not a cigarette is smoked; (2) brand switching or tapering: reducing nicotine levels to wean oneself from nicotine addiction; (3) building aversion: providing aversive outcomes associate with moking to cue negative outcome expectations; and (4) setting a quit date: making a commitment to stop smoking at a definite time.

Cessation—Just Doing It

According to the transtheoretical model of change, the smoker can move from the preparation stage to the stage of action, defined as the period ranging from 0 to 6 months after successful cessation. It is for this minority of smokers that most cessation programs are designed. The typical smoking cessation program employs a multicomponent approach in which several strategies and quitting techniques are combined to increase the likelihood of success. These programs generally assume the smoker is motivated to quit and ready to try and so do not tend to include a great deal of motivation or preparation activity. The strategies commonly included in smoking cessation programs are described later in this chapter.

Maintaining Abstinence and Preventing Relapse

Initial quitting is difficult, but remaining abstinent is the primary task for quitters. According to the transtheoretical model of change, smokers who remain abstinent for 6 months enter the maintenance stage. Although problem-solving and coping techniques to deal with urges and withdrawal symptoms are taught in cessation programs, a broader view of relapse prevention has been described by Marlatt and Gordon (1985). This model outlines the determinants of relapse from a cognitive–behavioral viewpoint. Basically, the relapse prevention model includes both coping skills to avoid or deal with danger situations plus techniques to deal with "lapses" (giving in to the urge to smoke) so that they do not become full relapses into regular smoking. The key to preventing a lapse from becoming a relapse is to avoid the "abstinence violation effect" in which the smoker views the slip as having "blown it" and gives up trying to remain abstinent (Marlatt & Gordon, 1985). The primary method of avoiding the abstinence violation effect is self-talk to counter the all-or-nothing thinking and guilt that occur after a slip. This self-talk centers on thinking of a slip as a learning opportunity and a natural part of becoming a nonsmoker. As with much of the smoking cessation research, the results of studies that evaluate relapse prevention techniques have been mixed (Lando, 1993; AHCPR, 1996). A very intensive approach in which quitters' danger situations were individually diagnosed and appropriate coping responses practiced produced relatively high sustained quit rates (Stevens & Hollis, 1989), but other studies have been less successful (Curry, Marlatt, & Gordon, 1987; Curry, Marlatt, Gordon, & Baer, 1988).

Progression through the stages stages of change from being a smoker to a nonsmoker is often not linear; people often backslide to earlier stages. Within the transtheoretical model of change, relapse is viewed as a normal part of the change process as opposed to a failure. Treatment must be matched to a smoker's stage of readiness for optimal results (DiClemente & Prochaska, 1982; Prochaska, DiClemente, Velicer, & Rossi, 1993).

Processes of Change

A unique contribution of the transtheoretical model of change is the acknowledgment that all stages of readiness are important, including the early (i.e., preaction) stages, and that smokers make use of specific processes of change at each stage (DiClemente et al., 1991; Prochaska & DiClemente, 1983, 1984). Ten processes of change may be utilized by smokers as they progress through the stages of change: consciousness raising, dramatic relief, environmental reevaluation, self-reevaluation, self-liberation, helping relationships, contingency management, counterconditioning, stimulus control, and social liberation (Prochaska & DiClemente, 1986; Prochaska, Di-Clemente, Velicer, & Fava, 1988). Detailed descriptions of these processes are found in another chapter of this volume. In the earlier stages, individuals tend to emphasize the cognitive–affective processes of change labeled "experiential," whereas in the later stages, the "behavioral" processes are emphasized by individuals (Prochaska & DiClemente, 1992; Prochaska, Norcross, & DiClemente, 1994a). The treatment strategy is to facilitate use of the "right" processes at the "right" stages in order to help individuals progress more quickly through the stages.

Predictors of Cessation

Behavioral scientists have collected and analyzed data on smokers and quitters to determine factors that are associated with successful quitting. In general, people who have better personal and socioeconomic resources, such as higher education, income, and coping skills, are more successful at quitting (Fisher, Lichtenstein, & Haire-Joshu, 1993). These factors, or predictors of cessation, fall into two categories: factors that can be changed, such as knowledge of the harms of smoking and factors that are not amenable to change, such as gender and age. Further, the patterns of causality among the factors is unclear. For example, in the Lung Health Study, Bjornson and colleagues (1995) initially reported that, compared to women, men had higher rates of sustained abstinence from smoking after 12 and 36 months, but when they controlled for selected baseline variables, the association between gender and sustained abstinence was reduced (i.e., differences were detected at 36 months only). These researchers concluded that other demographic and smoking history variables were more important than gender *per se* in sustained abstinence. Similarly, African Americans have less success at quitting but are also more affected by stress and fewer socioeconomic resources. Older age is more clearly associated with cessation success, even after the presence of illness has been accounted for (Ward, Klesges, & Halpern, 1997). Different health problems are associated in different ways with cessation. Cardiovascular disease correlates with higher success rates (Ockene, 1987), but pulmonary disease and depression are associated with less success (Fisher *et al.*, 1993; AHCPR, 1996). Negative mood states and stress have been shown to predict relapse to smoking after cessation (Fisher *et al.*, 1993).

Other factors that predict successful abstinence are more amenable to change. A higher nicotine-dependence level has been associated with quitting difficulty (Orleans, 1993). Two sociocognitive factors—decisional balance and perceived self-efficacy—are frequently associated with cessation. Research conducted in the context of the transtheoretical model of change suggests that cessation is, in part, a function of making the benefits of smoking less salient than the cons for individuals trying to quit (DiClemente *et al.*, 1991; Prochaska *et al.*, 1994b; Velicer, DiClemente, Prochaska, & Brandenburg, 1985). Similarly, beliefs about the dangers of smoking have been associated with quitting (Ward *et al.*, 1997). Perceived self-efficacy is a widely studied theoretical construct that is predictive of a number of health behaviors (Bandura, 1997). Smokers who feel little confidence in their ability to quit are much less likely to try, and those that do try are less likely to persist in the face of obstacles (Bandura, 1997). Across the stages of smoking cessation, self-efficacy (confidence) scores increase almost linearly from precontemplation to maintenance.

Cessation Strategies

Early Tobacco Control Measures

Early efforts to reduce smoking initiation and motivate people to quit assumed that if the public was aware of the health risks associated with smoking, they would quit. This assumption was the basis of early mass media campaigns to inform the public about the dangers of smoking. These campaigns apparently were successful at communicating health risks: Recent surveys suggest that 80% of current smokers know that smoking is harmful to their health. However, these campaigns were less successful in decreasing the prevalence of smoking. Mass media campaigns in the 1950s and 1960s were associated with millions of people quitting; however, millions more did not succeed (US DHHS, 1991).

Other early tobacco control activities focused on the individual smoker to motivate and help him or her to quit. In addition to education, early approaches focused on behavioral therapies of conditioning and self-control (Lichtenstein, 1982). Cognitive components, such as those aimed at changing outcome and efficacy expectations, were later added; currently, cognitive–behavioral strategies comprise the major nonpharmacological approaches to cessation.

Current Approaches to Smoking Cessation

In addition to formal cessation programs, smoking and quitting have become the focus of clinical interventions delivered in the context of usual medical care (Glynn, 1988; US DHHS, 1991). In recognition of the strong link between smoking and health problems and the multiple opportunities for health care providers to interact with smokers, a number of agencies have begun promoting strategies to address smoking as a routine part of medical care. The National Cancer Institute recommends the "4A's" approach to treating smokers: (1) Ask about smoking at every visit; (2) advise all smokers to quit; (3) assist those who agree to try; and (4) arrange follow-up for all smokers (Glynn & Manley, 1993) Building on this framework, the clinical practice guideline on smoking cessation includes several recommendations for clinicians, smoking cessation specialists, and administrators of health care systems aimed at improving efforts to help smokers quit (AHCPR, 1996).

Published analyses of smoking cessation studies indicates that the more intense the smoking cessation treatment, the more effective it is in producing long-term abstinence (AHCPR, 1996). Formal smoking cessation programs include the most intensive approaches to smoking treatment. The typical smoking cessation program employs a multicomponent approach in which several strategies and quitting techniques are combined to increase the likelihood of success. Such programs will often include specific quitting activities, instruction on coping with urges and withdrawal symptoms and on using problem-solving techniques to avoid or resist temptation. In addition, many programs also have included components such as dealing with nutrition and weight, exercise and fitness, and dealing with depression.

The following is a summary of strategies commonly employed by formal smoking cessation programs:

- The quit date: Setting a quit date is a preparatory activity that is aimed at strengthening commitment to follow through with quitting plans. Often, the smoker will sign a pledge or contract to quit on a specific date. When the quit day arrives, smokers are instructed to get rid of all smoking materials (e.g., cigarettes, lighters, ashtrays) and to begin nicotine replacement therapy if used. Quit day can be timed to coincide with a special day such as a birthday, but it is often advised to avoid trying to quit during stressful periods, such as holidays.

- Coping with urges and withdrawal: Methods for coping with urges and withdrawal symptoms are important for users of nicotine replacement therapy as well as other quitters. Deep breathing exercises are often recommended to help the quitter get past the urge. Also, informing people that urges last only about 5 minutes helps them persevere. Finally, quitters can use oral and tactile substitutes, such as chewing on straws, carrot sticks, or gum, or sucking on hard candy (Benowitz & Fredericks, 1993). To cope with the stress, irritability, and other physical symptoms associated with nicotine withdrawal, quitters are advised to use relaxation techniques and to increase physical exercise. However, the empirical evidence that this increases cessation rates is relatively weak (AHCPR, 1996)

- Cue exposure (stimulus control): In addition to managing urges to smoke, it can be helpful to address the cues that trigger the urges. Smokers light up in response to a variety of internal and environmental stimuli. Use of self-monitoring techniques can help quitters identify the stimuli and plan to avoid the cues or to use alternative responses to them, such as self-talk. Cue exposure methods to extinguish the association between the stimulus and the smoking response provide the smoker with practice in resisting cigarettes that are smoked in response to certain cues until the smoking response fades away or is replaced by another response. There is little published research on these techniques; strong evidence that these techniques are either effective or ineffective is not currently available (AHCPR, 1996).

- Aversive therapy: Especially prior to the availability of nicotine replacement, many programs employed aversive smoking procedures with some success. Aversive smoking procedures are used under the guidance of a trained facilitator and involve intensive smoking to the point of feeling sick. Two types of aversive smoking are rapid smoking and rapid puffing. Rapid smoking involves smoking and inhaling continuously for a period of time and is potentially dangerous to the smoker (AHCPR, 1996). Rapid puffing does not involve inhalation and so is considered safer. Smoke holdling is an even less intense technique in which smokers must hold the smoke in their mouths while breathing through their noses. This technique has also met with some success in research trials (Lando, 1993).

- Social support: Many smoking cessation programs include the smoker's choice of support person or include activities for the smoker to enlist social support from their social networks. Common sense tells us that when one's social network is supportive, one is more likely to cope with the stress of quitting; however, research on smoking cessation techniques aimed at bolstering social support has failed to show improved quit rates, possibly because one's social support system is extremely difficult to manipulate as a study variable (Lando, 1993). However, the social support a smoker receives from treatment personnel does seem to have an effect on quitting, and it has been recommended that clinicians take advantage of this by communicating care and conern (AHCPR, 1996).

- Problem solving and coping with stress: A major objective of most smoking cessation programs is to teach smokers how to cope with the stress of quitting, often by employing problem-solving techniques. The *Smoking Cessation Clinical Guideline* (AHCPR, 1996) provides a summary of the common elements of problem solving and coping skills training: (1) identification of danger situations, such as specific events, mental–emotional states, or specific activities that produce a strong urge to smoke; (2) learning and practicing cognitive and behavioral activities that distract attention from smoking urges and/or reduce negative moods; (3) anticipating the danger situation and avoiding it or using the practiced distraction activity; and (4) providing realistic expectations for stress and withdrawal associated with quitting.
- "Alternative" techniques: A number of other techniques have been tried by smokers, usually as alternatives to the more common methods described above. These include hypnosis, acupuncture, and medication other than nicotine replacement. Hypnosis is widely advertised as a smoking cessation method and often is associated with "charlatan" practices, although it has been used as a legitimate tool of therapy for a number of psychological problems. Acupuncture is used to counter the symptoms of withdrawal, but, like hypnosis, is often questioned as a legitimate therapy. Unfortunately, there is no research evidence that suggests either hypnosis or acupuncture is effective in helping people quit. A number of medications thought to mediate the effects of withdrawal, such as antidepressants, have been evaluated in controlled studies. Generally, none have been shown to increase quitting success. However, there are few data available, especially on newer forms of antidepressants, making it inappropriate to rule out these medications as potentially useful.

An analysis of the smoking cessation research published over the last decade has shown that there is a dose-response relationship between the number of techniques used to quit and the likelihood of success (AHCPR, 1996; Kottke, Battista, DeFriese, & Brekke, 1988). The more techniques that are employed by a smoker, the better the chances of quitting. In addition to the known effectiveness of nicotine replacement therapy, two of the components typically used in smoking cessation programs are most consistently associated with significant rates of quitting (AHCPR, 1996): (1) general problem-solving and coping skills, especially those focused on identifying and preparing for times when the desire to smoke will be high, and (2) availability of social support from the health care provider or smoking cessation counselor.

The program components above can also be included in formats other than formal classes or group sessions, such as individual clinical (medical or psychological) counseling, self-help programs in the form of books or computer programs, and mass media programs.

While the evidence is clear that smoking interventions have played a significant role in helping a portion of smokers to quit (most studies report a quit rate in the 20 to 40% range), it should be noted that the vast majority of smokers who quit do so in the absence of a formal cessation program (Fiore *et al.*, 1990). With the availability of nicotine replacement therapy without a prescription, it is likely that "self-quitting" will continue to be the norm. However, there also will continue to be a significant minority of smokers who desire and use the more structured approaches seen with the cognitive–behavioral techniques that have been described here.

Treatment Matching

Many researchers and clinicians are beginning to recognize that a single intervention approach may not be appropriate for all individuals who smoke. As with other health-related problems, intervention efforts have evolved to identify the "best fit" between an individual's characteristics and intervention strategies.

It seems important to distinguish the difference between the concepts of "tailoring" and "matching" intervention strategies. First, tailoring entails designing interventions according to specific demographic variables such as age, gender, education, racial–ethnic composition, culture, geographic location, or other subjective characteristics such as existing comorbidities (e.g., illness or pregnancy). Treatment matching, on the other hand, usually involves implementing interventions strategies that correspond to a person's motivation and readiness for change. Many smoking cessation programs and techniques were designed with an explicit action-oriented strategy that assumed the individual smoker was ready to quit and by simply following the guidelines of the cessation program would soon be a successful nonsmoker (Fava, Velicer, & Prochaska, 1995). Moreover, many smoking cessation programs have been tailored to age and/or gender of specific smoking populations, but continue to provide "one-size-fits-all" interventions by not considering people's readiness to follow such advice (Prochaska, 1994).

However, due to the addictive nature of nicotine, matching nicotine replacement therapies such as nicotine gum, the patch, or nasal spray with a person who is a heavy smoker and motivationally ready to change holds promise by helping to reduce physical withdrawal symptoms. Behavior change programs that are both matched *and* tailored are more likely to be efficacious and cost-effective.

Smoking cessation researchers have attempted to identify which cognitive variables are associated with which stage of quitting smoking. For example, expectations have been linked to prequitting stages and the decision to quit, while self-efficacy has been thought to be more important in relapse prevention (Baer, Holt, & Lichtenstein, 1986). Both the stage theories, which emphasize the processes of behavior change, and the behavioral theories, which emphasize the determinants and mechanisms of a particular behavior, are useful for informing smoking cessation research and treatment.

Summary and Conclusions

Tobacco smoking represents a prevalent problem with major health consequences, including economic and quality of life consequences for large segments of the population. Although the United States has seen a decline in smoking since the first Surgeon General's report, nearly one in four people continue to smoke. Current public health efforts are directed at both the prevention of smoking behavior in youth and the cessation of smoking behavior among those who smoke. Both initiation and cessation behaviors can be categorized as processes in which one passes through several stages. Behavioral research on smoking behavior has focused on the correlates of smoking initiation and cessation that predict who will start and who will quit. Smoking prevention and cessation intervention research combines the predictors of smoking with sociocognitive models and theories of behavior to develop and evaluate the efficacy of strategies aimed at changing the determinants of these behaviors. New pharmacological treatments have increased the chances for remaining abstinent among many quitters. Tobacco control efforts overall include interventions aimed at individuals and more broadly based public health interventions, including those targeting policy rather than behavior. As the ill effects of tobacco smoke and secondhand smoke are increasingly made public knowledge and the nature of nicotine dependence becomes better understood, public health practitioners can look forward to more and better avenues to reducing this important public health problem.

References

Agency for Health Care Policy and Research (AHCPR). (1996). *Smoking Cessation Clinical Guideline.* DHHS Publication No. (AHCPR) 96-0692.

Baer, J. S., & Lichtenstein, E. (1988). Cognitive assessment. In D. M. Donovan & G. A. Marlatt (Eds.), *Assessment of addictive behaviors* (pp. 161–201). New York: Guilford Press.

Baer, J. S., Holt, C. S., & Lichtenstein, E. (1986). Self-efficacy and smoking re-examined. Construct validity and clinical utility, *Journal of Consulting and Clinical Psychology, 54,* 846–852.

Bandura, A. (1986). *Social foundations of thought and action: A social cognitive theory.* Englewood Cliffs, NJ: Prentice-Hall.

Bandura, A. (1977). Self-efficacy: Toward a unifying theory of behavior change. *Psychological Review, 84,* 191–215.

Bandura, A. (1982). Self-efficacy mechanism in human agency. *American Psychologist, 37,* 122–147.

Bandura, A. (1997). *Self efficacy. The exercise of control.* New York: W. H. Freeman.

Beck, A. T. (1976). *Cognitive Therapy and the Emotional Disorders.* New York: New American Library.

Benowitz, N. L., & Fredericks, A. B. (1993). *Clinical management of smoking cessation.* Caddo, OK: Professional Communications, Inc.

Best, J. A., Thompson, S. J., Santin, S. M., Smith, E. A., & Brown, K. (1988). Preventing cigarette smoking among school children. In L. Breslow, J. E. Fielding, & L. B. Lave (Eds.), *Annual Review of Public Health* (vol. 9, pp. 161–209). Palo Alto, CA: Annual Reviews.

Bjornson, W., Rand, C., Connet, J. E., Lindgren, P., Nides, M., Pope, F., Buist, A. S., Hoppe-Ryan, C., & O'Hara, P. (1995). Gender differences in smoking cessation after three years in the Lung Health Study. *American Journal of Public Health, 85,* 223–230.

Botvin, G. J., & Wills, T. J. (1985). Personal and social skills training: Cognitive–behavioral approaches to substance abuse prevention. In C. S. Bell & R. Battjes (Eds.), *Prevention research: determining drug abuse among children and adolescents* (pp. 8–49). Monograph No. 63. US DHEW, PHS, Alcohol, Drug Abuse, and Mental Health Administration, National Institute on Drug Abuse. Bethesda, MD: DHHS Publication No. (ADM) 85-1334.

Bruvold, W. H. (1992). A meta-analysis of adolescent smoking-prevention programs. *American Journal of Public Health, 83*(6), 872–880.

Centers for Disease Control and Prevention (CDC). (1993). Cigarette-smoking attributable mortality and years of potential life lost—United States, 1990. *Morbidity and Mortality Weekly Report, 42,* 645–649.

CDC. (1994a). Cigarette smoking among adults—United States, 1992, and changes in the definition of current cigarette smoking. Morbidity and Mortality Weekly Report, 43, 342–346.

CDC (1994b). Cigarette smoking among adults—United States, 1993. *Morbidity and Mortality Weekly Report, 43,* 925–930.

CDC. (1994c). Medical-care expenditures attributable to cigarette smoking—United States, 1993. *Morbidity and Mortality Weekly Report, 43*(26), 469–471.

Conrad, K., Flay, B., & Hill, D. (1992). Why children start smoking cigarettes: Predictors of onset. *British Journal of Addiction, 87,* 1711–1724.

Crawford, M., Winders, S., & Kohler, C. (1996). Evaluating tobacco use among teens: A deep south perspective. Presented at the 124th annual meeting of the American Public Health Association, New York, NY.

Curry, S. Marlatt, G. A., & Gordon, J. R. (1987). Abstinence violation effect: Validation of an attributional construct with smoking cesssation. *Journal of Consulting and Clinical Psychology, 55,* 145–149.

Curry, S. J., Marlatt, G. A., Gordon, J., & Baer, J. S. (1988). A comparison of alternative theoretical approaches to smoking cessation and relapse. *Health Psychology, 7,* 5545–5566.

Dawson, J., Henderson, M. (1987). Living with risk: A report of the British Medical Association, *Preventive Medicine, 20,* 279–291.

DiClemente, C. C. (1986). Self-efficacy and the addictive behaviors. *Journal of Social and Clinical Psychology, 4,* 302–315.

DiClemente, C. C, & Prochaska, J. O. (1982). Self-change and therapy change of smoking behavior: A comparison of processes of change in cessation and maintenance. *Addictive Behaviors, 7,* 133–142.

DiClemente, C. C., Prochaska, J. O., Fairhurst, S. K., Velicer, W. F., Velasquez, M. M., & Rossi, J. S. (1991). The processes of smoking cessation: An analysis of precontemplation, contemplation and preparation stages of change. *Journal of Consulting and Clinical Psychology, 59,* 295–304.

Duncan, C. L., Cummings, S. R., Hudes, E. S, Zahnel. E., & Coates, T. J. (1992). Quitting smoking: Reasons for quitting and predictors of sensation among medical patients. *Journal of General Internal Medicine, 7,* 398–409.

Durell, J., & Bukoski, W. (1984). Preventing substance abuse: The state of the art. *Public Health Reports, 99*(1), 23–31.

Eneroth, M., & Persson, B. M. (1993). Risk factors for failed healing in amputation for vascular disease. A prospective, consecutive study of 177 cases. *Acta Orthopaedica Scandinavica, 64,* 369–372.

Evans, R. I. (1976). Smoking in children: Developing a social psychological strategy of deterrence. *Preventive Medicine, 5,* 122–127.

Evans, R. I., Rozelle, R. M., Mittlemark, M. B., Hanseb, W. B., Bane, A. I., & Havis, J. (1978). Deterring onset of smoking in children: Knowledge of immediate physiologic effects and coping with peer pressure, media pressure, and parent modeling. *Journal of Applied Social Psychology, 8,* 126–135.

Evans, R. I., Rozelle, R. M., Maxwell, S. E., Raines, B. E., Dill, C. A., Guthrie, T. J., Henderson, A. H., & Hill, P. C. (1981). Social modeling films to deter smoking in adolescents: Results of a three-year field investigation. *Journal of Applied Psychology, 66*(4), 399–414.

Fava, J. L., Velicer, W. F., & Prochaska, J. O. (1995). Applying the transtheoretical model to a representative sample of smokers. *Addictive Behaviors, 20,* 189–195.

Fiore, M. C., Novotny, T. E., Pierce, J. P., Giovino, G. A., Hatziandreu, E. J., Newcomb, P. A., Surawicz, T. S., & Davis R. M., (1990). Methods used to quit smoking in the United States. Do cessation programs help? *Journal of the American Medical Association, 263,* 2760–2765

Fisher, E. B., Jr., Lichtenstein, E., & Haire-Joshu, D. (1993) Multiple determinants of tobacco use and cessation. In C. T. Orleans & J. Slade (Eds.), *Nicotine addiction: Principles and management* (pp. 59–88). New York: Oxford University Press.

Flay, B. R. (1985). Psychosocial approaches to smoking prevention: A review of findings. *Health Psychology, 4*(5), 449–488.

Flay, B. R. (1993). Youth tobacco use: Risks, patterns, and control. In J. Slade & C. T. Orleans (Eds.), *Nicotine addiction: Principles and management* (pp. 365–384). New York: Oxford University Press.

Flay, B. R., D'Avernas, J. R., Best, J. A., Kersell, M. W., & Ryan, K. B. (1983). Cigarette smoking: Why young people do it and ways of preventing it. In P. J. McGrath & P. Firestone (Eds.), *Pediatric and adolescent behavioral medicine* (pp. 257–323). New York: Springer Verlag.

Gilchrist, L. D., Schinke, S. P., & Blythe, B. J. (1979). Self-control skills for smoking prevention. In P. F. Engstrom, P. N.Anderson, & L. E. Mortenson (Eds.), *Advances in cancer control* (pp. 125–30). New York: Alan Liss.

Giovino, G. A., Henningfield, J. E., Tomar, S. L., Escobedo, L. G., & Slade, J. (1995). Epidemiology of tobacco use and dependence. *Epidemiologic Reviews, 17*(1), 48–65.

Giovino, G. A., Schooley, M. W., Zhu, B-P, Chrismon, J. H., Tomar, S. L., Peddicord, J. P., Merritt, R. K., Husten, C. G., & Eriksen, M. P. (1994). *Morbidity and Mortality Weekly Report, 43*(SS-3), 1–43.

Glanz, K., Lewis, F. M., & Rimer, B. K. (Eds.). (1997). *Health behavior and health education theory, research and practice* (2nd ed). San Francisco: Josey & Bass.

Glynn, T. J. (1988). Physicians and a smoke free society. *Archives of Internal Medicine, 148,* 1013–1016.

Glynn, T. J., & Manley, M. W. (1993). *How to help your patients stop smoking. A National Cancer Institute manual for physicians.* US DHHS: National Cancer Institute. Washington, DC: Government Printing Office.

Goodstadt, M. S. (1978). Alcohol and drug education: models and outcomes. *Health Education Monographs, 6*(3), 263–79.

Hansen, W. B., Johnson, C. A., Flay, B. R., Graham, J. W., & Sobel, S. (1988). Affective and social influence to the prevention of multiple substance abuse among seventh grade students: Results from Project SMART. *Preventive Medicine, 17,* 135–154.

Herdman, R., Hewitt, M., & Laschober, M. (1993). *Smoking-related deaths and financial costs: Office of technology and assessment estimates, 1990.* Congress of the United States. Office of Technology and Assessment. Washington, DC: Government Printing Office.

Higgins, M. W., Enright, P. L., Kronmal, R. A., Schenker, M. B., Anton-Culver, H., & Lyles, M. (1993). Smoking and lung function in elderly men and women: The cardiovascular health study. *Journal of the American Medical Association, 269,* 2741–2748.

Jones, E. E., Kanouse, D. E., Kelly, H. H., Nisbett, R. E., Valins, S., & Weiner, B. (1971). *Attribution: Perceiving the causes of behavior.* Morristown, NJ: General Learning Press.

Kiesler, C. A. (1971). *The psychology of commitment: Experiments linking behavior to beliefs.* New York: Academic Press.

Kottke, T. E., Battista, R. N., DeFriese, G. H., & Brekke, M. L. (1988). Attributes of successful smoking cessation interventions in medical practice. A meta-analysis of 39 controlled trials. *Journal of the American Medical Association, 259*(19), 2882–2889.

Lando, H. (1993). Formal quit smoking treatments. In C. T. Orleans and J. Slade (Eds.), *Nicotine addiction: Principles and management* (pp. 221–244). New York: Oxford University Press.

Leventhal, H., & Cleary, P. D. (1980). The smoking problem: A review of the research and theory on behavioral risk modification. *Psychological Bulletin, 88*(2), 370–405.

Leventhal, H., Fleming, R., & Glynn, T. (1988). A cognitive-developmental approach to smoking intervention: In S. Maes, C. D. Spielberger, P. B. Defares, & I. G. Sarason (Eds.), *Topics in health psychology: Proceedings of the first annual expert conference in health psychology.* New York: John Wiley & Sons.

Lichtenstein, E. (1982). The smoking problem: A behavioral perspective. *Journal of Consulting and Clinical Psychology, 50,* 804–819.

Marlatt, G. A., & Gordon, J. R. (Eds.). (1985). *Relapse prevention. Maintenance strategies in the treatment of addictive behaviors.* New York: Guilford Press.

McGuire, W. J. (1969). The nature of attitudes and attitude change. In G. Lindzay & E. Aaronson (Eds.), *Handbook of Social Psychology* (2nd ed., vol. 3). Reading, MA: Addison-Wesley.

McNeill, A. D. (1990). The development of dependence on smoking in children. *British Journal of Addiction, 86,* 589–592.

McNeill, A. D., West, R. J., Jarvis, M., Jackson, P., & Bryant, A. (1986). Cigarette withdrawal symptoms in adolescent smokers. *Psychopharmacology, 90,* 533–536.

Miller, W. R., & Rollnick, S. (Eds.). (1991). *Preparing people to change. Motivational interviewing.* New York: Guilford Press.

Morris, J. F., & Temple, W. (1985). Spirometric "lung age" estimation for motivating smoking cessation. *Preventive Medicine, 14,* 665–662.

Ockene, J. K. (1987). Clinical perspectives: Physician delivered interventions for smoking cessation: Strategies for increasing effectiveness. *Preventive Medicine, 16,* 723–737.

Orleans, C. T. (1993). Treating nicotine dependence in medical settings: A stepped care model. In C. T. Orleans & J. Slade (Eds.), *Nicotine addiction: Principles and management* (pp. 145–161). New York: Oxford University Press.

Pierce, J. P., & Gilpin, E. (1996). How long will today's adolescent smoker be addicted to cigarettes? *American Journal of Public Health, 86*(2), 253–256.

Prochaska, J. O. (1994, April). *Staging: A revolution.* Master scientific lecture presented at the annual meeting of the Society of Behavioral Medicine, Boston, MA.

Prochaska, J. O., & DiClemente, C. C. (1983). The stages and processes of self-change of smoking: Toward an integrative model of change. *Journal of Consulting and Clinical Psychology, 51,* 390–395.

Prochaska, J. O., & DiClemente, C. C. (1984). *The transtheoretical approach: Crossing the boundaries of therapy.* Homewood, IL: Irwin.

Prochaska, J. O., & DiClemente, C. C. (1986). Toward a comprehensive model of change. In W. Miller & N. Heather (Eds.), *Treating addictive behaviors* (pp. 3–27). New York: Plenum Press.

Prochaska, J. O., & DiClemente, C. C. (1992). Stages of change in the modification of problem behaviors. In M. Herson, R. M. Eisler, & P. M. Miller (Eds.), *Progress in behavior modification* (pp. 39–46). Sycamore, IL: Sycamore Publishing.

Prochaska, J. O., DiClemente, C. C., Velicer, W., & Fava, J. S. (1988). Measuring processes of change: Applications to the cessation of smoking. *Journal of Clinical and Consulting Psychology, 56,* 520–528.

Prochaska, J. O., Velicer, W. F., DiClemente, C. C., Guadagnoli, E., & Rossi, J. (1991). Patterns of change: Dynamic topology applied to smoking cessation. *Multivariate Behavioral Research, 26,* 83–107.

Prochaska, J. O., DiClemente, C. C., & Norcross, J. C. (1992). In search of how people change: Application to addictive behaviors. *American Psychologist, 47,* 1102–1114.

Prochaska, J. O., DiClemente, C. C., Velicer, W. F., & Rossi, J. S. (1993). Standardized, individualized, interactive, and personalized self-help programs for smoking cessation. *Health Psychology, 12,* 399–405.

Prochaska, J. O., Norcross, J. C., & DiClemente, C. C. (1994). *Changing for good.* New York: William Morrow.

Renwick, D. S., & Connelly, M. J. (1996). Prevalence and treatment of chronic airways obstruction in adults over the age of 45. *Thorax, 51,* 164–168.

Rooney, B. (1992). A meta-analysis of smoking-prevention programs after adjustment for study design [dissertation]. Minneapolis: University of Minnesota.

Rundall, T. G., & Bruvold, W. H. (1988). A meta-analysis of school-based smoking and alcohol use prevention programs. *Health Education Quarterly, 15*(3), 317–334.

Schinke, S. P., & Blythe, B. J. (1981). Cognitive–behavioral prevention of children's smoking. *Child Behavior Therapy, 3*(4), 25–42.

Seddon, J. M., Willett, W. C., Speizer, F. E., & Hankinson, S. E. (1996). A prospective study of cigarette smoking and age-related macular degeneration in women. *Journal of the American Medical Association, 276,* 1141–1146.

Seeman, T., Mendes de Leon, C., Berkman, L., & Ostfeld, A. (1993). Risk factors for coronary heart disease among older men and women: A prospective study of community-dwelling elderly. *American Journal of Epidemiology, 138,* 1037–1049.

Sherman, S. J., Presson, C. C., Chassin, L., Bensenberg, M., Corty, E., & Olschavshky, R. W. (1982). Smoking intentions in adolescents: Direct experience and predictability. *Personality and Social Psychology Bulletin, 8,* 376–383.

Shinton, R., & Beevers, G. (1989). Meta-analysis of the relation between cigarette smoking and stroke. *British Medical Journal, 298,* 789–794.

Stevens, V. J., & Hollis, J. F. (1989). Preventing smoking relapse using an individually tailored skills training technique. *Journal of Consulting and Clinical Psychology, 57,* 420–424.

Thompson, E. A. (1978). Smoking education programs 1960–1976. *American Journal of Public Health, 68*(3), 250–257.

Tobler, N. S. (1986). Meta-analysis of 143 adolescent drug prevention programs: Quantitative outcome results of program participation compared to a control comparison group. *Journal of Drug Issues, 17,* 537–567.

US Department of Health and Human Services (US DHHS). (1990). *Health people 2000: National health promotion and disease prevention objectives.* United States Department of Health and Human Services, Public Health Service (PHS), Centers for Disease Control, Center for Health Promotion and Education, Office on Smoking and Health. DHHS Publication No. (PHS), 91-50212. Washington, DC: Government Printing Office.

US DHHS. (1991). *Strategies to control tobacco use in the United States: A blueprint for public health action in the 1990s.* US DHHS, PHS, National Institutes of Health, National Cancer Institute. NIH Publication No. 92-3316. Washington, DC: Government Printing Office.

US DHHS. (1994). *Preventing tobacco use among young people: A report of the Surgeon General.* US DHHS, PHS, CDC, S/N 0/7 001-00491-0. Washington, DC: Government Printing Office.

US Public Health Service. (US PHS). (1964). *Smoking and health. A report of the advisory committee to the Surgeon General of the Public Health Service.* US DHEW, Public Health Service. PHS Publication No. 1103. Washington, DC: Government Printing Office.

Velicer, W. F., DiClemente, C. C., Prochaska, J. O., & Brandenburg, N. (1985). Decisional balance measure for assessing and predicting smoking status. *Journal of Personality and Social Psychology, 48,* 1279–1289.

Ward, K. D., Klesges, R. C., & Halpern, M. T. (1997). Predictors of smoking cessation and state-of-the-art smoking interventions. *Journal of Social Issues, 53,* 129–145.

CHAPTER 9

Obesity and Nutrition

Bonnie A. Spear and Christopher Reinold

Introduction

Obesity in America has reached epidemic proportions. It has been called a major health care crisis. In little over a decade, between 1971–1980 and 1988–1991, the prevalence of significantly overweight adults in the United States rose by 33%, far from the decrease of 23% targeted by the US Public Health Service. Currently, 20% of adolescent children and approximately one third of all adults in America are defined as obese. Minority populations, especially minority women, are disproportionately affected; nearly 50% of African-American women are overweight. Overweight and obese adults are at increased risk for morbidity and mortality associated with acute and chronic medical conditions including hypertension, elevated serum lipid levels, coronary artery disease, diabetes mellitus, respiratory disease, certain types of cancer, gout, and arthritis (American Dietetic Association, 1997).

While a few overweight individuals are fortunate enough not to display the adverse health risks that are associated with increased weight, the majority of Americans do, and it is evident that the main effect of weight gain on mortality is its affect in promoting the rise in blood pressure and the rise in blood cholesterol levels, particularly the low-density lipoprotein fraction. In terms of public health, it is the underlying effects of weight gain with age that increase the risks of high cholesterol and hypertension (James, 1995).

The prevalence of obesity in Americans is at its highest at precisely the same time that our life expectancy is at its highest. In America and many European countries (e.g., Britain and Finland) there is an escalating problem of obesity and at the same time a significant reduction in mortality rates from cardiovascular diseases (CVD). This situation demonstrates that factors other than obesity influence our health. One such explanation is the decline in smoking.

Some of the gains made in CVD prevention have to do with nutritional interactions. Fat intake has decreased but an even more significant change is the types of fat

Bonnie A. Spear and Christopher Reinold • Department of Pediatrics, School of Medicine, University of Alabama at Birmingham, Birmingham, Alabama 35294.

Handbook of Health Promotion and Disease Prevention, edited by Raczynski and DiClemente. Kluwer Academic/Plenum Publishers, New York, 1999.

ingested. It is clear that the general trend in food preparation is shifting away from saturated fat and toward unsaturated. This may not result in a reduction in weight, but it will improve cardiac outcomes.

Health care expenditures could be decreased by reducing the prevalence of obesity. In the United States alone, we could have saved approximately $45.8 billion or 6.8% of the health care expenditures in 1990 alone if obesity were prevented. Similarly, 52.9 million days of lost productivity would have been averted, saving employers nearly $4 billion (Wolf & Golditz, 1996).

The prevalence of obesity in children is also on the rise, and the numbers of overweight children and adolescents are higher than at any time in the past. Reasons for increased weights among children and adolescents may include eating while doing homework, eating in their bedrooms, excessive televission watching (>2 hours/day), eating alone (lack of family meals), large helpings, large number of snack foods, fast food more than four times per week, and a decrease in physical activity. Studies clearly suggest that obese subjects tend to eat more fast foods than nonobese subjects and more frequently skip early morning meals.

It is clear that the problem of obesity affects all age levels and that an approach geared toward both the treatment and prevention of obesity is necessary. What is unclear is why there has been such a rapid rise in the prevalence of obesity. There are many current hypotheses to suggest reasons for the rise, but there is no clear consensus. It is possible that social conditions such as stress and isolation may contribute to the problem. A clear link has been found between abdominal fat and cortisol responses to stress testing (James, 1995). They propose that constant stress-induced cortisol secretion will promote channeling of fat stores to abdominal tissues.

There is now an emerging link between low birth weight and the future likelihood of high adult waist-to-hip ratio; a baby's weight and body proportions are also increasingly being linked to maternal nutrition (James, 1995). For many years we have known that obese pregnant women tend to have big babies and this is particularly true if they have significant glucose intolerance or gestational diabetes during pregnancy. Though not inevitable, there is a tendency for large babies to retain their percentile positions during growth and to become tall and plump children. James (1995) proposes an interesting consideration that because we have populations with young women becoming progressively heavier, we may be in the process of inducing major intergenerational changes because of the reprogramming of the genotype. From his own research it appears that maternal nutrition has a profound effect on the early responses of the ovum, and that fetal growth and size may be programmed very early (James, 1995). The conclusion that James makes is that gene–environmental interactions underlie almost all genetically related disorders, including obesity, and there is now evidence that environmental reprogramming of genetic traits may be profoundly impacting the prevalence of obesity in our young children. This evidence coupled with the poor eating habits and lack of physcial activity of so many young children and adolescents are likely to be working together to cause the intergenerational amplification of the prevalence of obesity.

Kelly Brownell (1997) describes the availability of high-fat foods in the United States today as a toxic environment. He points out that there is now an unprecedented availability of poorly nutrient-dense food. Americans have ready access to foods that are inexpensive, high in fat, and good tasting. In fast-food restaurants, quick-stop food marts, and 24-hour gas stations highly fattening food is readily available even in the poorest neighborhoods.

All these problems, from changing eating habits, decreasing physical activity, increased societal stress, and increased influence from marketing and advertising, demonstrate the difficulties in dealing with the problem of obesity. It is clear that primary prevention in addition to determining the best method for treatment of obesity is the key. We will not be effective in dealing with the crisis of obesity without addressing both its prevention and treatment.

Epidemiology of Obesity

According to findings from the Third National Health and Nutrition Examination Survey (NHANES III), substantial proportions of the US population at all age levels are overweight. Specifically, among women, 34% of non-Hispanic whites, 52% of non-Hispanic blacks, and 50% of Hispanics are overweight. Among men the overall average is approximately 33% (NCHS, 1997).

Racial Differences

In comparing racial differences, black women are at greater risk for developing obesity than white women. While black women are overweight more frequently than white women in adulthood, the prevalence in infancy and early childhood has been reported to be less than or equal to that of whites. This suggests that during the preadolescent period and the adolescent years, racial differences in obesity emerge. In a study conducted by McNutt, Hu, and Schriber (1997), over the age span of 9 to 14 years, black girls more frequently engage in eating practices that are believed to be associated with weight gain than do whites, even when controlling for parental income, education, and number of parents or guardians in the household. These eating practices are clearly associated with weight gain and are frequently the targets of behaviorally based weight management programs. These findings suggest that other influences such as cultural factors may affect behavior.

Not only are adult black females less concerned about their own weight and weight reduction, they also appear more tolerant of obese individuals compared to black males and whites. In a study of 1000 teenagers, black girls had a higher desired weight, were more concerned about being underweight, and generally seemed more satisfied with their figures than did white girls (McNutt *et al.*, 1997). Kumanyika and Wilson (1993) suggest that there is a greater tolerance and perhaps acceptance of obesity in the black culture. In one study she found that only 36% of severely overweight black women reported their husband or boyfriend thought they were very overweight.

The limited data available indicate that proportionally more overweight adolescents, principally females, are found in Native American and Hispanic groups. Among Native America tribes, there are a range of levels of overweight individuals. The trends in overweight from compilation of data, however, indicate a rapidly increasing prevalence of overweight in adults and children. The trends are especially striking among southwestern Native Americans and somewhat less among native Alaskans. Data from the NHANES national survey afford an opportunity to compare Mexican Americans, Cuban Americans, and Puerto Rican Americans from one year and older. Cuban Americans have slightly lower proportions of overweight obese males and females than other Hispanic groups; this difference is consistent among adults. For children and adolescents, the proportion of overweight individuals is greater than for white, non-Hispanic groups. Throughout the age range and across all Hispanic groups, females have proportionally greater overweight and obese categorization than do males (Braussard, Johnson, & Himes, 1991; Knowler *et al.*, 1991; Pawson, Martorell, & Mendoza, 1991).

Although the behaviors associated with increased weight gain are more prevalent in some minority populations, there are behaviors that are occurring in all population groups and causing an estimated 1% per year increase in the incidence of obesity. The prevention of obesity has become a high priority. Physicians approaching the subject of prevention may feel detached because they see little role for themselves other than as health educators and prescribers of obesity drugs. We have become accustomed to thinking of obesity in terms of one patient and his responsibility for his health. To reverse the trends, we must begin to ask why obesity rates have increased with age and why there has been such a profound increase in the past 10 years.

Defining Obesity

The exact definition of obesity has always been somewhat difficult to determine and, indeed, somewhat controversial. Professionals are coming to a closer consensus through the use of the body mass index (BMI). BMI is a weight-for-height index expressed as kg/m^2. This relationship between weight and height is now being used to help assess a person's health. This definition is now recognized, because although obesity is an excess in body fat, it is difficult to measure body fat directly. The BMI usually predicts body fat well except in pregnant women, highly muscular individuals, and young children.

Overweight Prevalence of Children and Adolescents

From 1988 to 1991, the prevalence of overweight in children and adolescents was 10.9% based on the 95th percentile and 22% based on the 85th percentile cutoff points from cycles II and III of the NHANES. During that time, overweight prevalence increased during the period examined among all sex and age groups (Troiano, Flegal, Kuczmarski, Campbell, & Johnson, 1995).

The Framingham Children's Study, a longitudinal study of childhood cardiovascular risk behaviors, was conducted beginning in 1987. When age, television viewing, energy intake, and parent's BMIs were controlled for, inactive preschoolers were 3.8 times as likely as active preschoolers to have an increasing triceps skin fold measurements during follow up, rather than stable or decreasing triceps skinfold. This estimate was slightly higher for children with more body fat at baseline. Perhaps more importantly from a health risk standpoint, preschool children with low physical activity levels gained substantially more subcutaneous fat than did more active children (Moore, Nguyen, Rothman, Cupples, & Ellison, 1995).

Consequences of Obesity in Childhood

The most prevalent immediate consequences of overweight during childhood and adolescence are psychosocial. Beginning as young as 6 years of age, peers described overweight children as ugly, dishonest, lazy, and even stupid (Must, 1996).

Cultural messages regarding obesity are internalized by adolescence and often produce a lasting and distorted self-image.

A greater long-term health concern is the risk that adolescent's overweight persists into adulthood. Longitudinal studies tracking overweight trends suggest that 25–50% of adolescents who are overweight become overweight or obese adults. The percentage of overweight persisting into adulthood is even greater when tracking is restricted to adolescents who were measured above the 95th percentile for BMI (Must, 1996).

Weight Control Practices in America

In a study by Serdula *et al.* (1994) of nearly 61,000 adults, approximately 38% of women and 24% of men reported that currently they were trying to lose weight. Methods of weight loss reported included counting calories (24% of women and 14% of men), participating in organized weight-loss programs (10%, 3%), taking special supplements (10%, 7%), taking diet pills (4%, 2%), and fasting for 24 hours or longer (5%, 5%). Among both males and females, only half of those trying to lose weight reported using the recommended methods of caloric restriction combined with increased physical activity.

The question of whether intentional weight loss increases longevity of obese individuals is important, given the fact that the prevalence of obesity is currently so high. A number of studies published recently suggest that both weight loss and weight fluctuation are associated with increased mortality; however, in many of these studies factors such as smoking and preexisting illness are not considered in relation to the findings. A study in the United States (Williamson, 1997), controlling for confounding factors, found that intentional weight loss by overweight, white women consistently reduced mortality in those with obesity-related comorbidities. Those losing > 5 kg had the greatest reduction in both total and cardiovascular mortality. Weight loss was approximately 10% of initial body weight.

Theoretical Models

Although numerous theoretical models can be used in developing and implementing obesity prevention and intervention programs, three models appear to be the most commonly used. These are the health belief model, transtheoretical model or stages of change model, and relapse prevention model.

Health Belief Model

Health educators and health professionals who are planning programs in obesity prevention or intervention need to make use of the health belief variables, with special attention to self-efficacy and perceived barriers. Information should be obtained on the extent to which members of the target population feel competent in implementing the prescribed action over the time of the intervention. In the planning stages, data should be collected on health belief including self-efficacy. This would permit planning of more effective programs than otherwise would be possible. Interventions then can be targeted to the specific needs identified by such assessment. Additionally, program planners utilizing the health belief model should provide more emphasis on skills training to enhance self-efficacy. This can be done by breaking down the needed behavior changes in to short-term, easily managed target behavioral components. This requires a careful examination of the target behavior and identification of the specific aspects of the behavior that call for skill development. For example, in obesity management, dietary changes would be necessary. Skill development of decreasing the fat content would include skills in the area of choosing correct foods, label reading, proper cooking techniques, and menu planning. Specific tasks could be arranged in a specific sequence to that they can be consecutively mastered, with beginning tasks being easier than subsequent tasks. In addition, setting short-term goals may be more helpful than setting long-term goals that the client feels are unreachable.

Transtheoretical Model or Stages of Change Model

A weight management program for an adult or adolescent who is not ready to change not only may be futile but also harmful because an unsuccessful program may diminish the individual's self-esteem and prevent future efforts to improve weight. If a younger child is not ready for change, the parent who is ready can successfully modify diet and activity. Families who are not ready to change may express a lack of concern about the child's obesity, may believe the obesity is inevitable and cannot be changed, or are not interested in modifying activity or eating. The provider-based assessment and counseling for exercise (PACE), a program cosponsored by the Centers for Disease Control and Prevention and the Association for Teachers of Preventive Medicine, guide clinicians as they counsel adult patients to improve activity and includes questions about patient readiness (Long *et al.*, 1996). An adolescent program is under development. Depending on the severity of the obesity, families who are not ready for change may benefit from counseling to improve motivation or from deferral of obesity therapy until they are ready for action. Motivation interviewing (Rollnick, Healther, & Bell, 1992), a technique used with adults to prepare them to change addictive behavior, may have applications in obesity treatment.

A study by Campbell *et al.* (1994) demonstrated that messages individually tailored to a person's stage of change generated a significantly greater reduction in dietary fat intake than nontailored messages. Interventions based on a stages of change model could help professionals use this model to target interventions to reduce dietary fat intakes more effectively. The Campbell study developed an algorithm for classifying person's stages of change using the action criterion of fat intake $\leq 30\%$ of energy. This algorithm is a rapid, self-administered instrument that can be used to tailor interventions to a person's stage of change. Future research is needed to determine which strategies are most effective in helping individuals accelerate their rate of change in reducing dietary fat intake.

Relapse Prevention

The effort to improve the maintenance of weight loss will be aided by increased understanding of the behavioral, cognitive, emotional, physiological, and social factors associated with regaining lost weight. There is little information about how these factors interact to cause weight regain. The reason for this lack of knowledge is clear: Weight regain usually occurs after patients have finished treatment and no longer are seen in the clinic. Only after relapse do we see again patients. Although many programs have extended the duration of treatment that has decreased the amount of relapse, relapse is still a critical problem in obesity management. In relapse prevention training, patients need to be taught to identify high-risk situations and learn skills to cope with such situations.

Primary Prevention

Prevention can be divided into primary prevention and secondary and tertiary prevention. Primary prevention is designed to intervene before the start of the problem, thereby preventing obesity in the population. There have been numerous successful community-based primary prevention programs. Unfortunately, the programs can be expensive and prevention efforts stop when funding stops. The key to primary prevention is to develop prevention strategies that will continue once funding has ceased. A discussion of community-based programs that have been successful follows.

School-Based Primary Prevention Programs

The fact that pediatric obesity has increased dramatically over the last two decades is well known. Since 40–80% of obese adolescents become obese adults, many of the primary prevention programs have concentrated on the pediatric population.

More than 90% of the nation's children and adolescents are in school. The schools are the primary educating facilities and major socializing environments. Young people's experiences in school help to determine their vulnerability to health problems during adolescence. Today, more than 25 million children participate in the National Child Nutrition Program daily. Therefore, schools appear to be the prime setting for health promotion and obesity prevention programs.

Research during the 1980s, sponsored by the National Heart, Lung and Blood Institute (NHLBI) (Stone, 1985; Stone, Perry, & Luepker, 1989), tested components of the social learning model of intervention with children and have reported favorable results for knowledge and attitudes and modest improvements on behavior and physiological measures. The majority of the school-based health promotion studies do not focus only on prevention of obesity, but concentrate on overall health promotion as well. Recently, there have been several programs incorporating the multicomponent prevention model, beginning in elementary and extending to high school. Three such programs are included here.

The Health Ahead/Health Smart elementary health promotion program funded by NHLBI incorporated all aspects of the school environment and encouraged elementary schoolchildren, beginning in kindergarten, to adopt healthy lifestyles by promoting realistic judgments of personal ability and self-esteem (Berenson, Arbeit, Hunter, Johnson & Nicklas, 1991). The program incorporated classroom, physical education, food service, and the family into the prevention activity.

The K–6 classroom curriculum covered (1) cardiovascular health, anatomy and physiology, infectious disease, and injury prevention; (2) nutrition and eating behavior; (3) physical activity and exercise behavior; and (4) behavioral and coping skills. The physical education component included a 12–lesson curriculum and aerobic activities integrated into the physical education program. The goals of the school food service program were to modify school meals for total fat, saturated fat, and sodium through menu planning, food purchasing, recipe modification, and food preparation and production techniques. To complete the program, there was a parent support program that not only kept parents informed through newsletters but also included popular school health fairs.

Results of this program showed that school lunch choices were successfully altered and children whose lunch choices were healthy showed the greatest cholesterol reduction. Improvements in run–walk performance were associated with overall risk reductions. Additionally, increases in high-density lipoprotein-cholesterol (HDL-C) were observed at all intervention schools.

The Child and Adolescent Trial for Cardiovascular Health (CATCH) is an NHLBI-sponsored multisite longitudinal field trial for a multidisciplinary primary prevention intervention for children in grades 3, 4, and 5 from culturally diverse populations. The primary goal was to assess the effects of the intervention on changing the environment of schools (food service and physical education) and lifestyles of children (eating and physical activity behaviors) to reduce subsequent cardiovascular disease risk (Perry *et al.*, 1992). CATCH also included activities for the classroom, physical education, and food service as well as with the family. The classroom curriculum focused on eating patterns and physical activity patterns. The physical education component sought to increase the amount of moderate-to-vigorous physical activity to 40% of the class period at school and to encourage these activities outside of school. The food service component was designed to provide children with tasty meals lower in fat (<30% of calories), saturated fat (<10% of calories), and sodium (600–1000 mg/serving) while maintaining adequate calories and essential nutrients. Only certain schools were randomized to the family intervention component. This included activity packets that were sent home and family night at school (games, healthy snacks, contests, and awards).

CATCH demonstrated that a school-based program involving school food service, physical education, classroom curricula, and the family could be successfully implemented in diverse populations in four areas of the country. The school environment can be changed to allow children the practice of healthful behaviors without adding substantial cost and time to the busy school schedule. These changes, when continued for several years, have considerable potential for altering behaviors long term and perhaps for producing cardiovascular health benefits (Luepker *et al.*, 1996).

The most recent nutritional primary prevention program has been the National Cancer Institute's 5-a-Day program. This has been a merger of public and private groups, and for the first time has included the point of sale food industry as well as a national marketing campaign. The message from 5-a-Day is to include five fruits and vegetables each day in the diet in order to reduce risk of cancer as well as to improve the overall nutrition quality of the diet. Diets high in fruits and vegetables are lower in calories and fat and can have direct effects on achieving healthy weights. The majority of the programs have been school-based programs where the school food service increased the availability, variety, and types of fruits and vegetables meeting 5-a-Day standards. There was also an increased emphasis on improving the choices in vending machines in the schools. A family component of flyers and home activities have also been included in the programs. Results indicate that through environmental changes (food service) and education, children and adolescents improve their intakes of fruits and vegetables.

This is in agreement with a study by Story and Resnick (1986) in which they determined that adolescents' perceived barriers toward improving their diets were (1) lack of time, (2) inconvenience of eating properly, (3) lack of urgency, and (4) cost. When fresh fruits, fruit juice, and vegetables were made conveniently available in the school cafeteria and in the vending machines at a lower cost than the higher fat and calorie snacks, there was a significant increase in these foods being purchased. When the cost returned to normal, the rate of consumption went down.

Barriers to Primary Interventions in the Schools

Many barriers exist in the school setting that hinder effective health promotion. These include: (1) limited resources including staff, space, and school scheduling; (2) declining health education and physical education programs; and (3) difficulty in making changes in school food service due to staff resistance to change and the role of "competitive foods" within the school. An increasing number of programs aimed at reaching parents are being developed. But this too has its limitations. The trend of both parents working and the increasing prevalence of single-parent families could account for a large proportion of the lack of parental involvement in school-based health education programs. In the CATCH program, in-school family activities that were successful at the third grade level were less attended as the children progressed to higher grade levels.

Community-Based Health Promotion Programs

It is estimated that overweight employees cost business more than any other health risk, including smoking. Health insurance claims of overweight employees are about 37% higher than their slimmer counterparts and the number of days spend in hospitals are 143% greater. Thus, companies are attempting to offer health promotion activities to address employees' needs.

Studies (Crump, Ear, Chiasma, & Hertz-Paced, 1996; Lemer & Shemer, 1996) assessing work site health promotion showed that overall, employees on average participated in fewer than two agency-supported health-related activities per year. Minority employees and employees in lower-level positions were more likely to participate in fitness activities when organizations had a more comprehensive program structure, engaged in more marketing strategies, gave time off to employees to participate, or had on-site facilities. Results also indicate that programs often enrolled people who already were committed to healthy lifestyles and did not reach the high-risk segments of the work force. More research is needed on how to reduce the barriers and design programs to reach the obese and high-risk individuals who could benefit from work site wellness activities.

Four large-scale, community-based health promotion programs—the Stanford Three-Community Study, the Stanford Five-City Study, the North Karelia Study, and the Minnesota Heart Health Program—have evaluated programs aimed at weight. The results have been discouraging. Although prevention of obesity was not the sole focus of the programs, each included projects targeting weight using multiple channels of intervention (media, physicians, work sites, etc.). The results in each case indicated that the trend of obesity was not slowed even though there were improvements in other areas such as smoking and blood pressure (Stunkard, 1995).

With the high competition of health care plans, a recent study by Schauffler and Rodriques (1994) showed that the persons enrolled in health maintenance organizations (HMOs) that offered stop-smoking programs, stress management programs, weight control programs, cholesterol and blood pressure screening, or any health promotion program were more satisfied with their health plan than those who did not have these services available. Additionally, employees who participated in a health promotion program were more satisfied than employees who had not participated in a structured program. These findings have important implications for designing and restructuring health plans to better meet consumer preferences.

In summary, nutrition primary prevention programs have been targeted primarily at school-aged children. During this age, health behavior habits are formed that will affect the individual for a lifetime. Studies in this age group have shown that intervention can change or improve behaviors to healthier ones. Major health initiatives are addressing this population but sustaining the programs once the funding has stopped is critical. This may require policy or political changes that often are not addressed. Intervention programs for adults are targeted at more of an individual level, addressing areas of perceived susceptibility such as cancer and cardiovascular disease. Weight management, improving dietary intake, and prevention of obesity are often several of the many components of these interventions. Until health insurers recognize the benefit of health promotion and primary prevention, there will be few programs for adults.

Secondary and Tertiary Prevention

Secondary prevention focuses on reducing the duration or ill effects of the disorder through early recognition and effective treatment. Secondary prevention may be a promising approach to obesity, especially if children are the focus (Battle & Brownell, 1996). Additionally, secondary and tertiary prevention methods should be targeted at the individual as well as at the environmental level.

Intervention in Children and Adolescents

School-based interventions designed for obese children appear to have mixed results. Foster, Wadden, and Brownell (1985) implemented a school-based, peer-led program for treatment and prevention of obesity in second through fifth graders. Results showed significant differences in weight loss and self-concept between intervention and control groups, with program children reducing and control subjects increasing their percentage overweight. However, there was only partial maintenance at an 18-week follow-up.

A 2-year program by Donnelly et al. (1996) used nutrition education, physical activity, and modification of the school lunch in rural schools to address obesity issues and promote physical and metabolic fitness. The program improved the diets of intervention compared to control children in school, but not outside of school. However, improved physical activity in school was associated with less activity outside of school and had no effect on weight. Williams et al. (1997) advocates that secondary prevention should be based on attention to the obese child, presumably in the clinical setting.

A 10–year follow-up study conducted by Epstein, Valoski, Wind, and McCurley (1990) of a family-based intervention program showed that interventions need to focus on reinforcing weight loss and behavior change for both parent and child. In this study, obese children, 6 to 12 years of age, from two-parent, mostly white, middle-class families in which at least one parent was obese, were treated with their parents for 8 months in weekly meetings, followed by monthly meeting. They were randomized into three behavior treatment groups. Group 1 focused on and rewarded weight loss and behavior change for both parent and child; group 2 focused on weight loss and behavior change only for the child; and group 3 reinforced attendance at meetings only. At the end of 8 months, weight loss in the three groups were similar, with a decrease in weight by about 17%. At 21 months, again there was no difference. But by 5 years the differences were striking. Children in group 1 had maintained their relative weight change, and 42% were no longer obese. Children in group 2 had regained to baseline, with only 19% not obese. Group 3 were heavier than at baseline, with only 5% not obese. These authors state that many benefits may be gained from treating childhood obesity. They suggest, however, that negative side effects of dieting or dieting inappropriately may include eating disorders, poor nutrition, and less than expected growth.

In the pediatric population, treatment programs should provide weight management that ideally has the child within 20% of the average weight for height; teach appropriate eating and exercise habits so the child can maintain a lower relative weight while getting appropriate nutrition for growth and development, be appropriate for child's age, developmental capabilities, and parental influence; and incorporate a diet that lowers weight/height, a maintenance program that promotes growth, and an exercise program that the child finds fun and that is realistic for the child to follow.

Epstein (1986) has developed a multiple-stage model for the treatment of obesity. This model shifts the responsibility for habit change from the parent to the child based on the child's developmental capabilities. Although these can be used as a guide, the interventionist must evaluate the child's cognitive ability and tailor the program to meet the family/individual's needs. These guidelines include:

1. Age 1–5 years: The program must focus on parent management, as parents are the major influences on child eating and activity. Children of this age are most likely not motivated.
2. Age 5–8 years: A program in this age group must focus on parent management, but the child must be trained to handle social situation in which food is offered. The child can learn to solicit parental cooperation so that reciprocal reinforcement occurs with the parent or significant adult.
3. Age 8–12 years: Although children are still responsive to parent management methods, they can take greater responsibility for weight loss. Reading and writing skills are more advanced and children are capable of self-monitoring and goal setting. Children in this age group are more motivated to lose weight to improve athletic performance, look better, and avoid criticism from peers.
4. Age 13 and older: Children in this age group possess the motivation and capability of managing their program with appropriate support from their parents. Behavior management programs for adolescents must be carefully planned, because conflict can arise when parents are involved as the adolescent is struggling for independence.

Adult Interventions

Shape Up America and the American Obesity Association (1996) have sponsored the development of a document, "Guidance for Treatment of Adult Obesity," as well as a treatment model. The document provides the first comprehensive medical guidelines for the treatment of obesity and was developed by a seven-member expert panel composed of clinical and basic scientists, practicing physicians and surgeons, and specialist in psychology, nutrition, and epidemiology.

Both the assessment of recommended risk and treatment decisions are outlined in the document. The determination of the patient's BMI-related health risk using BMI alone and adjusted in combination with the presence of comorbid conditions and/or other risk factors are important. Until recently, a major criterion for measuring successful weight loss was the attainment of ideal body weight. However, the calculation of BMI-based targets is replacing ideal body weight as a primary means of evaluating the degree of overweight obesity and weight-associated health risks. A BMI of >27 has been used by many investigators as a starting point for obesity. BMI is a useful index in the assessment of weight because it has been related to disease risks. It relates weight to height and eliminates the measure of frame size. It is the same for men and women aged 19–70 years. For children, new soon to be released BMI guidelines will have tables by age and gender. One advantage of the BMI is that it deemphasizes ideal weight and presents a healthy range for each height.

The American Health Foundation (Meisler, 1996) recommends a healthy weight of a BMI between 19 and 25 for everyone over the age of 20. Table 1 shows treatment strategies with level of BMI.

The recommended focus of weight loss efforts should be a loss of 10% of initial body weight and for long-term changes necessary to sustain this degree of weight loss. For example, modest weight losses of 5–10% have been shown to decrease total cholesterol by approximately 16%, decrease low-density lipoprotein (LDL)–cholesterol by 12%, increase HDL–cholesterol by 18%, and improve the LDL–HDL ratio (Institute of Medicine, 1996). In obese person with diabetes, weight losses of 5–10% increases glycemic control and reduces hyperinsulinemia (Kanders, 1992).

The treatment model developed by Shape Up America and the American Obesity Association (1996) guides the practitioner or counselor on how to assess and treat the obese adult. A key component is assessing the individuals readiness to change. This critical component is often missed in weight management programs and often labels the individual as noncompliant and/or frustrates the practitioner. This model

Table 1. Treatment Strategies for Different Levels of BMI

BMI category	Health risk based solely on BMI	Risk adjusted for presence of comorbid conditions and/or risk factors	Treatments
<25	Minimal	Low	Healthy eating plan, moderate, increased
25–<27	Low	Moderate	Behavior modification
27–<30	Moderate	High	May add: low-calorie diets
30–<35	High	Very high	May need to add:
35–<40	Very high	Extremely high	Pharmacotherapy and/or surgical
> 40	Extremely high	Extremely high	interventions

allows for individuals in different stages of readiness but still provides them information and guidance in all stages.

Of interest is preliminary work being done by Pronk *et al.* (1998) regarding telephone counseling. In a trial project funded by a managed care organization, 30 adults were counseled for weight loss over the telephone. The intervention lasted greater than six months and each participant averaged 11.6 calls from the counselor. Results measured in the office of their primary care physician showed a mean weight loss of 11.4 pounds, a mean decrease in BMI by 1.85, and an increase in VO_2 Max by 1.2 ml/kg/min. Although, still in progress, this type of work may show the future of nutrition counseling for weight loss.

Currently, there are many national secondary and tertiary intervention programs. Noncommercial weight loss/support organizations include:

1. TOPS Club, Inc. (Take Off Pounds Sensibly) is an international, nonprofit, noncommercial weight loss support group. Members obtain an exercise and food plan and a goal weight from their personal physicians. TOPS provides a supportive environment in which an individual can make the slow, steady, permanent lifestyle changes necessary to reach and maintain their personal goals. There are no data on the amount of weight loss or reduction in comorbidities in this program.
2. Overeaters Anonymous (OA) is a nonprofit international organization that provides volunteer support groups worldwide patterned after 12-step Alcoholics Anonymous program. Members are encouraged to seek professional help for individualized diet–nutrition plan and for emotional or physical problems. This program makes no exercise or food recommendations.

Physical Activity

The 1996 Surgeon General's Report on Physical Fitness and Health (US Department of Health and Human Services, 1996) identified inactivity as a significant health problem for Americans. The report concluded that Americans can substantially improve their health and quality of life by including moderate amounts of physical activity in their daily lives. The Surgeon General's report found that more than 60% of American adults practice no regular physical activity. One quarter of adults are not active at all. Additionally, almost half of all young people aged 12 to 21 years are not vigorously active on a regular basis and 14% are completely inactive. Girls are twice as likely as boys to be inactive. In the 1990s alone, daily participation in physical education classes by high school students dropped dramatically, form 42% in 1991 to 25% in 1995.

Increasing physical activity behavior will be one of the most important behavioral changes targeted in a weight management problem. Engaging in physical activity on a regular basis reduces the risk of developing the comorbidities of obesity including coronary heart disease, hypertension, and diabetes. Additionally, regular physical activity can build and maintain healthy bones, muscles, and joints. Adults who engage in moderate physical activity, such as walking and gardening, four or more times a week are 33% less likely to die than those who are inactive during the same period of time. By recognizing that some physical activity is better than none and that every movement counts toward reducing obesity and preventing the development of chronic disease, the President's Council on Physical Fitness has many programs that target increasing the amount of physical activity. These include the President's Council Physical Fitness Test conducted with children in grade school. All children who participate are given a participation certificate and those who exceed the minimum standards are given certificates of achievement. The council also has programs as well as media campaigns targeted to adults. The impact of these programs in reducing the amount of physical inactivity on weight loss is unknown.

Television and computer use have a major impact on inactivity. Dietz and Gortmaker (1985) examined the association of television viewing and obesity in data collected using NHANES II and III. Results showed significant associations between time spent watching televison and the prevalence of obesity. In 12- to 17-year-old adolescents, the prevalence of obesity increased by 2% for each additional hour of television viewed. The associations persisted when prior obesity, region, season, population density, race, socioeconomic class, and a variety of other family variables were controlled for. The strength of the association suggests that televison viewing may contribute to obesity in at least some children and adolescents. The potential effects of obesity on activity and the consumption of calorically dense foods are consistent with this hypotheses.

Environmental Level

In the United States today, there is an unprecedented availability of nutritionally poor food. More than any other populations in the world, Americans have ready access to foods that are relatively inexpensive, high in fat, and good tasting. In addition to fast food restaurants, food courts, and vending machines, service stations are now equipped with 24-hour markets that concentrate on the sale of high-fat foods.

Fast-Food Franchises

Increasing numbers of Americans are eating in fast-food restaurants. Seven percent of the US population eats at McDonald's every day; 75% of the firm's business consists of people who eat there at least twice a week (Brownell, 1997). Although restaurants are responding to consumer demand with lower-fat foods, the majority of the foods in all fast-food restaurants derive greater than 40% of calories from fat.

Serving Sizes

Visitors from other countries often marvel at the serving sizes of food in American restaurants and indeed at the size of our meals in general. Consider, for example, fast-food meals that offer a burger, fries, and a drink at a cost lower than the individual items sold separately. Because of the perceived bargain, many people select these meals and as a result consume extra fat and extra calories. The fast-food establishment is now so much a part of American culture that the word "supersize" has entered our vocabulary as a verb (Brownell, 1997).

Food Advertising

Food advertisements can be both beguiling and deceptive. Examples include calling pork "the other white meat," packaging yogurt in 6 rather than 8 ounce containers and calling it "lower fat," or putting the label "no cholesterol " on a bag of potato chips. Most consumers consider that products labeled "low fat" are also low calorie. But, in fact, many of the "low-fat" foods have the same calories as the regular food of that product. Such claims contribute to the difficulties people have in maintaining their weight (Brownell, 1997).

Environmental factors are major contributors to the failure of weight loss and maintenance programs. From a very young age, people are exposed to powerful messages about how they can and should look. As a result, people aspire to unrealistic ideals of how much weight they can lose and what they will ultimately look like. Health professionals must understand the impact of culture on body image before they can appreciate the importance and difficulty of helping people accept that modest weight losses are beneficial.

One example of this is the analysis of the change in the average weights of Miss America contestants between 1960 and 1988. In 1960, the average Miss America contestant was 11% below healthy weight; in 1988, the average was 16% below healthy weight. One diagnostic criterion for anorexia nervosa is weight 15% or more below ideal. Similarly, the average fashion model has a BMI of 16, while clinicians begin to worry about eating disorders when the BMI falls below 19. This idealization of women who are extemely thin results in unrealistic and unhealthy weight goals for most American women (Brownell, 1997).

Health education initiatives must focus on addressing this environmental and communicative elements to aid in the prevention of obesity in the American population. Without this intervention, Americans will continue to be misled and receive potentially dangerous health messages.

Summary

In summary, secondary and tertiary interventions must address obesity at the individual as well as the environmental level. Without both, the prevalence of obesity will continue to increase, placing a further strain on the health care dollar. Addressing intervention and prevention strategies in the pediatric population appears to be the most promising, because if children enter adulthood in a healthy weight range, this will greatly reduce the incidences of adult obesity. Additionally, emphasis and education needs to be placed on increasing the physical activity of the American population. Nutrition education is beginning to work by reducing the dietary fat, but health education must emphasis physical activity to decrease the rise in obesity.

Future Research Directions

Presently, there are a scant number of preventive programs that work effectively in the schools. It will be necessary to pilot different ways of increasing moderate activity among our children as well as to continue to improve the child nutrition programs. The schools need to be rewarded (e.g., grant money or donations at the local level to purchase athletic equipment) for being innovative, and the successes need to be marketed effectively to other schools. These programs will target the primary prevention of obesity.

To reverse the current trends, we must begin to think in terms of community and what can be done locally to help reverse the trends of our sedentary lifestyles. We need to develop a completely new series of schemes, not only to affect the whole community, but to deal effectively with high-risk patients. We must combine health promotion and obesity management in the same forum. At the health care provider level, doctors need to be able to relate to their patients in regard to their diets as well as the importance of activity. Clinical studies of the use of "Guidance for Treatment of Adult Obesity" (Shape Up America and American Obesity Association, 1996) need to be completed to determine the effectiveness of this model in a primary care setting. Families need to understand the importance of preventive behaviors like increasing activity, family meals, less dependance on fast and convience foods, playing with your kids, walking the dogs, and so on.

We also must reach people at the consumer level. There is currently so much information available that consumers are tired of trying to sift through all of our recommendations. What is worthwhile and what is hype? The American Dietetic Association (1997) has a new campaign to reach the consumer with meaningful health messages. The authors want to encourage people to make healthy lifestyle choices so they can do the things they want to do. This includes staying active, feeling healthy, and so forth. Future research goals should include the addition of these recommendations and how best to "market" them to the consumer.

While we encourage people, we should think in terms of messages that will be helpful to them and also get our health messages across. These recommendations were formed by an alliance of differing interests including the Food Marketing Institute, National Cattlemen's Beef Association, National Pork Producers Council, the Produce Marketing Association, and many other varied alliance members. This team–community marketing approach has the potential to serve as a model for future interventions that directly target obesity. The recommendations from the alliance are designed to be simple and effective.

First, be realistic. Make small changes over time in what you eat and your physical activity. Second, be adventurous. Expand your tastes to enjoy a variety of foods. Third, be flexible. Go ahead and balance what you eat and your physical activity over several days. Fourth, be sensible. Enjoy all your favorite foods, just pay attention to your hunger cues and do not overdo it. Finally, be active. Walk the dog, don't just watch the dog walk. These recommendations will work because consumers find the messages simple, clear, positive, and humorous (The Dietary Guidelines Alliance, 1997).

Future studies need to determine the most effective tertiary treatment based on patients' risk categories. It will be necessary in the future to design very individualized treatment protocols in concert with primary interventions beginning in childhood and community programs that include neighborhood planning with local and regional community health goals. We must wed individualism with a sense of community health that will be seen as empowering to individuals and not as stifling to their freedoms.

Summary and Conclusions

The recent increase in the prevalence of overweight seen in all age groups reflects a population shift toward positive energy balance. Data from NHANES II and III suggest that a dramatic increase in energy intake alone does not explain the rapid increase in prevalence, particularly in adolescents and children. Concurrent with the increased availability of energy-dense foods is the move of the US population toward a sedentary lifestyle. Secular trends suggest parents perceive less time available for relaxation and family activities. The proportion of food expenditures spent on meals outside the home has increased since the 1970s, but has experienced more rapid increase during the past several years.

There has been a steady decline in physical education in the schools at the elementary and secondary levels. This is particularly troubling because school-based, health-oriented physical education provides both immediate beneficial health effects and serves to pique children's interest and affect lifelong activity patterns. It is clear that an effective program to target obesity must work on several levels within society.

First, it is crucial to focus on the prevention of overweight among our youth. Improvements in the child nutrition program that allows children appropriate choices of food that meet the dietary guidelines of < 30% of calories from fat but are also adequate in calories to promote growth are critical in health promotion activities. Nutrition professionals should become involved in the planning of menus, purchasing of food, and training of child nutrition workers. For physical education programs to contribute to the public health goal of lifelong activity, they should include moderate-intensity activities and should not focus exclusively on team-oriented sports activities and competitive sports. These play an important role in our society, but the weight competitive sports have at the elementary and secondary school level must be moderated to allow all students, regardless of skill level, to experience the benefit of moderate activity.

Second, our public health campaign must focus on the family and community. Individuals must be given the correct nutrition information and how to interpret nutrition advertising. Additionally, we must begin a campaign to help people realize and experience the benefits of physical activity. This has not been necessary in the past but is now, because our society is now so highly automated that it is possible and even preferable to move very little each day as part of our careers and daily activities. This trend, which can rightly be attributed to affluence, is one of the main reasons for the dramatic increased prevalence of obesity in the past several years. Concurrent to this campaign, we must raise the awareness of the importance of healthy body weight versus ideal body weight as well as the reasons (i.e., sedentary lifestyle, increased caloric intake) why our societal trends need to be redirected.

Third, we must approach the patient currently interested in weight loss in an individual, specialized way that complements the goals of our public health interventions, but also appropriately teaches behavior modification and realistic health-related goals. We must empower patients struggling to lose weight, particularly those with a great deal of weight to lose, with the belief that small losses have a significant health benefit. We must teach them to have realistic expectations and we must base our efforts on their health-related risks and monitor their success based on their ability to reduce that risk.

References

American Dietetic Association (ADA). (1997). Weight management: A position of the American Dietetic Association. *Journal of the American Dietetic Association, 97,* 71–74.

Battle, E. K., & Brownell, K. D. (1996). Confronting a rising tide of eating disorders and obesity: Treatment vs. prevention and policy. *Addictive Behaviors, 21,* 755–765.

Berenson, G. S., Arbeit, M. L., Hunter, S. M., Johnson, C. C., & Nicklas, T. A. (1991). Cardiovascular health promotion for elementary school children. *Annals of the New York Academy of Science, 623,* 299–313.

Braussard, B. A., Johnson, A., & Himes, J. H. (1991). Prevalence of obesity in American Indians and Alaska Natives. *American Journal of Clinical Nutrition, 53,* 1535s–1542s.

Brownell, K. D. (1997). Managing patient expectations for weight loss. In *New multidisciplinary strategies in obesity management.* Clark, NJ: Health Learning Systems.

Campbell, M. C., DeVellis, B. M., Strecher, V. J., Ammerman, A. S., DeVellis, R. E., & Sandler, R. S. (1994). The impact of message tailoring on dietary behavior change for disease prevention in primary care settings. *American Journal of Public Health, 84,* 739–787.

Crump, C. E., Ear, J. A., Chiasma, C. M., & Hertz-Paced, I. (1996). Effects of organization-level variable on differential employee participation in 10 federal work site health promotion programs. *Health Education Quarterly, 23(2),* 204–223.

The Dietary Guidelines Alliance. (1997). Reaching consumers with meaningful health messages: It's all about you. *Journal of the American Dietetics Association, 97,* 249.

Dietz, W. H., & Gortmaker, S. L. (1985). Do we fatten our children at the television set? Obesity and television viewing in children and adolescents. *Pediatrics, 75,* 807–812.

Donnelly, J. E., Jacobsen, D. J., Whatley, J. E., Hill, J. O., Swift, L. L., Cherrington, A., Polk, B., Tran, S. V., & Reed, G. (1996). Nutrition and physical activity program to attenuate obesity and promote physical and metabolic fitness in elementary school children. *Obesity Research, 4,* 229–243.

Epstein, L. (1986). Treatment of childhood obesity. In K. D. Brownell & J. P. Foreyt (Eds.), *Handbook of eating disorders* (pp. 157–179). New York: Basic Books.

Epstein, L. A., Valoski, R., Wind, & McCurley, J. (1990). The effects of a family based obesity treatment in children. *Journal of the American Medical Association, 264,* 2519–2523.

Foster, G. D., Wadden, T. A., & Brownell, K. D. (1985). Peer-led program for the treatment and prevention of obesity in the school. *Journal of Consulting and Clinical Psychology, 53,* 538–540.

Institute of Medicine. (1996). *Weighing the options: Criteria for evaluating weight-management programs.* Washington, DC: National Academy Press.

James, W. P. (1995). A public health approach to the problem of obesity. *International Journal of Obesity, 19,* 37S–45S.

Kanders, B. S., & Blackburn, G. L. (1991). Reducing primary risk factors by therapeutic weight loss. In T. A. Waddesk & T. B. Van Itallie (Eds.), *Treatment of the seriously obese patient* (pp. 213–230). New York: Guilford Press.

Knowler, W. C., Pettitt, D. J., Saad, M. F., Charles, M. A., Nelson, R. G.,. Howard, B. V., Bogardus, C., & Bennett, P. H. (1991). Obesity in Pima Indians: Its magnitude and relationship ship with diabetes. *American Journal of Clinical Nutrition, 53(6 Suppl),* 1543S–1551S.

Kumanyika, S., & Wilson, J. F. (1993). Weight-related attitudes and behaviors of black women. *Journal of the American Dietetic Association, 93,* 416–422.

Lemer, Y., & Shemer, J. (1996). Epidemiological characteristic or participants and nonparticipants in health promotion programs. *Journal of Occupational and Environmental Medicine, 38(5),* 535–538.

Long, B. J., Calfas, K. J., Wooten,W., Sallis, J. F., Patrick, K., Goldstein, M., Marcus, B. H., Schwenk,T. L., Chenoweth, J., Carter, R., Torres, T., Plalinkas, L. A., & Heath, G. (1996). A multisite field test of the acceptability of physical activity counseling in primary care: Project PACE. *American Journal of Preventive Medicine, 12,* 73–81.

Luepker, R. V., Perry, C. L., McKinlay, S. M., Nader, P. R., Parcel, G. S., Stone, E. J., Webber, L. S., Elder, J. P., Feldman, A. H., Johnson, C. C., & Kelder, S. H. for the CATCH Collaborative Groups. (1996). Outcomes of a field trial to improve children's dietary patterns and physical activity: The Child and Adolescent Trial for Cardiovascular Health (CATCH). *Journal of the American Dietetic Association, 275,* 768–776.

McNutt, S. W., Hu,Y., & Schriber, G. B. (1997). A longitudinal study of the dietary practices of black and white girls 9 and 10 years at enrollment: The NHLBI growth and health study. *Journal of Adolescent Health, 20,* 27–37.

Meisler, J. R., St. Jeor, S., Shapior, A., & Wynder, E. L. (1996). American Health Foundation Roundtable on health weight. *American Journal of Clinical Nutrition, 63,* 409s–477s.

Moore, L. L., Nguyen, U. S., Rothman, K. J., Cupples, L. A., & Ellison, R. C. (1995). Preschool physical activity levels and change in body fatness in young children: The Framingham children's study. *American Journal of Epidemiology, 142,* 982–988.

Must, A. (1996). Morbidity and mortality associated with elevated body weight in children and adolescents. *American Journal of Clinical Nutrition, 63,* 445s–447s.

National Center for Health Statistics (NCHS). (1997). Division of Health Examination Statistics, National Center for Health Statistics Update: *Prevalence of overweight among children, adolescents, and adults— United States, 1988–1994* (vol. 277, p. 1111).

Pawson, I. G., Martorell, R., & Mendoza, F. E. (1991). Prevalence of overweight and obesity in U.S. Hispanic populations. *American Journal of Clinical Nutrition, 53,* 1552w–1585s.

Perry, C. L., Parcel, G. S., Stone, E. J., Nader, P. H., McKinlay, S. M., Luepker, R. V., & Webber, L. S. (1992). The Child and Adolescent Trial for Cardiovascular Health (CATCH): Overview of the intervention program and evaluation methods. *Cardiovascular Risk Factors, 2(2),* 36–44.

Pronk, N. Telephone counseling for weight loss. (1997). Personal communication.

Rollnick, S. N., Healther, A., & Bell, A. (1992). Negotiating behavior change in medical settings: the development of brief motivational interviewing. *Journal of Mental Health, 1,* 25–37.

Schauffler, H. H., & Rodriques, T. (1994). Availability and unitization of health promotion programs and satisfaction with health plans. *Medical Care, 32(12),* 1182–1196.

Serdula, M. K., Williamson, D. F., Anda, R. F., Levy, A., Heaton, A., & Byers, T. (1994). Weight control practices in adults: Result of a mulitstate telephone survey. *American Journal of Public Health, 84*(11), 1821–1824.

Shape Up America. American Obesity Association. (1996). *Guidance for treatment of adult obesity.* Bethesda, MD: Shape Up America.

Stone, E. J. (1985). School-based health research funded by the National Heart, Lung and Blood Institute. *Journal of School Health, 55,* 168–174.

Stone, E. J., Perry, C. L., & Luepker, R. V. (1989). Synthesis of cardiovascular behavioral research for youth health promotion. *Health Education Quarterly, 16,* 155–169.

Story, M., & Resnick, M. J. (1986). Adolescent's perceived barriers towards improving their diets. *Journal of Nutrition Education, 18,* 125–128.

Stunkard, A. J. (1995). The prevention of obesity. In K. D. Brownell & C. G. Fairburn (Eds.), *Eating disorders and obesity: A comprehensive handbook* (pp. 572–576). New York: Guilford Press.

Troiano, R. P., Flegal, K. M., Kuczmarski, R. J., Campbell, S. M., & Johnson, C. L. (1995). Overweight prevalence and trends for children and adolescents. *Archives of Pediatrics and Adolescent Medicine, 149,* 1085–1091.

U.S. Department of Health and Human Services, Centers for Disease Control and Prevention, National Center for Chronic Disease Prevention and Health Promotion, President's Council on Physical Fitness and Sports. (1996). *Physical activity and health: A report of the Surgeon General.* Washington, DC: U.S. Government Printing Office.

Williams, C. L., Campanaro, L. A., Squillace, M., & Bollella, M. (1997). Management of childhood obesity in Pediatric Practice. In M. S. Jacobson, J. M. Rees, N. H. Golden, & C. E. Irwin (Eds.), *Adolescent nutritional disorders: Prevention and treatment* (pp. 225–240). Annals of the New York Academy of Sciences, Volume 817. New York: The New York Academy of Sciences.

Williamson, D. F. (1997). Intention weight loss: Patterns in the general population and its association with morbidity and mortality. *International Journal of Obesity and Related Metabolic Disorders, March,* s14–s19.

Wolf, A. M., & Golditz, G. A. (1996). Social and economic effects of body weight in the United States. *American Journal of Clinical Nutrition, 63,* 466S–469S.

CHAPTER 10

Physical Activity

Bonnie K. Sanderson and Herman A. Taylor, Jr.

Introduction

Physical activity is regarded as an essential component of a healthy lifestyle. The beneficial impact of regular physical activity on various diseases and physical and mental conditions varies widely. Evidence links regular physical activity to reducing the risk of all-cause mortality primarily due to lowered rates of cardiovascular disease (CVD) (Fig. 1) (Blair *et al.*, 1989; Paffenbarger, Hyde, Wing, & Hsieh, 1986). Unfit men who increase their physical activity patterns from sedentary to higher levels of physical activity and fitness reduce their risk of mortality from 24% to 44% (Blair *et al.*, 1995; Paffenbarger *et al.*, 1993). Regular physical activity impacts psychological health, which promotes health and disease resistance (Dishman, 1992), reduces stress and improves mood (Stephens, 1988), and enhances productivity and increases energy levels (Brown, 1990). There is an abundance of evidence that links regular physical activity with other positive health aspects on a variety of diseases and conditions (Bouchard, Shepard, & Stephens, 1994). The most striking health promotion evidence is the association of regular physical activity and its positive impact on CVD. Physical activity can lower mortality from CVD (Morris, Clayton, Everitt, Semmence & Burgess, 1990), and physically active people have about half the risk of developing coronary artery disease (CAD) compared to inactive people (Powell, Thompson, Caspersen & Kendrick, 1987). Physical inactivity is now recognized by the American Heart Association (AHA) as a major, independent risk factor for the development of CAD (Fletcher *et al.*, 1992). An active lifestyle also favorably modifies other CAD risk factors including hypertension, hyperlipidemia, insulin resistance, and obesity (Bouchard *et al.*, 1994; Chandrashekhar & Anand, 1991). Despite the increasing evidence of the health benefits of physical activity, the majority of the population in the United States remain physically inactive.

Bonnie K. Sanderson • Division of Cardiovascular Disease, School of Medicine, UAB Center for Health Promotion, University of Alabama at Birmingham, Birmingham, Alabama 35294. *Herman A. Taylor, Jr.* • University of Mississippi Medical Center, Jackson, Mississippi 39216.

Handbook of Health Promotion and Disease Prevention, edited by Raczynski and DiClemente. Kluwer Academic/Plenum Publishers, New York, 1999.

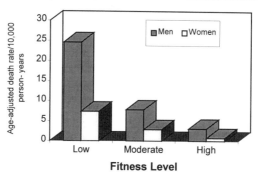

Figure 1. Age-adjusted CVD death rates per 10,000 person-years for men and women by low, moderate, and high levels of physical fitness, Aerobics Center Longitudinal Study. Data from Blair *et al.*, 1989.

Due to the continuing and increasing trend of sedentary lifestyles among most Americans, national health agencies have released statements to provide the general public and health professionals with the latest scientific evidence about the relationship between physical activity and health. The first report of the Surgeon General of the US Public Health Service presented on physical activity and health was released on the eve of the Centennial Olympic Games in Atlanta, Georgia (US Dept. of Health and Human Services, 1996). Based on the comprehensive literature review on physical activity and health, the message about the importance of physical activity and health was directed to individuals, families, health professionals, businesses, communities, schools, and others to make it a national commitment to include physical activity in daily life. Another statement was published by the National Institutes of Health (NIH) on physical activity and cardiovascular health to provide physicians and the general public with a scientific-based consensus statement about the recommendations for physical activity (NIH Consensus Development Panel, 1996). The conclusion on physical activity and cardiovascular health by the NIH panel is quoted in a consensus statement:

> All Americans should engage in regular physical activity at a level appropriate to their capacity, needs, and interests. Children and adults alike should set a goal of accumulating at least 30 minutes of moderate-intensity physical activity on most, and preferably all, days of the week. Most Americans have little or no physical activity in their daily lives, and accumulating evidence indicates that physical inactivity is a major risk factor for cardiovascular disease. However, moderate levels of physical activity confer significant health benefits. Even those who currently meet these daily standards may derive additional health benefits by becoming more physically active or including more vigorous activity. For those with known cardiovascular disease, cardiac rehabilitation programs that combine physical activity with reduction in other risk factors should be more widely used. (p. 241)

The NIH statement reinforces the earlier recommendations from the Centers for Disease Control and Prevention (CDCP) and the American College of Sports Medicine (ACSM) that advised every US adult to accumulate 30 minutes or more of moderate-intensity physical activity on most days of the week (Pate *et al.*, 1995). Previous physical activity guidelines recommended adults to engage in 20 to 60 minutes of moderate-to-high-intensity aerobic exercise (60 to 90% of maximum heart rate) three or more times a week (ACSM, 1990). These recommendations were based on evidence of improved fitness or aerobic capacity derived from physical activity participation at that level. However, evidence now indicates that substantial health benefits are accrued by performing moderate-intensity physical activity that can be performed outside of structured exercise programs. The high prevalence of physical inactivity may be due in part to the misperception of many people that they must engage in vigorous, continuous exercise to gain health benefits (Pate *et al.*, 1995). The latest recommendation recognizes the dose–response relationships between physical activity and a variety of health outcomes and makes an important distinction between physical activity as it relates to health versus fitness (Haskell, 1994). From a public health perspective, encouraging the least fit of our nation to increase their physical activity beyond the sedentary category would decrease the health burden of our nation while promoting individual well-being (McGinnis, 1992).

This chapter summarizes information about physical activity as an important factor influencing health with a specific emphasis on its positive health relationship with CVD. An overview of the current prevalence of physical inactivity as a risk behavior in the United States affecting our population and subgroups within our population provides an epidemiologic summary and the potential impact of physical inactivity on public health. A discussion of selected theoretical models that are commonly applied in promoting physical activity to individuals, groups, and communities provides a summary of some successful approaches to changing physical activity patterns. In conjunction with other risk-reducing behaviors, regular physical activity helps prevent initial cardiac events (primary prevention), reduces the risk of recurrent cardiac events (secondary prevention), and aids in the recovery of patients following cardiac events (rehabilitation). An overview of some current physical activity interventions that target primary and secondary prevention of CVD describes a variety of approaches applied in different settings that include community and clinical interventions. Last, a discussion of identified research needs provides direction for the future in the design and the implementation of effective physical activity interventions for primary and secondary prevention of CVD.

Epidemiology

Despite evidence of the positive health aspects of physical activity, the majority of people in the United States remain sedentary. The promotion of physical activity and fitness is a priority for preventive action in the Healthy People 2000 National Health Promotion and Prevention Objectives (US Dept. of Health and Human Services, 1991). Specific physical activity objectives have been set in the areas of health status, risk reduction, and services and protection (Table 1). There have been positive national trends observed with cigarette smoking, hypertension, and hyperlipidemia, but the prevalence of obesity and physical inactivity has not improved (NIH Consensus Development Panel, 1996). The relative risk of physically inactive adults is nearly twice that of their more active counterparts on the development of CVD (Powell et al., 1987). This is comparable to the relative risks of other major CVD risk factors of smoking (2.5), hypertension (2.1), and hyperlipidemia (2.4). Although the relative risk of physical inactivity is slightly less than the other major risk factors, the prevalence of physical inactivity is much greater in the US population. Nearly 60% of the adult pop-

Table 1. Healthy People 2000 Physical Activity Objectives[a]

Objective	Year 2000 target	Baseline
Health status		
CHD deaths	≤100 per 100,000	135 per 100,000
Overweight	≤20% of adults	26% aged 20–74
Risk reduction		
Regular physical activity	≥30% aged 6+	22% aged 18+
Vigorous physical activity	≥20% aged 18+	12% aged 20–74
Sedentary lifestyle	≤15% aged 6+	24% aged 18+
Strength/flexibility activity	≥40% aged 6+	Unknown
Overweight reduction	≥50% aged 12+	30% women aged 18+
		25% men aged 18+
Services and protection		
Daily PE[b] in school	≥50% grades 1–12	36% grades 1–12
PE class time exercising	≥50% PE class time	27% PE class time
Work site fitness programs	≥50% work sites 250– 749 employees	32% work sites
Outdoor fitness trails	≥1 per 10,000 people	1 per 71,000 people
Routine counseling on exercise	≥50% primary care providers	30% primary care providers

[a] From US Dept. of Health and Human Services (1991).
[b] PE, physical education.

ulation is relatively inactive. This compares to the prevalence of other attributable risk factors in the adult population: 25% currently smoking, 30% with elevated cholesterol of >200 mg/dl, and 30% with hypertension defined by a systolic blood pressure >140 mm/Hg (CDCP, 1993). Since the prevalence of physical inactivity is almost doubled compared to other major CVD risk factors, increasing physical activity patterns can have a significant public health impact on reducing the incidence of CVD.

The prevalence of physical inactivity among US adults aged 18 years and older is summarized by various demographic characteristics in the Surgeon General's Report on Physical Activity in Table 2. Using data from the National Health Interview Survey (NHIS), the Third National Health and Nutrition Survey (NHANES III), and the Behavioral Risk Factor Surveillance System (BRFSS), the Surgeon General's Report reveals approximately 25% of adults report no leisure-time physical activity (LPTA), which is far above the 15% target of the Healthy People 2000 risk reduction objective. The prevalence of physical inactivity is reported highest among women when compared to men and there is an inverse relationship to physical activity according to age, education, and income levels. Among the ethnic and sex-specific groups, white men were the least likely to report no LPTA, while white women and black men reported similar percentages of inactivity. The prevalence of physical inactivity is reported to be highest in black and Hispanic women, at approximately 33%. The geographic distribution of physical inactivity tends to be higher in the southern and northeastern states compared to the north central and western states.

Reports leading up to the Surgeon General's Report on Physical Activity supported the growing concerns about the prevalence of physical inactivity in our nation. Caspersen and Merritt (1995) analyzed data from the BRFSS and reported that approximately 60% of the respondents were physically inactive or irregularly active. Al-

Table 2. Proportion of Adults Reporting No Leisure-Time Physical Activity within the
Last Month, 1991 Behavioral Risk Factor Surveillance System[a]

Demographic group	Sedentary (%)	95% CI
Sex		
Male	27.89	27.18–28.60
Female	31.48	30.85–32.11
Race		
White	27.75	27.24–28.26
Nonwhite	37.52	36.27–38.77
Age, year		
18–34	23.77	23.01–24.53
35–54	29.50	28.70–30.30
$\geq$55	38.00	37.10–38.90
Annual income, $		
<14,999	40.14	39.06–41.22
15,000–24,999	32.00	30.90–33.10
25,000–50,000	25.43	24.63–26.23
>50,000	18.64	17.60–19.68
Education		
Some high school	48.06	46.75–49.37
High school/tech school graduate	33.57	32.79–34.35
Some college/college graduate	20.16	19.55–20.77

[a] From US Dept. of Health and Human Services (1996).

most 40% of the respondents were regularly active, but less than 10% of those responding to be active participated in physical activity at the intensity level recommended to promote or maintain cardiorespiratory fitness. This report supports another study (DiPietro & Caspersen, 1991) that compared physical activity patterns among African Americans and other ethnic minorities with white Americans. In this report, African-American women were least active compared to white men and women and African-American men. A report from NHANES III data examined the prevalence of physical inactivity among adults 20 years or older from 1988 through 1991 (Crespo, Keteyian, Heath, & Sempos, 1996). The overall prevalence of no LPTA was 22% with a higher rate in women (27%) compared to men (17%). The rate of no LTPA was higher among older age groups when compared to younger age groups in both men and women. Among ethnic minorities, the prevalence of no LTPA was even more striking: Mexican-American men (33%), Mexican-American women (46%), and non-Hispanic black women (40%) had the highest rate of sedentary lifestyles. The results of these studies suggest that specific activity patterns and behavioral determinants of physical activity should be examined among population subgroups, especially women, older persons, some ethnic minorities, and individuals with lower education and economic status. There also is a need to enhance the efforts of physical activity interventions that target those groups that are least active and who may derive the most health benefits from increasing physical activity patterns.

The public health burden of physical inactivity can be related to an economic burden on our nation. The cost of newly diagnosed CVD in approximately 1.5 million individuals accounts for an estimated $47 billion in direct and indirect health care costs (American Heart Association, 1991). A report (CDCP, 1993) that summarizes the potential efficacy and cost-effectiveness of physical activity promotion in preventing CVD estimates the extrapolated cost of physical inactivity at $5.7 billion. The only higher estimated cost was elevated serum cholesterol at $7 billion. Promoting physical activity for the prevention of CVD has both health and economic implications in saving lives and dollars.

Theoretical Models in Promoting Physical Activity

Understanding the determinants of exercise adoption and adherence are fundamental for promoting the health potential of physical activity (Dishman, 1994). The lack of a theoretical approach to the study of exercise and physical activity behavior may have hampered efforts in designing more effective physical activity interventions for our sedentary populations. This may explain some of the cause for a poor understanding and consequently a low level of physical activity adherence among North Americans (Godin, 1994). Two theoretical models that show promising results in promoting exercise adoption in the sedentary adult include: (1) social learning theory with a specific emphasis on the self-efficacy concept, and (2) transtheoretical or stages of change model.

Social learning theory provides a theoretical basis for the planning, development, and implementation of programs designed to assist individuals in the process of behavior change. Major concepts of the social learning theory emphasize the importance of the following factors: environment, situation, behavioral capability, expectations, expectancies, observational learning, reinforcements, self-control and self-efficacy, emotional coping responses, and reciprocal determinism. Examples of the major concepts of the social learning theory and the implications for physical activity interventions are outlined in Table 3. Among the social learning variables, self-efficacy is found to be a powerful determinant of exercise change (Sallis, Hovell & Hofstetter, 1992) and is acquired from primarily four sources of information: (1) performance accomplishment, (2) vicarious experiment, (3) persuasion, and (4) physiological states (Bandura, 1986; King et al., 1992; Sallis et al., 1992; Marcus, Shelby, Niauru, & Rossi, 1992c). Performance accomplishment is based on mastery experience and provides the most dependable source of self-efficacy information. Realistic goal setting, log or record keeping, constructive feedback, and identifying meaningful rewards or incentives are examples of providing performance accomplishment feedback in physical activity interventions. The provision of physical activity role-modeling by identifying an exercise partner or teaching self-imagery techniques to individuals desiring to increase their physical activity levels are examples of providing vicarious experiments. Seeing others or visualizing self-success in performing physical activity may raise exercise self-efficacy. The techniques of persuasion are only effective if the expectations are within realistic bounds and the persuader is perceived to be credible and trustworthy by the person attempting to adopt or increase physical activity. Last, physiological states refer to aversive arousal and individuals are more inclined to expect success if aversive arousal is minimized. It is important for individuals to choose an activity that is personally enjoyable and to be aware of negative feelings that may be associated with different aspects of physical activity. For example, if a person is not a "morning person," that individual may be more successful in planning physical activities in the evening rather than in the morning. The social cog-

Table 3. Major Social Learning Theory Concepts, Definitions, and Implications for
Physical Activity Interventions

Concept	Definition	Implication
Environment	Physical and social factors that are external to the person	Provide convenient opportunities and social support that promotes physical activity
Situation	Person's perception of the environment	Correct misconceptions about physical activity and promote active norms
Behavior capability	Knowledge and skill necessary to perform a specific behavior	Promote mastery learning of physical activity through education, skills training, and practice
Expectations	Person's anticipated outcomes of a behavior	Model and provide examples of a physically active lifestyle
Expectancies	Person's values placed on a given outcome	Present outcomes of physical activity that have functional meaning to the person
Observational learning	Behavioral acquisition that occurs by watching the actions and outcomes of others' behavior	Include credible and similar-to-self role models performing desired physical activity behaviors
Reinforcements	Responses to a person's behavior that increase or decrease the likelihood of recurrence of the behavior	Promote self-initiated incentives and rewards for physical activity; identify and reduce barriers and negative influences on physical activity
Self-Control	Personal regulation of goal-directed behavior or performance	Provide opportunities for goal-setting, self-monitoring, and contracting for physical activity
Self-Efficacy	Personal confidence in performing a particular behavior	Approach increase in physical activity in small, manageable steps; seek specificity in goal setting; guarantee success
Emotional coping responses	Strategies or tactics that are used by a person to deal with emotional stimuli	Provide skills training in problem solving, stress management, and relapse prevention
Reciprocal determinism	The dynamic interaction between the person, behavior, and the environment	Consider multiple strategies to increase physical activity including internal and external tactics to promote behavior change

nitive models have been used most frequently to analyze exercise behavior and the most popular theoretical frameworks related to exercise behavior are reviewed more extensively elsewhere (Godin, 1994).

The transtheoretical or stages of change model by Prochaska *et al.* (1992) describes different phases involved in the acquisition and maintenance of behavior. The stages include: (1) precontemplation (no intention to change behavior), (2) contemplation (intention to change behavior), (3) action (involved in behavior change), (4) maintenance (sustained behavior change), and (5) termination (cessation of behavior). This model has been helpful in guiding research in the cessation of addictive behavior, such as smoking, and shows promising help in guiding research in exercise behavior, since the process of adopting physical activity can be conceptualized as the cessation of a sedentary lifestyle (Marcus & Simkin, 1994). A strength in applying the transtheoretical model to physical activity behavior is its dynamic nature and the opportunity to tailor interventions based on different stages of change. The processes in behavior change are emphasized differently according to the transitions of behavior varying from adoption through maintenance of physical activity behavior. Since the majority of our population remain sedentary, there may be a mismatch between the availability of action-oriented programs and interventions that target precontemplators who may have little interest in starting to exercise. The transtheoretical model has been applied to physical activity inventions in the community (Marcus et al., 1992a), clinical settings (CDCP, 1992), and worksite health promotion programs (Marcus, Rossi, Selby, Niaura & Abrams, 1992b). Interest in applying the transtheoretical model in physical activity interventions has accelerated in recent years. Limitations using the transtheoretical model in exercise behavior still exist. More research is needed in the determinants of exercise behavior at different stages and with the inclusion of a more representative and diverse sample. More objective measures of physical activity (compared to self-report) need to be used and the use of more longitudinal and efficacy studies in matching treatment to stage interventions (Marcus & Simkin, 1994).

Primary Prevention and Community Interventions

The consequences on health of the current trends of physical inactivity in our population appear ominous. The majority of exercise adherence literature and interventions targeting the promotion of physical activity has been directed toward the individual with limited and often short-lived success (Dishman, 1994). While most physical activity promotion strategies rely primarily on convincing the individual to become more active, the advances in labor-saving equipment and entertainment technology are bombarding our population with devices and messages that ultimately decrease energy expenditure. With the current negative trends in physical activity and obesity in our population, it becomes more convincing for us to broaden the scope of our physical activity interventions. The application of community-based and other higher-level approaches, such as environmental, organizational, and policy-level strategies, may be more effective in promoting physical activity to larger segments of the population (King, 1994). Community-based and other societal approaches to promoting physical activity provide opportunities to influence a greater proportion of the inactive who may derive the most health benefits from increasing physical activity. Broader-based physical activity promotion approaches also may provide an opportunity to influence future generations to perceive an active lifestyle as the norm compared to the current societal norm of a sedentary lifestyle.

Community-based approaches to promoting physical activity require different perspectives when compared to individual approaches. The comparison of the two physical activity promotion approaches contrasts the traditional medical, or clinical, model to a public health model (King, 1994). The different perspectives are summarized in Table 4. In the medical model, the individual is the target for change and the structure and function of the interventions are usually designed for the convenience of the provider. Potential participants are required to seek out such programs, and they are usually offered in specific settings such as gyms, health clubs, wellness centers, or clinics. This is referred to by King (1994) as a "waiting" stance, and the out-

Table 4. Comparison of Intervention Approaches When the Target Is the Individual versus the Community[a]

Target	Individual	Community
Initial goal	Individual behavior change	Community change in behaviors, social networks/milieu, organizational norms and policies, physical environment, laws
Long-term goal	Individual maintenance of target behavior	Institutionalization of programs; structural or environmental change
Level of intervention	Personal, interpersonal	Personal, interpersonal, organizational, environmental, institutional, societal
Theories/perspectives	Psychosocial, behavioral (focused on the person or small groups)	Psychosocial, behavioral; public health (who to reach); social marketing (how to reach); communication, diffusion, systems approaches
Professional stance	Waiting	Seeking
Location	Setting-based	Settings; nonsetting specific
Type of activity targeted	Programmed, leisure	Programmed, leisure; household-related (e.g., yardwork, use of appliances); routine activity (taking stairs, walking); transportation activities (bicycling, walking)
Method	Health professional (face-to-face)	Health professional, community agencies or organizations, legislators, mass media
Intervention time frame	Usually time-limited	Usually long term

[a] Reprinted with permission from King (1994).

come of this approach often reaches those who may already be reasonably active and healthy.

The public health perspective encompasses a "seeking" stance in community-based physical activity interventions. The goals are typically designed to reach beyond individual behavior change and promote changes that enhance the promotion of physical activity in the environment. Physical activity interventions are designed to influence organizational norms, regulatory policies, social structures, and the provision of structural facilities that promote physical activity in the community. Providers of the community-based physical activity strategies go beyond targeting health professionals in clinical settings to provide the message but encourage a collaborative network of other community professionals and organizations in a larger environment to communicate the importance of behavior change. This allows a systematic approach to the promotion of total physical activity that encompasses usual activity (e.g., taking stairs, walking instead of driving short distances, gardening, etc.) and is not limited to leisure-time or structured exercise programs (King, 1994). Theories relevant to community change such as social marketing, communication theories, diffusion, community organization, and systems approaches are integrated within planned physical activity interventions in conjunction with individual behavior change theories (King, 1991).

Community-based approaches to promoting physical activity can include interpersonal approaches to access individuals directly rather than rely on impersonal approaches that focus on group or class format. There are potential advantages to this format including cost-effectiveness, instructor modeling, supervision, encouragement, and potential peer support and modeling (King, 1994). However, interpersonal approaches have a primary focus on individual change unless measures are used to promote social forces that promote a more widespread community involvement. An effective example of promoting social influence for physical activity was used in the Zuni Indian Diabetes Project (Heath, Leonard, Wilson, Kendrick, & Powell, 1987) that trained exercise instructors who were culturally and demographically similar to the target population. A similar strategy was used in the Physical Activity for Risk Reduction (PARR) project designed to promote physical activity among low-socioeconomic status, African-American residents of a public housing community (Lewis, Raczynski, Heath, Levinson, & Cutter, 1993). PARR employed and trained community residents as exercise group leaders, and although statistically significant changes were not observed in intervention communities, there was some success in delivering interventions to promote physical activity.

The Community Health Assessment and Promotion Project (CHAPP), supported by CDCP, was a comprehensive community-based organizational strategy that targets environmental change in order to promote physical activity. The goal of CHAPP was to modify dietary and exercise behaviors of predominately obese women in an African-American community (Lasco et al., 1989). Specific strategies employed by this project included the formation of a community coalition that encouraged a variety of organizations to work together in maintaining programs, providing security escorts to walking groups, and providing free transportation and child care to promote program participation. Other organizational approaches used to promote physical activity include work site programs, senior centers and senior residential homes, schools, and churches (King, 1994). The effectiveness of these programs in promoting sustained physical activity participation varies and many lack systematic program design and evaluation. Although environmental and organizational approaches to the promotion of physical activity appear promising, the majority of interventions in institutions remain focused on the personal and interpersonal approaches to promoting physical activity.

Several demonstration research projects were designed to evaluate the effectiveness of communitywide health education interventions that targeted the reduction of multiple CVD risk factors. Three of the most notable communitywide CVD risk reduction projects included: (1) Stanford Five-City Project (Farquhar et al., 1990), (2) Minnesota Heart Health Program (Mittelmark et al., 1986), and (3) Pawtucket Heart Health Program (Elder et al., 1986). All these demonstration research projects included physical activity educational messages and will have sufficient data to assess the effectiveness of interventions on physical activity behavior. A report that summarized the effectiveness of the Stanford Five-City Project on changes in physical activity knowledge, attitudes, self-efficacy, and behavior was recently published (Young, Haskell, Taylor & Fortmann, 1996). There was not a significant impact of the educational effort on the knowledge, attitude, and self-efficacy in women or men. Physical activity behavior in men showed a positive effect by an increased percent participation in vigorous activities and estimated energy expenditures. Physical activity behavior in women showed a positive effect by an increased percent participation in moderate-level activities. This report emphasized the importance of targeting specific subgroups and designing physical activity interventions accordingly. Another report on the Stanford Five-City Project (Winkleby, Flora & Kraemer, 1994) provided a prospective examination of predictors of change based on subgroups in the multiple risk factor intervention study. Sixty-nine percent of the respondents showed a positive change in the risk factor score during the community-based intervention. Among the subgroup of positive changers, 83% were older adults ($\geq$ 55 years) with the highest perceived CVD risk. The subgroup with the lowest percentage of positive changers was the least educated, most likely to be Hispanic, and had the lowest health knowledge and self-efficacy scores. This finding is additional reinforcement of the need to develop specific interventions that target subgroups within our population that include individuals at different ages, education levels, and socioeconomic status.

It is important to review the physical activity choices of our more active population when we are attempting to convince those least active to change their behavior. Walking appears to be an acceptable and accessible type of physical activity for those population subgroups that report a low prevalence of leisure-time physical activity. An analysis of the 1990 BRFSS revealed the overall percentage of leisure-time physical activity participation rates lower among low-income, unemployed, and obese persons compared to the total adult population, but the prevalence of walking among these groups was similar (Siegel, Brackbill, & Heath, 1995). Similar results were reported by Ford et al. (1991) when physical activity behaviors in lower and higher socioeconomic status populations were analyzed. Gardening was another common leisure-time activity reported most frequently among men and women, regardless of socioeconomic status. Analysis of the NHANES III reported similar trends when comparing leisure-time physical activities among different ethnic and age groups (Crespo et al., 1996). Rates of inactivity are greater for women, older persons, non-Hispanic blacks, and Mexican Americans. Walking and gardening ranked first and second as the most frequently reported leisure-time activities for all groups except for non-Hispanic black women. Black women reported dancing (other than aerobic dancing) as second and gardening as third in the most frequently reported leisure-time activity. Due to the beneficial effects on health of these types of moderate-intensity physical activity, community and individual efforts may be more successful if they are directed toward reducing the barriers for our predominately sedentary population in adopting and maintaining consistent behavior in these types of physical activities.

Secondary Prevention and Cardiac Rehabilitation

Secondary prevention for CVD relates to the medical treatment recommended for patients who have experienced a clinical event such as acute myocardial infarction (AMI), coronary artery bypass graft surgery (CABG), angina pectoris, or percutaneous transluminal coronary angioplasty (PTCA). Treatment includes a systematic approach of applying both pharmacological and nonpharmacological strategies to achieve the following outcomes: (1) reducing the recurring incidence of cardiovascular events and mortality; (2) decreasing potential complications such as cardiac arrhythmias, heart failure, and other manifestations of atherosclerosis; and (3) improving general health and quality of life (Pearson, 1996). The risk factors that are most strongly associated with development and progression of CVD include cigarette smoking, abnormal blood lipids, hypertension, diabetes mellitus, and physical inactivity. In secondary prevention, the nonpharmacological approaches to risk reduction (behavioral approaches to smoking cessation, diet, and physical activity) may not be sufficient to achieve the desired outcome (Smith *et al.*, 1995).

Pharmacological therapy, such as the use of antihypertensive or lipid-lowering drugs, may be needed to supplement the traditional risk reduction strategies. Since these "prevention" strategies are clearly within the more formal clinical setting, it may be preferable to describe these risk reduction activities as "optimal medical management" of coronary atherosclerosis (Swan, Gersh, Graboys, & Ullyot, 1996). Although risk reduction interventions are demonstrated to improve clinical outcomes in patients with CVD, current medical management often does not reflect the advances in current knowledge of the effectiveness of risk factor modification (Swan *et al.*, 1996). The American Heart Association released a consensus panel statement (Smith *et al.*, 1995) urging a comprehensive application of risk reduction in all eligible patients across medical care settings and patient groups. The consensus panel published a guide to comprehensive risk reduction for patients with coronary and other vascular disease encouraging a team approach (physicians, nurses, dietitians, exercise specialists, etc.) to manage risk reduction therapy.

Cardiac rehabilitation provides a structured approach in providing comprehensive secondary prevention services to patients with CVD. The earlier programs in the 1960s enrolled patients recovering from uncomplicated AMIs with a primary focus of providing medically supervised exercise programs. These programs did show effectiveness in improving physical activity in a safe manner (DeBusk, Houston, Haskell, Fry, & Parker, 1979; Van Camp & Peterson, 1986). Today's cardiac rehabilitation programs serve a much larger and diverse coronary population compared to the earlier programs. The treatment of CVD has changed drastically with the advanced technologies and acute interventions such as CABG, PTCA, and thrombolytic therapy. Often these therapies are successful in preventing or limiting cardiac muscle damage that previously hindered the recovery of patients with AMI in the past. With these new therapies, more cardiac patients are surviving heart disease who may have died in the past and may have residual myocardial ischemia, congestive heart failure, cardiac arrhythmias, or other complications. The delivery of cardiac rehabilitation services reflects the change in the demographics and characteristics of the coronary population and includes patients who are older, sicker, and with more complications compared to the patients with uncomplicated cardiac disease.

As the scientific evidence increased on the benefits of other secondary prevention measures, most cardiac rehabilitation programs expanded their services to include risk factor modification counseling, but the majority retained their primary focus on exercise training. Since the provision of cardiac rehabilitation services varied widely, the Agency for Health Care Policy and Research (AHCPR) and the NHLBI convened a panel of experts to use science-based methodology and expert clinical judgment to develop a guideline for health practitioners using cardiac rehabilitation services (US DHHS, 1995). The definition of cardiac rehabilitation by the panel states:

> Cardiac rehabilitation services are comprehensive, long-term programs involving medical evaluation, prescribed exercise, cardiac risk factor modification, education, and counseling. These programs are designed to limit the physiologic and psychological effects of cardiac ill-

ness, reduce the risk of sudden death or reinfarction, control cardiac symptoms, stabilize or reverse the atherosclerotic process, and enhance the psychosocial and vocational status of selected patients. (p. 3)

Based on reports in the scientific literature reviewed by the panel, the most substantial benefits of cardiac rehabilitation include: (1) improvement in exercise tolerance, (2) improvement in symptoms, (3) improvement in blood lipid levels, (4) reduction in cigarette smoking, (5) improvement in psychosocial well-being and reduction of stress, and (6) reduction in mortality.

The AHCPR panel emphasized the added effectiveness of multifactorial cardiac rehabilitation services integrated in a comprehensive approach involving exercise training and education, counseling, and behavioral interventions. On the basis of the scientific literature review, the panel concluded that cardiac rehabilitation services are an essential component of the contemporary management of patients with multiple presentations of CVD and with heart failure. The challenge to existing cardiac rehabilitation programs is to extend their exercise-focused therapy to include more comprehensive risk reduction education and counseling; the challenge to health care payors is to extend their reimbursement to be more inclusive of multifactorial services.

Summary: Future Directions and Research Needs

Despite the growing body of knowledge on physical activity and its effects on health and well-being, data are still limited. Mounting evidence supports the common knowledge that exercise is healthful, yet the majority of Americans are not regular in physical activity. It becomes clear that studying the processes of health behavior in physical activity equals the importance of understanding how physical activity affects physiological function. The behavioral and physiological approach to studying physical activity must encompass an adequate representation of our population according to age, gender, ethnicity, geographic location, and socioeconomic status and must include individuals with specific disease states and/or disabilities. We need to determine the minimal, optimal, and most important features or combination of features of physical activity (intensity, duration, frequency, type, total amount, pattern) that offer specific health benefits for varying subgroup populations. Better methods of measuring total physical activity, inclusive of work and leisure time activity, need to be developed and evaluated that provide improved quantitative estimates. This may allow more flexibility in developing and evaluating physical activity interventions that will reduce barriers and enable our current sedentary population to adopt and maintain more active lifestyles.

Behavioral and social science research on physical activity is a relatively new endeavor and includes the study of determinants of physical activity as well as behavioral responses to physical activity interventions. If we are to increase our effectiveness in the promotion of physical activity, we need to better understand the determinants of physical activity behavior so more effective interventions can be planned. We need to assess the determinants of physical activity patterns among those that are regularly active, intermittently active, and inactive for various population subgroups. Although individual counseling on physical activity has shown some success, we need to move beyond the singular approach and develop and evaluate interventions that include policy and environmental supports. Individual barriers that challenge physical activity patterns have been studied, but little attention has been devoted to the interactive effects of cultural, environmental, and public policy barriers to an active lifestyle. Research conducted in a broader context may help us understand the influences on individuals, communities, and government policies that result in specific physical activity patterns.

Last, there needs to be collaborative research among exercise scientists, behavioral and social scientists, health professionals, city planners, and government officials to better understand how to remove barriers and create opportunities in promoting physical activity. The importance of promoting physical activity in combination with other desired health practices, such as diet and smoking cessation, needs to be communicated in a simple, unified message. Urging our nation's population to make healthier behavior choices in general is a concept to portray in broad-based public health messages to reach large segments of the population. Research in social marketing and dissemination of health messages needs to develop and reach the level of accomplishment achieved in commercial advertising. By working together, multidisciplinary groups can develop, implement, and evaluate interventions that may simultaneously promote physical activity in schools, communities, work sites, and health care systems. The synergistic efforts of multidisciplinary groups at multiple sites may have the potential to influence individuals as well as community organizations and government policies. This approach may optimize our success in achieving the public health goal of reducing the prevalence of physical inactivity, thus leading to a healthier nation.

References

American College of Sports Medicine (ACSM). (1990). Position stand on the recommended quantity and quality of exercise for developing and maintaining cardiorespiratory and muscular fitness in healthy adults. *Medicine and Science in Sports and Exercise, 22,* 265–274.

American Heart Association. (1991). *1992 Heart and stroke facts.* Dallas: Author.

Bandura, A. (1986). *Social foundations of thought and action.* Englewood Cliffs, NJ: Prentice Hall.

Blair, S. N., Kohl, H. W., Paffenbarger, R. S. Jr., Clark, D. G., Cooper, K. H., & Gibbons, L. W. (1989). Physical fitness and all-cause mortality: a prospective study of healthy men and women. *Journal of the American Medical Association, 273,* 1179–1184.

Blair, S.N., Kohl, H.W., Barlow, C.E., Paffenbarger, R.S. Jr. Gibbons, L.W., & Macera, C.A. (1995). Changes in physical fitness and all-cause mortality: A prospective study of healthy and unhealthy men. *Journal of the American Medical Association, 273,* 1093–1098.

Bouchard, C., Shepard, R. J., & Stephens, T. (Eds.). (1994). *Physical activity, fitness, and health.* Champaign, IL: Human Kinetics.

Brown, C. R. (1990). Exercise, fitness, and mental health. In C. Bouchard, R.J. Shepard, T. Stephens, J.R. Sutton, & B.D. McPherson (Eds.), *Exercise, fitness, and health: A consensus of current knowledge* (pp. 607–626). Champaign, IL: Human Kinetics.

Caspersen, C. J., & Merritt, R. K. (1995). Physical activity trends among 26 states, 1986–1990. *Medicine and Science in Sports and Exercise, 27,* 713–720.

Centers for Disease Control and Prevention (CDCP). (1992). *Project PACE: Physician's manual: Physician-based assessment and counseling for exercise.* Atlanta, GA: Author.

Centers for Disease Control and Prevention (CDCP). (1993). Public health focus: Physical activity and the prevention of coronary heart disease. *Morbidity and Mortality Weekly Report, 43,* 669–672.

Chandrashekhar, Y., & Anand, I. S. (1991). Exercise as a coronary protective factor. *American Heart Journal, 122,* 1723–1739.

Crespo, C. J., Keteyian, S. J., Heath, G. W., & Sempos, C. T. (1996). Leisure-time physical activity among U.S. adults: Results from the third national health and nutrition exmination survey. *Archives of Internal Medicine, 156,* 93–98.

DeBusk, R. F., Houston, N., Haskell, W., Fry, F., & Parker, M. (1979). Exercise training soon after myocardial infarction. *American Journal of Cardiology, 44,* 1223–1229.

DiPietro, L., & Caspersen, C. J. (1991). National estimates of physical activity among white and black Americans. *Medicine and Science in Sports and Exercise, 23* (suppl.), S105.

Dishman, R. K. (1992). Psychological effects of exercise for disease resistance and health promotion. In R. R. Watson & M. Eisinher (Eds.), *Exercise and disease* (pp. 179–207). Boca Raton, FL: CRC Press.

Dishman, R. K. (Ed.). (1994). *Advances in exercise adherence.* Champaign, IL: Human Kinetics.

Elder, J. P., McGraw, S. A., Abrams, D. B., Ferreira, A., Lasater, L. M., Longpre, H., Peterson, G. S., Schwertfezes, R., & Carleton, R. A. (1986). Organizational and community approaches to community-wide prevention of heart disease: the first two years of the Pawtucket Heart Health Program. *Preventive Medicine, 15,* 107–117.

Farquhar, J. W., Fortmann, S. P., Flora, J. A., Taylor, C. B., Haskell, W. L., Williams, P. T., Maccoby, N., & Wood, P. D. (1990). The Stanford Five-City Project: Effects of communitywide education on cardiovascular disease risk factors. *Journal of the American Medical Association, 264,* 359–365.

Fletcher, G. F., Blair, S. N., Blumenthal, J., Caspersen, C., Chaitman, B., Epstein, S., Falls, H., Froelicher, E. S., Froelicher, V. C., & Pina, I. L. (1992). AHA medical/scientific statement on exercise. *Circulation, 86,* 340–344.

Fletcher, G. F., Balady, G., Blair, S. N., Blumenthal, J., Caspersen, C. Chaitman, B., Epstein, S., Froelicher, E. S., Froelicher, V. F., Pina, I. L., & Polloci, M. L. (1996). Statement on exercise: Benefits and recommendations for physical activity programs for all Americans. *Circulation, 96,* 857–862.

Ford, E. S., Merritt, R. K., Heath, G. W., Powell, K. E., Washburn, R. A., Kriska, A., & Haile, G. (1991). Physical activity behaviors in lower and higher socioeconomic status populations. *American Journal of Epidemiology, 133,* 1246–1256.

Godin, G. (1994). Theories of reasoned action and planned behavior: usefulness for exercise promotion. *Medicine and Science in Sports and Exercise, 26,* 1391–1394.

Haskell, W. L. (1994). Health consequences of physical activity: understanding and challenges regarding dose–response. *Medicine and Science in Sports and Exercise, 26,* 649–660.

Heath, G. W., Leonard, B. E., Wilson, R. H., Kendrick, J. S., & Powell, K. E. (1987). Community-based exercise intervention: Zuni diabetes project. *Diabetes Care, 10,* 579–583.

King, A. C. (1991). Community intervention for promotion of physical activity and fitness. *Exercise and Sport Sciences Review, 19,* 211–259.

King, A. C. (1994). Community and public health approaches to the promotion of physical activity. *Medicine and Science in Sports and Exercise, 26,* 1405–1412.

King, A. C., Blair, S. N., Bild, D., Dishman, R. K., Dubbert, P. M., Marcus, B. H., Oldridge, M., Paffenbarger, R. S., Powell, K. E., & Yeager, K. (1992). Determinants of physical activity and interventions in adults. *Medicine and Science in Sports and Exercise, 24,* S221–S236.

Lasco, R. A., Curry, R. H., Dickson, V. J., Powers, J., Menes, S., & Merritt, R. K. (1989). Participation rates, weight loss, and blood pressure changes among obese women in a nutrition-exercise program. *Public Health Reports, 104,* 640–646.

Lewis, C. E., Raczynski, J. M., Heath, G. W., Levinson, R., & Cutter, G. (1993). Physical activity of public housing residents in Birmingham, Alabama. *American Journal of Public Health, 83,* 1016–1020.

Marcus, B. H., & Simkin, L. R. (1994). The transtheoretical model: applications to exercise behavior. *Medicine and Science in Sports and Exercise, 26,* 1400–1404.

Marcus, B. H., Banspach, S. W., Lefebvre, R. L., Rossi, J. S., Carleton, R. A., & Abrams, D. B. (1992a). Using the stages of change model to increase the adoption of physical activity among community participants. *American Journal of Health Promotion, 6,* 424–429.

Marcus, B. H., Rossi, J. S., Selby, V. C., Niaura, R. S., & Abrams, D. B. (1992b). The stages and processes of exercise adoption and maintenace in a work site sample. *Health Psychology, 11,* 386–395.

Marcus, B. H., Selby, V. C., Niaura, R. S., & Rossi, J. S. (1992c). Self-efficacy and the stages of exercise behavior change. *Research Quarterly for Exercise and Sport, 63*(1), 60–66.

McGinnis, J. M. (1992). The public health burden of a sedentary lifestyle. *Medicine and Science in Sports and Exercise, 24,* S196–S200.

Mittelmark, M. B., Luepker, R. V., Jacobs, D. R., Bracht, N. F., Carlaw, R. W., & Crow R. S. (1986). Community-wide prevention of cardiovascular disease: education strategies of the Minnesota Heart Health Program. *Preventive Medicine, 15,* 1–17.

Morris, J. N., Clayton, D. G., Everitt, M. G., Semmence, A. M., & Burgess, E. H. (1990). Exercise in leisure time: coronary attact and death rates. *British Heart Journal, 63,* 325–334.

NIH Consensus Development Panel on Physical Activity and Cardiovascular Health. (1996). Physical activity and cardiovascular health. *Journal of the American Medical Association, 276,* 241–246.

Paffenbarger, R. S., J., Hyde, R. T., Wing, A. L., & Hsieh, C. C. (1986). Physical activity: All-cause mortality and longevity of college alumni. *New England Journal of Medicine, 314,* 605–613.

Paffenbarger, R. S., Hyde, R. T., Wing, A. L., Lee, I. M., Jung, D. L., & Kampert, J. B. (1993). The association of changes in physical activity level and other lifestyle characteristics with mortality among men. *New England Journal of Medicine, 328,* 538–545.

Pate, R. R., Pratt, M., Blair, S. N., Haskell, W. L., Macera, C. A., Bourchard, C., Buchner, D., Ettinger, W., Heath, G. W., King, A. C., Kriska, A., Leon, A. S., Marcus, B. H., Morris, J., Paffenbarger, R. S., Patrick, K., Pollock, M. L., Rippe, J. M., Sallis, J., & Wilmore, J. H. (1995). Physical activity and health: A recommendation from the Centers for Disease Control and Prevention and the American College of Sports Medicine. *Journal of the American Medical Association, 273,* 402– 407.

Pearson, T. A., & Fuster, V. (1996). Executive summary: Task force on the management of cardiovascular risk factors. *Journal of the American College of Cardiology, 27,* 961–963.

Powell, K. E., Thompson, P. D., Caspersen, C. J., & Kendrick, J. S. (1987). Physical activity and the incidence of coronary heart disease. *Annual Review of Public Health, 8,* 253–287.

Prochaska, J. O., DiClemente, C. C., & Norcross, J. C. (1992). In search of how people change: Application to addictive behaviors. *American Psychologist, 47,* 1102–1111.

Sallis J. F., Hovell, M. F., & Hofstetter, C. R. (1992). Predictors of adoption and maintenance of vigorous physical activity in men and women. *Preventive Medicine, 21,* 237–251.

Siegel, P. Z., Brackbill, R. M., & Heath, G. W. (1995). The epidemiology of walking for exercise: Implications for promoting activity among sedentary groups. *American Journal of Public Health, 85,* 706–710.

Smith, S. C., Blair, S. N., Criqui, M. H., Fletcher, G. F., Fuster, V., Gersh, B. J., Gotto, A. M., Gould, K. L., Greenland, P., Grundy, S. M., Hill, M. N., Hlatky, M. A., Houston-Miller, N., Krauss, R. M., LaRosa, J., Ockene, I. S., Oparil, S., Pearson, T. A., Rapaport, E., & Starke, R. D. (1995). AHA Consensus Panel Statement: Preventing heart attack and death in patients with coronary disease. *Circulation, 92,* 2–4.

Stephens, T. (1988). Physical activity and mental health in the United States and Canada: Evidence from four population surveys. *Preventive Medicine, 17,* 35–47.

Swan, H. J., Gersh, B. J., Graboys, T. B., & Ullyot, .D. J. (1996). Task force 7: Evaluation and management of risk factors for the individual patient (case management). *Journal of the American College of Cardiology, 27,* 1030–1039.

U.S. Dept. of Health and Human Services (US DHHS). (1991). *Healthy People 2000: National health promotion and disease prevention objectives.* Washington, DC: US Dept. of Health and Human Services.

US DHHS. (1995). *Clinical practice guideline: Cardiac rehabilitation.* Rockville, MD: Agency for Health Care Policy and Research.

US DHHS. (1996). *Physical activity and health: A report of the Surgeon General.* Atlanta, GA: Centers for Disease Control and Prevention, National Center for Chronic Disease Prevention and Health Promotion.

Van Camp, S. P., & Peterson, R. A. (1986). Cardiovascular complications of outpatient cardiac rehabilitation programs. *Journal of the American Medical Association, 256,* 1160–1163.

Winkleby, M. A., Flora, J. A., & Kraemer, H. C. (1994). A community-based heart disease intervention: Predictors of change. *American Journal of Public Health, 84,* 767–772.

Young, D. R., Haskell, W. L., Taylor, C. B., & Fortmann, S. P. (1996). Effect of community health education on physical activity knowledge, attitudes, and behavior. *American Journal of Epidemiology, 144,* 264–274.

CHAPTER 11

Alcohol and Drug Abuse

Joseph E. Schumacher and Jesse B. Milby

Introduction

The use, abuse, and dependency of substances includes a wide variety of compounds consisting of tobacco, alcohol, illicit drugs, prescription medications, inhalants, and designer drugs. No sex, race, social strata, or culture are immune to the effects of drug abuse and dependency. Exposure and experimentation with mood-altering substances occurs in some unfortunate individuals as early as before birth, *in utero,* from drug-using mothers, but more frequently among youth in their early teens. Peer group and media are powerful influences for the initiaton of drug use and abuse. Physiological, sociological, and psychological determinants pave the path to dependence. The negative effects of drug abuse and dependence are widespread. Drugs affect psychological, family, friends, work, health, legal, and social functioning in destructive ways. Treatment approaches are varied and can be matched to clients according to beliefs, severity, drug type, stage of recovery, motivation, and comorbidity.

However, there is no question that treatment works. David Mactus, Director of the Center for Substance Abuse Treatment, compares the effectiveness of drug treatment to diabetes; the disorder of diabetes can be controlled or "cured" as long as the patient takes his insulin. Drug dependence is also a chronically relapsing disorder that can be controlled with appropriate intervention and maintenance. A 12-Step saying, "It works if you work it," exemplifies the effectiveness of drug treatment. The challenge to researchers and practitioners of drug treatment now is to enhance motivation to initiate change in addictive behaviors and maintain compliance with aftercare and relapse prevention interventions.

This chapter reviews the prevalence of substance abuse in the United States according to substance type, substance use disorder, historical trends, age, gender, and ethnicity and socioeconomic variables. A brief analysis of substance abuse etiology and associated risk factors and theoretical models of addiction are presented. Effective pri-

Joseph E. Schumacher and Jesse B. Milby • Behavioral Medicine Unit, Division of Preventive Medicine, Department of Medicine, School of Medicine, UAB Center for Health Promotion, University of Alabama at Birmingham, Birmingham, Alabama 35294.

Handbook of Health Promotion and Disease Prevention, edited by Raczynski and DiClemente. Kluwer Academic/Plenum Publishers, New York, 1999.

mary prevention programs are reviewed including school-based educational projects, family involvement, and multiagency collaborations. Common threads, cultural and gender issues, and future directions for prevention research are presented. A wide range of secondary and tertiary prevention interventions are presented including innovative stage of change-based motivational interviewing, traditional counseling and methadone maintenance approaches, and recent effective outpatient contingency management treatments for cocaine dependence. Common aspects and gender and ethnic issues related to drug treatment are discussed. The chapter concludes with an overview of the substance abuse problem in the United States and directions for the future.

Epidemiology

Prevalence

Prevalence and incidence of substance use are not static and are subject to effects of the substance type, time, age, gender, ethnicity, region, and socioeconomic status. It is important to consider not only each of these variables in any analysis of the occurrence of substance use, but their interactions as well. Drug use and abuse is a cultural phenomenon that spans temporal, demographic, socioeconomic, ethnic, and drug-type influences. A person who uses or abuses substances can be a regular cigarette smoker, a problem drinker, a high school marijuana user, a white, homeless crack smoker, an impaired professional, or an employed opiate injector. Tendencies to categorize drug abuse as a minority or a poverty problem is an overgeneralization and should be cautioned in any analysis of prevalence reports. The following summary of substance use prevalence data is organized by a nonexhaustive list of important variables to consider when discussing prevalence.

Much of the following prevalence data is summarized from the 1990, 1992, and 1994 National Household Surveys on Drug Abuse (NHSDA) [National Institute on Drug Abuse (NIDA), 1991; Substance Abuse and Mental Health Services Administration (SAMHSA), 1993, 1995]. The NHSDA surveys were designed to measure the prevalence of illicit drug use, prescription drugs used nonmedically, alcohol, and tobacco products in the United States. In the most recent 1994 survey, a total of 22,181 eligible household members were contacted through personal visits. It is important to note that the NHSDA data was obtained from self-report, utilized small samples for some specific subgroups, relied on population census projections subject to error, and most importantly, surveyed noninstitutionalized civilians living in households, college dormitories, and on military installations. Therefore, the NHSDA does not report present estimates for some segments of the US population that may contain a substantial proportion of drug users such as persons without homes or those hospitalized, institutionalized, or incarcerated.

Substance Type

Prevalence rates from the 1994 NHSDA for any illicit drug use was 34.4% ever used, 10.8% used in the past year, and 6.0% used in the past month. The pattern, of approximately twice as many drugs used in the past year as in the past month and three times as many ever used as used in the past year, is generally true for most drugs of abuse presented below.

The prevalence in the past year of substance use for nine classifications including any illicit substances, alcohol, and cigarettes by sex and age groups were reviewed from the 1994 NHSDA. Alcohol use was reported among 66.9% of the population and cigarettes among 31.7% over the past year. Marijuana was the most prevalently used illicit substance (8.5%), with cocaine, crack cocaine, inhalants, hallucinogens, and any psychotherapeutics ranging from 0.6 to 2.9% used within the last year. Crack cocaine (0.6%) has been distinguished from the general cocaine category because of its distinguishing reinforcing, addictive, and lifestyle characteristics. Prevalence rates in the past year for other categories of substances were: smokeless tobacco (4.8%), phencyclidine (PCP) (0.1%), lysergic acid diethylamide (LSD) (0.8%), heroin (0.1%), and anabolic steroids (0.1%). Needle use was present in 0.1% of the population. In estimating alcohol and other drug use among the homeless, the rate of alcohol abuse is reliably estimated to exceed 40% and an additional 15 to 20% also abuse other drugs (Wright, 1989a,b). It is also estimated that as many as 75% of those arrested in the criminal justice system were using alcohol or other drugs upon arrest.

Substance Use Disorders

Substance Use Disorders is a category of mental disorders in the American Psychiatric Association Diagnostic and Statistical Manual of Mental Disorders, fourth edition (DSM-IV) (American Psychiatric Association, 1994). This manual is an empirically based classification system by which substance abuse, substance dependence, or substance-induced disorders are classified. DSM-IV substance use disorders go beyond experimental or moderate use resulting in significant substance-related life and health problems.

The DSM-IV reports lifetime Substance Abuse or Dependency prevalence information for the following specific substances: alcohol (14%); amphetamine (2% of the adult population); cannabis (4%); cocaine (0.2%); hallucinogens (0.3%); inhalants (abuse/dependence appear to occur in only a small proportion of users); nicotine (20%); opiates (0.7%); phencyclidine (3% of high school seniors in 1990); and sedatives, hypnotics, or anxiolytics (1.1%). Nicotine and Alcohol Dependence and Abuse are the most prevalent Substance Use Disorders in the general population.

The prevalence of Alcohol and Drug Abuse/Dependency disorders from the Epidemiologic Catchment Area Study (Robbins & Reiger, 1991), a large-scale study of almost 20,000 Americans, was sponsored by the National Institute of Mental Health. They reported the following lifetime prevalence rates: Alcohol Abuse/Dependence (13.8%), Drug Abuse/Dependence (6.2%), Any Substance Use Disorder (17.0%), Alcohol Abuse/Dependence only (10.7%), Drug Abuse/Dependence only (3.2%), and Alcohol and Drug Abuse/Dependence (3.0%). It is important to note that while many persons have a drug of choice, use of multiple substances including alcohol is quite common for purposes of compensating for withdrawal symptoms, obtaining unique euphoria, "triggers" for use of harder drugs, and use during periods of unavailability of a preferred substance.

Historical Trends

Substance use has changed throughout the years in accordance with shifting societal standards, discovery of new compounds, and drug availability. Drug use may have begun as early as 4000–7000 BC with use and cultivation of opium poppies (Maurer & Vogel, 1973). Coca use can be traced back to 600 AD. Archeological digs have revealed South American Indian mummies buried with supplies of coca leaves. Pottery from this period has been recovered portraying the characteristic cheek bulge of the coca leaf chewer (see review by Milby, 1981). Cocaine, derived from coca, is just a little more than 100 years old. Crack cocaine, a smokable form of crystal cocaine, however, has reached epidemic proportions among economically disadvantaged populations in metropolitan areas only in the last few decades.

Trends in lifetime and past month use of any illicit drugs, alcohol, and cigarettes from the 1970s to 1990 suggested that the use of illicit drugs, alcohol, and cigarettes peaked during the late 1970s and declined thereafter as shown in the highlights report of the 1990 NHSDA. Further decline in the past year of any illicit drug use for all age groups (except youth aged 12–17) was seen from 1990 to 1994 (13% to 10.8%), as shown in the 1994 NHSDA. An increase in past month use of cigarettes for youth aged 12–17 was revealed from 1990 to 1994 (13% to 18.9%). An increase in any illicit drug use was revealed for youth aged 12–17 from 16.5% to 20.3% (ever used), 11.7% to 15.5% (used past year), and 6.1% to 8.2% (used past month) as shown in the 1992 and 1994 NHSDA surveys. Marijuana use remained relatively consistent from 1990 to 1994.

Lifetime use of cocaine among adults aged 26 and older increased steadily during the 1980s to a peak of approximately 11% in 1990. Crack cocaine use specifically has increased slightly between 1990 and 1994 for those sampled in the NHSDA surveys. The use of crack cocaine among the economically disadvantaged not surveyed may have shown greater increases.

Age

Research suggests the most vulnerable period for initiation to illicit drugs occurs before age 30 (Chen & Kandel, 1995). In a cross-sectional study of 1108 12th graders from New York State public schools, Kandel, Yamaguchi, and Chen (1992) confirmed that the developmental pattern of drug involvement identified in the 1970s still characterizes adolescent patterns of drug use progressing to abuse. Age of first use of licit drugs was a strong predictor of further progression to illicit use, but most drug users do not become chronic abusers. Virtually no systematic longitudinal research has been conducted to clarify the association between age of drug abuse onset and progression to Substance Use Disorders (Tarter & Mezzich, 1992) and should be considered when interpreting age trends and prevalence data.

Comparisons of trends in prevalence of use of any illicit drugs, alcohol, and cigarettes in the lifetime and past month among age groups from the 1990 NHSDA from 1974 to 1990 supported the following conclusions. Young adults (aged 18–25) were consistently more likely than youth (aged 12–17) or older adults (26 and older) to have used illicit drugs in the past month. Prevalence rates of lifetime use of illicit drugs in the 1994 NHSDA was 46.3% among young adults, 56.1% among older adults, and 20.3% among youth. In 1994, the rates of lifetime use of any illicit drugs dropped for young and older adults. There was, however, a 4% increase in any illicit drug from 1992 to 1994 for youth aged 12–17.

Youth were the least likely of all the age groups to have ever used alcohol in their lifetime or in the past month across all NHSDA surveys. In 1994, 41.7% of youth and over 80% of all adults used alcohol in their lifetime; 21.6% and over 60%, respectively, used in the past month. Young adults and older adults were about equally likely to have used cigarettes in their lifetime (70%) and were much more likely than youth to have ever smoked (37.6%) according to the 1992 and 1994 NHSDA surveys.

Gender

For alcohol and most drugs, abuse and dependence disorders are more prevalent in men than women. The DSM-IV reports that Alcohol Abuse and Dependence has a male-to-female ratio as high as 5:1. However, this ratio varies depending on the age group. Intravenous amphetamine use has a male–female ratio of 3 or 4:1. The male–female ratio is more evenly divided among those with nonintravenous use. Cannabis Use Disorders appear more often in males and hallucinogen abuse is three times more common in males than females. Males account for 70-80% of inhalant-related and three quarters of phencyclidine-related emergency room visits. Males are more commonly affected by opiate addiction, with a male-to-female ratio typically being 3 to 4:1. The prevalence of cigarette smoking is slightly higher in males than in females. However, the prevalence of smoking is reportedly decreasing more rapidly in males. Finally, the use of caffeine is greater in males than in females (APA, 1994).

Recently, gender has begun to receive research and clinical attention as a useful grouping variable because of the increasing numbers of women presenting for alcohol and drug treatment over the last 20 years (Denier, Thevos, Latham, & Randall, 1991). The National Pregnancy and Health Survey by NIDA gathered self-report data from a sample of 2613 women who delivered babies in 52 urban and rural hospitals during 1992. More than 5% of the 4 million women who gave birth in the United States in 1992 used illegal drugs while they were pregnant (Mathias, 1995). Marijuana and cocaine were the most frequently used, 2.9% and 1.1%, respectively. At some point in their pregnancy, 20.4% of the women smoked cigarettes and 18.8% drank alcohol.

Ethnicity and Socioeconomics

According to the DSM-IV (APA, 1994), in the United States, whites and African Americans have nearly identical rates of Alcohol Abuse and Dependence. Latino males reportedly have somewhat higher alcohol disorder rates, although prevalence is lower among Latina females than among females from other ethnic groups. In a review of recent studies, however, whites were found to have higher rates of drug and alcohol use, abuse, and dependence than other racial and ethnic groups despite the perception that drug and alcohol abuse is a "minority problem" (Smith, 1993).

Cocaine use and disorders affect all race, socioeconomic, age, and gender groups in the United States. Cocaine use has shifted from more affluent individuals to include lower socioeconomic groups living in large metropolitan areas (APA, 1994). Since the 1920s in the United States, members of minority groups living in poverty have been overrepresented among persons with Opiate Dependence (APA, 1994). However, in the late 1800s and early 1900s, Opiate Dependence was seen more often among white middle-class individuals, suggesting that differences in use reflect the availability of opiate drugs and other social factors (APA, 1994).

It should be noted that basic subgroup or descriptive data, like race, are not sufficient and are not intended to identify underlying etiologic processes (Gfroered,

1993). Findings of race-associated differences in substance abuse research are often presented as if the person's race has intrinsic explanatory power (Lillie-Blanton, Anthony, & Schuster, 1993). These authors offer strong evidence that race-specific explanations of crack cocaine use may obscure, in fact, the role that environmental and social characteristics play in the epidemiology of crack use. In Lillie-Blanton and colleagues' reanalysis of data from the 1988 NHSDA, once respondents were grouped into neighborhood clusters, crack use did not differ significantly for African Americans or for Hispanic Americans as compared to white Americans. The authors called for future studies of drug use prevalence that seek to include epidemiologic analyses of neighborhood-level social conditions. Ethnicity is a multidimensional concept. Using only one dimension, as in the case of many alcohol/drug use studies, is inadequate (Cheung, 1993).

Substance Abuse Etiology and Theoretical Models

Etiology and Risk Factors

Drug abuse is a multifaceted problem. It includes biological, pharmacological, sociopsychological, and socioecological phenomena. Research has shown that animals with no prior exposure to drugs will self-administer psychoactive drugs and their drug-seeking behavior patterns are similar to human users. These findings suggest that psychoactive drugs can exert their abuse and dependence properties on a human biological system with no preexisting psychopathology or addictive liability required to establish initial use and self-administration. Understanding the etiology of drug abuse requires recognizing that basic biological and molecular mechanisms underlie the reinforcing effects of psychoactive substances. These mechanisms provide foundations for other etiologic factors operating at the intrapersonal, interpersonal, and social levels, which together provide a more complete understanding of well-established precursors for drug abuse and variables known to contribute to individual and subpopulation vulnerability.

In a cross-sectional study of 1108 12th graders from New York State public schools by Kandel *et al.* (1992) reported earlier, age of first use of licit drugs was a strong predictor of further progression to illicit use. They found compelling evidence for a sequential pattern of drug involvement in adolescence. The best-fitting model for males described alcohol use preceding marijuana, marijuana and cigarettes preceding cocaine and crack, and powder cocaine preceding crack use. It most parsimoniously classified 93.4%. A similar best-fit model for females classified 94.2% of females. Even though experimentation with many drugs is the statistical norm among US adolescents (Johnston, O'Malley, & Bachman 1993), early use and use of multiple drugs are not sufficient to predict with any certainty the small proportion of early users who become chronic abusers in young adulthood. This phenomenon of widespread experimentation in the young but with selected vulnerability to chronic abuse has been a challenge for theories of addiction etiology.

Murray and Perry (1985) reviewed 12 studies conducted from 1977 and identified social and environmental factors associated with increased drug use. They included family–peer approval or tolerance for drug use, family–peers as models for use, pressure from family–peers to use drugs, greater influence by peers than parents, incompatibility between parents and peers, greater involvement in peer-related activities such as dating or parties, greater reliance on peers than parents, low educational aspiration for children by parents, lack of parental involvement in their children's activities, weak parental controls and discipline, and ready access to drugs. Correlations were fairly constant across gender and ethnic groups. Also, many factors predicted future drug usage with predictive strength varying as a function of the different substances used. Results from these studies of antecedents of later use and abuse suggest that future users live in an environment peopled by multiple models for drug use, significant others who tolerate or even encourage drug use, and an environment where drugs are readily available. Adolescents who spend most of their time with peers are more likely to experience an environment that supports drug use than those who spend their free time with their family or alone.

Theoretical Models of Addiction

It is possible to divide theories of addiction into two broad types: (1) circumscribed theories that aim to explain a limited domain such as the development of heroin addiction or tolerance and (2) comprehensive theories that attempt to explain the broad spectrum of phenomena from initiation of use to maintenance of abuse or dependence (Milby, 1981). Types of circumscribed theories include psychoanalytic, metabolic disease, moral models, and learning theories. Several theorists have focused on relapse and have postulated useful constructs from which practical interventions for relapse prevention have been derived (Marlatt & Gordon, 1985; Carroll *et al.*, 1994). Generally, the more rigorous scientific theories from which testable hypotheses can be drawn are found among circumscribed theories.

Most rigorous scientific theories have postulated mechanisms underlying physical dependence and tolerance and base their explanatory concepts on varieties of evidence that physical dependence and tolerance generally develop and decay on a similar time course. Solomon and Corbit (1974) explain tolerance and dependence by postulating opponent-adaptive biological processes that seek to return the system to its predrug state. This homeostatic process opposes the drug action and becomes a disruptive state itself when drug administration ceases and it remains unopposed. Until relatively recently, these explanatory mechanisms remained hypothetical constructs. Recent research now indicates, however, that tolerance and dependence are not only separable processes (Ternes, Ehrman, & O'Brien, 1985) but have reliably identifiable brain sites and measurable molecular mechanisms of action. Recent brain scan research has also identified specific brain areas activated by abused drugs, especially cocaine, and that cues associated with cocaine administration activate similar areas in the absence of the drug (Childress *et al.*, 1995). Thus, neural substrates of addiction are being identified and neural bases for conditioning effects of cues associated with drug use support conditioning and learning theories of addiction (Solomon and Corbit, 1974; Wikler, 1973). A recent comprehensive theory postulates a neurobiological basis for drug dependence that utilizes known and postulated linkages between cellular and behavioral effects of three classes of drugs: opiates, psychostimulants, and alcohol (Koob & Bloom, 1988).

Associated with research on precursors of abuse in adolescence, several theories on the etiology of abuse have been developed. These focus on how drug use is initiated and maintained in adolescence and propose social phenomena in adolescence to explain development of abuse. Two recently proposed theories receiving considerable attention in the literature are self-medication theory, perhaps best articulated by Khantzian (1985), and the social stress model of substance abuse recently reviewed by Lindenberg, Gendrop, and Reiskin (1993).

Though self-medication theory originally was proposed from the psychoanalytic tradition, it is also espoused by biological researchers. It proposes that individuals abuse drugs to obtain relief from aversive emotional states in an attempt to regulate, that is, self-medicate, intolerable affect. An individual's drug of choice is not seen as accidental, but chosen for its pharmacological properties to relieve specific affective symptoms and feeling states. One of the theory's main attractive features is its parsimonious explanation of abuse and dependence. Opponents of the theory have criticized it because it has been based mostly on anecdotal data. However, there is at least one large empirical study that provided mostly supportive evidence for the theory. Weis, Griffin, and Mirin (1992) examined a group of 494 hospitalized drug abusers. They focused on possible self-medication for depression. They found 63% of patients reported drug use in response to depressive symptoms and experienced mood elevation regardless of the type drug abused.

The social stress model of substance abuse explains the contribution of variables that influence initiation of drug abuse, especially for urban adolescents (Lindenberg *et al.*, 1993). The model proposes that initiation of drug abuse is a function of the stress level experienced by the individual, which is buffered by three social modifier variables. These modifiers are social networks, social competencies, and community resources. These social modifiers interact with each other and together buffer the impact of stress. Lindenberg *et al.* (1993), in their recent review, found 35 studies that assessed one or more of the model's constructs. Though their review found many studies flawed by inconsistent operational definitions of constructs and resulting noncomparability of findings among the studies, findings showed a consistent relationship of the model's constructs with drug use.

Space does not permit a more detailed review of theories of etiology. The interested reader will find excellent reviews in Milby (1981), where 63 different theories are compared and contrasted. Murray and Perry (1985) summarize nine models of etiology in adolescence, and an excellent exposition of self-medication theory is found in Khantzian (1985). A learning model of addictioin is described by O'Brien *et al.* (1992). Last, a summary and review of research on the social stress model is found in Lindenberg *et al.* (1993).

Substance Abuse Prevention

Primary Prevention

Effective Programs

A comprehensive approach to understanding drug abuse prevention programming and research relies on four interrelated areas: descriptive epidemiology, etiology, intervention development, and evaluation (Hansen, 1994). Descriptive epidemiology provides the field with information about the nature, prevalence, incidence, and developmental course of the problem. These data help target high-risk populations, age of onset, developmental patterns, and provide a measure of success. Etiology refers to knowledge of the cause or history of drug initiation or misuse. Identification of risk and protective factors help provide clues for interventions. Interventions range from policy centered to program development to individual based. Educational prevention programs are the most common because of the accessability of the target population. Finally, evaluation provides the evidence needed to disseminate effective programs (Hansen, 1994).

In Hansen's (1994) review, specific areas of prevention research have shown potential to prevent alcohol use, alcohol abuse, and its effects. For example, descriptive epidemiology has shown a general trend toward reduced alcohol consumption and a major related outcome: alcohol-related fatal automobile accidents. While the specific policy and programmatic events responsible for these outcomes are impossible to identify, Hansen posits great impact of policy-related prevention approaches, such as increasing the minimum drinking age, lowering the legal blood alcohol content level for minors, laws that allow police to administer immediate punishment to motorists who test above the minimum blood alcohol level, and alcohol-server interventions and liability.

School-based educational strategies that have been found to be effective have utilized social influences, skills acquisition for resisting peer pressure, and correction of erroneous perceptions of social norms. In one review, school prevention programs were taught in middle or junior high school. They focused on counteracting social influences to use drugs, including standardized teacher or staff training, multiple class sessions, boosters, student peer leaders, and active social learning methods. These prevention programs showed 20% or larger net reductions in rates of drug use onset (Pentz, 1994).

Hansen (1994) concluded that many prevention measures have not yet been evaluated that show promise like student assistance programs, school-based clubs, and family interventions. Multichannel community programs—those that include multiple program components and channels for program delivery in addition to the school—were found to reduce the rate of drug use prevalence early on and produce early delays in experimental or initiation that could reduce progression to more regular or harder drug use (Pentz, 1994). The efficacy of primary prevention programs directed at elementary grade schoolchildren is often limited by exaggerated emphasis of negative long-term consequences of drug taking, too much focus on general coping skill development and not on particular drug-specific situations, and lack of subcultural forces on children (including families, friends, and mass media) (van Heeringen, 1995).

Eight models of preventing substance involvement were reviewed by Lorion and Ross (1992). These community-based programs were a part of the Office for Substance Abuse Prevention's high-risk youth initiative in 1987 and are summarized below.

The Substance Use Prevention and Education Resource II in Atlanta, Georgia, was targeted to minority youth from economically disadvantaged, single-parent families and designed to deter alcohol and drug use by increasing resources available to these youth and involving parents in preventive interventions (Bruce & Emshoff, 1992). While few parents participated in all sessions, significant increases were found in both parents and youth in their knowledge of drugs and good communication, family functioning and parental esteem for their children, and decreases in the frequency of substance use of youths at 3–month follow-up.

An after-school program on precursors of substance abuse for primary grade latchkey students was a large-scale intervention targeted to latchkey children in New Orleans (Ross, Saavedra, Shur, Winters, & Felner, 1992). The program collaborated with local schools and developed after-school programs in two dozen sites. The program focused on improving children's self-esteem and academic performance with a balance of recreation, homework support, and self-esteem-building exercises. Despite reluctance by program staff to randomize students to nonintervention groups and parental refusal to allow some selected students to participate, which in effect denied them access to various publicly funded services, the program demonstrated significant effects on children's academic performance, limited to children who were exposed to the self-esteem-building component.

The Child and Family Options Project was a primary drug and alcohol prevention program for kindergarten-aged children and their mothers, primarily single, low-income, African Americans, located in a large public housing project in Chicago (Ruch-Ross, 1992). The primary components of the program were structured, center-based, parent–child activities, parent meetings and training, and monthly family outings. The results of a quasi-experimental, nonequivalent control group design included positive but nonstatistically significant trends in children returning to school and mothers seeking drug and alcohol treatment.

CODA, a creative therapy program for children in families affected by abuse of alcohol or other drugs, was conducted and evaluated in California using art and play therapy as an intervention (Springer, Phillips, Phillips, Cannady, & Kerst-Harris, 1992). Evaluation findings revealed success in recruiting and maintaining participation by youth and parents in chemically dependent families and pre- and postcomparisons showed significant gains in competencies and reductions in identified behavior problems.

A psychoeducational and substance abuse risk reduction intervention for children of substance abusers conducted in inner city East Baltimore targeted urban, primarily minority public school adolescent children (Gross & McCaul, 1992). Using a social support and social-skills-building model of drug abuse prevention, there was little evidence at posttest and at 1–year follow-up to support the effectiveness of the intervention for reducing substance abuse risk factors.

A study of multiagency collaborative strategies between substance abuse and juvenile justice agencies was conducted with juvenile delinquents in the Colorado Office of Substance Abuse Prevention (OSAP) Project (Stein et al., 1992). The services provided focused on affective education, drug-free alternatives, prosocial bonding, self-competency development, and transition skills within a wilderness program. Multiple agencies were able to collaborate, resulting in a temporary decrease of alcohol and drug use, positive behavior change, increases in prosocial choices, peer bonding, learning new academic skills, and tremendous cost savings.

An early intervention program comparing an adaptation of the Botvin Life Skills Training model and a combined program of an antiviolence model and a values clarification model were conducted with a population of high-risk adolescents in Philadelphia (Friedman & Utada, 1992). Several improvements in behavior and attitudes were significant for the total sample. The values clarification–antiviolence intervention combination fared better than the Botvin Life Skills Training program.

Boys and girls clubs within residential public housing developments in 15 sites across the country were evaluated on their effectiveness in reducing substance abuse and other problem rates among children (Schinke, Orlandi, & Cole, 1992). Findings revealed that public housing developments with boys and girls clubs had less drug-related activity, measurably fewer damaged and unoccupied units, and increased parental involvement in youth activities than housing developments without these clubs.

Common Threads

Lorion and Ross (1992) describe three main lessons from their review of these eight model prevention demonstration projects. First, prevention interventions seemed to work best when targeted toward youth with a cooccurrence of individual, familial, peer, and community risk factors. The "shotgun" approach toward addressing multiple risk factors was common among these high-risk youth demonstration projects. Second, the development and implementation of community-based prevention programs was complicated and difficult. Multiple, interacting steps were involved in the development and implementation of these programs: selecting the target population, defining the planned intervention, reaching the target population, gaining their trust, securing active participation, and choreographing the delivery of the interventions. Third, evaluating the process and outcome of the programs was a special challenge. Issues revolved around program readiness to be evaluated, balancing accountability demands with the reluctance of many providers to be evaluated, provider resistance to random assignment of participants to comparison or no treatment conditions, choosing meaningful outcomes in addition to the impact on rates of alcohol and drug use, and difficulty conducting longitudinal confirmation studies to differentiate substance avoidance from simple postponement.

Additional common threads of effective primary prevention programs have been identified in the literature. First, interest has shifted from larger groups to children at high risk for developing drug abuse. As the knowledge about genetic predisposition and earlier age of drug use onset increases, recent preventive efforts focus on high-risk children (van Heeringen, 1995). Second, identification of protective factors (individual or environmental variables that inhibit, reduce, or buffer the probability of drug use or abuse) as well as risk factors (individual or environmental factors that increases the probability of drug use) is now considered in the development and implementation of effective prevention programs (Clayton, 1992). Third, teaching particular drug-specific coping skills as well as general coping skills and self-esteem, such as strategies to resist prodrug pressures from friends or the mass media, is now common among effective prevention programs (van Heeringen, 1995). Finally, ethnic, cultural, and gender influences and factors involved in the initiation of drug use is considered in any effective prevention effort, especially involving ethnic populations.

Cultural and Gender Issues

Enculturation is the process by which a cultural or ethnic group prescribe, proscribe, or tolerate the use of destructive substances for social or personal purposes (Westermeyer, 1995). For example, family and peer influences dominate initiation of alcohol or drug use through value development, social acceptance, and modeling. Parents who use alcohol to excess but caution their children not to drink are likely to raise substance-abusing children (Westermeyer, 1995). Children also may be enticed by the glamorized lifestyle of drug using and dealing presented by their peers.

Ethnic enculturation also may decrease the risk of becoming involved in drug abuse within a population as a protective factor (Westermeyer, 1995). Religious and church experiences support drug-free lifestyles and preach the hazards of drug abuse to congregations. All cultures have resiliency or protective factors that guard against initiation encompassed in education, religion, socialization, or athletics. Many persons who grow up in disadvantaged, drug-involved environments avoid involvement with drugs and succeed in life. Primary prevention and early recognition efforts should reflect both risk and protective cultural, ethnic, economic, and religious factors that influence substance use and abuse (Westermeyer, 1995).

A review of 19 Office of Substance Abuse Prevention-funded drug abuse prevention demonstration projects was conducted that targeted significant populations of African-American youth (Courtney, 1993). Common program themes were an emphasis on cultural specificity, for example, Afrocentric principles guiding program development and implementation. Most programs tried to incorporate values of African-American institutions, including an emphasis on the extended family and spirituality. Many projects noted that extreme exposure to environmental stress like crime and poverty contributed to threats to personal safety. Most programs believed that providing a sense of safety and protection was a key to successful program implementation. Measurements of outcome were culturally specific and sensitive to Afrocentric characteristics of the population, environment, and culture. Reductions in alcohol and drug experimentation and/or abuse were found. Three ingredients were reported to contribute to successful prevention efforts: (1) adherence to a structured curriculum with clear objectives; (2) minimum service contact of 20 hours over approximately 6 weeks; and (3) visibility and involvement of program staff with African-American heritage.

Prevention of drug and alcohol abuse during pregnancy is a prevention effort specifically relevant to women. Significant numbers of women use and abuse alcohol and other substances during pregnancy, which results in immediate or long-term negative effects on the pregnancy and the fetus, such as intrauterine growth retardation, preterm labor, fetal alcohol syndrome, and neonatal abstinence syndrome. The Center for Substance Abuse Treatment treatment improvement protocol on pregnant substance-abusing women recommended guidelines for comprehensive preventive care for pregnant women (Mitchell, 1993). It suggests early intervention during the prenatal period, focus on education about the dangers of drug and alcohol abuse during pregnancy rather than criminal prosecution of substance-abusing pregnant women, gender-specific and culturally relevant treatment opportunities, comprehensive medical care, and training for obstetric health care providers in the area of substance abuse and pregnancy. An innovative obstetric practice substance use training program called OBIWOM (obstetrics and substance use among women) is presently being evaluated by M. Engle and J. E. Schumacher and colleagues in Birmingham, Alabama. The cost-benefit of a perinatal intervention is unquestionable. A cost-benefit analysis conducted by James G. Haughton, policy advisor to the Los Angeles County Department of Health Services, supported the hypothesis that perinatal substance abuse intervention prevents drug-related fetal problems by reporting significant cost reductions of postnatal care among women receiving substance use prevention interventions (Center for Substance Abuse Prevention, 1994).

Future Directions

Genetic research in the last two decades has revealed heritability estimates indicating an association between the distribution of genotypes in the population and the distribution of certain observable characteristics or phenotypes such as use or misuse of drugs (Tater, 1995). The author comments that the results from these investigations do not allow extrapolation of genetic effects operating at the individual level. Thus, the opportunity to use genetic information for primary prevention depends on the result of advances in molecular genetics. The potential hazards (labeling, confidentiality protection, the unknown genetic–environment interaction, and separating families based on genetic testing at birth) of uncovering underlying behavioral traits related to drug abuse must be guarded against. However, the potential benefits (predisposing predictions based on saliva DNA analyses, the marshaling of environmental resources for high-risk babies, and cost-effective prevention targeted at those at high risk are worth considering in the field of prevention as we near the year 2000.

Parental involvement with children is a necessary and effective component to academic performance, social development, and self-esteem building. It also can be an effective primary prevention measure to avoiding experimentation and initiation of drug use. Parental use of alcohol or drugs may conflict with abstinence or controlled use messages to children. In a study linking parental illicit drug and tobacco use to three health belief model constructs (susceptibility, seriousness, and health motivation), Hahn (1993) found that parent drug and tobacco users tended to view their children as more susceptible to future drug or alcohol use, but they were less likely to perceive alcohol or drug use by their children as serious as compared to nonusers. Smokers were less likely to value early prevention activities with their children than the total sample. The author suggests that primary prevention providers can build on the psychological readiness of parents who use alcohol or drugs by teaching them ways to help their children avoid experimentation and initiation. Providers can also refer alcohol- and drug-using parents for treatment to increase their insight about the harms of use and address smokers' lack of health motivation for early prevention activities (Hahn, 1993).

An analysis of prevention programs by Pentz (1994) revealed the following concerns and needs of current prevention efforts: (1) most prevention programs are based on demand reduction strategies (i.e., the greater avoidance of drugs, the less the demand), but little is known about the relative effectiveness of this approach since avoidance and demand have not been compared in the same studies; (2) most prevention programs are aimed at school-attending populations of youth and to a lesser extent dropouts, homeless, or other high-risk children; (3) little is known about the synergistic effect of school programs and multiple program channels within the community on prevention, since these programs are evaluated separately; (4) the extent to which prevention components found to be effective in the laboratory are generalizable to the community is limited due to few technology transfer studies; and (5) too little interface between basic and social science approaches to drug abuse prevention is occurring with the intent of integrating both biological and social behavioral intervention methods. Pentz (1994) offers a comprehensive view of the future of drug prevention research in terms of current developments, research needs/gaps, and potential for basic/social science interface for the following research directions: integrated supply and demand reduction, strategic prevention, comprehensive prevention, technology transfer, and prevention research methods development.

Secondary and Tertiary Prevention

Effective Programs and Interventions

Contrary to public knowledge, over the last two decades a variety of secondary and tertiary substance abuse prevention programs have been demonstrated to be effective in reducing or eliminating substance abuse and associated health risks in a variety of settings with different types of abuse populations (Miller & Hester, 1986; Hubbard *et al.*, 1990). However, relatively high relapse rates are common to most types of addiction (Hunt, Barnett, & Branch, 1971) and remain a challenge to the field. Several effective drug treatment models and programs are discussed below.

Motivational interviewing (Miller & Rollnick, 1991) is based on Prochaska and DiClemente's theory of behavior change which postulates that change occurs in stages during which more or less resistance to change is expected and more or less compliance and motivation for change occurs. Motivational interviewing assesses the person with regard to where they are in the change process, then targets an interviewing intervention to the stage of change identified. Motivational interviewing strategies are directed to increase the probability that a person will enter into, continue, and comply with change-directed behavior. Assessments are often utilized to provide personalized, nonjudgmental feedback to the person to help them move along the continuum of change. This approach has been highly effective in reducing alcohol intake in problem drinkers relative to controls in a brief two session intervention with assessment for self-identified problem drinkers. The Drinkers Checkup (DCU; Miller & Marlatt, 1987) has demonstrated success in attracting alcohol-impaired people who do not think of themselves as problem drinkers and who otherwise would not seek treatment. Research has shown the DCU to yield an average 50% reduction in alcohol consumption within 6 weeks after the brief intervention, whereas waiting list controls showed such a marked reduction only after receiving the DCU as a delayed treatment. Suppression of drinking lasted over 18 months follow-up (Miller & Rollnick, 1991).

The efficacy of drug counseling and psychotherapy for drug abusers has been established in well-controlled outcome research. For example, Woody and colleagues (1983) randomly assigned methadone maintenance patients to drug counseling alone or with additional psychotherapy that employed manualized treatments. Results showed that counseling alone was associated with significant gains, especially for patients with little or no psychopathology in addition to their Substance Use Disorder. However, those patients with multiple mental disorders improved substantially beyond therapeutic benefits from drug counseling alone with additional psychotherapy (Woody *et al.*, 1984).

The community reinforcement model (Hunt & Azrin, 1972) has been demonstrated to be an effective program for chronic alcoholics referred for inpatient treatment. The original study developed a procedure to rearrange community reinforcers such as job, family, and social relations of the alcoholic such that drinking produced timeout from high-density reinforcement. The procedure used innovative job finding and counseling and a community tavern turned into an nonalcohol recreation center for families. Alcoholics who received this treatment were compared against matched controls who received institutional usual care. Results showed that community reinforcement counseling clients drank less, worked more, and spent more time with their families and out of institutions than controls. This approach has been replicated several times since the original study and adapted for different locations and populations with similar success.

Controlled drinking, as opposed to an abstinence-based approach, when first tried as an intervention was quite controversial. Sobel and Sobel (1976) based a behavioral intervention for problem drinkers on the research showing that most people who undergo treatment for alcohol problems return to some drinking, even after treatment that established abstinence for a time. Their approach used behavioral principles to analyze and intervene with alcohol approach and consummatory behaviors, teaching controlled volume (sip volume), frequency, and beverage choice behaviors. Their early results were quite encouraging and persisted beyond 1 year follow-up. In spite of intense criticism from the 12-Step movement and other alcohol researchers, some of whom contested their findings, an independent panel validated their methods and reported results and follow-up outcomes. This useful intervention is probably more appropriate for problem social drinkers and alcohol abusers who would resist intervention efforts to force abstinence treatment goals. For individuals who are dependent on alcohol, it is less likely to be effective and could set up unrealistic expectations for controlling an addiction that has a strong physiological component. Thus, for the appropriate target population and if conceptualized as a harm reduction secondary prevention intervention, it is more likely to be accepted as one intervention technique among many for clinicians who intervene with alcohol abuse, especially for those clients who are resistant to typical abstinence oriented and 12-Step programs.

Several effective outpatient interventions for cocaine abuse have emerged from the recent clinical research on treatment: an outpatient day treatment model like that reported by O'Brien, Alterman, Walter, Childress, and McLellan (1989) and Washton and Stone-Washton (1990); a contingency management behavioral therapy program (Raczynski et al., 1993); and a relapse prevention model that can be incorporated as a major day treatment component (Carroll et al., 1994). The Higgins et al. (1991) study provided clients with reinforcement contingencies for consecutive clean urines, that is, sustained abstinence, and counseled them to develop new recreational activities or reinvolve themselves with previously enjoyed nondrug-related recreational activities.

Until recently, no programs have designed interventions for cocaine- and alcohol-abusing homeless persons, especially for those who have coexisting mental disorders. O'Brien et al. (1989) reported they were uniformly unsuccessful in treating their homeless cocaine abusers since 100% dropped from the program before completing treatment. The above-listed programs that have reported successful outcome, given reasonable control or comparison conditions (Higgins et al., 1991; Washton & Stone-Washton, 1990; O'Brien et al., 1989), all included common similar elements. Two of the three involved intense daily contact 4–5 days per week (Washton & Stone-Washton, 1990; O'Brien et al., 1989). All involved at least once weekly urine surveillance with feedback to clients and an emphasis on relapse prevention by avoiding drug-using friends and associates and developing new nondrug-related sources of gratification, although Higgins et al. (1991) emphasized this more than the others.

The Birmingham 1991 and 1993 substance abuse treatments for the homeless projects, the most recent of which incorporated elements of Higgins' voucher system

(Higgins *et al.*, 1991) and relapse prevention (Milby *et al.*, 1996a,b) have developed an innovative day treatment model that has been relatively successful in engaging homeless alcohol and substance abusers and in producing positive outcomes of reduced substance use, increased employment, improved habitat status, and improved depressive symptomatology and self-esteem (Raczynski *et al.*, 1993). However, the 1991 Birmingham project was originally conceived for alcoholism intervention and had to intervene with a patient population with coexisting alcohol and cocaine abuse–dependence and underlying mental illness (mostly affective and personality disorders). Thus, the successful outcomes were obtained in spite of an absence of specially designed interventions for those abusing cocaine and those with associated mental disorders.

Since the literature described there are successful interventions for cocaine and combined cocaine–alcohol abuse as reported earlier, and that contingencies requiring abstinence are effective in other contexts (Milby, Garrett, English, Fritschi, & Clarke, 1978; Milby *et al.*, 1996b) incorporated and elaborated on the reinforcement procedures of Higgins *et al.* (1991) and maximized them within a behavioral social reinforcement day treatment program, while measuring the adjunctive efficacy of a potentially potent treatment contingency for substance-abusing homeless and abstinent-contingent work and housing. Preliminary results with 6-month follow-up show that abstinent-contingent work and housing as an adjunct to day treatment was significantly more effective than day treatment alone, with significant differences observed on average weeks and consecutive weeks of abstinence at 2 and 6 months and on homelessness severity at 2 months and days employed at 6 months.

Methadone maintenance involves substituting a pharmacologically pure, long-acting, orally consumed, synthetic opiate—methadone—for adulterated street opiates that are typically used intravenously. Prospective patients for this treatment are carefully examined to meet Food and Drug Administration (FDA) criteria for chronic opiate addiction. Treatment involves daily dosing and usually involves a time course of one or more years before detoxification is recommended. Because detoxification is more often than not followed by relapse to opiate use, especially since the acquired immunodeficiency syndrome (AIDS) epidemic, there has been less emphasis on preparing patients for eventual detoxification and more emphasis on engaging and maintaining patients in treatment and use of sufficiently high enough methadone doses to prevent continued illicit intravenous opiate use.

Despite enduring criticism that methadone maintenance simply substitutes one addiction for another, it has been found to be a safe and effective maintenance treatment to temper illicit drug use and help addicts return to productive activity without the need to support an illegal drug habit via criminal activities (Connell, 1975; Gossop, 1978; Milby, 1981, 1988). A recent multicenter follow-up study 6.5 years after identification of a methadone maintenance cohort, found that more than half of followed patients were functioning drug-free except for prescribed methadone (Milby *et al.*, 1994).

Common Aspects of Effective Programs

There are several common aspects of effective substance abuse treatment programs. Effective programs provide a therapeutic focus on problem behaviors that are changeable. The therapeutic programs are organized in such a way to provide regular and meaningful contact with the patients. Effective programs regularly use urine and breath testing to objectively assess progress of the patient and to provide feedback to the patient and information on which program changes are made. Effective programs and the most effective counselors can be discriminated by documentation in the record reflecting a logical intervention plan, treatment goals formulated with the patient, activities that derive from the plan, and changes in the plan in response to patient's progress or lack of progress.

Another common aspect of effective treatment programs are the use of naturally occurring or contrived contingencies to promote therapeutic progress. For example, a consecutive period of urine tests free of drugs has successfully been imposed as a contingency for take-home doses of methadone in methadone maintenance programs (Milby *et al.*, 1978; Stitzer *et al.*, 1977). Higgins *et al.* (1991) have utilized vouchers worth money for the purchase of recreational items as a reinforcer with contingencies for consecutive urine tests free of cocaine. This procedure, along with behavioral counseling that targeted specific behavior changes, led to impressive abstinence rates and consecutive weeks abstinent relative to usual care control treatment where patients from the same pool of subjects where randomized to a community 12-Step program. Milby and colleagues (1996a,b) effectively used work and housing to reinforce abstinence among primarily crack-cocaine-abusing homeless. The community reinforcement model (Hunt & Azrin, 1972) as noted above successfully identified and altered contingencies for naturally occurring reinforcers for chronic alcoholics and obtained substantial outcomes relative to usual care matched controls. Nationwide, treatment alternatives to street crime and drug court programs have effectively utilized legal sanctions and incentives to control drug use among offenders.

For cocaine addicts, several common elements of effective programs can be identified. Successful programs require attendance several times per week, if not daily, in highly structured activities that focus on and measure behavior change with regularly scheduled urine testing. Further positive outcomes can be established by incorporating the use of therapeutic contingencies to target and reinforce rehabilitation behaviors that are objectively defined and monitored on a weekly basis with feedback to patients. Innovative pharmacological agents for the treatment of cocaine dependency are being tested (Kosten, 1992).

Gender and Ethnic Issues

Women face unique barriers to effective drug and alcohol treatment as a function of their sex. First, most drug treatment programs are based on models devised for men. Male and female treatment centers rarely focus on relationship issues that contribute to relapse rates for women. Second, women have multiple needs of housing, employment, child care, and treatment for depression at greater rates than men, which require special attention in drug treatment programs. Finally, many women are unable to engage in treatment that requires most of the day or residential stay due to lack of child care support. These barriers in addition to others are particularly powerful when added to the stigmatizing effect of poverty and racial discrimination. Gender-specific treatment requires programming that eliminates these barriers for women and focuses on women's issues in drug treatment like relationship triggers to relapse and gender-relevant issues related to human immunodeficiency virus (HIV) risk. Any drug treatment program should incorporate child care services and provide services related to pre- and postnatal exposure issues. One program in Birmingham, Alabama, called Olivia's House, is a center for substance abuse treatment-funded demonstration of women's-specific drug treatment that strives to reduce the above-mentioned barriers and provide drug treatment to women with children by supporting up to three preschool-aged children who live with their mothers and participate in a child development program while in treatment (Schumacher, Siegal, Socol, Harkless, & Freeman, 1996).

Treatment programs should first take into consideration differential prevalence rates of specific substances and related etiology when creating or modifying treatment to be ethnic specific. Ethnic groups have differing views about drug abuse and drug-abusing lifestyles that should be incorporated into the treatment process. Afrocentric drug treatment models have been proposed for African Americans that take into consideration important treatment issues related to relationships, the extended family, and religious affiliation and background.

Limitations for Targeted Behaviors and Subpopulations

Even though Substance Use Disorders are among the most common mental disorders in the United States, a recent large epidemiologic catchment area study of several communities, which included almost 20,000 people, found that 85–90% of persons with these disorders had never been exposed to treatment (Robbins & Reiger, 1991). Thus, it appears that only a small and probably select subpopulation of all persons with Substance Use Disorders, find their way into treatment and receive professional assistance or treatment. Clearly, the United States has a major public health problem for which its current prevention and treatment programs are inadequate to the population's need. If close to one half of all those who had a Substance Use Disorder presented for treatment, our treatment resources would be overwhelmed and they would not be able to offer treatment to most of the people who presented for assistance. Thus, the United States could benefit from increased attention to prevention efforts that would reduce exposure to substance abuse and by making available more treatment slots.

Prevention messages on the dangers of alcohol and drug use that currently appear infrequently on national television reach a much larger segment of the population than local prevention interventions. If research shows these to have positive impacts, prevention messages and other interventions that are targeted to known at-risk populations and individuals, especially at the community and school levels, could have a significant impact on the problem.

Conclusions

The epidemiology of drug use reflects demonstrable portions of the US population affected. The last two decades have documented an epidemic related to crack cocaine use among economically disadvantaged in metropolitan areas. The rise in HIV infection and AIDS is significantly greater among drug users. There is a rise in cigarette and illicit drug use among youth. Survey research has shown that there are significantly more persons in need of treatment than treatment capacity available. The problem of drug use, abuse, and dependency is all but obvious. There is, however, a bright side.

Drug and alcohol abuse is less a moral problem and more a health concern today than historically. Congressional support exists for drug abuse science and empirically based treatment approaches among a lowering of priorities for social services and human welfare. Effective prevention models have been developed that target protective as well as risk factors as predictors of drug-free lifestyles. Parental support and involvement and peer mentor programs provide key strategies in preventing drug initiation and maladaptive involvement. Drug treatment strategies continue to evolve and target specific populations and drug types better than ever. Contingency management interventions for cocaine addiction hold great promise as innovative and effective empirically based treatments for this most destructive and addictive substance. The shift of focus from punishment to treatment by the criminal justice system and the effectiveness of contingency management programs like treatment alternatives to street crime and drug courts across the country have begun to effectively address the association between addiction and criminal behavior.

Remaining concerns include challenges to initiate motivation, prevent relapse, involve parents, and rehabilitate neighborhoods. Continued investigation of new models of prevention and treatment, gender-specific and culturally relevant treatment programs, and new medications to reduce cravings will require congressional support and funding. Attention to the reduction of crime and drug abuse and the risk of HIV among drug abusers will be priorities of the future. With improved societal acceptance, empirical research, and compassionate treatment, we are likely to shift priorities and make needed changes.

References

American Psychiatric Association (APA). (1994). *Diagnostic and statistical manual of mental disorders* (4th ed.). Washington, DC: Author.

Bruce, C., & Emshoff, C. (1992). The SUPER II program: An early intervention program. *Journal of Community Psychology (OSAP Special Issue)*, 10–21.

Carroll, K. M., Rounsaville, B. J., Nich, C., Gordon, L. T., Wirtz, P. W., & Gawin, F. (1994). One-year follow-up of psychotherapy and pharmacotherapy for cocaine dependence: Delayed emergence of psychotherapy effects. *Archives of General Psychiatry, 51,* 989–997.

Center for Substance Abuse Prevention. (1994). *Cost-benefit issues in programs for prevention of alcohol and other drug abuse.* Washington, DC: US Department of Health and Human Services.

Chen, K., & Kandel, D. B. (1995). The natural history of drug use from adolescence to the mid-thirties in a general population sample. *American Journal of Public Health, 85,* 41–47.

Cheung, Y. W. (1993). Approaches to ethnicity: Clearing roadblocks in the study of ethnicity and substance use. *The International Journal of the Addictions, 28,* 1209–1226.

Childress, A. R., Mozley, P. D., Fitzgerald, J., Reiuich, M., Jaggi, J., & O'Brien, C. P. (1995). *Regional brain blood flow during cue induced cocaine craving.* NIDA Research Monograph No. 162. Problems of Drug Depencence: Proceedings of the 57th Annual Scientific Meeting. Rockville, Maryland: National Institute on Drug Abuse.

Clayton, R. R. (1992). Transitions in drug use: Risk and protective factors. In M. Glanz & R. Pickens (Eds.), *Vulnerability to drug abuse* (pp. 15–52). Washington, DC: American Psychological Association.

Connell, P. H. (1975). Review of methadone maintenance schemes. In *Skandia International Symposium on Drug Dependence: Treatment and evaluation* (pp. 133–146). Stockholm: Almquist & Wiksell International.

Courtney, R. J. (1993). Prevention and intervention programs targeted toward African-American youth at high risk. In L. L. Goddard (Ed.), *An African-American centered model of prevention for African-American youth at high risk.* Rockville, MD: US Department of Health and Human Services.

Denier, C. A, Thevos, A. K., Latham, P. K., & Randall, C. L. (1991). Psychosocial and psychopathology differences in hospitalized male and female cocaine abusers: A retrospective chart review. *Addictive Behaviors, 16,* 489–496.

Friedman, A. S., & Utada, A. T. (1992). Effects of two group interaction models on substance-using adjudicated adolescent males. *Journal of Community Psychology (OSAP Special Issue)*, 106–117.

Gfroered, J. (1993). Race and crack cocaine. *Journal of the American Medical Association, 270,* 45–46.

Gossop, M. (1978). A review of the evidence for methadone maintenance as a treatment for narcotic addiction. *Lancet, 1,* 812–815.

Gross, J., & McCaul, M. E. (1992). An evaluation of a psychoeducational and substance abuse risk reduction intervention for children of substance abusers. *Journal of Community Psychology (OSAP Special Issue),* 75–87.

Hahn, E. J. (1993). Parental alcohol and other drug (AOD) use and health beliefs about parent involvement in AOD prevention. *Issues in Mental Health Nursing, 14,* 237–247.

Hansen, W. B. (1994). Prevention of alcohol use and abuse. *Preventive Medicine, 23,* 683–687.

Higgins, S., Delaney, D., Budney, A., Bickel, W. K., Hughes, J. R., Foerg, F., & Fenwick, J. W. (1991). A behavioral approach to achieving initial cocaine abstinence. *American Journal of Psychiatry, 148*(9), 1218–1224.

Hubbard, R. L., Marsden, M. E., Rachal, J. V., Harwood, H. J., Cavanough, E. R., & Ginzburg, H. M. (1990). *Drug abuse treatment; A national study of effectiveness.* Chapel Hill: The University of North Carolina Press.

Hunt, G. M., & Azrin, N. H. (1972). A community-reinformcement approach to alcoholism. *Behavioral Research and Therapy, 11,* 91–104.

Hunt, W. A., Barnett, W., & Branch, L. G. (1971). Relapse rates in addiction programs. *Journal of Clinical Psychology, 27,* 455–456.

Johnston, L. D., O'Malley, P M., & Bachman, J. G. (1993). *Smoking, drinking, and illicit drug use among American high school students, college students and young adults, 1975–1991,* vol. 1. NIH Publication No. (ADM) 93-3481. Washington, DC: US Government Printing Office.

Kandel, D. B., Yamaguchi, K., & Chen, K. (1992). Stages of progression in drug involvement from adolescence to adulthood: Further evidence for the gateway theory. *Journal on Studies of Alcoholism, 53,* 447–457.

Khantzian, E. J. (1985). The self-medication hypothesis of addictive disorders: Focus on heroin and cocaine dependence. *American Journal of Psychiatry, 142,* 1259–1264.

Koob, G. F., & Bloom, F. E. (1988). Cellular and molecular mechanisms of drug dependence. *Science , 242,* 715–723.

Kosten T. (1992, June). *Diverse pharmacological agents for possible treatment of cocaine dependency.* Paper presented at the 54th annual scientific meeting of the College on Problems of Drug Dependence, Keystone, CO.

Lillie-Blanton, M., Anthony, J. C., & Schuster, C. R. (1993). Probing the meaning of racial/ethnic group comparisons in crack cocaine smoking. *Journal of the American Medical Association, 269,* 993–997.

Lindenberg, C. S., Gendrop, S. C., & Reiskin, H. K. (1993). Empirical evidence for the social stress model of substance abuse. *Research in Nursing and Health, 16,* 351–362.

Lorion, R. P., & Ross, J. G. (1992). Programs for change: A realistic look at the nation's potential for preventing substance involvement among high-risk youth. *Journal of Community Psychology (OSAP Special Issue),* 3–9.

Marlatt, G. A., & Gordon, J. R. (1985). *Relapse prevention: maintenance strategies in the treatment of addictive behaviors.* New York: Guilford Press.

Mathias, R. (1995, January/February). NIDA survey provides first national data on drug use during pregnancy. In *NIDA Notes* (pp. 6–7). Washington, DC: National Institute on Drug Abuse.

Maurer, D. W., & Vogel, V. H. (1973). *Narcotics and narcotic addiction* (4th ed.). Springfield, IL: Charles C. Thomas.

Milby, J. B. (1981). *Addictive behavior and its treatment.* New York: Springer.

Milby, J. B. (1988). Methadone maintenance to abstinence: How many make it? *The Journal of Nervous and Mental Disease, 176*(7), 409–422.

Milby, J. B., Garrett, C., English, C., Fritschie, O., & Clarke, C. (1978). Take-home methadone: Contingency effects on drug-seeking and productivity of narcotic addicts. *Addictive Behaviors, 3,* 215–220.

Milby, J. B., Hohman, A. H., Gentile, M., Huggins, N., Sims, M. K., McLellan, A. T., Woody, G., & Haas, N. (1994). Methadone maintenance outcome as a function of detoxification phobia. *American Journal of Psychiatry, 151*(7), 1031–1037.

Milby, J. B., Schumacher, J. E., Raczynski, J. M., Caldwell, E., Engle, M., Michael, M., & Carr, J. (1996a). Sufficient conditions for effective treatment of substance abusing homeless persons. *Drug and Alcohol Dependence, 43,* 39–47.

Milby, J. B., Schumacher, J. E., McNamara, C., Wallace, D., McGill, T., Stange, D., & Michael, M. (1996b). Abstinence contingent housing enhances day treatment for homeless cocaine abusers. Paper presented at the Annual Scientific Meeting of the College for Problems of Drug Dependence, San Juan, Puerto Rico, June 23.

Miller, W. R., & Marlatt, G. A. (1987). The drinker's check-up. Odessa, Florida: Psychological Assessment Resources, Inc.

Miller W. E., & Rollnick, S. (1991). *Motivation interviewing: Preparing people for change.* New York: Guilford Press.

Miller, W. R., & Hester, R. K. (1986). The effectiveness of alcoholism treatment: What research reveals. In W. Miler & N. Hester (Eds.), *Treating addictive behaviors: Processes of change* (pp. 121–174). New York : Plenum Press.

Mitchell, J. L. (1993). *Pregnant substance-using women.* Rockville, MD: US Department of Health and Human Services.

Murray, D. M., & Perry, C. L. (1985). The prevention of adolescent drug abuse: Implications of etiological, developmental, behavioral, and environmental models. In C. L. Jones & R. J. Battjes (Eds.), *Etiology of drug abuse: Implications for treatment* (pp. 111–121). National Institute on Drug Abuse. DHHS Pub. No. (ADM) 85-1335, Washington, DC: Government Printing Office.

National Institute on Drug Abuse. (1991). *National household survey on drug abuse: Highlights 1990.* Rockville, MD: US Department of Health and Human Services.

O'Brien, C. P., Alterman, A., Walter, D., Childress, A. R., & McLellan, A. T. (1989). *Evaluation of treatment for cocaine dependence.* NIDA Research Monograph No. 95. Rockville, MD: Department of Health and Human Services.

O'Brien, C. D., Childress, A. R., McLellan, A. T., & Ehrman, R. (1992). A learning model of addiction. In C. P. O'Brien & J. H. Jaffe (Eds), *Addictive states* (pp. 45–61). New York: Raven Press.

Pentz, M. A. (1994). Directions for future research in drug abuse prevention. *Preventive Medicine, 23,* 646–652.

Raczynski, J. M., Schumacher, J. E., Milby, J. B., Michael, M., Engle, M., Lerner, M., & Wooley, T. (1993). Comparative substance abuse treatments for the homeless: The Birmingham project. *Alcoholism Treatment Quarterly, 10*(3/4), 217–233.

Robbins, L. M., & Reiger, D. A. (1991). (Eds.). *Psychatric disorders in America: The Epidemiologic Catchment Area Study.* New York: Free Press.

Ross, J. G., Saavedra, P. J., Shur, G. H., Winters, F., & Felner, R. D. (1992). The effectiveness of an after-school program for primary grade latchkey students on precursors of substance abuse. *Journal of Community Psychology (OSAP Special Issue),* 22–38.

Ruch-Ross, H. S. (1992). The child and family options program: Primary drug and alcohol prevention for young children. *Journal of Community Psychology (OSAP Special Issue),* 39–54.

Schinke, S. P., Orlandi, M. A., & Cole, K. C. (1992). Boys and girls clubs in public housing developments: Prevention services for youth at risk. *Journal of Community Psychology (OSAP Special Issue),* 118–128.

Schumacher, J. E., Siegal, S. H., Socol, J. C., Harkless, S., & Freeman, K. (1996). Making evaluation work in a substance abuse treatment program for women with children: Olivia's House. *Journal of Psychoactive Drugs, 28,* 73–83.

Smith, E. M. (1993). Race or racism? Addiction in the United States. *Annals of Epidemiology, 3,* 165–170.

Sobel, M. B., & Sobel, L. C. (1976). Second-year treatment outcome of alcoholics treated by individualized behavior therapy: Results. *Behavior Research and Therapy, 14,* 195–215.

Solomon, R. L., & Corbit, J. D. (1974). An opponent-process theory of motivation: I. Temporal dynamics of affect. *Psychological Review, 81*(2), 119–145.

Springer, J. F., Phillips, J. L., Phillips, L., Cannady, L. P., & Kerst-Harris (1992). CODA: A creative therapy program for children in families affected by abuse of alcohol or other drugs. *Journal of Community Psychology (OSAP Special Issue),* 55–74.

Stein, S. L., Garcia, F., Marler, B., Embree-Bever, J., Garrett, C. J., Unrein, D., Burdick, M. A., & Fishburn, S. Y. (1992). A study of multiagency collaborative strategies: Did juvenile deliquents change? *Journal of Community Psychology (OSAP Special Issue),* 88–105.

Stitzer, M., Bigelow, G., Lawrence, C., Cohen, J., D'Lugoff, B., & Hawthorne, J. (1977). Medication take-home as a reinforcer in a methadone maintenance program. *Addictive Behaviors, 2,* 9–14.

Substance Abuse and Mental Health Services Administration. (1993). *National Household Survey on Drug Abuse: Population estimates 1992.* Rockville, MD: US Department of Health and Human Services.

Substance Abuse and Mental Health Services Administration. (1995). *National Household Survey on Drug Abuse: Population estimates 1994.* Rockville, MD: US Department of Health and Human Services.

Tater, R. E. (1995). Genetics and primary prevention of drug and alcohol abuse. *International Journal of the Addictions, 30,* 1479–1484.

Tarter, R. E., & Mezzich, A. C. (1992). Ontogeny of substance abuse: Prespectives and findings. In M. Glantz & R. Pickins (Eds.), *Vulnerability to drug abuse* (pp. 149–177). Washington, DC: American Psychological Association.

Ternes, J. W., Ehrman, R. N., & O'Brien, C. P. (1985). Nondependent monkeys self-administer hydromorphone. *Behavioral Neuroscience, 99*(3), 583–588.

van Heeringen, K. C. (1995). The prevention of drug abuse—State of the art and directions for future actions. *Clinical Toxicology, 33,* 575–579.

Washton, A. M., & Stone-Washton, N. (1990). Abstinence and relapse in outpatient cocaine addicts. *Journal of Psychoactive Drugs, 22*(2), 135–147.

Weis, R. D., Griffin, M. L., & Mirin, S. M. (1992). Drug abuse as self-medication for depression: An empirical study. *American Journal of Drug and Alcohol Abuse, 18*(2), 121–129.

Westermeyer, J. (1995). Cultural aspects of substance abuse and alcoholism: Assessment and management. *Psychiatric Clinics of North America, 18,* 589–605.

Wikler, A. (1973). Dynamics of drug dependence: Implications of a conditioning theory for research and treatment. *Archives of General Psychiatry, 28,* 611–616.

Woody, G. E., Luborsky, L., McClellan, A. T., O'Brien, C. P., Beck, A. T., Blaines, J., Aerman, I., & Hole, A. (1983). Psychotherapy for opiate addicts: Does it help? *Archives of General Psychiatry, 40,* 639–645.

Woody, G. E., McLellan, A. T., Luborsky, L., O'Brien, C. P., Blaine, I., Fox, S., Herman, I., & Beck, A. T. (1984). Psychiatric severity as a predictor of benefits from psychotherapy: The Penn VA study. *American Journal of Psychiatry, 141*(10), 1172–1177.

Wright, J. D. (1989a). *Address unknown: The homeless in America.* Hawthorne, NY: Aldine de Gruyter.

Wright, J. D. (1989b). *Correlates and consequences of alcohol abuse in the national "health care for the homeless" client population: Final results.* Washington, DC: National Institute on Alcohol Abuse and Alcoholism.

PART V

Behavior Change for Preventing Disease and Disability Outcomes

CHAPTER 12

Cardiovascular Diseases

James M. Raczynski, Martha M. Phillips, Carol E. Cornell,
M. Janice Gilliland, Bonnie Sanderson, and Vera Bittner

Introduction

Cardiovascular diseases (CVD) include a broad variety of diseases of the heart and blood vessels. Among others, CVD includes coronary heart disease [(CHD) also known as ischemic heart disease and coronary artery disease (CAD)], strokes of different types (including thrombotic, embolic, and hemorrhagic stroke), hypertension, and congenital heart defects. CHD mortality rates have declined in recent years as a result of modifications in risk factors through both early medical intervention and lifestyle changes as well as through newer treatment methods. Nonetheless, CHD remains the leading cause of mortality among both men and women of all ethnic groups in the United States [American Heart Association (AHA), 1998; Ayanian & Epstein, 1991] with rates that are higher than in other industrialized countries (Uemura & Pisa, 1988; World Health Organization, 1988). An estimated 1.1 million Americans will have acute myocardial infarctions (AMIs) resulting from CHD in 1998, with about one third of these resulting in death and an estimated 250,000 of those deaths occurring out of a hospital (AHA, 1998). Of 35 countries ranked by the World Health Organization (WHO), the United States had the 15th and 9th highest age-standardized CHD death rates for men and women, respectively (Uemura & Pisa, 1988); as a result of declines in CHD mortality, recent data suggest that the United States ranks 16th for both men and women in CHD mortality rates (AHA, 1998). Given the mor-

James M. Raczynski and M. Janice Gilliland • Behavioral Medicine Unit, Division of Preventive Medicine, Department of Medicine, School of Medicine, Department of Health Behavior, School of Public Health, UAB Center for Health Promotion, University of Alabama at Birmingham, Birmingham, Alabama 35294. *Martha M. Phillips* • UAB Civitan International Research Center, Department of Epidemiology, School of Public Health, UAB Center for Health Promotion, University of Alabama at Birmingham, Birmingham, Alabama 35294. *Carol E. Cornell* • Behavioral Medicine Unit, Division of Preventive Medicine, Department of Medicine, School of Medicine, UAB Center for Health Promotion, University of Alabama at Birmingham, Birmingham, Alabama 35294. *Bonnie Sanderson and Vera Bittner* • Division of Cardiovascular Disease, School of Medicine, UAB Center for Health Promotion, University of Alabama at Birmingham, Birmingham, Alabama 35294.

Handbook of Health Promotion and Disease Prevention, edited by Raczynski and DiClemente. Kluwer Academic/Plenum Publishers, New York, 1999.

tality risks associated with CHD, this disorder has been the primary focus among cardiovascular disorders of health promotion and disease prevention research and will be the primary focus of this chapter.

CHD actually includes several disorders that reduce blood flow to the heart. This reduced blood flow is most commonly attributable to narrowing of the coronary arteries due to atherosclerosis. The most common manifestations of CHD are angina pectoris (chest pain and tightness, which may be accompanied by pain radiating to the left arm or jaw, neck, or back), AMI or heart attack, and sudden death (Smith & Pratt, 1993).

Strategies to reduce CHD morbidity and mortality have been directed at the prevention of risk factors largely through what have often been termed "lifestyle" changes in populations that have not yet developed early stages of the disease (primary prevention), the pharmacological and behavioral control of risk factors as early disease stages emerge (secondary prevention), and the medical and behavioral factors that influence morbidity and mortality outcomes as CHD events occur. As our understanding of the role of primary risk factors has improved, primary prevention approaches have been modified. For example, as blood cholesterol was recognized as an independent risk factor for CHD, prevention strategies began to focus on dietary approaches to lower hypercholesterolemia (Blackburn, 1985; Harlan & Stross, 1985; Lenfant, 1986; Levy, 1985; Lowering Blood Cholesterol to Prevent Heart Disease Consensus Conference, 1985).

Behavioral issues have always been prominent in medical approaches to CHD prevention and treatment, not only because of a focus on modification of prominent lifestyle and psychosocial risk factors for CHD, but also because of the inherent issues of adherence with medical, behavioral, and psychosocial approaches. Additionally, innovations in medical therapies also have often raised new behavioral issues. For instance, medical innovations have resulted in reperfusion therapies to restore blood flow to the heart during an AMI, through either mechanical means, such as angioplasty or coronary artery bypass grafting surgery, or pharmacologically with thrombolytic agents; these reperfusion approaches only recently have been shown to lead to decreased CHD morbidity and mortality *if* treatment is delivered within the first few hours of symptom onset [AIMS Trial Study Group, 1990; Cannon, Antman, Walls, Braunwald, 1994; Every *et al.*, 1997; Fibrinolytic Therapy Trialists' Collaborative Group, 1994; Groupo Italiano per lo Studio della Streptochinasi nell'Infarto Miocardico (GISSI), 1986; Hennekens, O'Donnell, Ridker, & Marder, 1995; ISIS-2 Collaborative Group, 1988; Lee *et al.*, 1995; Marrugat *et al.*, 1997; O'Keefe *et al.*, 1989; Van de Werf & Arnold, 1988]. However, delay in seeking and obtaining treatment for AMI is unacceptably prolonged (Uemura & Pisa, 1988), severely limiting both the number of AMI patients who may benefit from reperfusion therapies and the effectiveness of therapy. Hence, medical care improvements in reperfusion therapies have resulted recently in greater attention being focused on behavioral issues involved in promoting people to recognize symptoms of AMI and to seek prompt medical treatment (Dracup *et al.*, 1997).

Finally, as our understanding of the role that behavioral and psychosocial factors play in influencing morbidity and mortality outcomes for CHD has improved, new directions for behavioral therapies have emerged. For instance, depression only recently has been recognized as a major predictor of morbidity and mortality after an AMI (Carney *et al.*, 1988; Frasure-Smith, Lesperance, & Talajic, 1993; Kennedy, Hofer, & Chen, 1987; Ladwig, Kiesert, Konig, Breithardt, & Borggrefe, 1991; Silverstone, 1990;

Sloan & Bigger, 1991), even after adjustment for disease severity (Frasure-Smith *et al.*, 1993; Sloan & Bigger, 1991), and social isolation (Berkman & Breslow, 1983; Berkman & Syme, 1979; Blumenthal *et al.*, 1987; Ruberman, Weinblatt, Golberg, & Chaudhary, 1984; Seeman & Syme, 1987). These data have led to recent interest in determining the degree to which pharmacological and nonpharmacological approaches to ameliorate depression and social isolation can impact on CHD morbidity and mortality.

Epidemiology

CVD has been the leading cause of death in the United States in almost every year since 1900 (AHA, 1998). The epidemic rise in CVD mortality rates that began earlier this century in the United States slowed and even began reversing in the 1960s. CVD mortality declined 37% between 1963 and 1982, with accelerated decline since the early 1970s (Kannel & Thom, 1984). CVD mortality rates continued to decline through 1994 [National Heart, Lung, and Blood Institute (NHLBI),1994], a trend that was likely due both to changes in lifestyle habits and to advances in medical treatments (Goldman & Cook, 1984). However, the number of CVD deaths rose in 1995 for both men and women (AHA, 1998), and CVD is still the leading cause of death in the United States, accounting annually for more than 960,000 deaths or 41.5% of all deaths. Over half the deaths due to CVD result from CHD, principally from AMI (AHA, 1998); this accounts for more than one fifth (21%) of the deaths from all causes (AHA, 1998). About 6 million US citizens were recently estimated to be living with CHD or about 25 per 1000 when adjusted for age (DeStefano, Merritt, Anda, Casper, & Eaker, 1993).

Women and CHD

Certainly, much more is known about CHD risk factors and prevention and treatment of CHD among men than among women. This situation has arisen because many studies either excluded women or failed to examine gender differences (e.g., Holme, Helgeland, Hjermann, Leren, & Lund-Larsen, 1980; Kagan, Gordon, Rhoads, & Schiffman, 1975; Mosca *et al.*, 1997; Rose & Shipley, 1986; Shaper & Elford, 1991; Shekelle *et al.*, 1981; Stamler, Wentworth, & Neaton, 1986; Yarnell *et al.*, 1991). Largely resulting from the paucity of data among women (Fields, Savard & Epstein, 1993; Lerner & Kannel, 1986) and the later onset of CHD among women (AHA, 1988), CHD was often thought of as a disease affecting primarily men. In fact, this opinion was so prevalent that the American Heart Association conducted a campaign during the 1960s and early 1970s to educate women about reducing the risk of heart disease *for the men in their lives,* virtually ignoring the risk of the women themselves (Wenger, 1994).

Recent data, however, provide some evidence of the incidence and prevalence of CHD and risk factors among women. These data suggest differences between men and women in patterns of CHD incidence and prevalence as well as risk factors (Legato, 1996; Lloyd *et al.*, 1996; Mosca *et al.*, 1997). Despite lower overall rates of CHD among young women when compared to men due to CHD being less common in younger, premenopausal women, the occurrence of CHD quickly accelerates after menopause to approximate the rates found among men (AHA, 1998). These incidence rates lead to an estimated 6.8 million women in the United States who have CHD (AHA, 1998).

Once CHD develops, it is the major source of mortality and morbidity among women. CVD is responsible for more than 500,000 deaths among women each year (compared with some 250,000 deaths attributed to all cancers), and the American Heart Association estimates that one in two women will die of heart disease (AHA, 1998). Early data suggested that women were at a survival disadvantage relative to men, suffering higher mortality and morbidity following AMI (Knopp, 1990; Wenger, 1990). Although the short-term survival of women appears lower, the long-term survival after medical or surgical treatment is comparable between gender groups (Davis, Chaitman, Ryan, Bittner, & Kennedy, 1995). The greater morbidity and mortality seen among women in the immediate period after having an AMI is thought to be due to technical difficulties encountered during angioplasty and coronary artery bypass grafting, such as those that result from smaller vessel size, more common comorbidities, and more advanced age of women at the time of their AMIs (Knopp, 1990; Wenger, 1990). These mortality gender patterns may also be related to women being referred for surgical treatment at a later disease stage than men (Khan *et al.*, 1990; Steingart *et al.*, 1991) or from women delaying longer in seeking treatment (Mosca *et al.*, 1997), although this area remains an active area of research.

In addition to CHD being a disease that prominently affects women, there are disturbing trends in the rates of CHD morbidity and mortality among women, relative to men, which highlight the importance of CHD for women. During the 1980s, among men and women 45- to 54-years old, prevalence of CHD, that is, patients who reported having an AMI, angina pectoris, or CHD, decreased and the overall incidence rate, or new cases within each year, of nonfatal CHD remained relatively flat at about 3 per 1000 per year after 1983 (DeStefano *et al.*, 1993). Yet, during this same 10-year period, the CHD incidence rate among white women doubled, going from 1.4 to 2.8 per 1000, and by the end of the decade it nearly equaled the incidence rate among white men (DeStefano *et al.*, 1993). While the declining CHD prevalence rates among both gender groups are encouraging, the apparent increasing CHD incidence rate among surviving women is a source of great concern; these patterns clearly suggest the need for greater attention to the identification of risk factors for CHD among women and more aggressive approaches to reduce these risk factors with methods that reach and support risk factor change among women.

CHD among Minority Populations

CHD mortality patterns differ significantly among various ethnic groups. Mortality rates for African Americans exceed those of whites until approximately age 60 (Castaner, Simmons, Mar, & Cooper, 1988; Gillum, 1982; Watkins, 1984), and age-adjusted CHD mortality rates are approximately one third lower for Hispanics than for whites or African Americans (Smith & Pratt, 1993). Although prevalence rates of risk factors (e.g., hypertension, diabetes) appear to differ between some ethnic groups, these risk factor differences are often offset by lower risk in other risk factors such that risk factors alone do not appear to account for the mortality rate differences between some ethnic groups. These CHD mortality patterns have led working groups (e.g., Johnson & Payne, 1984) and others (e.g., Department of Health and Human Services, 1985; Watkins, 1984) to call for investigations of factors affecting

CHD in minority groups (e.g., Adams *et al.*, 1984; Caldwell *et al.*, 1984; James, 1984; Kasl, 1984).

A variety of factors may account for ethnic disparities in CHD prevalence and mortality. Among these, the disproportionately lower socioeconomic status (SES) level of some ethnic groups undoubtedly is a factor accounting for some ethnic differences in CHD mortality patterns and risk factors (e.g., Bucher & Ragland, 1995; Luepker *et al.*, 1993). SES, as assessed with a variety of proxy measures such as education and occupation, consistently has been inversely associated with CHD prevalence (Bucher & Ragland, 1995; Kaplan & Keil, 1993; Luepker *et al.*, 1993). Additionally, SES also has been inversely associated with other CHD risk factors, including hypertension, cigarette smoking, obesity, and physical inactivity (Luepker *et al.*, 1993; Smith & Pratt, 1993). Krieger (1994) has proposed that oppression and discrimination may be a contributing factor in the development of hypertension for ethnic minorities. A variety of other factors are also likely to contribute to the increased CHD incidence, morbidity, and mortality for those who are in lower SES groups, such as limitations in access to routine as well as specialized care, limitations in the information they are provided to reduce risk factors, and increased barriers to adherence with risk reduction methods.

Aside from SES, a variety of other influences associated with ethnic group may affect CHD patterns. For instance, knowledge of heart disease symptoms and risk factors has been reported to differ between minority and nonminority groups, a factor that may contribute to morbidity and mortality differences through effects on care-seeking behaviors (Folsom, Sprafka, Luepker, & Jacobs, 1988; Hazuda, Stern, Gaskill, Haffner, & Gardner, 1983; Kumanyika *et al.*, 1989). Differences in symptom patterns between African Americans and whites have also been noted, with African Americans reporting fewer painful symptoms than their white counterparts, possibly due to differences in the prevalence of physiological risk factors (e.g., hypertension and diabetes) or due to cultural influences determining symptom perception and reporting (Raczynski *et al.*, 1994b). Knowledge disparities and/or patterns of symptom perception may, in turn, lead to greater attributions of acute AMI symptoms to noncardiac sources among African Americans relative to whites (Raczynski *et al.*, 1994b). Differences in symptom reporting also may account for subsequent disparities in medical management (Raczynski *et al.*, 1994a).

Differences in the utilization of diagnostic and treatment procedures among ethnic groups also has been an area of active research. Disparities among ethnic groups in procedure utilization may lead to differences in CHD medical management as well as recommendations about behavioral or lifestyle changes to reduce risks of clinical outcomes (Feinleib *et al.*, 1989; Jenkins, Stanton, Savageau, Denlinger, & Klein, 1983; Mark *et al.*, 1994; Parisi, Folland, & Hartigan, 1992). Some studies have suggested that cardiac procedures are used less frequently among African-American patients compared to white patients (Ferguson *et al.*, 1997; Ford, Cooper, Castaner, Simmons, & Mar, 1989; Maynard, Fisher, Passamani, & Pullum, 1986; Oberman & Cutter, 1984; Sanderson, Raczynski, Cornell, Hardin, & Taylor, 1998; Wenneker & Epstein, 1989). A variety of potential explanations for ethnic disparities in cardiac procedure use have been suggested, including: (1) health care providers' perceptions about ethnic differences in risk factors and disease severity (Cooper & Ford, 1992; Gordon & Kannel, 1982; Hannan, Kilburn, O'Donnel, Lukacik, & Shields, 1991; Keil *et al.*, 1993); (2) health care systems' delivery of services based on procedure volume, payment method, and regional location (Ayanian, Udvarhelyi, Gatsonis, Pashos, & Epstein, 1993; Carlisle, Leake, & Shapiro, 1995; Goldberg, Hartz, Jacobsen, Krakauer, & Rimm, 1992; Mirvis, Burns, Gaschen, Cloar, & Graney, 1994; Whittle, Conigliaro, Good, & Lofgreen, 1993); (3) accessibility of services among population subgroups (Aday & Anderson, 1984; Keil, Sutherland, Knapp, & Tyroler, 1992; Mutchler & Burr, 1991; Penchansky & Thomas, 1981; Raczynski *et al.*, 1994a; Strogatz, 1990); (4) patients' health-care-seeking behavior, symptom perception, and symptom attribution (Blustein & Weitzman, 1995; Crawford, McGraw, Smith, McKinlay, & Pierson, 1994; Raczynski *et al.*, 1994a,b; Rose, 1962; Strogatz, 1990; Weissman, Stern, Fielding, & Epstein, 1991); and (5) physicians' patterns of diagnosing coronary disease when patients present with suspected signs and symptoms (Ayanian, Hauptman, & Guadagnoli, 1994; Birdwell, Herbers, & Kroenke, 1993; Epstein, Taylor, & Seage, 1985; Goldman & Braunwald, 1991; Pryor, Harrell, Lee, Califf, & Rosati, 1983; Pryor *et al.*, 1993; Sox *et al.*, 1990). Additional research is clearly needed in this area to determine the specific reasons for procedure use variations so that attempts may be made to address these disparities.

Risk Factors for CHD

There are a variety of risk factors for CHD. Although as the disease develops and progresses, physiological predictors of disease outcome begin to emerge; generally, the risk factors remain comparable across stages of the disease, that is, factors that predict the development of the disease (which might consequently be those targeted for primary prevention) are the same as those that will predict later disease outcomes (which might, in turn, be the focus for secondary prevention) as well as predict event outcomes, for example, death or reinfarction after AMI. Although there are different ways in which these risk factors may be classified, it is useful to consider them within categories of nonmodifiable, medical, lifestyle or behavioral, and psychosocial risk factors.

Nonmodifiable Risk Factors

Some factors have been identified that clearly increase the risk for CHD but are not readily amenable to change, and hence are not a behavioral target for intervention in risk reduction programs. Even though they are not specifically modifiable, they may serve as a means of targeting individuals at the greatest risk or motivating adherence to risk reduction interventions. The nonmodifiable risk factors for CHD include age, gender, ethnicity, family history, and menopause without hormone replacement therapy for women. Older age is associated with increased CHD risk and is also associated with changes in a number of the behavioral risk factors for CHD; for example, weight increases and physical activity decreases are often associated with increased age. Approximately 55% of all AMIs occur in people aged 65 and older, and four out of five fatal heart attacks occur in this age group (AHA, 1998). As mentioned earlier, risk is also associated with gender and ethnicity. Younger men are at greater risk than younger women, although this risk advantage for women almost disappears after menopause in the absence of hormone replacement therapy. Young African Americans also are at greater risk for CHD mortality than their white counterparts. Finally, family history of CHD and/or family history of some other medical risk factors for CHD, for example, hypertension and diabetes, are strongly related to risk for CHD.

Medical Risk Factors

Although classification as a medical versus lifestyle or behavioral risk factor is somewhat arbitrary, medical risk factors here are considered to be those that have resulted in physiological changes, which, in turn, place the individual at increased risk for CHD. These factors include hypertension, hyperlipidemia, diabetes, and obesity. Hypertension, especially high systolic blood pressure, increases CHD risk (e.g., Bittner & Oparil, 1997; Stokes, Kannel, & Wolf, 1989) and has been estimated by the American Heart Association to affect nearly one fourth of the adult US population (AHA, 1998). Serum lipid levels, in particular elevated total cholesterol and low-density lipoprotein (LDL), are strong predictors of CHD for all gender and ethnic groups (NHLBI, 1994). Some gender differences exist for risk associated with different lipid fractions. LDL does not predict risk as strongly in women as it does in men (Bass, Newschaffer, Klag, & Bush, 1993; Bittner, 1996; Eaker & Castelli, 1987), but low levels of high-density lipoproteins (HDL), associated with higher risk for CHD, appear to be a stronger risk factor for women than men (Bittner, 1996; Brunner *et al.*, 1987).

Diabetes increases risk of CHD twofold relative to that of nondiabetics. Diabetics have an increased incidence of AMI, larger infarct size (Cohn, 1989), more silent myocardial ischemia (Muller *et al.*, 1985), and higher rates of major cardiac complications, such as congestive heart failure (Biegon, Israeli, Elizur, Bruch, & Bar-Nathan, 1990; Crowley, Dempsey, Horwitz, & Horwitz, 1994; Malone *et al.*, 1993; Pandey, Pandey, Janicak, Marks, & Davis, 1990). Diabetics are also more likely to develop medical problems, such as hypertension and dyslipidemia, that are themselves risk factors for CHD (NHBLI, 1994). Family history of diabetes, some ethnic minority groups, age, being a woman, weight, and physical inactivity are all associated with increased risk for diabetes.

Finally, obesity is associated with elevations in other CHD risk factors, including diabetes, hypertension (e.g., Kannell & Gordon, 1979; National Institutes of Health Consensus Development on the Health Implications of Obesity, 1985; Stamler *et al.*, 1975a,b; The Lipid Research Clinics Population Studies Data Book, 1980; Van Itallie, 1979, 1985), and high-risk lipid profiles (Levy & Kannel, 1988; National Institutes of Health Consensus Development Panel on the Health Implications of Obesity, 1985; Van Itallie, 1979; Wood, Stefanick, Williams, & Haskell, 1991), as well as having a likely independent effect on CHD risk (Bild, 1994; Manson *et al.*, 1990; Hubert, Feinleib, McNamara, & Castelli, 1983). A fat distribution pattern in which fat is more centrally located is more predictive of CHD risk than one in which fat is more distributed throughout the body (Lapidus *et al.*, 1984; Spelsberg, Ridker, Manson, 1993).

Lifestyle or Behavioral Risk Factors

Lifestyle or behavioral risk factors, such as diet, smoking, and physical inactivity, are demonstrated independent risk factors for CHD. They also are related to CHD through their impact on some medical, that is, physiological, risk factors, including obesity, diabetes mellitus, dyslipidemia, and hypertension. Diets high in cholesterol and certain fats have been associated with increased CHD risk (NHLBI, 1994; Rich-Edwards, Manson, Hennekens, & Buring, 1995). In particular, diets high in saturated fats and cholesterol have been shown to adversely affect lipid profiles. Other dietary components, most notably antioxidants (e.g., beta carotene, vitamin E, and vitamin C) and possibly fish oils, may be beneficial in protecting against CHD (NHLBI, 1994; Rich-Edwards *et al.*, 1995). The evidence is strong in demonstrating that a diet that is low in saturated fats and high in fiber, whole grains, fruits, and vegetables lowers CHD risk (Mosca *et al.*, 1997; Willett & Lenart, 1996). In addition to the impact of high-fat diets on cholesterol, these diets, probably due to their increased caloric content, may be associated with obesity, diabetes mellitus, and hypertension.

Smoking increases the risk of CHD and AMI substantially, with data indicating risk for smokers two to six times that for those who have never smoked (LaCroix, Guralnik, & Curb, 1990; LaCroix, Lang, & Scherr, 1991; Willett, Green, & Stampfer, 1987). For women, the cardiovascular dangers of smoking are increased even further in those who both smoke and use oral contraceptives (AHA, 1998; NHLBI, 1994; Smith & Pratt, 1993).

Physical inactivity appears to be an independent risk factor for CVD (NHLBI, 1994). The evidence is strong in demonstrating decreased risk for CHD with even low levels of physical activity (Leon, Connett, Jacobs, & Rauramaa, 1987; Morris, Clayton, Everitt, Semmence, & Burgess, 1990; Paffenbarger, Hyde, Wing, & Hsieh, 1986; Pate et. al., 1995 for review; Powell, Thompson, Caspersen, & Ford, 1987). Prospective investigations have indicated that physical inactivity is an important risk factor for women as well as men (Blair *et al.*, 1989). Only about 22% of the US population is sufficiently active to meet the *Healthy People 2000* recommendation for "light to moderate physical activity for at least 30 minutes per day" (US Department of Health and Human Services, 1991). Women are even more physically inactive than men, and the disparity in physical activity between the gender groups increases with age (Caspersen, Christenson, & Pollard, 1986; Pate *et al.*, 1995). Physical inactivity likely contributes to other risk factors in both gender groups, although in a greater manner among women since physical inactivity is more common among women, such as obesity (e.g., King & Tribble, 1990; Owens, Matthews, Wing, & Kuller, 1990), hypertension (e.g., Blair, Goodyear, Gibbons, & Cooper, 1984), unfavorable lipid profiles (e.g., Leon, 1989), diabetes (e.g., Helmrich, Ragland, Leung, & Paffenbarger, 1991; Laws & Reaven, 1991), and possibly stress (e.g., Crews & Landers, 1987; Dimsdale, Alpert, & Schneiderman, 1986), although the data to support stress as a risk factor are equivocal and it is not an established risk factor.

Several studies suggest that daily consumption of low to moderate amounts of alcohol is associated with lower CHD risk relative to nondrinkers (Fuchs *et al.*, 1995; Gordon & Kannel, 1983; Kuller, 1991; Rosenberg *et al.*, 1981; Scragg, Stewart, Jackson, & Beaglehole, 1987; Stampfer, Colditz, Willett, Speizer, & Hennekens, 1988). In contrast, heavy alcohol intake has been associated with increased mortality from all causes (e.g., Fuchs *et al.*, 1995), and even moderate alcohol intake may increase the risk of other health problems such as hypertension (Klatsky, Friedman, Siegelaub & Gerard, 1977) and cancer (Smith-Warner *et al.*, 1998). Additional research is needed to determine the relative benefits–risks of alcohol intake for all health problems, including CHD, and to determine the physiological mechanisms by which alcohol impacts on CHD risk.

In addition to the interactions among lifestyle–behavioral and medical risk factors, evidence exists for relationships between lifestyle–behavioral factors and non-modifiable risk factors. For instance, family history may predispose people who are physically inactive, consume too many calories, and become overweight to develop diabetes mellitus and/or hypertension. There may also be relationships between lifestyle and behavioral risk factors and psychosocial risk for CVD, including depression, stress, and anxiety (e.g., King, Taylor, Haskell & DeBusk, 1989; Taylor, Sallis, & Needle, 1985).

Psychosocial Risk Factors

The type A behavior pattern, consisting of a pattern of time urgency, verbal aggressiveness, impatience, and hostility, was early identified as a risk factor for CHD (see Haynes & Matthews, 1988; Manuck, Kaplan, & Matthews, 1986; Matthews & Haynes, 1986). As research progressed, it was evident that not all type A behaviors are related to risk (Dembroski, MacDougall, Costa, & Grandits, 1989; Haynes & Matthews, 1988; Matthews, 1988; Matthews & Haynes 1986), and hostility emerged as the primary component associated with increased risk. Some evidence suggests that the relationship between hostility and CHD is stronger among women than men (Helmers *et al.*, 1993). Hostility has been found to be associated with a variety of other factors, including lower levels of education and social support (Scherwitz, Perkins, Chesney, & Hughes, 1991), cardiovascular reactivity to stress (Durel *et al.*, 1989; Suarez & Williams, 1990), negative health behaviors (Houston & Vavak, 1991; Leiker & Hailey, 1988), and unfavorable lipid profiles (Dujovne & Houston, 1991; Lundererg, Hendman, Melin, & Frankenhaeuser, 1989; Siegler *et al.*, 1990; Weidner, Sexton, McLellarn, Connor, Matarazzo, 1987). Thus, hostility may interact with other psychosocial and physiological factors to affect CHD risk (Weidner, 1994).

A number of studies have reported that negative affective changes, such as increased depression and anxiety, accompany myocardial infarction (MI) for many patients (Cay, Vetter, Philip, & Dugard, 1972a,b; Cleophas *et al.*, 1993; Forrester *et al.*, 1992; Lloyd & Cawley, 1978; Lloyd & Cawley 1982a,b; Schleifer *et al.*, 1989; Stern, Pascale, Ackerman, 1977; Stern, Pascale, McLoone, 1976). In some cases, depression in patients following AMI is associated with experiences of depression prior to MI (Cay *et al.*, 1972a,b; Stern *et al.*, 1976, 1977), but most patients studied have no history of depressive disorders (Forrester *et al.*, 1992; Schleifer *et al.*, 1989). Depression and anxiety are, in turn, associated with diminished short-term improvement following AMI (Pancheri *et al.*, 1978; Stern *et al.*, 1977), with increased time to return to work (Hlatky *et al.*, 1986; Schleifer *et al.*, 1989), and with increased reporting of cardiac symptoms (e.g., Coombs, Robert, Crist, & Miller, 1989; Costa *et al.*, 1985). Importantly, depression is also associated with greater cardiac mortality and morbidity, even after adjustment for disease severity (Ahern *et al.*, 1989; Frasure-Smith *et al.*, 1993; Sloan & Bigger, 1991). Little is known about the relationships between depression and CHD in women (Carney, Freedland, Smith, Lustman, & Jaffer, 1991). Two studies have shown higher levels of depression in women than in men following MI (Forrester *et al.*, 1992; Schleifer *et al.*, 1989). In general, the incidence of depression is higher in women than men (e.g., Cleary, 1987; Weissman & Klerman, 1977), so gender differences following MI are not unexpected. However, no studies have specifically reported on the relationship between depression or anxiety and CHD endpoints in women.

Social support also has been implicated as a risk factor for CHD, although it is not yet clear which aspect of social support is the major one related to risk. Individuals who are tense, suspicious, and isolated have been found to be at increased risk for CHD development (Ostfeld, Lebovits, Shekelle, & Paul, 1964). A number of studies have suggested that aspects of social support are related to outcomes after having an AMI. Low levels of integration into a social support system have been associated with increased CHD mortality, even after controlling for other risk factors (Berkman & Syme, 1979; House, Robbins, & Metzner, 1982; Schoenvack, Kaplan, Freman, & Kleinbaum, 1986), and social isolation has been associated with increased mortality after an AMI (Case, Moss, Case, McDermott, & Eberly, 1992; Fiebach, Viscoli, & Horwitz,

1990; Ruberman, 1992; Williams, Barefoot, Califf, 1992). Marital status and/or having a close confident has also been predictive of survival following an AMI, even after adjusting for other risk factors (Chandra, Szklo, Goldberg, & Tonascia, 1983) and disease severity (Williams *et al.*, 1992). Lack of emotional support has been related to mortality within the first 6 months after an AMI (Berkman, Leo-Summers, & Horowitz, 1992), and perceptions of support has predicted mortality even when other factors were controlled (Gorkin *et al.*, 1993). Social support has also been related to CHD morbidity and associated with extent of CAD (Blumenthal *et al.*, 1987; Seeman & Syme, 1987), degree of ST segment depression (Hedblad, Ostergren, Hanson, Janzon, Johansson, & Juul-Moller, 1992), and fibrinogen concentration (Rosengren *et al.*, 1990).

Physiological changes associated with stress have been suggested to contribute to the development and worsening of CHD (e.g., Keys *et al.*, 1971; Manuck, Kaplan, & Clarkson, 1983; Stoney, Matthews, McDonald & Johnson, 1988; Williams, 1989), although the evidence is not strong enough to consider stress as an established risk factor for CHD. Stress is a generic term that may be a common component of all psychosocial factors associated with CHD and/or may interact with other psychosocial risk factors. The evidence of associations between many of the possible psychosocial mediators of CHD is strong. Depression and social isolation have been found to commonly occur with AMI (e.g., Cleophas *et al.*, 1993), and social support is often identified as a stress buffer (e.g., Johnson, 1987; Medalie & Goldbourt, 1976). Similarly, social support has been associated with less anxiety and depression (Kulik & Mahler, 1993) and less stress and negative affect among CHD patients, which, in turn, were associated with lower morbidity and prevalence (Johnson, 1987; Medalie & Goldbourt, 1976), although negative findings have been reported (Reed, McGee, & Yano, 1984). Finally, greater hostility is associated with lower social support (Scherwitz *et al.*, 1991).

The interaction among psychosocial risk factors may mediate CHD risk through a final common physiological pathway. Evidence suggests that hostility, depression, and stress are all associated with increased catecholamine levels (Barefoot, Haney, Hershkowitz, & Williams, 1991; Potter & Manji, 1994), which are known to increase heart rate and blood pressure. Increased cardiovascular stimulation may contribute in turn to the development and worsening of CHD. The manner in which psychosocial risk factors interact and mediate CHD risk through physiological mechanisms is an area of active investigation, which may lead not only to our better understanding of this constellation of risk factors but also to improved means to identify patients at high psychosocial risk and to improved methods to treat these patients to reduce their psychosocial risk, reducing their morbidity and mortality.

Risk Factors: Putting It All Together

Within the four risk factor categories addressed in the brief review above (i.e, nonmodifiable, medical, lifestyle or behavioral, and psychosocial risk factors), substantial overlap occurs, such that many of the medical risk factors may be considered as resulting from the impact of one or more behavioral risk factors or psychosocial risk factors or from the interaction of behavioral or psychosocial risk factors and nonmodifiable risk factors, such as family history or genetic risk factor. For example, hypertension is now commonly thought of as a medical risk factor for CHD that results from the interaction of genetic predisposition with behavioral factors, such as diet, exercise, and possibly alcohol intake, as well as psychosocial factors, such as possibly stress

(Joint National Committee on Prevention, Detection, Evaluation, and Treatment of High Blood Pressure, and the National High Blood Pressure Education Program Coordinating Committee, 1997). Although substantial research continues to examine risk factors, their relationship to one another, their impact on physiological mechanisms, and their variation within gender and ethnic groups, some attempt at present can be made in attempting to relate variables across categories. Although not depicting the associations between all possible risk factors, Table 1 represents an effort to show some of the estimated relationships between the behavioral and psychosocial risk factors and the risk factors in the other categories considered in this review as well as the possible interaction among the risk factors in determining overall risk for CHD.

The top portion of Table 1 attempts to describe both the interaction of behavioral risk factors with risk factors in the other three categories as well as the strength of the interaction on CHD risk, while the bottom portion attempts to similarly describe interactions and interactive risk between psychosocial risk factors and risk factors in the other categories. It should be noted that the estimates of association are based on impressions of complex data, in some cases, and few data, in other cases. Nonetheless,

Table 1. Estimated Associations among Risk Factors

Associations/interactions between risk factors in categories (estimated strength of relationship between risk factors/estimated strength of interaction between risk factors in determining risk)

Each cell is given as association/interaction.

Behaviors	Nonmodifiable — Age	Gender	Ethnicity	Family hx	Menopause w/out HRT[a]	Medical — Hypertension	Hyperlipidemia	Diabetes	Obesity	Psychosocial — Oral contraceptives	Hostility	Depression	Anxiety	Social support	Behavioral — Diet	Smoking	Physical inactivity
Diet	+/0	0/0	+/+	0/+	0/0	++/++	+++/+++	+++/+++	+++/+++	0/0	0/0	++/0	+/0	0/0			
Smoking	+/0	+/0	+/0	0/0	0/+	+/++	+/++	0/++	0/+++	++/0	0/0	+/0	0/0	0/0			
Physical inactivity	+/0	++/0	++/0	0/0	0/+	++/++	++/++	+++/++	+++/+++	0/0	0/0	++/0	++/0	0/0			
Psychosocial hostility	0/0	+/0	0/0	0/0	0/0	+/+	0/+	0/+	0/0	0/0					0/0	0/0	0/0
Depression	0/0	+/0	0/0	++/0	0/0	+/++	+/++	0/++	0/0	0/0					0/0	+/0	++/0
Anxiety	0/0	0/0	0/0	0/0	0/0	+/+	0/0	0/0	0/0	0/0					0/0	0/0	++/0
Social support	+/0	+/0	+/0	0/0	0/0	0/0	0/0	0/0	0/0	0/0					0/0	0/0	0/0

[a] HRT, hormone replacement therapy.

0, no interaction; +, some association/interaction; ++, moderate association/interaction; +++, strong association/interaction.

several observations may be made from this table, including: (1) behaviors are often associated with other risk factors, such that this information may be used to define groups at increased risk for more aggressive prevention efforts; (2) the interactive or additive effect of behavioral risk factors with other risk factors suggests that the risk faced by individuals who have behavioral risk factors along with other risk factors is probably greater than the simple additive risk of the separate factors, again suggesting that individuals with multiple risk factors are at particularly high risk and may benefit from more aggressive efforts to control modifiable risk factors (not only behavioral risk factors, but medical and psychosocial risk factors as well); and (3) psychosocial risk factors, while not associated as strongly with other risk factors as behavioral risk factors, do have some associations to other risk factors, particularly for depression. Information concerning associations between risk factors and their interaction in determining risk are valuable in identifying not only populations that are at particular risk for CHD but also for educating people about the degree of their risk as a means to improve motivation and readiness to change and to affect adherence to risk reduction programs.

Theoretical Models Commonly Associated with CHD Interventions

As mentioned previously, CHD interventions have spanned from primary to secondary and even tertiary approaches. However, the models used by researchers have usually depended more on whether the intervention targets involved attempt to create changes in individuals or communities rather than the fact that the interventions have been focused on CHD risk reduction. For example, primary intervention approaches have involved efforts to change both the behaviors of communities through impersonal methods involved in media campaigns (e.g., Mittelmark *et al.*, 1986; Farquhar, Fortmann, Wood, & Haskell, 1983) or other approaches designed to impact on the community (e.g., Lasater *et al.*, 1984) as well as through methods to impact on individuals through interpersonal interventions in provider settings (e.g., Ockene, Ockene, Kabat-Zinn, Greene, & Frid, 1990). Efforts to impact on behaviors associated with secondary and tertiary intervention more commonly have adopted theories appropriate for the more interpersonal approaches needed to impact on identified individuals' behaviors, although impersonal media campaigns have also been used, for example, to impact during secondary prevention efforts such as with hypercholesterolemia (Lenfant, 1986) and even to promote rapid medical care seeking in response to AMI symptoms (Simons-Morton *et al.*, 1998). Thus, the major factor determining the theoretical models adopted to guide the development of CHD interventions has been the targeted methods of reaching either individuals through community-level approaches by impersonal means or through individually directed approaches by interpersonal means.

Examples of Current CHD Research

The demarcation between what constitutes primary versus secondary prevention is somewhat arbitrary, since it involves a determination of when in the course of a slowly developing disease a physiological change has occurred that is sufficient to warrant a diagnosis of CHD. Given that behavioral and psychosocial risk factors remain very similar across the development and progression of the disease and to a large extent the intervention programs that might be implemented to assist individuals in modifying their risk factors remain the same, it is not necessary to make fine distinctions between interventions to address risk factors across the course of disease. Some differences do emerge, however, since programs that target primary prevention can be delivered through population-directed methods more readily than programs that address more aggressive methods of lowering risk among patients who have more definitive disease; in the latter case, more aggressive methods can be more readily delivered through interpersonal approaches. Although the field of CHD risk reduction programs is large, below we discuss some of the current issues in the prevention of CHD.

Current Issues in Primary Prevention of CHD

Cardiopulmonary, community-based primary prevention trials were the focus of a recent conference sponsored by the National Heart, Lung, and Blood Institute, which was then summarized in an issue of the *Annals of Epidemiology* (1997, Volume 7, Number 7, Supplement), and the interested reader is referred to the excellent summaries of this conference. Primary prevention is generally focused on communities in order to reach populations large enough to demonstrate a change. The nature of the "community" has been varied, however, ranging from those defined by geographic regions to those that have focused on particular populations that are defined by access channels, such as schools, work sites, and churches.

Although some early community prevention trials were conducted starting in the mid-1970s (cf. Schooler, Farquhar, Fortmann, & Flora, 1997), the largest and more recent multifactor studies to target primary CHD risk reduction included the Minnesota Heart Health Project (Mittelmark *et al.*, 1986), the Pawtucket Heart Health Program (Carleton, Lasater, Assaf, Lefebvere, & McKinlay, 1987; Lefebvre, Lasater, Carleton, & Peterson, 1987), the Stanford Five-City Project (Farquhar *et al.*, 1985), and the earlier North Karelia Project conducted in Finland (Puska, 1973). Differences exist between these studies in their emphasis on specific intervention methods, such as extent of community organization, use of mass media and direct behavior change methods, focus on environmental changes, and use of volunteers (cf. Schooler *et al.*, 1997). Interpreting the results of these long-term studies is complicated by many factors such as the quasi-experimental nature of the study designs in which only a few communities were being randomized to intervention and usual care conditions (Schooler *et al.*, 1997). In addition, the three US projects encountered significant secular trends during this time in which the population, including those in the usual care communities, were being better educated and provided with better methods to facilitate reducing risk factors for CHD, an international trend that is accounting for the entire population reducing risk factors; in essence, these studies had to accomplish greater changes in their intervention communities than were occurring anyway in the usual care communities. Nonetheless, despite these limitations, the results of community risk reduction programs can be viewed as cautiously optimistic in reducing risk factors for CHD (Schooler *et al.*, 1997), the benefits of which undoubtedly account for reducing trends in CHD morbidity and mortality as considerable diffusion of primary risk reduction efforts has occurred worldwide.

Despite this optimistic view of primary prevention for CHD, as this chapter has noted, disturbing trends in CHD risk factors are occurring in some subgroups, and some subgroups are lagging behind others in the rate of risk factor and morbidity and mortality reductions. This argues for increased attention to methods to reach these special populations with efficacious primary prevention programs. In addition, it is important to realize that CHD is still the principal cause of death for all gender and ethnic groups in the United States, highlighting the need to further emphasize risk reduction efforts rather than being satisfied with recent trends, trends that already show some evidence of not continuing (AHA, 1998).

Current Issues in Secondary and Tertiary Prevention for CHD

Methods of lowering the risk of patients who have definitive medical risk factors for CHD have been addressed in a number of studies, including the Oslo Heart Study (Hjermann, Welve Byrne, Holme, & Leren, 1981), the Multiple Risk Factor Intervention Trial (Multiple Risk Factor Intervention Trial Research Group, 1982), the European Collaborative Trial of Multifactoral Prevention of Coronary Heart Disease (Levy, 1985), and the Lipid Research Clinics Coronary Primary Prevention Trial (The Lipid Research Clinics Coronary Primary Prevention Trial Group, 1984). The results of these and other studies strongly suggest the benefits of lowering behavioral risk factors for reducing risk of CHD. Clinical trial results, particularly those that deal with behavioral factors, are frequently not incorporated into clinical practice, emphasizing the need to address methods of promoting provider practice change and facilitating providers in incorporating effective methods to change patient behavioral and psychosocial risk factors. This emphasizes the provider and patient adherence as critical issues in achieving further reductions in CHD risk factors and morbidity and mortality (Schrott, Bittner, Vittinghoff, Herrington, & Hulley, 1997).

Among the most recent areas of development in risk reduction for the secondary and tertiary prevention of CHD are developing tested methods of encouraging people who are experiencing AMI symptoms to seek treatment quickly so that they may be eligible for reperfusion therapies, and examining the efficacy of psychosocial treatment of post-AMI patients who are at elevated risk due to being depressed and/or socially isolated. Efforts to develop efficacious programs in both of these areas are discussed below.

Treatment Seeking for AMI

A major thrust of prevention efforts to reduce morbidity and mortality from CHD currently involves efforts to encourage people to seek treatment quickly for AMI symptoms. As mentioned earlier, new developments in reperfusion therapies with thrombolytic or "clot-busting" drugs or through balloon angioplasty can decrease morbidity and mortality if treatment is delivered within the first few hours of symptom onset (AIMS Trial Study Group, 1990; Cannon et al., 1994; Every et al., 1997; Fibrinolytic Therapy Trialists' Collaborative Group, 1994; Groupo Italiano per lo Studio della Streptochinasi nell'Infarto Miocardico (GISSI), 1986; Hennekens et al., 1995; ISIS-2 Collaborative Group, 1988; Lee et al., 1995; Marrugat et al., 1997; O'Keefe et al., 1989; Van de Werf & Arnold, 1988). However, delay in seeking treatment is unacceptably great, resulting in most patients being ineligible for these treatments or reducing the effectiveness of treatment for those who are eligible but may have responded sooner to their symptoms (Uemura & Pisa, 1988). In an effort to promote a concerted and coordinated effort to reduce AMI mortality and morbidity, the National Heart, Lung, and Blood Institute (NHLBI) in 1991 initiated the National Heart Attack Alert Program (NHAAP). Although many hospitals and other advocates have believed, without empirical support, that delay can be reduced and have initiated a variety of efforts to educate people to seek treatment quickly, the NHAAP acknowledged the lack of empirical support for the benefits of a public education campaign. Initial delay-reducing efforts by the NHAAP were directed specifically toward assessment, diagnosis, and treatment in the emergency department (Dracup *et al.*, 1997; National Heart Attack Alert Program (NHAAP) Coordinating Committee 60 Minutes to Treatment Working Group, 1994). Concurrently, based on recommendations by the NHAAP, the NHLBI initiated planning and funding for the Rapid Early Action for Coronary Treatment (REACT) trial to better inform the NHAAP about the effectiveness of methods for a national campaign to reduce delay in seeking treatment for AMI symptoms (Feldman *et al.*, 1998; Simons-Morton *et al.*, 1998).

REACT is presently an ongoing multisite collaborative community trial with 20 communities randomized to either the intervention or a comparison group (Simons-Morton *et al.*, 1998). The 18-month intervention was developed based on: (1) the current research literature; (2) social cognitive theory (Bandura, 1986) and self-regulatory theory (Leventhal, Meyer, & Nerenz, 1980; Leventhal & Nerenz, 1985; Cameron, Leventhal, & Leventhal, 1993), which were used to guide the development, implementation, and evaluation of the intervention; (3) focus group and key informant interview formative research undertaken to understand better the decision-making processes as well as barriers and facilitators to seeking medical care as perceived by AMI patients, their families, and medical care professionals; (4) the synthesis of data sources in developing the intervention; and (5) the focus of the outcome, impact, and process measurement based on the intervention components and theories on which they were developed. A four-component intervention was designed for REACT to address different target audiences: a community organization component was incorporated to mobilize the community and to enlist support of key medical and nonmedical leaders and agencies; community education was used to target changes in attention/awareness, knowledge, beliefs, skills, and behavioral intentions of high-risk individuals, spouses of high-risk individuals, and community residents at large; professional education was developed to increase providers' knowledge, behavioral capacity and self-efficacy, and their behaviors for educating patients about methods to reduce delay in seeking treatment for AMI; and patient education was used for high-risk patients and their family members to alter their knowledge, behavioral capacity and self-efficacy, and behaviors for increasing quick action in seeking treatment for AMI. These components were conceptualized as a comprehensive, multifaceted intervention hypothesized to be necessary to reduce overall community delay in seeking treatment for AMI. For three components (community education, provider education, and patient education), both interpersonal and impersonal strategies were incorporated to reflect state-of-the-art educational standards (Glanz, Lewis, & Rimer, 1997; Windsor, 1984).

While REACT results have not yet been published, this research program exemplifies an important area of research that has the potential to impact to a significant degree in reducing morbidity and mortality from CHD. Additionally, the program demonstrates the manner in which a theory-based community intervention can be developed, implemented, and evaluated. In addition, it may serve to guide research and community programs in efforts to address other critical issues of health care seeking for CHD, such as those that may be associated with ethnic differences in CHD morbidity and mortality patterns.

Depression and Social Isolation

As mentioned earlier, depression (Carney *et al.*, 1988; Frasure-Smith *et al.*, 1993; Kennedy *et al.*, 1987; Ladwig *et al.*, 1991; Silverstone, 1990; Sloan & Bigger, 1991) and social isolation (Berkman & Breslow, 1983; Berkman & Syme, 1979; Blumenthal *et al.*, 1987; Ruberman *et al.*, 1984; Seeman & Syme, 1987) have only recently been recognized as a major predictor of morbidity and mortality after an AMI. These data thus suggest that treatment either through pharmacological or nonpharmacological approaches might benefit the morbidity and mortality of patients who have had AMIs. Studies of social and psychosocial support interventions for cardiac patients date back to the 1960s (Adsett & Bruhn, 1968). An early impressive demonstration of the effect of social support on cardiac outcome was reported by Frasure-Smith and Prince (1989). In this study, a large group of post-MI patients were randomly assigned to no treatment or a supportive treatment intervention consisting of regular telephone contact with a nurse augmented by an individually tailored program of home visits designed to provide support and reduce stress. At 1 year after treatment, there was a reduction in cardiac death rates by about 50%, but this effect disappeared with additional follow-up. A significant decrease in rates of recurrent MI, however, emerged when long-term follow-up data were examined. Not all studies, however, have detected beneficial effects of psychosocial intervention (Mayou, MacMahon, Sleight, & Florencio, 1981; Naismith, Robinson, Shaw, & MacIntyre, 1979). The benefit of group interventions aimed at reducing type A behavior pattern (TABP) at least partially may be due to increased availability of social support (Mendes deLeon, Powell, & Kaplan, 1991; Orth-Gomer & Unden, 1990). A meta-analysis of the available literature on psychological treatments for TABP found evidence of a reduction in incidence of cardiac events (3–year combined mortality and myocardial infarction) of approximately 50% in therapy-treated patients compared with controls (Nunes, Frank, & Kornfeld, 1987). Although there are very few studies of antidepressant efficacy in cardiac patients, preliminary evidence combined with clinical experience indicates that the majority of medically ill depressed patients respond favorably to antidepressants (Rodin, Craven, & Littlefield, 1991).

It is clear from this research that depression and social isolation are major risk factors for AMI patients. While the mediators of this increased risk need to be identified, it is likely that these mediators affect not only AMI patients but also patients who have CHD but have not experienced an AMI; relationships among recent AMI patients were identified first probably due to the very high morbidity and mortality rates among these patients.

Nonetheless, the exciting result of identifying depression and social isolation as risk factors is that efforts are underway to examine whether or not attempting to ameliorate depression and social isolation results in corresponding reductions in risk. Preliminary studies suggest that pharmacological interventions may be effective, despite serious concerns about adverse cardiovascular side effects associated with antidepressant medications. For example, a multicenter medication trial (Roose *et al.*, 1998) recently tested the relative efficacy of a specific serotonin reuptake inhibitor (SSRI) and a tricyclic antidepressant (TCA) in depressed CHD patients, finding that both drugs ameliorated depression. The SSRI medication was associated with significantly fewer adverse cardiac side effects than the tricyclic medication, adding to the body of evidence that suggests that SSRIs may be safer for use with depressed CHD patients than TCAs (Roose *et al.*, 1998). Unfortunately, recent early findings in the area of psychosocial interventions have been disappointing. A recent trial by Frasure-Smith and colleagues (1997) randomized nearly 1400 post-MI men and women to usual care or to a supportive home nursing intervention that included specific attention to depression, anxiety, and other psychosocial stress. After 1 year, analyses indicated that the program had no survival benefit and little impact on depression or anxiety; in fact, both cardiac and all-cause mortality were increased among the women in the intervention group, compared to women in the usual care group (Frasure-Smith *et al.*, 1997). However, the ability of the Frasure-Smith and colleagues study (1997) to reduce these psychosocial risk factors has been called into question, and concerns have been raised about the study lacking sufficient group sizes and power to detect a treatment effect.

At least some of the answers about the impact of psychosocial interventions on morbidity and mortality outcomes among post-AMI patients who are depressed and/or socially isolated may come from an ongoing study currently funded by the National Heart, Lung, and Blood Institute. This study, called Enhancing Recovery in CHD Patients (ENRICHD), is a multicenter study involving eight clinical centers (Raczynski, 1997). The goal is to recruit a total of 3000 patients who meet eligibility criteria of being depressed and/or socially isolated after having a documented AMI. Patients are randomized either to a psychosocial treatment, based on cognitive behavioral treatment with adjunctive pharmacotherapy if indicated, or to a usual care condition (Raczynski, 1997). The outcomes of this study, if demonstrable benefits are seen for the psychosocial treatment, have the potential for dramatically affecting care of cardiological patients and significantly impacting on CHD morbidity and mortality patterns.

Summary and Conclusions

Despite declines in CHD mortality rates as well as AMI rates in the United States since the 1960s, CHD is the leading source of mortality for all gender and ethnic groups in this country. Further, although the United States is a technological leader, mortality rates in this country exceed those of many other industrialized countries. Women and many ethnic groups have not benefited with as great a decline in CHD mortality rates as men and whites, respectively, emphasizing the need for increased attention to methods that may lead to improved CHD reductions among women and minorities. Additionally, our understanding of risk factors is improving, such as with the recent identification of depression and low social support as major risk factors for AMI, which should lead to new approaches to control of these risk factors and probably reductions in CHD morbidity and mortality. Further, with the advancement of new medical therapies, for example, the development of thrombolytic therapies, which, in turn, have led to the focus on new behavioral issues, that is, rapid health care seeking and treatment for AMI symptoms, progress is being made to ensure that community behavioral interventions are developed to complement medical advancements. Finally, it should be noted that there is a strong "secular trend" in this country that may pose challenges to community-focused researchers attempting to mount programs to outpace this national trend, but it portends well for the receptivity of the US public to behavioral approaches for further risk factor reductions. With the community intervention methods that have been built on over the past 20 years, substantial progress has been made in developing behavioral theories to provide the continuing programs that the US public clearly eagerly awaits.

References

Adams, L., Africano, E., Doswell, W., Frate, D., Gillum, R., Havlik, R., Langford, H., Mebane, I., Neser, W., Potts, J., Saunders, E., Savage, D., Schachter, J., Stamler, J., Tillotson, J., Watkins, L., & Williams, R. (1984). Summary of workshop I: Working group on epidemiology. *American Heart Journal, 108,* 699–702.

Aday, L., & Anderson, R. (1984). The national profile of access to medical care: Where do we start? *American Journal of Public Health, 74,* 1331–1339.

Adsett, C. A., & Bruhn, J. G. (1968). Short-term group psychotherapy for post-myocardial infarction patients and their wives. *Canadian Medical Association Journal, 99,* 577–584.

Ahern, D. K., Gorkin, L., Anderson, J. L., Tierney, C., Hallstrom, A., & Ewat, C., for the Cardiac Arrhythmia Pilot Study (CAPS) Investigators. (1989, November). *Behavioral variables and mortality or cardiac arrest in the CAPS.* Papers presented at the annual meeting of the American Heart Association, New Orleans.

AIMS Trial Study Group. (1990). Long-term effects of intravenous anistreplase in acute myocardial infarction: final report of the AIMS Study. *Lancet, 335,* 427–431.

American Heart Association (AHA). (1998). *Heart attack and stroke facts,* Dallas, TX: American Heart Association.

Ayanian, H., & Epstein, A. (1991). Differences in the use of procedures between women and men for coronary artery disease. *New England Journal of Medicine, 325,* 221–225.

Ayanian, J., Hauptman, P., & Guadagnoli, E. (1994). Knowledge and practice of generalist and specialist physicians regarding drug therapy for acute myocardial infarction. *New England Journal of Medicine, 331*(17), 1136–1142.

Ayanian, J. Z., Udvarhelyi, I. S., Gatsonis, C. A., Pashos, C. L., & Epstein, A. M. (1993). Racial differences in the use of revascularization procedures after coronary angiography. *Journal of the American Medical Association, 269,* 2642–2646.

Bandura, A. (1986). *Social foundation of thought and action: A social cognitive theory.* Englewood Cliffs, NJ: Prentice-Hall.

Barefoot, J. C., Haney, T. L., Hershkowitz, B. D., & Williams, R. B. (1991, March). *Hostility and coronary artery disease in women and men.* Presented at the annual meeting of the Society of Behavioral Medicine, Washington, DC.

Bass, K. M., Newschaffer, C. J., Klag, M. J., & Bush, T. L. (1993). Plasma lipoprotein levels as predictors of cardiovascular death in women. *Archives of Internal Medicine, 153,* 2209–2216.

Berkman, L., & Breslow, L. (1983). *Health and ways of living: Findings from the Alameda County Study.* New York: Oxford University Press.

Berkman, L.F., & Syme, S. L. (1979). Social networks, host resistance, and mortality: A nine year follow-up study of Alameda County residents. *American Journal of Epidemiology, 109*(2), 186–204.

Berkman, L. F., Leo-Summers, L., & Horowitz, R. I. (1992). Emotional support and survival after myocardial infarction: A prospective, population based study of the elderly. *Annals of Internal Medicine, 117,*1003–1009.

Biegon, A., Israeli, M., Elizur, A., Bruch, S., & Bar-Nathan, A. A. (1990). Serotonin 5–HT_2 receptor binding on blood platelets as a state dependent marker in major affective disorder. *Psychopharmacology, 102,* 73–75, 149.

Bild, D. E., (1994). Overview of cardiovascular disease risk factors in women. In S. M. Czajkowski, D. R. Hill, & T. B Clarkson (Eds.), *Women, behavior, and cardiovascular disease* (pp. 37–46). Washington, DC: US DHHS, NIH Publication No. 94-3309.

Birdwell, B., Herbers, J., & Kroenke, K. (1993). Evaluating chest pain: The patient's presentation style alters the physician's diagnostic approach. *Archives of Internal Medicine, 153,* 1991–1995.

Bittner, V. (1996). Hyperlipidemia. In R. E. Blackwell (Ed.), *Women's medicine* (pp. 4–65). Cambridge, MA: Blackwell Science.

Bittner, V., & Oparil, S. (1997). Hypertension. In D. G. Julian & N. K. Wenger (Eds.), *Women and heart disease* (pp. 299–327). United Kingdom: Martin Dunitz.

Blackburn, H. (1985). Public policy and dietary recommendations to reduce population levels of blood cholesterol. *American Journal of Preventive Medicine, 1*, 3–10.

Blair, S. N., Goodyear, N. N., Gibbons, L. W., & Cooper, K. H. (1984) . Physical fitness and incidence of hypertension in healthy normotensive men and women. *Journal of American Medical Association, 252*, 487–490.

Blair, S. N., Kohl, H. W. III, Paffenbarger, R. S., Jr., Clark, D. G., Cooper, K. H., & Gibbons, L. W. (1989). Physical fitness and all-cause mortality: A prospective study of healthy men and women. *Journal of American Medical Association, 262*, 2395–2401.

Blumenthal, J. A., Burg, M. M., Barefoot, J. Williams, R. B., Haney, T., & Zimet, G. (1987). Social support, type A behavior and coronary artery disease. *Psychosomatic Medicine, 49*, 331–339.

Blustein, J., & Weitzman, B. (1995). Access to hospitals with high-technology cardiac services: How is race important? *American Journal of Public Health, 85*, 345–351.

Brunner, D., Weisbort, J., Meschulam, N., Schwartz, S., Gross, J., Saltz-Rennert, H., Altman, S., & Loebl, K. (1987). Relation of serum total cholesterol and high density lipoprotein cholesterol perentage to the incidence of definite coronary events: Twenty-year follow-up of the Donolo-Tel Aviv Prospective Coronary Artery Disease Study. *American Journal of Cardiology, 59*, 1271–1276.

Bucher, H. C., & Ragland, D. R. (1995). Socioeconomic indicators and mortality from coronary heart disease and cancer: A 22-year follow-up of middle-aged men. *American Journal of Public Health, 85*, 1231–1239.

Caldwell, J., Cooper, R., Eaker, E., Edozien, J., Harburg, E., Hayden, G., Hedeger, M., Hullettt, S., James, S., Kasl, S., Keil, J., Maloy, J., McDonald, R., McLarin, W., Myers, H., Pierce, C., Schoenberger, J., Shapiro, A., Thomson, G., Wallace, J., Wellons, R., & Wright, J. (1984). Summary of workshop III: Working group on socioeconomic and sociocultural influences. *American Heart Journal, 108*, 706–710.

Cameron, L., Leventhal, E. A., & Leventhal, H. (1993). Emotional and behavioral processes. In J. Johnston & L. Wallace (Eds.), *Stress and medical procedures* (pp. 7–30). New York: Pergamon.

Cannon, C. P., Antman, E. M., Walls, R., & Braunwald, E. (1994). Time as an adjunctive agent to thrombolytic therapy. *Journal of Thrombosis and Thrombolysis, 1*, 27–34.

Carleton, R .A., Lasater, T. M., Assaf, A., Lefebvere, R. C., & McKinlay, S. M. (1987). The Pawtucket Heart Health Program. I. An experiment in population based disease prevention. *Rhode Island Medical Journal, 70*, 533–538.

Carlisle, D., Leake, B., & Shapiro, M. (1995). Racial and ethnic disparities in the use of invasive cardiac procedures among cardiac patients in Los Angeles County, 1986 through 1988. *American Journal of Public Health, 85*, 345–51.

Carney, R. M., Rich, M. W., Freedland, K. E., Saini, J., teVelde, A., Simeone, C., & Clark, K. (1988). Major depressive disorder predicts cardiac events in patients with coronary artery disease. *Psychosomatic Medicine, 50*, 627–633.

Carney, R. M., Freedland, K. E., Smith, L., Lustman, P. J., & Jaffe, A. S. (1991). Relation of depression and mortality after myocardial infarction in women. *Circulation, 84*, 1876–1877.

Case, R. B., Moss, A. J., Case, N., McDermott, M., & Eberly, S. (1992). Living alone after myocardial infarction: Impact on prognosis. *Journal of the American Medical Association, 267*, 515–519.

Caspersen, C. J., Christenson, G. M., & Pollard, R. A. (1986). Status of the 1990 physical fitness and exercixe objectives: Evidence from NHIS 1995. *Public Health Report, 101*, 587–592.

Castaner, A., Simmons, B. E., Mar, M., & Cooper, R. (1988). Myocardial infarction among black patients: Poor prognosis after hospital discharge. *Annals of Internal Medicine, 109*, 33–35.

Cay, E. L., Vetter, N., Philip, A. E., & Dugard, P. (1972a). Psychological reactions to a coronary care unit. *Journal of Psychosomatic Research, 16*, 437–447.

Cay, E. L., Vetter, N., Philip, A. E., & Dugard, P. (1972b). Psychological status during recovery from an acute heart attack. *Journal of Psychosomatic Research, 16*, 425–435.

Chandra, V., Szklo, M., Goldberg, R., & Tonascia, J. (1983). The impact of marital status on survival after an acute myocardial infarction: A population-based study. *American Journal of Epidemiology, 117*, 320–325.

Cleary, P. D. (1987). Gender difference in stress-related disorders. In R.C. Barnett, L.Biener, & G.K. Baruch (Eds.), *Gender and stress* (pp. 39–72). New York: Free Press.

Cleophas, T. J., deJong, S., Niemeyer, M., Tavenier, P., Zwinderman, K., & Kuypers, C. (1993). Changes in life-style in men under sixty years of age before and after acute myocardial infarction: A case-control study. *The Journal of Vascular Diseases. 44*, 761–768.

Cohn, J. N. (1989). Sympathetic nervous system activity and the heart. *American Journal of Hypertension, 2*, 353S–356S.

Coombs, D. W., Robert, R. W., Crist, D. A., & Miller, H. L. (1989). Effects of social support on depression following coronary artery bypass graft surgery. *Psychology and Health, 3,* 29–35.

Cooper, R., & Ford, E. (1992). Comparability of risk factors for coronary heart disease among blacks and whites in the NHANES-I epidemiological follow-up study. *Annals of Epidemiology, 2,* 637–645.

Costa, P. T., Zonderman, A. B., Engel, B. T., Bails, W. F., Brimlow, D. L., & Brinker, J. (1985). The relation of chest pain symptoms to angiographic findings of coronary artery stenosis and neuroticism. *Psychosomatic Medicine, 47,* 285–293.

Crawford, S. L., McGraw, S. A., Smith, K. W., McKinlay, J. B., & Pierson, J. E. (1994). Do blacks and whites differ in their use of health care for symptoms of coronary heart disease? *American Journal of Public Health, 84,* 957–964.

Crews, D. J., & Landers D. M. (1987). A meta-analytic review of aerobic fitness and reactivity to psychosocial stressors. *Medicine and Science in Sports and Exercise, 19,* S114–S120.

Crowley, S. T., Dempsey, E. C., Horwitz, K. B., & Horwitz, L. D. (1994). Platelet-induced vascular smooth muscle cell proliferation is modulated by the growth amplification factors serotonin and adenosine diphosphate. *Circulation, 90,* 1908–1918.

Davis, K. B., Chaitman, B., Ryan, T., Bittner, V., & Kennedy, J. W. (1995) Comparison of 15-year survival for men and women after initial medical or surgical treatment for coronary artery disease: A CASS Registry study. *Journal of the American College of Cardiology, 25,* 1000–1009.

Dembroski, T. M., MacDougall, J. M., Costa, P. T., & Grandits, G. A. (1989). Components of hostility as predictors of sudden death and myocardial infarction in the Multiple Risk Factor Intervention Trial. *Psychosomatic Medicine, 51,* 514–522.

Department of Health and Human Services. (1985). Report of the Secretary's task force on black and minority health. Washington, DC: US Government Printing Office (GPO #017-090-00078-0).

DeStefano, F., Merritt, R. K., Anda, R. F., Casper, M. L., & Eaker, E.D. (1993). Trends in nonfatal coronary heart disease in the United States, 1980 through 1989. *Archives of Internal Medicine, 153,* 2489–2494.

Dimsdale, J. E., Alpert, B. S., & Schneiderman, M. (1986). Exercise as a modulator of cardiovascular reactivity In K. A. Matthews, S. M. Weiss, T. Detre, T. M. Dembroski, B. Falkner, S. B. Manuck, & R. B. Williams, Jr.. (Eds.),. *Handbook of stress, reactivity, and cardiovascular disease* (pp. 365–384). New York: John Wiley & Sons.

Dracup, K., Alonzo, A. A., Atkins, J. M., Bennett, N. M, Braslow, A., Clark, L. T., Eisenberg, M., Ferdinand, K. C., Frye, R., Green, L., Hill, M. N., Kennedy, J. W., Kline-Rogers, E., Moser, D. K., Ornato, J. P., Pitt, B., Scot, J. D., Selker, H. P., Silva, S. J., Thies, W., Weaver, W. D., Wenger, N. K., & White, S. K. (1997). The physician's role in minimizing prehospital delay in patients at high risk for acute myocardial infarction: Recommendations from the National Heart Attack Alert Program. *Annals of Internal Medicine, 126,* 645–651.

Dujovne, V. F., & Houston, B. K. (1991). Hostility-related variables and plasma lipid levels. *Journal of Behavioral Medicine, 14,* 555–565

Durel, L. A., Carver, C. S., Spitzer, S. B., Llabre, M. M., Weintraub, J. K., Saab, P. G., & Schneiderman, N. (1989). Associations of blood pressure with self-report measure of anger and hostility among black and white men and women. *Health Psychology, 8,* 557–575.

Eaker, E. D., & Castelli, W. P. (1987). Coronary heart disease and its risk factors among women in the Framingham Study. In E. D. Eaker, B. Packard, N. Winger, T. B. Clarkson, & H. A. Taylor (Eds.),. *Coronary heart disease in women* (pp. 122–130). New York: Haymarket Doyma.

Epstein, A., Taylor, W., & Seage, G. (1985). Effects of patients' socioeconomic status and physicians' training and practice on patient-doctor communication. *American Journal of Medicine, 78,* 101–106.

Every, N. R., Parsons, L. S., Fihn, S.D., Larson, E. B., Maynard, C., Hallstrom, A. P., Martin, J. S., & Weaver, W. D. (1997). Long-term outcome in acute myocardial infarction patients admitted to hospitals with and without on-site cardiac catheterization facilities. MITI Investigators. Myocardial infarction triage and intervention. *Circulation 96,* 1770–1775.

Farquhar, J. W., Fortmann, S. P., Wood, P. D., & Haskell, W. L. (1983). Community studies of cardiovascular disease prevention. In N. Kaplan, J. J. Stamler (Eds.), *Prevention of Coronary Heart Disease* (pp. 170–181). Philadelphia: W.B. Saunders.

Farquhar, J. W., Fortmann, S. P., Macccoby, N., Haskell,W. L., Williams, T.P. Flora, J. A., Taylor, C. B., Brown, B. W., Solomon, D. S. & Hulley, S. B. (1985). The Stanford Five-City Project: Design and methods. *American Journal of Epidemiology, 122,* 323–334.

Feinleib, M., Havlik, R. J., Gillum, R. F., Pokras, R., McCarthy, E., & Moien, M. (1989). Coronary heart disease and related procedures: National Hospital Discharge Survey data. *Circulation, 79,* 1–13.

Feldman, H. A., Proschan, M. A., Murray, D. M., Goff, D. C., Stylianou, M., Dulberg, E., McGovern, P. G., Chan, W., Mann, N. C., & Bittner, V. (1998). Statistical design of REACT (Rapid Early Action for Coronary Treatment), a multisite community trial with continual data collection. *Controlled Clinical Trials, 19*(4), 391–403.

Ferguson, J., Tierney, W., Westmoreland, G., Mamlin, L. A., Segar, D. S., Eckert, G. J., Zhou, X. H., Martin, D. K., & Weinberger, M. (1997). Examination of racial differences in management of cardiovascular disease. *Journal of the American College of Cardiology, 30*, 1707–1713.

Fibrinolytic Therapy Trialists' (FFT) Collaborative Group. (1994). Indications for fibrinolytic therapy in suspected acute myocardial infarction: Collaborative overview of early mortality and major morbidity results from all randomized trials of more than 1000 patients. *Lancet, 343*, 311–322.

Fiebach, N. H., Viscoli, C. M., & Horwitz, R. I. (1990). Differences between women and men in survival after myocardial infarction: Biology or methodology? *Journal of the American Medical Association, 263*, 1092–1096.

Fields, S. K., Savard, M. A., & Epstein, K.R. (1993). The female patient. In P. S. Douglas (Ed.), *Cardiovascular health and disease in women* (pp. 3–21). Philadelphia: W.B. Saunders.

Folsom, A. R., Sprafka, M., Luepker, R. V., & Jacobs, D. R. (1988). Beliefs among black and white adults about causes and prevention of cardiovascular disease: The Minnesota Heart Survey. *American Journal of Preventive Medicine, 4*, 121–127.

Ford, E., Cooper, R., Castaner, A., Simmons, B., & Mar, M. (1989). Coronary arteriography and coronary bypass surgery among whites and other racial groups relative to hospital-based incidence rates for coronary artery disease: Findings from NHDS. *American Journal of Public Health, 79*, 437–440.

Forrester, A., Lipsey, J., Teitelbaum, M., DePaulo, J. R., Andrzejewski, P., & Robinson, R. (1992). Depression following myocardial infarction. *International Journal of Psychiatry in Medicine, 22*(1), 33–46.

Frasure-Smith, N., & Prince, R. (1989). Long-term follow-up of the Ischemic Heart Disease Life Stress Monitoring Program. *Psychosomatic Medicine, 51*, 485–513.

Frasure-Smith, N., Lesperance, F., & Talajic, M. (1993). Depression following myocardial infarction: Impact on 6–month survival. *Journal of the American Medical Association, 270*, 1819–1825.

Frasure-Smith, N., Lesperance, F., Prince, R. H., Verrier, P., Garber, R. A., Juneau, M., Wolfson, C., & Bourassa, M. G. (1997). Randomised trial of home-based psychosocial nursing intervention for patients recovering from myocardial infarction. *Lancet, 350*, 473–479.

Fuchs, F. C., Stampfer, M. J., Colditz, G. A., Giozannucci, E. L., Manson, J. E., Kawachi, I., Hunter, D. J., Hankinson, P. E., Hennekens, C. H., Rosner, B., Speizer, F. E., & Willett, W. C. (1995). A prospective study of alcohol consumption and mortality among women. *New England Journal of Medicine, 332*, 1245–1250.

Gillum, R. F. (1982). Coronary heart disease in black populations. I: Mortality and morbidity. *American Heart Journal, 104*(4 Pt 1), 839–851.

Glanz, K., Lewis, F. M., & Rimer, B. K. (1997). *Health behavior and health education; Theory research and practice.* San Francisco: Jossey-Bass.

Goldberg, K. C., Hartz, A. J., Jacobsen, S. J., Krakauer, H., & Rimm, A. A. (1992). Racial and community factors influencing coronary artery bypass graft surgery rates for all 1986 Medicare patients. *Journal of the American Medical Association, 267*, 1473–1477.

Goldman, L., & Braunwald, E. (1991). Chest discomfort and palpitations. In A. S. Sauci, E. Braunwald, K. J. Isselbacher, J. D. Wilson, J. B. Martin, D. L. Kaspers, S. L. Hauser, & D. L. Longo (Eds.), *Harrison's principles of internal medicine* (pp. 98–105). New York: McGraw-Hill.

Goldman, L., & Cook, E. F. (1984). The decline in ischemic heart disease mortality rates: An analysis of the comparative effects of medical interventions and changes in life style. *Annals of Internal Medicine, 825*, 101–106.

Gordon, T., & Kannel, W. (1982). Multiple risk functions for predicting coronary heart disease: The concept, accuracy, and application. *American Heart Journal, 103*, 1031–1039.

Gordon, T., & Kannel, W. B. (1983). Drinking habits and cardiovascular disease: The Framingham Study. *American Heart Journal, 105*, 667–673.

Gorkin, L., Schron, E. B., Brooks, M. M., Wiklund, I., Kellen, J., Verter, J., Schoenberg, J. A., Paitan, Y., Morrism M., & Shumaker, S., for the CAST Investigators. (1993). Psychosocial predictors of mortality in the Cardiac Arrhythmia Suppression Trial-1(CAST-1). *American Journal of Cardiology, 71*, 263–267.

Groupo Italiano per lo Studio della Streptochinasi nell'Infarto Miocardico (GISSI). (1986). Effectiveness of intravenous thrombolytic treatment in acute myocardial infarction. *Lancet,1*, 397–402.

Hannan, E. L., Kilburn, H., Jr., O'Donnel, J. F., Lukacik, G., & Shields, E. P. (1991). Interracial access to selected cardiac procedures for patients hospitalized with coronary artery disease in New York State. *Medical Care, 29*, 430–441.

Harlan, W. R., & Stross, J. K. (1985). An educational view of a national initiative to lower plasma lipid levels. *Journal of the American Medical Association* ,*253*, 2087–2090.

Haynes, S. G., & Matthews, K. A. (1988). Area review: Coronary-prone behavior: Continuing evolution of the concept. *Annals of Behavioral Medicine, 10*(2), 47–59.

Hazuda, H. P., Stern, M. P., Gaskill, S. P., Haffner, S. M., & Gardner, L. I. (1983). Ethnic differences in health knowledge and behaviors related to the prevention and treatment of coronary heart disease: The San Antonio Heart Study. *American Journal of Epidemiology, 117*, 717–728.

Hedblad, B., Ostergren, P. O., Hanson, B. S., Janzon, L., Johansson, B. W., & Juul-Moller, S. (1992). Influence of social support on cardiac event rate in men with ischaemic type ST segment depression during ambulatory 24-h long-term ECG recording: The prospective population study 'Men born in 1914,' Malmo, Sweden. *European Heart Journal. 13*(4), 433–439.

Helmers, K. F., Krantz, D. S., Howell, R. H., Klein, J., Bairey, C. N., & Rozanski, A. (1993). Hostility and myocardial ischemia in coronary artery disease pateints: Evaluation by gender and ischemic index. *Psychosomatic Medicine, 55*, 29–36.

Helmrich, S. P., Ragland, D. R., Leung, R. W., & Paffenbarger, R. S. (1991). Physical activity and reduced occurrence of non-insulin-dependent diabetes mellitus. *New England Journal of Medicine, 147*–152.

Hennekens, C. H., O'Donnell, C. J., Ridker, P. M., & Marder, V. J. (1995). Current issues concerning thrombolytic therapy for acute myocardial infarction. *Journal of the American College of Cardiology, 25*, 18S-22S.

Hjermann, I., Welve Byrne, K., Holme, I., & Leren, P. (1981). Effect of diet and smoking intervention on the incidence of coronary heart disease: Report from the Oslo Study Group of a randomized trial in health men. *Lancet, 2*, 1303–1310.

Hlatky, M. A., Haney, T., Barefoot, J. C., Califf, R. M., Mark, D. B., & Williams, R. B. (1986). Medical, psychological and social correlates of work disability among men with coronary artery disease. *American Journal of Cardiology, 58*, 911–915

Holme, I., Helgeland, A., Hjermann, I., Leren, P., & Lund-Larson, P. G. (1980). Four and two-thirds years incidence of coronary heart disease in middle-aged men. The Oslo Study. *American Journal of Epidemiology, 112*, 149–160.

House, J. S., Robbins, C., & Metzner, H. C. (1982). The association of social relationships and activities with mortality: Perspective evidence from the Tecumseh community health study. *American Journal of Epidemiology, 116*(1), 123–140.

Houston, B. K., & Vavak, C. R. (1991). Cynical hostility: developmental factors, psychological correlates, and health behaviors. *Health Psychology, 10*, 9–17.

Hubert, H. B., Feinleib, M., McNamara, P. M., & Castelli, W. P. (1983). Obesity as an independent risk factor for cardiovascular disease: A 26–year follow up of participants in the Framingham Heart Study. *Circulation, 67*, 970–1983.

ISIS-2 Collaborative Group. (1988). Randomized trial of intravenous streptokinase, oral aspirin, both, or neither among 17,187 cases of suspected acute myocardial infarction: ISIS-2. *Journal of the American College of Cardiology, 12*(6 Suppl.), 3A–13A.

James, S. A. (1984). Socioeconomic influences on coronary heart disease in black populations. *American Heart Journal, 108*, 669–672.

Jenkins, C. D., Stanton, B. A., Savageau, J. A., Denlinger, P., & Klein, M. D. (1983). Coronary artery bypass surgery: Physical, psychological, social and economic outcomes six months later. *Journal of the American Medical Association, 250*, 782–88.

Johnson, E. H. (1987). Behavioral factors associated with hypertension in black Americans. In S. Julius & D. R. Bassett (Eds.), *Handbook of hypertension, vol. 9: Behavioral factors in hypertension* (pp. 181–197). Amsterdam: Elsevier Sciences.

Johnson, K. W., & Payne, G. H. (1984). Report of an NHLBI working conference on coronary heart disease in black populations: Preface. *American Heart Journal, 108*, 633–634.

Joint National Committee on Detection, Evaluation, and Treatment of High Blood Pressure (JNC-V). (1993). Fifth report. *Archives of Internal Medicine, 153*, 154–183.

Kagan, A., Gordon, T., Rhoads, G. G., & Schiffman, J. C. (1975). Some factors related to coronary heart disease incidence in Honolulu Japanese men: The Honolulu Heart Study. *International Journal of Epidemiology, 4*, 271–279.

Kannell, W. B., & Gordon, T. (1979). *Physiological and medical concomittants of obesity: The Framingham study* (pp. 125–163) (in Publication NIH 79-359). Washington, DC: US Government Printing Office.

Kannel, W. B., & Thom, T. J. (1984). Declining cardiovascular mortality. *Circulation, 70*, 331–336.

Kaplan, G.A., & Keil, J.E. (1993). Socioeconomic factors and cardiovascular disease: A review of the literature. *Circulation, 88*(4 Pt 1), 1973–1998.

Kasl, S. V. (1984). Social and psychologic factors in the etiology of coronary heart disease in black populations: An exploration of research needs. *American Heart Journal, 108,* 660–669.

Keil, J., Sutherland, M., Knapp, R., & Tyroler, H. (1992). Does equal socioeconomic status in black and white men mean equal risk of mortality? *American Journal of Public Health, 82,* 1133–1136.

Keil, J. E., Sutherland, S. E., Knapp, R. G. Lackland, D. T., Gazes, P. C., & Tyroler, H. A. (1993). Mortality rates and risk factors for coronary disease in blacks compared with white men and women. *New England Journal of Medicine, 323,* 73–78.

Kennedy, G. J., Hofer, M. A., & Chen, D. (1987). Significance of depression and cognitive impairment in patients undergoing programmed stimulation of cardiac arrhythmias. *Psychosomatic Medicine, 49,* 410–421.

Keys, A., Taylor, H. L, Blackburn, H., Brozek, J., Anderson, J. T., & Comonson, E. (1971). Mortality and coronary heart disease among men studied for 23 years. *Archives of Internal Medicine, 128,* 201–214.

Khan, S. S., Nessim, S., Gray, R., Czer, L. S., Chaux, A., & Matloff, J. (1990). Increased mortality of women in coronary artery bypass surgery: Evidence for referral bias. *Annals of Internal Medicine, 112,* 561–567.

King, A. C., & Tribble, D. (1990). The role of exercise in weight maintenance in non-athletes. *Sports Medicine, 11,* 331–349.

King, A. C., Taylor, C. B. Haskell, W. L., & DeBusk, R. F. (1989). Influence of regular aerobic exercise on psychological health. *Health Psychology, 8,* 305–324.

Klatsky, A. L., Friedman, G. D., Siegelaub, A. B., & Gerard, M. J. (1977). Alcohol consumption and blood pressure: Kaiser-Permanente multiphasic health examination data. *New England Journal of Medicine, 296,* 1194–2000.

Knopp, R. H. (1990). Effects of estrogen on serum lipoproteins and significance for arteriosclerotic disease. *Cholesterol and Coronary Disease: Reducing the Risk, 2*(6), 8–10.

Krieger, N. (1994). Influence of social class, race, and gender on the etiology of hypertension among women in the United States. In S. M. Czajkowski, D. R. Hill, & T. B. Clarkson (Eds.), *Women, behavior, and cardiovascular disease* (pp. 191–206). Washington DC: US DHHS, NIH Publication No. 9-3309.

Kulik, J. A., & Mahler, H. I. M. (1993). Emotional support as a moderator of adjustment and compliance after coronary artery bypass surgery: A longitudinal study. *Journal of Behavioral Medicine 16*(1) 45–63.

Kuller, L. H. (1991). Epidemiologic data. Proceedings of interdepartmental dean's conference. Alcohol and atherosclerosis. *Annals of Internal Medicine, 114,* 967–976.

Kumanyika, S., Savage, D. D., Ramirez, A. G., Hutchinson, J., Trevino, F. M., Adams-Campbell, L. L., & Watkins, L. O. (1989). Beliefs about high blood pressure prevention in a survey of blacks and Hispanics. *American Journal of Preventive Medicine, 1,* 21–26.

LaCroix, A. Z., Guralnik, J. M., & Curb, J. D. (1990). Chest pain and coronary heart disease mortality among older men and women in three communities. *Circulation, 81,* 437–446.

LaCroix, A. Z., Lang, J., & Scherr, P. (1991). Smoking and mortality among older men and women in three communities. *New England Journal of Medicine, 324,* 1619–1625.

Ladwig, K. H., Kiesert, M., Konig, J., Breithardt, G., & Borggrefe, M. (1991). Affective disorders and survival after acute myocardial infarction: Results from the post-infarction late potential study. *The European Heart Journal, 12*(9), 959–964.

Lapidus, L., Bengtsson, C., Larsson, B., Pennert, K., Rybo, E., & Sjostrom, L. (1984). Distribution of adipose tissue and risk of cardiovascular disease and death: A 12-year follow-up of participants in the population study of women in Gothenburg, Sweden. *British Medical Journal, 289,* 1257–1263.

Lasater, T., Abram, D., Artz, L., Beaudin, P., Cabrera, L., Elder, J., Ferreira, A., Knisley, P., Peterson, G., Rodrigues, A., Rosenberg, P., Snow, R., & Carleton, R. (1984). Lay volunteer delivery of a community-based cardiovascular risk factor change program: The Pawtucket experiment. In J. D. Matarazzo, S. M. Weiss, J. A. Herd, N. E. Miller, & S. M. Weiss (Eds.), *Behavioral health: A handbook of health enhancement and disease prevention* (pp.1166–1170). New York: John Wiley & Sons.

Laws, A., & Reaven, G. M. (1991). Physical activity, glucose tolerance, and diabetes in older adults. *Annals of Behavioral Medicine, 13,* 125–132.

Lee, K. L., Woodlief, L. H., Topol, E. J., Weaver, W. D., Betriu, A., Col, J., Simmons, M., Aylward, P., Van de Werf, F., & Califf, R. M. (1995). Predictors of 30-day mortality in the era of reperfusion for acute myocardial infarction. Results from an international trial of 41,021 patients. GUSTO-I Investigators. *Circulation, 91,*1659–1668.

Lefebvre, R. C., Lasater, T. M., Carleton, R. A., & Peterson, G. (1987). Theory and delivery of health programming in the community. *Preventive Medicine, 16,* 80–95.

Legato, M. J. (1996). Coronary artery disease in women. *International Journal of Fertility and Menopausal Studies, 41*(2), 94–100.

Leiker, M., & Hailey, B. J. (1988). A link between hostility and disease: poor health habits. *Behavioral Medicine, 14,* 129–133.

Lenfant, C. (1986). The National Cholesterol Education Program. *Public Health Reports, 101,* 2–3.

Lerner, D. J., & Kannel, W. B. (1986). Patterns of coronary heart disease morbidity and mortality in the sexes: A 26-year follow up of the Framingham population. *American Heart Journal, 111,* 383–390.

Leon, A. S. (1989). Effects of physical activity and fitness on health. In National Center for Health Statistics. *Assessing physical fitness and physical activities in population-based surveys.* DHHS publication No. (Phs 89–1253). Hyattsville, MD: US Department of Health and Human Service.

Leon, A. S., Connett, J., Jacobs, D. R., & Rauramaa, R. (1987) . Leisure-time physical activity levels and risk of coronary heart disease and death: The Multiple Risk Factor Intervention trial. *Journal of American Medical Association, 258,* 2388–2395.

Leventhal, H., Meyer, D., & Nerenz, D. (1980). The common-sense representation of illness danger. In S. Rachman (Ed.), *Medical psychology* (pp. 7–30). New York: Pergamon.

Leventhal, H., & Nerenz, D. (1985). The assessment of illness cognition. In P. Karoly (Ed.), *Measurement strategies in health* (pp. 517–554). New York: John Wiley & Sons.

Levy, D., & Kannel, W. B. (1988). Cardiovascular risks: new insights form Framingham. *American Heart Journal, 116,* 2664–2667.

Levy, R. I. (1985). Cholesterol and cardiovascular disease: No longer whether but rather when, in whom, and how? *Circulation 72,* 686– 696.

The Lipid Research Clinics Population Studies Data Book. (1980). I. *The prevalence study.* US Department of Health, Education, and Welfare Publication (NIH 80-1527) Bethesda MD: National Institutes of Health.

The Lipid Research Clinics Coronary Primary Prevention Trial Group. (1984). The Lipid Research Clinics Coronary Primary Prevention Trial results. I. Reduction in incidence of coronary heart disease. *Journal of the American Medical Association, 251,* 351–164.

Lloyd, G. G., & Cawley, R. H. (1978). Psychiatric consultation in a coronary care unit. *Annals of Internal Medicine, 75,* 9–14.

Lloyd, G. G., & Cawley, R. H. (1982a). Psychiatric morbidity in men one week after first acute myocardial infarction. *British Medical Journal, 2,* 1453–1454.

Lloyd, G. G., & Cawley, R. H. (1982b). Distress or illness? A study of psychological symptoms after myocardial infarction. *British Journal of Psychiatry, 142,* 120–125.

Lloyd, C. E., Kuller, L. H., Ellis, D., Becker, D. J., Wing, R. R., & Orchard, T. J. (1996). Coronary artery disease in IDDM: Gender differences in risk factors but not risk. *Arteriosclerosis, Thrombosis, and Vascular Biology, 16*(6), 720–726.

Lowering Blood Cholesterol to Prevent Heart Disease Consensus Conference. (1985). *Journal of the American Medical Association, 253,* 2080–2086.

Luepker, R. V., Rosamond, W. D., Murphy R., Sprafka, J. M., Folsom, A. R., Mcgovern, P. G., & Blackburn, H. (1993). Socioeconomic status and coronary heart disease risk factor trends: The Minnesota Heart Survey. *Circulation, 88*(5 Pt 1), 2172–2179.

Lunderg, U., Hendman, M., Melin, B., & Frankenhaeuser, M. (1989). Type A behavior in healthy males and female as related to physiological reactivity and blood lipids. *Psychosomatic Medicine, 51,* 113–122.

Malone, K. M., Thase, M. E., Mieczkowski, T., Myers, J. E., Stull, S. D., Cooper, T. B., & Mann, J. J. (1993). Fenfluramine challenge test as a predictor of outcome in major depression. *Psychopharmacology Bulletin, 29,* 155–161.

Manson, J. E., Colditz, G. A., Stampfer, J. J., Willett, W. C., Rosner, B., Monson, R. R., Speizer, F. E., & Hennekens, C. H. (1990). A prospective study of obesity and risk of coronary heart disease in women. *New England Journal of Medicine, 32,* 882–889.

Manuck, S. B., Kaplan, J. R., & Clarkson, T. B. (1983). Behaviorally induced heart rate reactivity and atherosclerosis in cynomolgus monkeys. *Psychosomatic Medicine, 45,* 95–108.

Manuck, S. B., Kaplan, J. R., & Matthews, K. A. (1986). Behavioral antecedents of coronary heart disease and atherosclerosis. *Arteriosclerosis, 6*(1), 2–14.

Mark, D. B., Naylor, C. D., Hlatky, M. A., Califf, R. M., Topol, E. J., Granger, C. B., Knight, J. D., Nelson, C. L., Lee, K. L., & Clapp-Channing, N. E. (1994). Use of medical resources and quality of life after acute myocardial infarction in Canada and the United States. *New England Journal of Medicine, 331,* 1130–1135.

Marrugat, J., Sanz, G., Masia, R., Valle, V., Molina, L., Cardona, M., Sala, J., Seres, L., Szescielinski, L., Albert, X., Lupon, J., & Alonso, J. (1997). Six-month outcome in patients with myocardial infarction initially admitted to tertiary and nontertiary hospitals. *Journal of the American College of Cardiology, 30,* 1187–1192.

Matthews, K. A. (1988). Coronary heart disease and Type A behaviors: Update on and alternative to the Booth-Kewley and Friedman (1987) quantitative review. *Psychological Bulletin, 104,* 373–380.

Matthews, K. A., & Haynes, S. G. (1986). Type A behavior pattern and coronary disease risk. *American Journal of Epidemiology, 123,* 923–960.

Maynard, C., Fisher, L. D., Passamani, E. R., & Pullum, T. (1986). Blacks in the Coronary Artery Surgery Study (CASS): Race and clinical decision making. *American Journal of Public Health, 76,* 1446–1448.

Mayou, R., MacMahon, D., Sleight, P., & Florencio, M. J. (1981). Early rehabilitation after myocardial infarction. *Lancet, 2,* 1399–1404.

Medalie, J. H., & Goldbourt, U. (1976). Angina pectoris among 10,000 men: Psychosocial and other factors as evidenced by a multivariate analysis of a 5 year incidence study. *American Journal of Medicine, 60,* 910–921.

Mendes deLeon, C. F., Powell, L. H., & Kaplan, B. H. (1991). Change in coronary-prone behaviors in the Recurrent Coronary Prevention Project. *Psychosomatic Medicine, 53,* 407–419, 1991.

Mirvis, D. M., Burns, R., Gaschen, L., Cloar, F. T., & Graney, M. (1994). Variation in utilization of cardiac procedures in the Department of Veterans Affairs Health Care System: Effect of race. *Journal of the American College of Cardiology, 24,* 1297–1304.

Mittelmark, M. B., Leupker, R.V., Murray, D. M., Jacobs, D. R., Bracht, N., Carlaw, R., Crow, R., Elmer, P., Finnegan, J., & Folsom, A. R. (1986). Community education for cardiovascular disease prevention: Risk factor changes in the Minnesota Heart Health Program. *American Journal of Public Health, 84,* 1383–1393.

Morris, J. N., Clayton, D. G., Everitt, M. G., Semmence, A. M., & Burgess, E. H. (1990) . Exercise in leisure time: Coronary attack and death rates. *British Heart Journal, 63,* 325–334.

Mosca, L., Manson, J. E., Sutherland, S. E., Langer, R. D., Manolio, T., & Barrett-Connor, E. (1997). Cardiovascular disease in women: A statement for healthcare professionals From the American Heart Association. *Circulation, 96,* 2468–2482.

Muller, J. E., Stone, P. H., Turi, Z. G., Rutherford, J. D., Czeisler, C. A., Parker, C., Poole, W. K., Passamani, E., Roberts, R., Robertson, T., Sobel, B. E., Wilerson, J. T., Braunwald, E., & the MILLIS Study Group. (1985). Circadian variation in the frequency of onset of acute myocardial infarction. *New England Journal of Medicine, 313,* 1315–1322.

Multiple Risk Factor Intervention Trial Research Group. (1982). Multiple risk factor intervention trial: Risk factor changes and mortality results. *Journal of the American Medical Association, 248,* 1465–1477.

Mutchler, J. E., & Burr, J.A. (1991). Racial differences in health and health care service utilization in later life: The effects of socioeconomic status. *Journal of Health and Social Behavior, 32,* 342–356.

Naismith, L. D., Robinson, J. F., Shaw, G. B., & MacIntyre, M. M. (1979). Psychosocial rehabilitation after infarction. *British Medical Journal, 1,* 439–444.

National Heart Attack Alert Program (NHAAP) Coordinating Committee 60 Minutes to Treatment Working Group. (1994). Emergency department: Rapid identification and treatment of patients with acute myocardial infarction. *Annals of Emergency Medicine, 23,* 311–329.

National Heart, Lung, and Blood Institutes (NHLBI). (1994). *Report of the task force on research in epidemiology and prevention of cardiovascular diseases.* (1994). Washington, DC: US Department of Health and Human Services.

National Institutes of Health Consensus Development Panel on the Health Implications of Obesity. (1985). Health implications of obesity: National Institutes of Health Consensus Development Conference statement. *Annals of Internal Medicine, 103,* 1073–1077.

Nunes, E. V., Frank, K. A., & Kornfeld, D. S. (1987). Psychologic treatment for the type A behavior pattern and for coronary heart disease: A meta-analysis of the literature. *Psychomatic Medicine, 48,* 159–173.

Oberman, A., & Cutter, G. (1984). Issues in the national history and treatment of coronary heart disease in black population: Surgical treatment. *American Heart Journal, 108,* 688–694.

Ockene, J. K., Ockene, I. S., Kabat-Zinn, J., Greene, H. L., & Frid, D. (1990). Teaching risk-factor counseling skills to medical students, house staff, and fellows. *American Journal of Preventive Medicine, 6*(Suppl.), 35–42.

O'Keefe, J. H., Jr, Rutherford, B. D., McConahay, D. R., Ligon, R. W., Johnson, W. L., Jr., Giorgi, L. V., Crockett, J. E., McCallister, B. D., Conn, R. D., & Gura, G. M., Jr. (1989). Early and late results of coronary angioplasty without antecedent thrombolytic therapy for acute myocardial infarction. *American Journal of Cardiology, 64,* 221–230.

Orth-Gomer K., & Unden, A. L. (1990). Type A behavior, social support, and coronary risk: Interaction and significance for mortality in cardiac patients. *Psychosomatic Medicine, 52,* 59–72.

Ostfeld, A. M., Lebovits, B., Shekelle, R., & Paul, O. (1964) A prospective study of the relationship between personality and coronary heart disease, *Journal of Chronic Disease, 17,* 265–276.

Owens, J. F., Matthews, K. A., Wing, R. R., & Kuller, L. H. (1990) . Physical activity and cardiovascular risk: a cross-sectional study of middle-aged premenopausal women. *Preventive Medicine, 19,* 147–157.

Paffenbarger, R. S., Hyde, R. T., Wing, A. L., & Hsieh, C.-C. (1986) . Physical activity, all-cause mortality, and longevity of college alumni. *New England Journal of Medicine, 314,* 605–613.

Pancheri, P., Matteoli, S., Pollizzi, C., Bellaterra, M., Cristofari, M., & Pulleti, M. (1978). Infarct as a stress agent: Life history and personality characteristics in improved versus not-improved patients after severe heart attack. *Journal of Human Stress, 4,* 16–42.

Pandey, G. N., Pandey, S. C., Janicak, P. G., Marks, R. C., & Davis, J. M. (1990). Platelet serotonin-2 receptor binding sites in depression and suicide. *Biological Psychiatry, 28,* 215–222.

Parisi, A., Folland, E., & Hartigan, P. (1992). A comparison of angioplasty with medical therapy in the treatment of single-vessel coronary artery disease. *New England Journal of Medicine, 326,* 10–16.

Pate, R. R., Pratt, M., Blair, S. N., Haskell, W. L., Macera, C. A., Bouchard, C., Buchner, D., Ettinger, W., Heath, G. W., King, A. C., Kriska, A., Leon, A. S., Marcus, B. H. Morris, J., Paffenbarger, R. S., Patrick, K. Pollock, M. L., Rippe, J. M., Sallils, J., & Wilmore, J. H. (1995). Physical activity and public health: A recommendation from the Centers for Disease Control and Prevention and the American College of Sports Medicine. *Journal of the American Medical Association, 273,* 402–407.

Penchansky, R., & Thomas, J. (1981). The concept of access: definition and relationship to consumer satisfaction. *Medical Care, 19,* 127–140.

Potter, W. Z., & Manji, H. K. (1994). Catecholamines in depression: An update. *Clinical Chemistry, 40,* 279–287.

Powell, K. E., Thompson, P. D., Caspersen, C. J., & Ford, E. S. (1987) . Physical activity and the incidence of coronary heart disease. *Annual Review of Public Health, 8,* 253–287.

Pryor, D. B., Harrell, F. E., Jr., Lee, K. L., Califf, R. M., & Rosati, R. A. (1983). Estimating the likelihood of significant coronary artery disease. *American Journal of Medicine, 75,* 771–780.

Pryor, D. B., Shaw, L., McCants, C.B., Lee, K. L., Mark, D. B., Harrell, F. E., Jr, Muhlbaier, L. H., & Califf, R. M. (1993). Value of the history and physical in identifying patients at increased risk for coronary artery disease. *Annals of Internal Medicine, 118,* 81–90.

Puska, P. (1973). The North Karelia Project: An attempt at community prevention of cardiovascular disease. *The World Health Organization Chronicle, 27,* 55–58.

Raczynski, J. M. (1997, April) Basic structure of ENRICHD. In N. Schneiderman, R. Williams, J. Raczynski, C. Thorsen, B. Taylor, & S. Czajkowski (Eds.), *ENRICHD: New NHLBI multi-center trial for enhancing recovery after myocardial infarction.* Symposium presented at the meeting of the Society of Behavioral Medicine, San Francisco, CA.

Raczynski, J. M., Taylor, H., Cutter, G., Hardin, M., Rappaport, N., & Oberman, A. (1994a). Rose questionnaire responses among black and white inpatients admitted for coronary heart disease: Findings from the Birmingham-BHS Project. *Ethnicity and Disease, 3,* 290–301.

Raczynski, J. M., Taylor, H., Rappaport, N., Cutter, G., Hardin, M., & Oberman, A. (1994b). Diagnoses, acute symptoms and attributions for symptoms among black and white inpatients admitted for coronary heart disease: Findings of the Birmingham-BHS Project. *American Journal of Public Health, 84*(6), 951–995

Reed, D., McGee, D., & Yano, K. (1984). Psychosocial processes and general subseptibility to chronic disease. *American Journal of Epidemiology, 119,*356–370.

Rich-Edwards J., Manson, J. E., Hennekens, C. H., & Buring, J. E. (1995). The primary prevention of coronary heart disease in women. *The New England Journal of Medicine, 332*(26), 1758–1766

Rodin, G., Craven, J., & Littlefield, C. (1991). *Depression in the medically ill.* New York: Brunner/Mazel.

Roose, S. P., Laghrissi-Thode, F., Kennedy, J. S., Nelson, J. C., Bigger, J. T., Pollock, B. G., Gaffeny, A., Narayan, M., Finkel, M. S., McCafferty, J., & Gergel, I. (1998). Comparison of paroxetine and nortriptyline in depressed patients with ischemic heart disease. *Journal of the American Medical Association, 279*(4), 287–291.

Rose, G. (1962). The diagnosis of ischemic heart pain and intermittent claudication in field surveys. *Bulletin of the World Health Organization, 27,* 645–58.

Rose, G., & Shipley, M. (1986). Plasma cholesterol concentration and death form coronary heart disease: 10–year results of the Whitehall Study. *British Medical Journal, 293,* 306–307.

Rosenberg, L., Slone, D., Shapiro, S., Kaufman, D. W., Miettinen, O. S., & Stolley, P. D. (1981). Alcoholic beverages and myocardial infarction in young women. *American Journal of Public Health, 71,* 82–85.

Rosengren, A., Wilhelmsen, L., Welin, L., Tsipogianni, A., Teger-Nilsson, A. C., & Wedel, H. (1990). Social influences and cardiovascular risk factors as determinants of plasma fibrinogen concentration in a general population sample of middle aged men. *British Medical Journal, 300,* 634–638.

Ruberman, W. (1992). Psychosocial influence on patients with coronary heart disease. *Journal of the American Medical Association, 267,* 559–560.

Ruberman, W., Weinblatt, E., Golberg, J. D., & Chaudhary, B. S. (1984). Psychosocial influences on mortality after myocardial infarction. *New England Journal of Medicine, 311,* 552–559.

Sanderson, B. K., Raczynski, J. M., Cornell, C. E., Hardin, M., & Taylor, H. A., Jr. (1998). Ethnic disparities in patients' recall of physicians' recommending diagnostic and treatment procedures for coronary disease. *American Journal of Epidemiology, 148*(8), 741–749.

Scherwitz, L., Perkins, L., Chesney, M., & Hughes G. (1991). Cook–Medley Hostility Scale and subscales: Relationship to demographic and psychosocial characteristics in CARDIA. *Psychosomatic Medicine, 53,* 36–49.

Schleifer, S. J., Macari-Henson, M., Coyle, D. A., Slater, W., Kahn, M., Gorlin, R., & Zucker, H. (1989). The nature and course of depression following myocardial infarction. *Archives of Internal Medicine, 149,* 1785–1789.

Schoenbach, V. J., Kaplan, B. H., Freman, L., & Kleinbaum, D. G. (1986). Social ties and mortality in Evans County, Georgia. *American Journal of Epidemiology, 123,* 577–591.

Schooler, C. S., Farquhar, J. W., Fortmann, S. P., & Flora, J. A. (1997). Synthesis of findings and issues from community prevention trials. *Annals of Epidemiology, 7*(Suppl.), S54–S68.

Schrott, H., Bittner, V., Vittinghoff, E., Herrington, D.M., & Hulley, S. (1997). Adherence to National Cholesterol Education Program (NCEP) treatment goals in postmenopausal women with heart disease: The Heart and Estrogen/Progestin Replacement Study (HERS). *Journal of the American Medical Association, 277,* 1281–1286.

Scragg, R., Stewart, A., Jackson, R., & Beaglehole, R. (1987). Alcohol and exercise in myocardial infarction and sudden coronary death in men and women. *American Journal of Epidemiology, 126,* 77–85.

Seeman, T. E., & Syme, S. L. (1987). Social networks and coronary artery disease: A comparison of structure and function of social relations as predictors of the disease. *Psychosomatic Medicine, 49,* 340–353.

Shaper, A. G., & Elford, J. (1991). Place of birth and adult cardiovascular disease: The British Regional Heart study. *Acta Paediatrica Scandinavica, 373 (Suppl.),* 73–81.

Shekelle, R. B., Shyrock, A. M., Paul, O., Lepper, M., Stamler, J., Liu, S., & Raynor, W. J., Jr. (1981). Diet, serum cholesterol, and death from coronary heart disease. The Western Electric Study. *New England Journal of Medicine, 304,* 65–70.

Siegler, I. C., Peterson, B. L., Barefoot, J. C., Dahlstrom, W. G., Suarez, E. C., & Williams, R. B. (1990). Hostility levels at age 19 predict lipid risk profiles at age 42. *Circulation, 82* (suppl. IIII), 228.

Silverstone, P. H. (1990). Depression increases mortality and morbidity in acute life-threatening medical illness. *Journal of Psychosomatic Research, 34,* 651–657.

Simons-Morton, D. G., Goff, D. C., Osganian, S., Goldberg, R. J., Raczynski, J. M., Finnegan, J. R., Zapka, J., Eisenberg, M. S., Proschan, M. A., Feldman, H. A., Hedges, J. R., & Luepker, R. V. (1998). Rapid early action for coronary treatment: rationale, design, and baseline characteristics. *Academic emergency medicine, 5*(7), 726–738.

Sloan, R., & Bigger, J., Jr. (1991, April). Biobehavioral factors in Cardiac Arrhythmia Pilot Study (CAPS): Review and examination. *Circulation, 83* (Suppl. II), II-52–II-57.

Smith, C. A., & Pratt, M. (1993). Cardiovascular disease. In R. C. Brownson, P. L. Remington, & J. R. Davis (Eds.), *Chronic disease epidemiology and control* (pp. 83–107). Washington, DC: American Public Health Association.

Smith-Warner, S. A., Spiegelman, D., Yaun, S. S., van den brandt, P. A., Folsom, A. R., Goldbohm, R. A., Graham, S., Holmberg, L., Howe, G. R., Marshall, J. R., Miller, A. B., Potter J. D., Speizer, F. E., Willett, W. C., Wolk, A., & Hunter, D. J. (1998). Alcohol and breast cancer in women—A pooled analysis of cohort studies. *Journal of the American Medical Association, 279,* 535–540.

Sox, H. C., Jr., Hickman, D. H., Marton, K. I., Moses, L., Skeff, K. M., Sox, C. H., & Neal, E. A. (1990). Using the patient's history to estimate the probability of coronary artery disease: a comparison of primary care and referral practices. *American Journal of Medicine, 89,* 7–14.

Spelsberg, A., Ridker, P. M., & Manson, E. (1993). Carbohydrate, metabolism, obesity, and diabetes. In P. S. Douglas (Ed.), *Cardiovascular health and disease in women* (pp. 191–216). Philadelphia: W.B. Saunders.

Stamler, J., Rhomberg, P., Schoenberger, J. A., Shekelle, R. B., Dyer, A., Shekelle, S., Stamler, R., & Wanna-maker, J. (1975a). Multivariate analysis of the relationship of seven variables to blood pressure: Findings of the Chicago Heart Association Detection Project in Industry 1967–1972. *Journal of Chronic Diseases, 28*, 527–544.

Stamler, J., Stamler, R., Rhombery, P., Dyer, A., Berkson, D. M., Reedus, W., & Wannamaker, J. (1975b). Multivariate analysis of the relationship of six variables to blood pressure: Findings from the Chicago community surveys, 1965–1972. *Journal of Chronic Diseases, 28*, 499–526.

Stamler, J., Wentworth, D., & Neaton, J. D. (1986). Is the relationship between serum cholesterol and risk of premature death from coronary heart disease continuous and graded? Findings in 356,222 primary screenees of the Multiple Risk Factor Intervention Trial (MRFIT). *Journal of the American Medical Association 256*, 2823–2828.

Stampfer, M. J., Colditz, G. A., Willett, W. C., Speizer, F. E., & Hennekens, C. H. (1988). A prospective study of moderate alcohol consumption and the risk of coronary disease and stroke in women. *New England Journal of Medicine, 319*, 267–273.

Steingart, R. M., Packer, M., Hamm, P., Coglianese, M. E., Gersh, B., Geltman, E.M., Sollano, J., Katz, S., Moye, L., & Basta, L. L. (1991). Sex differences in the management of coronary artery disease. *New England Journal of Medicine, 325*, 226–230.

Stern, M. J., Pascale, L., & McLoone, J. B. (1976). Psychosocial adaptation following an acute myocardial infarction. *Journal of Chronic Disease, 29*, 513–526.

Stern, M. J., Pascale, L., & Ackerman, A. (1977). Life adjustment post-myocardial infarction. *Archives of Internal Medicine, 137*, 623–633.

Stokes, J., III, Kannel, W. B., & Wolf, P. A. (1989). Blood pressure as a risk factor for cardiovascular disease. The Framingham Study—30 years of follow-up. *Hypertension, 13* (Suppl. I), I13–I18.

Stoney, C. M., Matthews, KL. A., McDonald, R. H., & Johnson, C. A. (1988). Sex differences in lipid, lipoprotein, cardiovascular, and neuroendocrine responses to acute stresss. *Psychophysiology, 25*, 645–656.

Strogatz, D. (1990). Use of medical care for chest pain: differences between blacks and whites. *American Journal of Public Health, 80*, 290–294.

Suarez, E. C., & Williams, R. B., Jr. (1990). The relationships between dimensions of hostility and cardiovascular reactivity as a function of task characteristics. *Psychosomatic Medicine, 52*, 558–570.

Taylor, C. B., Sallis, J. F., & Needle, R. (1985). The relationship of physical activity and exercise to mental health. *Public Health Reporter, 100*, 195–201.

Uemura, K., & Pisa, Z. (1988). Trends in cardiovascular disease mortality in industrialized countries since 1950. *World Health Organization, 4*, 155–178.

US Department of Health and Human Services. (1991). *Healthy People 2000: National health Promotion and Disease Prevention Objectives.* (DHHS Publication No. PHS 91-50212). Washington, DC: US Dept. of Health and Human Services.

Van de Werf, F., & Arnold, A. E. R., for the European Cooperative Study Group for recombinant tissue type plasminogen activator. (1988). Intravenous tissue plasminogen activator and size of infarct, left ventricular function, and survival in acute myocardial infarction. *British Medical Journal, 297*, 1374–1379.

Van Itallie, T. B. (1979). Obesity: Adverse effects on health and longevity. *American Journal of Clinical Nutrition, 32*, 2723–2733.

Van Itallie, T. B. (1985). Health implications of overweight and obesity in the United States. *Annals of Internal Medicine, 103*, 983–988.

Watkins, L. O. (1984). Epidemiology of coronary heart disease in black populations: Methodologic proposals. *American Heart Journal, 108*, 635–640.

Weidner, G. (1994). In S. M. Czajkowski, D. R. Hill, & T. B. Clarkson (Eds.), *Women, behavior, and cardiovascular disease* (pp. 103–116). NIH Publication No. 94-3309. Washington, DC: US DHHS.

Weidner, G., Sexton, G., McLellarn, R., Connor, S. L., & Matarazzo, J. B. (1987). The role of type A behavior and hostility in an elevation of plasma lipids in adult women and men. *Psychosomatic Medicine, 48*, 136–145.

Weissman, J. S., Stern, R., Fielding, S. L., & Epstein, A. M. (1991). Delayed access to health care: Risk factors, reasons, and consequences. *Annals of Internal Medicine, 114*, 325–331.

Weissman, M. M., & Klerman, G. L. (1977). Sex differences in the epidemiology of depression. *Archives of General Psychiatry, 34*, 98–111.

Wenger, N. K. (1990). Gender, coronary artery disease, and coronary bypass surgery. *Annals of Internal Medicine, 112*, 557–558.

Wenger, N. K. (1994). Coronary heart disease in women: Needs and opportunities. In S. M. Czajkowski, D. R. Hill, & T. B. Clarkson (Eds), *Women, behavior, and cardiovascular disease* (pp. 7–15). Washington, DC: US DHHS, NIH Publication No. 94-3309.

Wenneker, M. B., & Epstein, A. M. (1989). Racial inequalities in the use of procedures for patients with ischemic heart disease in Massachusetts. *Journal of the American Medical Association, 261*, 253–257.

Whittle, J., Conigliaro, J., Good, C., & Lofgreen, R. (1993). Racial differences in the use of invasive cardiovascular procedures in the Department of Veterans Affairs Medical System. *New England Journal of Medicine, 329*, 621–627.

Willett, C. W., Green, A., & Stampfer, M. J. (1987). Relative and absolute excess risk of coronary heart disease among women who smoke cigarettes. *New England Journal of Medicine, 317*, 1303–1309.

Willett, W. C., & Lenart, E. B. (1996). Dietary factors. In J. E. Manson, P. M. Ridker, J. M. Gaziano, & C. H. Hennekens (Eds.), *Prevention of myocardial infarction* (pp. 351–383). New York: Oxford University Press.

Williams, R. B., Jr. (1989). Biological mechanisms mediating the relationship between behavior and coronary heart disease. In A. W. Siegman & T. M. Dembroski (Eds.), *In search of coronary-prone behavior* (pp. 195–205). New York: Erlbaum

Williams, R. B., Jr., Barefoot, J. C., Califf, R. M., Haney, T. L., Saunders, W. B., Pryor, D. B., Hlatkey, M. A., Siegler, I. C., & Mark, D. B. (1992). Prognostic importance of social and economic resources among medically treated patients with angiographically documented coronary artery disease. *Journal of the American Medical Association, 267*, 520–524.

Windsor, R. A. (1984). *Evaluation of health promotion and education programs.* Palo Alto, CA: Mayfield.

Wood, P. D., Stefanick, M. I., Williams, P. T., & Haskell, W. L. (1991). The effects of plasma lipoproteins of a prudent weight-reducing diet, with or without excercise, in overweight men and women. *New England Journal of Medicine, 325*, 461–466.

World Health Organization (WHO). (1988). Geographical variation in the major risk factors of coronary heart disease in men and women aged 35–64 years. The WHO MONICA Project. *World Health Statistics Quarterly, 41*, 115–140.

Yarnell, J. W., Baker, I. A., Sweetnam, P. M., Bainton, D., O'Brien, J. R., Whitehead, P. J., & Elwood, P. C. (1991). Fibrinogen, viscosity, and white blood cell count are major risk factors for ischemic heart disease. The Caerphilly and Speedwell Collaborative Heart Disease Studies. *Circulation, 83*, 836–844.

CHAPTER 13

Cancer Prevention and Control

Kim D. Reynolds, Polly P. Kratt, Suzan E. Winders,
John W. Waterbor, John L. Shuster, Jr., Marilyn Gardner,
and Renée A. Harrison

Introduction

This chapter reviews the role of health education and health promotion in cancer prevention and control by examining the epidemiology of cancer and by reviewing a number of risk factors for cancer that can be impacted through the implementation of behavioral interventions. In addition, the psychosocial aspects of cancer are addressed and are linked to treatment issues in cancer prevention and control. Within each section of this chapter, we have attempted to review the relationship between behaviors and cancer at specific sites. This review is followed in most sections by an examination of the role of primary, secondary, and, when appropriate, tertiary prevention as they relate to these cancers.

This chapter is not a comprehensive review of the literature on cancer prevention and control. However, the chapter does provide an overview of many important elements of cancer prevention and control, with a special emphasis on behavioral issues and interventions. As such, the chapter will help prepare health professionals to enact the various recommendations put forth for limiting the occurrence of cancer and controlling the health burdens it presents in the United States. For example, the National Cancer Institute (NCI) Working Group on Behavioral Research on Cancer Prevention and Control (Lerman, Rimer, & Glynn, 1997) recently identified six priority areas for research in cancer prevention and control including: (1) preventing tobacco use among children and teenagers; (2) enhancing risk communication, comprehension, and in-

Kim D. Reynolds • Center for Behavioral Studies, AMC Cancer Research Center, Lakewood, Colorado 80214.   *Polly P. Kratt and Suzan E. Winders* • Behavioral Medicine Unit, Division of Preventive Medicine, Department of Medicine, School of Medicine, UAB Center for Health Promotion, University of Alabama at Birmingham, Birmingham, Alabama 35294.   *John W. Waterbor and Renée A. Harrison* • Department of Epidemiology, School of Public Health, University of Alabama at Birmingham, Birmingham, Alabama 35294.   *John L. Shuster, Jr.* • Department of Psychiatry, School of Medicine, University of Alabama at Birmingham, Birmingham, Alabama 35294.   *Marilyn Gardner* • Department of Health Behavior, School of Public Health, University of Alabama at Birmingham, Birmingham, Alabama 35294.

Handbook of Health Promotion and Disease Prevention, edited by Raczynski and DiClemente. Kluwer Academic/Plenum Publishers, New York, 1999.

formed decision making under uncertainty; (3) integrating preventive and early detection services into changing health delivery systems; (4) improving the outcomes of
genetic testing for cancer susceptibility; (5) enhancing survivorship of cancer patients;
and (6) promoting a healthy diet and physical activity. In addition, the working group
has identified four crosscutting themes that were deemed relevant to all the priority
areas of research, including: (1) consideration of race, social class, and culture; (2) theory-driven research; (3) multiple-level interventions targeted to multiple risk factors;
and, (4) research settings, meaning that "behavioral research initiatives should span all
phases of cancer control research and take place in a variety of settings." The present
chapter complements efforts such as the recommendations of the NCI Working Group
by providing background on several risk factors for cancer and by further highlighting
ways that behavioral research and intervention can help target identified objectives for
cancer prevention and control.

Cancer Epidemiology

Cancer is a set of site-specific diseases characterized by uncontrolled cell
growth. Only cardiovascular disease accounts for more American deaths than cancer,
and for children under age 15, cancer is the second leading cause of death. An estimated 565,000 Americans were expected to die from cancer in 1998. Approximately
7.5 million Americans live with some form of cancer and an estimated 1.2 million new
cases were expected to be diagnosed during 1998.

The types of cancer and their rate of diagnosis and death vary by gender. More
men are diagnosed with cancer each year than women (Table 1), and more men die
from cancer each year than women (Table 2). The overall 1991–1993 mortality rates
(cases per 100,000 age-adjusted to 1970 US census population) are 219 for men and
142 for women, indicating that men are about 54% more likely than women to die
from the disease. Greater tobacco use by men is one reason for their greater cancer in-

Table 1. Ten Sites for Estimated 1997 Cancer Cases by Site by Gender[a,b]

Males		Females	
Site	Number cases	Site	Number cases
Prostate	209,900	Breast	180,200
Lung	98,300	Lung	79,800
Colorectal	66,400	Colorectal	64,800
Urinary bladder	39,500	Endometrium	34,900
Non-Hodgkin's Lymphoma	30,300	Ovary	26,800
Melanoma	22,900	Non-Hodgkin's Lymphoma	23,300
Oral cavity	20,900	Melanoma	17,400
Kidney	17,100	Urinary Bladder	15,000
Leukemia	15,900	Cervix	14,500
Stomach	14,000	Pancreas	14,200
All sites	661,200	All sites	596,600

[a] Adapted from American Cancer Society (1997), as modified.
[b] Excluding basal and squamous cell skin cancer and *in situ* carcinomas except bladder.

Table 2. Leading Sites for Estimated 1997 Cancer Deaths by Site by Gender[a,b]

Males		Females	
Site	Number cases	Site	Number cases
Lung	94,400	Lung	66,000
Prostate	41,800	Breast	43,900
Colorectal	27,000	Colorectal	27,900
Pancreas	13,500	Pancreas	14,600
Non-Hodgkins Lymphoma	12,400	Ovary	14,200
Leukemia	11,770	Non-Hodgkin's Lymphoma	11,400
Esophagus	8,700	Leukemia	9,540
Stomach	8,300	Corpus uteri	6,000
Urinary bladder	7,800	Brain	6,000
Liver	7,500	Stomach	5,700
All sites	294,100	All sites	265,900

[a] From American Cancer Society (1997).
[b] Excluding basal and squamous cell skin cancer and *in situ* carcinomas except bladder.

cidence and mortality rates. The recent upsurge in the number of young female smokers, which suggests a future increase in cancer diagnoses and deaths among women, therefore has been a cause for alarm among advocates for public health.

The burden of cancer also varies by ethnic background (Tables 3 and 4). African-American and Euro-American men have the highest overall incidence and Native American men and men from many Asian cultures have the lowest incidence. The rate of prostate cancer in African-American men is the highest in the world. Although the rates of diagnosis for women do not vary as much by ethnicity as for men, Alaskan Natives and Euro-Americans have the highest overall cancer incidence. Minority populations frequently do not survive cancer as long as their majority Euro-American counterparts. For example, as measured by relative 5-year survival rates, which compare survival of those within an ethnic group who have cancer to those within the group without cancer, African Americans have a substantially lower relative 5-year survival rate (44%) compared to Euro-Americans (59%). Hypotheses for the lower survival rate among African Americans include lower rates of adherence to cancer screening guidelines, resulting in diagnosis at a more advanced stage (Caplan, Wells, & Haynes, 1992; Cowen, Kattan & Miles, 1996; Kleinman & Kopstein, 1981;

Table 3. Cancer Burden by Ethnic Background—US Incidence Rates, 1988–1992[a,b]

Race or ethnicity[c]	Male rate	Female rate
African American	560	326
Whites	469	346
Alaska Natives	372	348
Hawaiians	340	321

[a] From American Cancer Society (1997).
[b] Incidence rates are per 100,000 and are age-adjusted to the 1970 US standard population.
[c] Only the four ethnicities with the greatest incidence rates are listed. Native Americans have the lowest incidence of 11 US ethnic backgrounds.

Table 4. Incidence Rates for the Five Most Frequently Diagnosed Cancers by Race/Ethnicity and Gender[a,b]

Cancer	African Americans	Whites	Alaska Natives	Hawaiians
Males				
Prostate	180.6	134.7	46.1	57.2
Lung	117.0	76.0	81.1	89.0
Colorectal	60.7	56.3	79.7	42.4
Urinary bladder		31.7		
Oral	20.4			
Stomach	17.9		27.2	20.5
Non-Hodgkins		18.7		12.5
Females				
Breast	95.4	111.8	78.9	105.6
Colorectal	45.5	38.3	67.4	30.5
Lung	44.2	41.5	50.6	43.1
Endometrium	14.4	22.3		23.9
Ovary		15.8		
Cervix	13.2		15.8	
Stomach				13.0

[a] From American Cancer Society (1997).
[b] Incidence rates are per 100,000 and are age-adjusted to the 1970 US standard population.

Richardson *et al.,* 1987), poor health-care-seeking practices (see Chapter 6, this volume), use of health care resources (USDHHS, 1985), and biological differences (Gregorio, Cummings, & Michalek, 1983). Poverty, which is prevalent among some ethnic groups and associated with a higher cancer incidence, also has been considered an independent risk factor for cancer (Sterling, Rosenbaum, & Weinkam, 1993).

The causes of cancer can be classified as external or internal to an individual. External causes are generally environmental or lifestyle related. Environmental carcinogens may be chemical carcinogens whose presence was not known at the time of exposure, such as dioxin in fish, or whose carcinogenic properties were not recognized at the time of exposure, such as benzene or asbestos, which were common in certain work sites until their causal links with cancer were verified. Some viruses, such as the human papilloma virus or the human immunodeficiency virus, have cancer sequelae. Lifestyle behaviors, however, comprise the largest classification of causes of cancer. Tobacco is considered causal in 30% of all cancer deaths and diet in 35% of all cancer deaths (Doll & Peto, 1981). Tobacco and dietary behavior accompanied by sedentary activity patterns are also associated with a third of deaths from all causes in this country (McGinnis & Foege, 1993). A number of other cancers have specific behavioral origins. Overexposure to the ultraviolet rays of the sun contributes to skin melanomas. Sexual intercourse with an infected man can transmit the HPV, which can contribute to a woman's development of cervical cancer. Alcohol misuse contributes to oral cancers such as cancers of the pharynx, larynx, and tongue.

Internal factors that can cause cancer are genes, hormones, and immune conditions. The identification of specific aberrant genes that predispose individuals to specific cancers continues at a rapid pace. However, it is believed that such genetic predisposition accounts for a rather small proportion of cancers [e.g., no more than 10-15% of breast cancer (Colditz & Frazier, 1995)]. Hormones, such as prolonged exposure to estrogen, can be causes of cancer, but the excess exposure may be part of a complex series of biological events. In general, a variety of external and/or internal causal factors may act together or in sequence to initiate or to promote cancer. Age is another and perhaps the predominant risk factor for cancer, although features of the aging process that cause cancer are not well understood.

Diet and Cancer

Diet is considered a causal factor in approximately one third of all cancers (Conney *et al.*, 1992) and in an estimated 85–90% of all colorectal cancers (Vargas & Alberts, 1991). The accumulating evidence linking diet and disease is reflected in the specific objectives set forth by the Public Health Service to improve the health of Americans. These objectives include a substantial reduction in the amount of fat in the diet, an increase in fruit and vegetable intake to five or more servings per day, and an increase in the number of daily servings of grain products (USDHHS, 1991). In addition to natural dietary intake, chemoprevention research, which typically administers micronutrients in pharmacologically sized doses, is being pursued in clinical trials to augment the preventive effects of a nutritious diet in persons at higher risk of cancer.

Dietary Risk Factors for Cancer

Ecological studies first highlighted discrepancies in cancer prevalence among various cultures and lifestyles. The Japanese, with a lower incidence of breast cancer in their homeland, assumed the higher incidence rate of Americans after immigrating to and living in the United States (Haenszel & Kunhara, 1968). The Mediterranean cultures experienced an increasing incidence in cancer as their traditional high vegetable intake has been supplanted by a more meat-oriented Western diet (Serra-Majem *et al.*, 1993). Studies with increasingly more scientific rigor have followed.

A review of the literature indicates that the cancer sites with an established etiologic link to diet are primarily those of the gastrointestinal (GI) tract and the reproductive system (Goldin-Lang, Kreuser, & Zunft, 1996). Within the GI tract, listed in order of the greatest causal attribution to diet, are cancers of the colon, esophagus, stomach, and oral cavity. Alcohol, although usually studied separately from "diet," is also considered a risk factor for GI tract cancers. Within the reproductive system, cancers of the prostate, breast, and endometrium have strong links to diet. In general, higher fat and lower fiber (lower amounts of grains, fruits, and vegetables) are considered risk factors for dietary-related cancers. The role of dietary fat has been somewhat controversial. Although a number of studies have implicated excess fat intake, clinical trials have not confirmed it as a significant risk factor in clinical trials for female reproductive cancers (Willett & Hunter, 1994).

The scientific understanding of cancer remains limited by our inability to specify the sequence of biological events and mechanisms involved in the initiation and progress of cancer. However, the evidence to date supports the continued investigation into the causal contribution of dietary fat and the related issues of excessive calorie consumption. Because a positive energy imbalance, created when energy (calorie) intake exceeds energy utilization, leads to weight gain, the relationship between obesity and cancer is also being examined. A severe overweight condition, or obesity, has been implicated in the dominant causal hypothesis for endometrial cancer. One of the body's metabolic responses to obesity is to produce additional insulin which, in turn, produces additional estrogen and less progesterone, creating the hormonal environment for endometrial cancer (Hill & Austin, 1996). Although a similar scenario has been proposed for breast cancer (Prentice *et al.*, 1990), the supporting evidence is not as strong as for endometrial cancer.

In addition to cancer causation, obesity is a risk factor for adverse cancer outcomes. Individuals weighing 40% more than the average participants in an American Cancer Society sample were reported to have a higher risk of death from any form of cancer than the participants that were not overweight (Garfinkle, 1985). Women who were overweight also had significantly higher death rates from cancers of the breast, cervix, endometrium, uterus, and ovary than women with these diseases who were not overweight. The risk of death for overweight males was also higher in colorectal and prostate cancer. Whether the type of dietary intake (high fat, high calorie) or the degree of obesity is the more important factor in this association is not known.

Higher levels of fruit and vegetable consumption have been linked to reduced risk for various forms of cancer (Block, Patterson, & Subar, 1992; National Research Council, 1989; Patterson & Block, 1991; Steinmetz & Potter, 1996; Ziegler, 1991). As a result, several national organizations have recommended increased consumption of fruit and vegetables for both adults and children (USDHHS, 1991; USDA & USDHHS, 1990; NCI, 1986) with the NCI advocating five servings or more per day (NCI, 1986). In addition, research continues on antioxidants (e.g., vitamins A, E, C, and beta-carotene) and other vitamins (folate) that may be protective against either specific cancers or, as in the case of folic acid, protective of an individual's DNA. However, for most Americans, supplements should not be considered a substitute for a healthy diet. In general, adherence to a healthy diet should be considered prudent behavior (USDHHS, 1991).

Diet as Primary Prevention

Primary prevention research on cancer has predominantly targeted increasing adherence to healthy lifestyle behaviors. Because the maximum potential for long-term health is achieved by an appropriate diet at an early age (Oliveria *et al.*, 1992; Willett *et al.*, 1987; Williams, 1992), a number of major interventions have focused on elementary school children. Schools provide an attractive arena for such interventions because they offer repeated access to populations of a certain age in centralized locations. Some of the major interventions include the Go for Health Program (Parcel, Simons-Morton, O'Hara, Baranowski, & Wilson, 1989), the Minnesota Heart Health Program (Luepker & Perry, 1991), the Child and Adolescent Trial for Cardiovascular Health (CATCH) (Luepker *et al.*, 1996), and various 5-a-Day site projects such as High 5 Alabama (Havas *et al.*, 1994, 1995; Reynolds *et al.*, 1997). The majority of such clinical trials are grounded in social cognitive theory (SCT) (Bandura, 1977, 1986), which is addressed in more detail in Chapter 3, this volume. A good review of research to enhance the diet of children of all ages can be found in Lytle and Achterberg (1995).

Adults are perhaps more difficult to reach in interventions because of their dispersed locations. Use of the work site as the intervention location, as was done in the Working Well Trial (Abrams *et al.*, 1994), has been one approach to adults.

The Women's Health Trial (WHT) indicated that older women could change their behavior to reduce fat in their diets and that there were measurable changes in physiological outcomes (Henderson *et al.*, 1990). The WHT feasibility study in minority populations (Bowen *et al.*, 1996) indicated that the intervention was effective for older minority women. The WHT feasibility studies paved the way for the 11-year, multicenter, randomized clinical trial—the Women's Health Initiative—which addresses the relationships between diet and breast cancer, colorectal cancer, and coronary heart disease in women.

Diet and Secondary Prevention

Little is known about delaying the progress of an existing cancer or preventing either a recurrence of cancer or a second malignancy. However, in existing breast cancer patients, high fat intake has been associated with poorer rates of survival (Gregorio, Emrich, Graham, Marshall, & Nemoto, 1985; Nomura, Marchand, Kolonel, & Hankin, 1991) and dietary interventions that emphasize lower fat dietary intake have been recommended (Rose, 1996). The Women's Intervention Nutrition Study (WINS) is a randomized clinical trial of postmenopausal women with breast cancer to evaluate the relative efficacies of dietary fat reduction and tamoxifin to decrease the recurrence of breast cancer and increase patient survival (Chlebowski & Grosvenor, 1994; Glanz, 1994). Other chemoprevention trials with antioxidants and beta-carotene are underway.

Diet and Tertiary Prevention

A primary role for diet in tertiary prevention has been in treating cachexia in the cancer patient. Cachexia is a complex syndrome frequently characterized by anorexia, progressive undernourishment, and severe changes in body composition. Because nonvolitional enteral and parenteral feeding methods are frequently used to treat cachexia, they will not be addressed here. The reader is directed to Davis and Hardy (1994) and Klein *et al.* (1997) for additional information.

Cancer and Tobacco Smoke

Health Consequences of Smoking

Smoking is the single-most important cause of premature death in the United States today (USDHHS, 1990). Approximately 400,000 US citizens die each year from tobacco-related diseases (CDC, 1993a). Worldwide, an estimated 3 million people die from smoking each year (American Cancer Society, 1997). In addition, passive exposure to someone else's tobacco smoke poses a threat to the lives of many nonsmokers. For example, each year environmental tobacco smoke accounts for 35,000 to 40,000 deaths from heart disease alone (American Cancer Society, 1997). Exposure to tobacco use is associated with a number of serious diseases that include cardiovascular, pulmonary, and a variety of cancers (*Guide to Clinical Preventive Services*, 1996).

Smoking and Cancer Risk

Tobacco smoke is a well-established carcinogen. In 1990 alone, smoking is thought to have caused more than 150,000 deaths from neoplasms (CDC, 1993a).

Smoking has been linked to a variety of cancers including lung cancer and cancers of the mouth, pharynx, larynx, esophagus, pancreas, uterine cervix, kidney, and bladder (USDHHS, 1989). Although nonsmokers contract these cancers, smokers are at considerably higher risk. For example, lung cancer mortality rates are 22.4 times higher for male smokers and 11.9 times higher for female smokers compared to nonsmokers (US-DHHS, 1989). Among US men who are current smokers, when compared to men who do not smoke, the relative risk for cancer of the bladder is 2.9, cancer of the esophagus 7.6, cancer of the larynx 10.5, and cancer of the lip, oral cavity, and pharynx 27.5 (US-DHHS, 1989). Overall, smoking accounts for 87% of lung cancer deaths and 29% of all cancer deaths (American Cancer Society, 1997). Passive smoking is also associated with an elevated risk of contracting cancer. Each year about 3000 nonsmoking adults die of lung cancer as a result of breathing smoke from other people's cigarettes.

Risk Factors

Not surprisingly, the magnitude of cancer risk is most closely related to the exposure to tobacco smoke. For smokers, exposure is affected by a number of variables, including number of years smoked, number of cigarettes smoked per day, depth of inhalation, use of nonfiltered cigarettes, tobacco blend and tar yield of the tobacco, and young age of smoking onset. All these factors are positively associated with the likelihood of developing cancer (USDHHS, 1989). However, duration of smoking and age of smoking initiation appear to be the most critical (USDHHS, 1989). For example, when duration of regular tobacco use is doubled from 15 to 30 years, lung cancer incidence increases about 20-fold (Peto, 1986).

The type and prevalence of various forms of tobacco-induced cancer vary by racial and ethnic group, gender, and age cohort (American Cancer Society, 1997). Much of the difference in carcinoma incidence between groups reflects differences in smoking habits (CDC, 1993a). For example, the incidence of most smoking-related cancers is higher among men compared to women (American Cancer Society, 1997). Until recently, more men have smoked than women. Thus, some of the differences in morbidity and mortality are definitely attributable to gender differences in the prevalence of smoking. However, men suffer disproportionately more smoking-related illnesses even after controlling for differences in the numbers of men and women who smoke in the population. These differences are thought to be related to differences in the way men smoke compared to women. Specifically, men smoke more cigarettes per day and are more likely to inhale, take more puffs, have a larger puffing volume and longer puff duration, and are more likely to smoke their cigarettes to the end and to smoke filterless cigarettes than women (Grunberg, Winders, & Wewers, 1991).

Higher incidence of various environmental and lifestyle cancer determinants also appear to contribute to some of the risk of smoking-related cancers among some groups. For example, in the United States, the prevalence of drinking is higher among blacks compared to whites. The results of several large-scale studies suggest that differences in the prevalence of alcohol consumption among black versus white smokers accounts for some of the higher oral cancer rates among African-American smokers (Brown *et al.*,1994; Day *et al.*, 1993). Poverty may also contribute to elevated risk of tobacco-induced cancer. Sterling *et al.* (1993) analyzed data from two large data sets to estimate standardized mortality ratios for all cancers associated with poverty. This study did not specifically examine smoking-induced cancers, but these cancers were among those considered. People with incomes below the poverty line had substantially elevated risk for cancer. Risks were not appreciably affected by adjustments for confounding by smoking, alcohol, or occupation. Unadjusted comparisons revealed elevated mortality risk for African Americans compared to whites. However, these differences disappeared after adjusting for income. To the extent that all cancer mortality risks generalize to tobacco-induced cancer risks, the results of this study suggest that (1) poverty, rather than race, may be the biggest factor contributing to between-group differences in tobacco-induced neoplasms, and (2) poverty confers some risk *in addition to* that caused by smoking, alcohol consumption, and exposure to work-related toxins.

Differences in biological susceptibility to tobacco carcinogens also may contribute to some of the difference in carcinogenic risk associated with tobacco smoke exposure. For example, women have increased risk of lung cancer compared to men, after controlling for exposure to tobacco smoke and other known cancer-causing agents (Zang & Wynder, 1996; Muscat, Richie, Thompson, & Wynder, 1996b). One study found female smokers were exposed to higher levels of tobacco carcinogens per cigarette than male smokers, suggesting a possible biological explanation for the higher risk of lung cancer observed in women (Muscat *et al.*, 1996a).

Primary Prevention: Preventing Youth Smoking Initiation

The typical smoker starts and stops smoking an average of five times before quitting permanently and many smokers never quit despite numerous attempts (US-DHHS, 1990). Thus, it has been suggested that the best way to decrease nationwide smoking prevalence rates is to prevent smoking initiation (USDHHS, 1989). Although there are ethnic and regional variations in the age of smoking onset, most people start smoking some time during early adolescence, typically by age 15 (USDHHS, 1994a). By the time they reach high school, approximately one third of adolescents are regular cigarette smokers (USDHHS, 1994a). Not surprisingly, the focus of our nation's primary prevention efforts has been on young children and adolescents. Available programs are typically school-based and include information about long- and short-term health consequences of smoking and provide children with the skills to resist pressures to smoke from peers, family, and media (Flay, 1993). Some programs also include general self-esteem enhancement and social skills development (Botvin & Wills, 1985). The reported success rate of available programs varies considerably with treatment–control differences in smoking prevalence ranging from 25 to 60% and lasting anywhere from 1–4 years (USDHHS, 1994a). Factors that appear to enhance the effectiveness of school-based prevention programs are sustained treatment (e.g., multiple sessions delivered over several years), complementary communitywide and/or mass media components, and incorporation of the antismoking intervention into a more comprehensive school health education program (USDHHS, 1994a). A more comprehensive discussion of primary prevention interventions for smoking can be found in Chapter 9 in this handbook.

Secondary Prevention: Getting Adult Smokers to Quit

Despite widely acknowledged health consequences associated with continued smoking, approximately one quarter of the adult population in the United States smokes. Since the early 1960s, a variety of smoking cessation approaches have been developed, evaluated, and refined. The most effective behavioral programs provide the smoker with a variety of cognitive–behavioral components in the context of multises-sion support groups. The various components are designed to increase motivation and impart skills and support needed to quit smoking and avoid relapse. These intensive programs typically achieve 1-year abstinence rates of 20 to 25% (Schwartz, 1987; US-DHHS, 1989); however, several programs have yielded long-term abstinence rates ap-proaching 50% (Lando, 1993). A variety of less intensive smoking cessation approaches also have been tested, including self-help materials, advice from medical personnel, and brief supportive phone calls. The cessation rates associated with low-intensity tech-niques are typically quite low (8–15%) (Orleans, Glynn, Manley, & Slade, 1993). How-ever, these approaches are easy to implement and could be widely disseminated (Orleans, 1993). Therefore, they have the potential to reach a large number of smokers and could dramatically reduce smoking prevalence. For example, if only *half* of U.S. physicians delivered a brief quitting message to their patients who smoked and were successful with only 1 in 10, this would yield 1.75 million new ex-smokers every year, which would more than double the annual quit rate (Fiore *et al.*, 1990). Pharmacological treatments are available as adjuncts to behavioral techniques. The best researched group of medications for smoking cessation are nicotine polacrilex (nicotine gum) and transdermal nicotine (nicotine patch). Both have been shown to increase cessation rates among patients enrolled in either high- or low-intensity behavioral programs (Hughes, 1993). For a more comprehensive discussion of behavioral and pharmacological smok-ing cessation treatments, see Chapter 9 in this book.

Skin Cancer

Ironically, the most preventable and detectable type of cancer is also the most common. Approximately one million new cases of skin cancer develop each year (Miller & Weinstock, 1994), and skin cancer affects as many as one in five persons over the course of a lifetime (Rigel, Friedman, & Kopf, 1996). Skin cancer rates are in-creasing more rapidly than any other cancer (Rigel, 1997), despite estimates that 80% could be eliminated through primary prevention (Stern, Weinstein, & Baker, 1986).

There are three common types of skin cancer, classified by the type of cells af-fected: basal cell carcinoma (BCC), squamous cell carcinoma (SCC), and melanoma. BCC and SCC are frequently referred to collectively as nonmelanomic skin cancers (NMSC) and account for approximately 96% of skin cancer cases. Reporting of NMSC to cancer registries is not required; therefore, accurate and current epidemiological trends and data are difficult to obtain. More than 2100 deaths annually in the United States are attributable to these cancers (American Cancer Society, 1997).

Melanoma accounts for only about 4% of skin cancer cases, yet is responsible for more than 75% of all skin cancer deaths (CDC, 1995). Of the more than 40,000 people diagnosed with melanoma each year, approximately 20% will die (Weinstock, 1993). It is estimated that by year 2000, 1 in 75 people will develop melanoma over the course of a lifetime (Friedman, Rigel, Silverman, Kopf, & Vossaert, 1991).

Risk Factors

The three major types of skin cancer share common behavioral and genetic pre-disposing risk factors. The most strongly associated behavioral risk factor for the development of skin cancer is overexposure to the sun's harmful ultraviolet (UV) rays (Dubin, Pasternack, & Moseson, 1990; Hurwitz, 1988; Rhodes, Weinstock, Fitzpatrick, Mihm, & Sober, 1987). An overwhelming majority of skin cancers—more than 90% of NMSC and 65% of melanoma—are thought to be attributable to this factor (Preston & Stern, 1992). The amount of UV exposure a person receives over the course of her or his lifetime is associated with each type of skin cancer (Drobetsky, Turcotte, & Chateaneuf, 1995), though the *type* of sun exposure received appears to contribute to the development of specific types of skin cancer. Steady, long-term sun exposure is associated with NMSC, while intense, intermittent sun exposure is associated with melanoma (Drobetsky *et al.*, 1995; Taylor & Sober, 1996). Evidence also strongly suggests that the pediatric years are critical to the future development of skin cancer (Hurwitz, 1988). Melanoma risk, for example, increases twofold with one or more blistering sunburns in childhood (Dubin *et al.*, 1990; Weinstock *et al.*, 1989).

Skin pigmentation is the most significant genetic risk factor for skin cancer, with risk being highest among those with fair skin (Elder, 1995). Dark skin pigmentation, however, does not preclude the development of skin cancer, as evidenced by its development in all ethnic and racial groups (Weinstock, 1997). Additional predisposing risk factors include the propensity to burn and freckle, light hair and eyes, family history of skin cancer, and a large number of moles (Dubin *et al.*, 1990; Rhodes *et al.*, 1987). Skin cancer risk increases with age as well, although melanoma tends to strike earlier in life and is in fact the leading type of cancer among women aged 25–29 (American Cancer Society, 1997).

Primary Prevention

Skin cancer is highly preventable. Healthy People 2000 identified the following goal in an effort to promote the prevention of skin cancer : "Increase to at least 60 percent the proportion of people of all ages who limit sun exposure, use sunscreens and protective clothing when exposed to sunlight, and avoid artificial sources of ultraviolet light" (USDHHS, 1991, p. 425). Guidelines for primary prevention have been issued by various medical and professional organizations and include (Hurwitz, 1988):

1. Minimizing midday sun exposure, between 10 AM and 4 PM, when the sun's rays are the strongest.
2. Wearing protective, tightly woven clothing, such as dark-colored long-sleeved shirts and pants.
3. Wearing a 4-inch wide, broad-brimmed hat.
4. Wearing sunglasses that protect against UV rays.
5. Applying sunscreen with a sun protective factor (SPF) of 15 or higher to all exposed areas of the body at least 20 minutes before going outdoors, and reapplying every 2 hours.
6. Avoiding intentional tanning from natural or artificial sources, such as sunlamps or tanning beds.

Much to the detriment of primary prevention efforts, a suntan is a highly valued social symbol associated with attractiveness and good health (Marks &Hill, 1988). Studies show that a majority of people feel healthier with a tan and believe that tanned skin looks healthier and more attractive than untanned skin (Brodstack, Borland, & Gason, 1992; Keesling & Friedman, 1987). These beliefs may motivate intentional tanning behaviors and prevent the adoption of primary prevention practices.

There is a strong link between sun exposure during the pediatric years and the future development of skin cancer that underscores the need for these preventive behaviors to be used consistently from birth [with the exception of sunscreen, which is not recommended for infants under 6 months of age (Hurwitz, 1988)]. It is the responsibility of parents, teachers, and adults who serve children and adolescents to ensure that these preventive behaviors are used consistently and correctly, and to serve as good role models by employing these guidelines in their own lives.

Secondary Prevention: Screening and Detection

Skin cancer is outwardly visible, making it the ideal candidate for screening efforts aimed at early disease detection. Knowing the signs of skin cancer and engaging in regular self-examinations and screenings can significantly improve mortality rates and reduce the morbidity and disfigurement associated with this disease. Melanoma survival rates, for example, have improved dramatically from approximately 50% in the 1950s to nearly 90% today, due largely to public health campaigns aimed at early detection and treatment through self-examination and screening behaviors (Rigel *et al.*, 1996).

Tertiary Prevention: Treatment and Rehabilitation

The most common treatment option for skin cancer is surgery, with approximately 90% of lesions being removed through this method (American Cancer Society, 1997). Other treatment methods include radiation therapy, electrodessication, cryosurgery, and laser therapy (American Cancer Society, 1997). Depending on the location and stage of lesions, treatment for each type of skin cancer can be costly, highly invasive, and result in loss of function and permanent disfigurement.

Despite the preventable and recognizable nature of skin cancer, many cases remain undetected during the early stages. The vast majority of those who are diagnosed and treated early, however, will be cured, thus emphasizing the importance of secondary prevention. As with any disease, the primary prevention of skin cancer is ideal for the health and well-being of our nation.

Cancer and Sexual Behavior

Epidemiological evidence has long suggested that certain anogenital cancers, including cervical cancer, were caused by viruses transmitted sexually. A clear etiology for cervical cancer, however, has been developed only recently. Whereas limited evidence exists that implicates sexual transmission in various cancers, particularly prostate cancer, the strongest evidence for a sexual linkage exists with cervical cancer. Therefore, only cervical cancer will be addressed in this section. Further, the sexually transmitted human immunodeficiency virus (HIV), which has been associated with cervical dysplasia, a precursor to invasive cancer as well as other cancer sequelae, is addressed in Chapter 18 and not in this section.

Although cancer of the cervix is one of the most prevalent cancers worldwide, its presence has been successfully reduced in the United States. The incidence rate declined from 14.2 per 100,000 in 1973 to 8.2 in 1993 and the mortality rate dropped from 5.6 per 100,000 to 2.9 over the same period (American Cancer Society, 1997). Although a number of ethnic groups in the United States have experienced similar declines over this period, the rates for many of these populations remain high. Cervical cancer is one of the five most frequently occurring cancers among African Americans and Alaskan natives and for many immigrant populations. The death rate for African Americans remains more than twice that of Euro-American women (American Cancer Society, 1997).

Sexual Behavior Risk Factors for Cervical Cancer

The primary risk factor for cervical cancer is infection with the oncogenic types of the human papilloma virus (HPV) (Brinton, 1992; Grimes & Economy, 1995; Schiffman *et al.*, 1993). HPV is resident in an estimated 24 million Americans and 500,000 to 1 million cases occur annually (CDC, 1994). Although HPV may intermittently or chronically cause genital warts, such visual manifestations are usually benign in nature, whereas the more common subclinical genital HPV infection is estimated to increase the risk of invasive cervical cancer tenfold (Schiffman, 1992). Similar to other viral agents that cause sexually transmitted diseases (STDs), no curative treatment exists that can eliminate HPV from the body. Further, available screening tests for HPV infection tend to have less than desirable accuracy or are not suitable for clinical use, as in STD clinics (CDC, 1993b).

Not surprisingly, behaviors that increase the risk of developing cervical cancer are similar to those for contracting HPV and other STDs. These risks include young age at first intercourse, multiple sexual partners (Ley *et al.*, 1991), or having a sexual partner who has had multiple sexual partners (Koutsky *et al.*, 1992; Schneider, Sawada, Gissmann, & Shah, 1987). According to one study of sexually active women aged 18 to 44 years, 14% had more than one sex partner in the previous year and an additional 12–24% had a partner who had multiple sex partners (Kost & Forrest, 1992). However, in one survey, cited in the *Guide to Clinical Preventive Services* (p. 724), higher-risk women reported limited knowledge about common STDs: fewer than one fourth of those at highest risk—younger women and those with multiple partners— believed they were at risk *(Guide to Clinical Preventive Services*, 1996). Further, reports from STD clinics indicated many women did not understand the purpose or importance of Pap tests, the screening test for cervical cancer (CDC, 1993b).

In addition to behavior, HPV is associated with the following demographic characteristics: low socioeconomic status (Morrison *et al.*, 1991) young age (Morrison *et al.*, 1991; Schiffman *et al.*, 1993), and race (Ley *et al.*, 1991). Women with a history of STDs are at increased risk of cervical cancer and women that attend STD clinics frequently have the additional demographic characteristics that place them at even higher risk (CDC, 1993b).

Behavioral Recommendations for Primary Prevention

Preventing cervical cancer is best accomplished by avoiding those behaviors that risk exposure to HPV. These behaviors—multiple sexual partners, or having a sexual partner who has had multiple sexual partners—are the same for all STDs in general. For women who continue risky sexual behaviors, barrier contraception (diaphragm and condoms) and spermicide (foam or contraceptive) have been reported to lower the risk of cervical cancer by 50% (Grimes & Economy, 1995), probably due to the lowering of HPV infection (*Guide to Preventive Clinical Services*, 1996). However, the direct evidence for contraception preventing HPV is limited (Cates & Stone, 1992). Further, newer barrier contraception methods such as the female condom have not been fully evaluated. Interventions that address behavior change related to STDs are addressed in other chapters of this volume.

Behavioral Recommendations for Secondary Prevention

Early detection is the most effective method for preventing cervical cancer from becoming a debilitating illness or leading to death. The current screening guidelines are for any woman who has been sexually active or who is over the age of 18 to have an annual Pap test by a health care professional as part of a regular pelvic exam (*Guide to Clinical Preventive Services*, 1996). Addressing the needs of the higher-risk population of women attending STD clinics, CDC guidelines for STD treatment now recommend that providers discuss the purpose and need for Pap tests and that they give or refer out Pap tests for their patients (CDC, 1993b; Kamb, 1995).

The increased prevalence of Pap testing is credited with the dramatic reduction in cervical cancer in the United States. However, it is clear that many low-income and minority woman have not been beneficiaries of screening. Examples of research projects that have sought to reach these populations and to understand their barriers to screening include research with older urban African-American women in public primary care settings (Mandelblatt *et al.*, 1993a, b); research with rural African Americans (Windsor *et al.*, 1981); and with rural Native American women (Dignan *et al.*, 1996). The research underscores the difficulties inherent in achieving screening among the medically underserved.

Psychological Aspects of Cancer

Behavioral Risk Factors

There is no consensus that psychological factors, such as stress, anger, depression, bereavement, or personality traits, are of substantial importance in the causation or primary prevention of cancer (Fox, 1995). These factors have certainly received considerable attention from researchers in psychosomatic medicine and from popular authors, but results of research in this area are conflicting. Despite this, many patients, clinicians, and researchers continue to hold very strong beliefs in the importance of this association. These beliefs themselves are of clinical importance in the psychological management of cancer patients. Feelings of self-blame can add to the burden of suffering compounded by cancer. Some psychological factors may indirectly influence the risk of developing cancer by their effect on some of the well-accepted risk factors for malignant disease (e.g., smoking, diet, alcohol, sexual behavior).

Psychological factors are much more important in the secondary and tertiary prevention of cancer, although indirectly so. Anxiety, pathological denial, paranoia, depression, extreme stress, and other mental symptoms or disorders may prevent the patient from coping well with the prospect of having cancer. When these factors prevent adherence to screening or treatment recommendations, lead to avoidance of fol-low-up care, or adversely influence the patient's judgment in informed decision mak-ing, the potential impact on the course of disease is clear.

Psychological factors and treatments aimed at these factors clearly have a role in the area of tertiary prevention of cancer. Depression, anxiety, isolation, pain, and nau-sea are among the complications of cancer that add substantially to the patient's suf-fering. Treatments, such as support, relaxation, hypnosis, psychotropic meditations, or individual, couples, or group psychotherapy, can provide relief, even in the setting of advanced or terminal illness.

Psychosocial Treatments for Cancer

Numerous studies have shown that psychosocial interventions have beneficial effects on coping, distress, anxiety, depression, specific physical symptoms, and over-all quality of life. In fact, there is general acceptance of the relationship between these beneficial outcomes and a variety of psychosocial treatments (Fawzy et al., 1990; Fer-lic, Goldman, & Kennedy, 1979; Greer et al., 1992; Spiegel & Bloom, 1983; Wood, Mil-ligan, Christ, & Liff, 1978). Many of these studies have demonstrated that the benefit is sustained long after completion of the intervention. Some studies have shown im-provements in pertinent immune system parameters. Results of the numerous stud-ies of psychosocial interventions for cancer have been reviewed elsewhere (Fawzy, Fawzy, Arndt, & Pasnau, 1995; Trijsburg, van Knippenburg, & Rijpma, 1992). Spiegel (1994) has summarized the clinical and medicoeconomic value of psychosocial inter-ventions for cancer patients.

Some of the most promising studies in the area of psychosocial interventions for cancer have shown beneficial effects on time to tumor recurrence and survival. These studies have used a variety of intervention techniques and outcome measures, mak-ing comparative conclusions difficult. Still, this research represents one of the most exciting areas of behavioral medicine. Grossarth-Maticek, Schmidt, Vetter, and Arndt (1984) randomized cancer patients to psychotherapy treatments of different types, in-cluding an intensive standard psychotherapy, a behavioral therapy treatment, and a modified cognitive behavioral treatment intervention. Treated patients lived longer that untreated patients, with the strongest apparent benefit seen in those who re-ceived the modified cognitive behavioral treatment. Those who combined group treatment with somatic cancer therapy (radiation or chemotherapy) responded best of all. However, this research has been criticized on methodological grounds, as sum-marized by Fawzy et al. (1995).

Spiegel, Bloom, Kraemer, and Gottheil (1989) randomized 86 women with metastatic breast cancer to a support group versus routine oncological care alone. Their intent was to reduce pain, psychological distress, and interpersonal problems and maximize quality of life during terminal illness. At follow-up, the investigators found that survival was significantly prolonged in treated patients (an average of 36.6 months compared to 18.9 months for controls).

Most recently, Fawzy et al. (1993) reported follow-up data on 68 patients with malignant melanoma, randomly treated with either a brief (six session) structured psychiatric group intervention or standard oncological care alone. Experimental pa-tients were less likely to have a recurrence and had a statistically significant lower rate of death. After analysis of multiple covariates and adjustment for Breslow depth, treatment effect remained significant. Baseline affective distress and coping style were also predictors of recurrence and survival, though the authors were surprised to find that higher baseline levels of distress were associated with better outcomes. Although the number of patients with disease above stage I was very small, their results suggest that the effect of group treatment may be even more powerful in patients with more advanced disease. Effects of treatment on immune function, as measured by natural killer cell activity, were equivocal.

The precise mechanism of action of these psychiatric interventions is unknown. A number of possible explanations have been offered. It may be that group patients become less depressed and/or more involved in their treatment, consequently becoming more compliant, becoming more physically active, or taking better care of themselves overall. They may simply develop better health habits due to the educational component of these treatments. They may come to interact with their treating physicians in a better, more engaging way as a result of improved coping skills, encouraging physicians to offer more aggressive treatments. There may be a psychoneuroimmunological effect on immune function as a consequence of decreased stress or some other factor, though these interrelationships have been difficult to demonstrate (Stein, Miller, & Trestman, 1991). Finally, the social benefits of group membership may include the repeatedly demonstrated correlation between density of social support network and desirable medical outcome (Case, Moss, & Case, 1992; Goodwin, Hunt, Key, & Samet, 1987; House, Landis, & Umberson, 1988; Spiegel, 1994).

The results reported by Spiegel *et al.* (1989) and Fawzy *et al.* (1993) are some of the most exciting and encouraging findings in psychosomatic medicine. They suggest that it may be possible to improve cancer survival as well as quality of life with a nontoxic, structured psychiatric intervention. If others can demonstrate similar results for psychotherapeutic interventions in patients with cancer, we will have a new and valuable tool in the comprehensible medical treatment of malignant disease, and one without significant side effects. Furthermore, if validation of these findings is possible, the next level of investigation could advance our understanding of the mechanisms by which mental processes affect physical function and disease. This would clearly be a great step forward for medicine.

Epidemiology and Control of Environmental Carcinogens

The etiologies of most cancers are associated with lifestyle practices including smoking, alcohol consumption, sun exposure, diet, and sexual behaviors (Vessey & Gray, 1985). Chemical carcinogens from environmental, occupational, or medical exposures are thought to be responsible for far fewer cancers than are lifestyle factors. In fact, only about 8% of cancer deaths are attributed to occupation, pollution, industrial products, and drugs combined (Higginson, 1993). Still, such exposures can be an important cause of cancer for people working in certain occupational groups, where high-dose and long-term exposures are possible. Here we summarize the epidemiology and control of environmental carcinogenesis, that is, cancers caused by nongenetic, non-lifestyle-related factors.

Twenty-four substances are identified by the National Toxicology Program (NTP) as known human carcinogens (Table 5) (USDHHS, 1994b). These are substances for which the evidence from human studies indicates a causal relationship between exposure and development of cancer. They have been banned or their use is severely restricted in the workplace. Table 6 lists cancers associated with occupation or occupational exposures, by cancer site (USDHHS, 1996). For most of these agents, control efforts have been aimed at primary prevention by reducing or eliminating exposures. Control measures are focused on behavior change by requiring that workers wear masks and other protective apparel and equipment (Landrigan, 1996), and through implementation of regulatory policies and laws to limit occupational exposures (Stellman & Stellman, 1996). Secondary prevention via screening for cancers known to be screen detectable (such as oral cavity and skin) also may be appropriate in certain occupational groups (Cole & Morrison, 1980).

Animal studies are sometimes used to assess the carcinogenicity of chemicals. However, it is difficult to extend such results to assess human cancer risk. Animals are typically subjected to greater doses and shorter durations of exposure than is typically experienced by humans. Nonetheless, there is an increasing demand by the public to quantify the impact of low-level chemical exposures and cancer risk. Even if there is only a slight elevation of risk, a common exposure could account for a large number of cancer cases.

In addition to the 24 known carcinogens, NTP lists 97 substances as reasonably anticipated human carcinogens (USDHHS, 1994b). For these substances there is limited evidence of carcinogenicity in humans or sufficient evidence of carcinogenicity in experimental animals. In general, studies of long-term human exposures and cancer incidence are not available to estimate cancer risk with any confidence, but avoidance of chronic exposures to these substances is advisable nevertheless.

Table 5. Substances Known to Be Carinogenic[a]

Aflatoxins
4-Aminobiphenyl
Analgesic mixtures containing phenacetin
Arsenic and certain arsenic compounds
Asbestos
Azathioprine
Benzene
Benzidine
Bis(chloromethyl) ether and technical-grade chloromethyl methyl ether
1,4-Butanediol Demethylsulfonate (Myleran)
Chlorambucil
1-(2-Chloroethyl)-3-(4-methylcyclohexyl)-1-nitrosourea (MeCCNU)
Chromium and certain chromium compounds
Conjugated estrogens
Cyclophosphamide
Diethylstilbestrol
Erionite
Melphalan
Methoxsalen with ultraviolet A therapy (PUVA)
Mustard gas
2-Naphthylamine
Radon
Thorium dioxide
Vinyl chloride

[a] From USDHHS (1994b).

Table 6. Cancers Associated with Various Occupations or Occupational Exposures[a]

Cancer	Substances or processes
Lung	Arsenic, asbestos, bis(chloromethyl)ether, chromium compounds, coal gasification, mustard gas, nickel refining, foundry substances, radon, soots, tars, oils, acrylonitrile, berylium, silica
Bladder	Aluminum production, auramine and magenta manufacture, rubber industry, leather industry, 4-aminobiphenyl, benzidine, naphthylamine
Nasal cavity and sinuses	Formaldehyde, isopropyl alcohol manufacture, mustard gas, nickel refining, leather dust, wood dust
Larynx	Asbestos, isopropyl alcohol, mustard gas
Pharynx	Formaldehyde, mustard gas
Mesothelioma	Asbestos
Lymphatic and hematopoietic system	Benzene, ethylene oxide, chlorophenols, chlorophenoxy herbicides, X-radiation
Skin	Arsenic, coal tars, mineral oils
Soft-tissue sarcoma	Chlorophenols, chlorophenoxy herbicides
Liver	Arsenic, vinyl chloride

[a] From USDHHS (1996, p. 97).

It is logical to assume that reduction of exposure to a carcinogen will lower cancer risk. However, the effect of risk reduction following chronic exposure has not been quantified for most chemicals listed in Table 5. The reason is largely that most efforts to regulate environmental carcinogens are fairly recent and because the time from first exposure to developing cancer (the induction period) is prolonged (Cole & Morrison, 1980). Thus, risk reduction effects are difficult to measure until years or decades have passed. Also, past exposure levels may not serve as reliable indicators for cumulative exposures, so that dose is sometimes difficult to estimate.

Another category of environmental carcinogenesis is radiation effects. Ionizing radiation may cause cancer at any site, but the bone marrow and thyroid seem most susceptible (American Cancer Society, 1997). Sources of ionizing radiation include atomic weapons, radiation therapy, and occupations such as uranium mining (American Cancer Society, 1997). Medical and dental X rays and mammograms are generally of sufficiently low dose that they do not increase cancer risk (USDHHS, 1996). Naturally occurring radiation from the earth's crust in the form of radon may cause a small percentage of lung cancers (Higginson, 1993). Ultraviolet radiation from the sun causes most basal and squamous cell skin cancers as well as most melanomas (USDHHS, 1996), as is discussed elsewhere in this chapter.

Environmental tobacco smoke, that is, smoke from a cigarette, cigar, or pipe smoked by another, may cause lung cancer as well as other respiratory problems (American Cancer Society, 1997). Please see the section in this chapter on "Cancer and Tobacco Smoke" for a fuller discussion of passive smoking.

An alternative approach to cancer control is based on the view that it may be possible to prevent cancer through drugs or chemicals (chemoprevention), decreasing the host's susceptibility to environmental and occupational carcinogens. Therefore, future research should be directed toward understanding carcinogenic mechanisms including the multistep process of carcinogenesis, that is, induction, promotion, and progression, so that new chemopreventive substances may be developed.

Finally, we mention a number of the public's concerns about causes of cancer that are as yet unfounded in that there is little or no evidence of carcinogenicity. Such concerns include consumption of accumulated pesticide and herbicide residues in the food chain, low-dose emissions from nuclear power plants, and nonionizing radiation such as microwaves, radio waves, radar, and electromagnetic fields (American Cancer Society, 1997). Further investigation may be necessary to conclusively rule out such exposures as cancer concerns.

Summary and Conclusions

A number of themes emerge from our review of the literature in these eight areas of cancer prevention and control research. Although environmental factors are important in the etiology and prevention of cancer, lifestyle remains the primary known influence on cancer rates in the United States. The use of tobacco and quality of diet are major factors that influence the risk for contracting cancer. Exposure to ultraviolet radiation, often through the free choice behavior of youth and young adults, is a major risk factor in the occurrence of skin cancer. In addition, sexual behavior has been linked to the incidence of cervical cancer in women. Because much of the occurrence of cancer is linked to behavior, cancer can be prevented and controlled in part through behavior change. Many behavioral intervention techniques have been developed that can be used to influence each of these risk factors. The degree to which these techniques have been tested varies by risk factor and target population. However, substantial evidence has been accumulated for the effectiveness of behavioral interventions with several of these behaviors such as tobacco and diet. Although effective interventions exist, much future work remains to be done to test new and potentially more effective interventions, to build interventions for populations that have been underserved in the past, and to explore methods for disseminating interventions that are known to be effective.

Despite widespread awareness of the harmful effects of tobacco use, its use remains a leading cause of cancer in our society. The prevalence of tobacco use has been dropping and is one reason cited for the recently reported reductions in cancer mortality in the United States. However, more work remains to be done to strengthen the prevention and cessation of tobacco use. This is particularly true for young women where cancer rates are rising and for youth where the use of tobacco remains high.

The importance of cancer prevention and control for young people is a striking crosscutting theme in this chapter. For two cancer-risk factors—tobacco use and exposure to ultraviolet radiation—youth should be the central focus of cancer prevention and control efforts. Rates of tobacco use remain high for high school students and the initiation of tobacco use most frequently occurs before the age of 18. Thus, the prevention of tobacco use will lead to long-term reductions in cancer morbidity and mortality rates. For skin cancer, particularly melanoma, exposure to ultraviolet radiation in youth is central to the etiology of the disease. Thus, efforts to prevent melanoma may be most effective if targeted toward children and adolescents. Interventions with youth also might be highly effective for establishing healthier eating habits. These behaviors established in youth may track into adulthood, leading to many potential years of reduced risk for cancer. The establishment of decision skills in adolescents and young adults regarding responsible intimacy and the use of preventive measures may also reduce risk for sexually linked cervical cancer.

The role of socioeconomic status and ethnicity in cancer rates and the influence of risk factors is a recurrent theme in our review of the behavioral aspects of cancer prevention and control. With few exceptions, those who have lower socioeconomic status are at higher risk for cancer. African Americans also seem to be at higher risk for several forms of cancer relative to other ethnic groups. It is important to recognize that the role of both socioeconomic status and ethnic background in cancer is complex and will require many years of additional research before this relationship is understood. However, the weight of the evidence suggests a need to target both people of low-socioeconomic status and minority groups for enhanced intervention efforts for cancer prevention and control. Both groups are traditionally "underserved," with fewer evaluated interventions available for these groups. Future work is needed in which interventions for low-socioeconomic status and minority populations are designed and tested.

In sum, many cancer researchers have built a large body of knowledge on cancer etiology and on the behavioral strategies required to modify cancer risk. What remains is the further conduct of good epidemiological research to better understand causal factors, the further development of high quality cancer prevention and control interventions including those targeting populations at higher risk, the dissemination of interventions known to be effective, and the aggressive execution of guidelines such as those proposed by the NCI Working Group on Behavioral Cancer Prevention and Control.

References

Abrams, D. B., Boutwell, W. B., Grizzle, J, Heimenndinger, J., Sorensen, G., & Varnes, J. (1994). Cancer control at the workplace: The Working Well Trial. *Preventive Medicine, 23*, 15–27.

American Cancer Society. (1997). *Cancer Facts and Figures—1997*. New York: American Cancer Society.

Bandura, A. (1977). *Social learning theory*. Englewood Cliffs, NJ: Prentice-Hall.

Bandura, A. (1986). *Social foundations of thought and action: A social cognitive theory*. Englewood Cliffs, NJ: Prentice-Hall.

Block, G., Patterson, B., & Subar, A. (1992). Fruit, vegetables, and cancer prevention: A review of the epidemiologic evidence. *Nutrition and Cancer, 18*, 1–29.

Botvin, G. J., & Wills, T. A. (1985). Personal and social skills training: Cognitive–behavioral approaches to substance abuse prevention. In C. S Bell & R. Battjes (Eds.), *Prevention research: Deterring drug abuse among children and adolescents* (pp. 8–49). NIDA Research Monograph 63. DHHS Publication No. (ADM) 85–1334. Washington, DC: USDHHS.

Bowen, D., Clifford, C. K., Coates, R., Evans, M., Feng, Z., Fouad, M., George, V., Gerace, T., Grizzle, J. E., Hall, W. D., Hearn, M., Henderson, M., Kestin, M., Kristal, A., Leary, E. T., Lewis, C.E., Oberman, A., Prentice, R., Raczynski, J., Toivola, B., & Urban, N. (1996). The Women's Health Trial Feasibility Study in minority populations: Design and baseline descriptions. *Annals of Epidemiology, 6*, 507–519.

Brinton, L. A. (1992). Epidemiology of cervical cancer—overview. In N. Munoz, F. X. Bosch, K. V. Shah, & A. Meheus (Eds.), *The epidemiology of cervical cancer and human papilloma virus* (pp. 3–23). Lyon, France: IARC.

Brodstack, M., Borland, R., & Gason, R. (1992). Effects of suntan on judgements of healthiness and attractiveness by adolescents. *Journal of Applied Social Psychology, 2*, 157–172.

Brown, L. M., Hoover, R. N., Greenberg, R. S., Schoenberg, J. B., Schwartz, A. G., Swanson, G. M., Liff, J. M., Silverman, D. T., Hayes, R. B., & Pottern, L. M. (1994). Are racial differences in squamous cell esophageal cancer explained by alcohol and tobacco use? *Journal of the National Cancer Institute, 86*, 1340–1345.

Caplan, L. S., Wells, B. L., & Haynes, S. (1992). Breast cancer screening among older racial/ethnic minorities and whites: Barriers to early detection. *Journal of Gerontology, 47*, 101–110.

Case, R. B., Moss, A. J., & Case, N. (1992). Living alone after myocardial infarction: Impact on prognosis. *Journal of the American Medical Association, 267,* 515–519.

Cates, W., & Stone, K. M. (1992). Family planning, sexually transmitted disseases and contraceptive choice: A literature update—Part I. *Family Planning Perspectives, 24,* 394–398.

Centers for Disease Control and Prevention (CDC). (1993a). Mortality trends for selected smoking-related cancers and breast cancer—United States, 1950–1990. *Morbidity and Mortality Weekly Report, 42,* 857, 863–866.

Centers for Disease Control and Prevention (CDC). (1993b). Sexually transmitted diseases treatment guidelines—1993. *Morbidity and Mortality Weekly Report, 422* (no. RR-14), 83-91.

Centers for Disease Control and Prevention (CDC). (1994). *Sexually transmitted disease surveillance, 1993.* US Department of Health and Human Services, Public Health Service. Atlanta: Author.

Centers for Disease Control and Preventtion (CDC). (1995). Deaths from melanoma—United States, 1973–1992. *Morbitiy and Mortality Weekly Report, 44,* 337, 343–347.

Chlebowski, R. T., & Grosvenor, M. (1994). The scope of nutrition intervention trials with cancer-related endpoints. *Cancer, 74* (Suppl.), 2734–2738.

Colditz, G. A., & Frazier, A. L. (1995). Models of breast cancer show that risk is set by events of early life: prevention efforts must shift focus. *Cancer Epidemiology, Biomarkers and Prevention, 4,* 567–571.

Cole, P., & Morrsion, A. S. (1980). Basic issues in population screening for cancer. *Journal of the National Cancer Institute, 64,* 1263–1272.

Conney, A. H., Adamson, R. H., Hart, R. W., Scheuplein, R. J., Somogyi, A., & Sugimura, T. (1992). Panel discussion: Nutrition and cancer conference. *Cancer Research, 52* (Suppl. 1), 2124s–2125s.

Cowen, M. E., Kattan, M. W., & Miles, B. J. (1996). A national survey of attitudes regarding participation in prostate cancer testing. *Cancer, 78,* 1952–1957.

Davis, C. L., & Hardy, J. R. (1994). Palliative care. *The British Medical Journal, 308,* 1359–1362.

Day, G. L., Blot, W. J., Austin, D. F., Bernstein, L., Greenberg, R. S., Preston-Martin, S., Schoenberg, J. B., Winn, D. M., McLaughlin, J. K., & Fraumeni, J. F. (1993). Racial differences in risk of oral and pharyngeal cancer: alcohol, tobacco, and other determinants. *Journal of the National Cancer Institute, 85,* 465–473.

Dignan, M., Michielutte, R., Blinson, K., Wells, H. B., Case, L. D., Sharp, P., Davis, S., Konen, J., & McQuellon, R. P. (1996). Effectiveness of health education to increase screening for cervical cancer among eastern-based Cherokee Indian women in North Carolina. *Journal of the National Cancer Institute, 88,* 1670–1676.

Doll, R., & Peto, R. (1981). *The causes of cancer: Quantitative estimates of avoidable risks of cancer in the United States today.* New York: Oxford University Press.

Drobetsky, E. A., Turcotte, J., & Chateaneuf, A. (1995). A role for ultraviolet A in solar mutagenesis. *Proceedings of the National Academy of Science USA, 92,* 2350–2354.

Dubin, N., Pasternack, B. S., & Moseson, M. (1990). Simultaneous assessment of risk factors for melanoma and non-melanoma skin lesions, with emphasis on sun exposure and related variables. *International Journal of Epidemiology, 19,* 811–819.

Elder, D. E. (1995). Skin cancer. Melanoma and other specific nonmelanoma skin cancers. *Cancer, 75,* 245–256.

Fawzy, F. I., Cousins, N., Fawzy, N. W., Kemeny, M. E., Elashoff, R., & Morton, D. (1990). A structured psychiatric intervention for cancer patients. *Archives of General Psychiatry, 47,* 720–725.

Fawzy, F. I., Fawzy, N. W., Hyun, C. S., Elashoff, R., Guthrie, D., Fahey, J. L., & Morton, D. L. (1993). Malignant melanoma: Effects of an early structured psychiatric intervention, coping, and affective state on recurrence and survival six years later. *Archives of General Psychiatry, 50,* 681–689.

Fawzy, F. I., Fawzy, N. W., Arndt, L. A., & Pasnau, R. O. (1995). Critical review of psychosocial interventions in cancer care. *Archives of General Psychiatry, 52,* 100–113.

Ferlic, M., Goldman, A., & Kennedy, B. J. (1979). Group counseling in adult patients with advanced cancer. *Cancer, 43,* 760–766.

Fiore, M. C., Novotnyu, T. E., Pierce, J. P., Giovino, G. A., Hatziandreu, E. J., Newcomb, P. A., Surawica, T. S., & Davis, R. M. (1990). Methods used to quit smoking in the United States: Do cessation programs help? *Journal of the American Medical Association, 263,* 2760–2765.

Flay, B. R. (1993). Youth tobacco use: risks, patterns, and control. In C. T. Orleans & J. Slade (Eds.), *Nicotine addiction: Principles and management* (pp 365–384). New York: Oxford University Press.

Fox, B. H. (1995). The role of psychological factors in cancer incidence and prognosis. *Oncology, 9,* 245–253.

Friedman, R. J., Rigel, D. S., Silverman, M. K., Kopf, A. W., & Vossaert, K. A. (1991). Malignant melanoma in the 1990s: The continued importance of early detection and the role of physician examination and self-examination of the skin. *CA: A Cancer Journal for Clinicians, 41,* 201–226.

Garfinkle, L. (1985). Overweight and cancer. *Annals of Internal Medicine, 103,* 1034–1036.

Glanz, K. (1994). Reducing breast cancer risk through changes in diet and alcohol intake: From clinic to community. *Annals of Behavioral Medicine, 16,* 334–346.

Goldin-Lang, P., Kreuser, E. D., & Zunft, H. J. (1996). Basis and consequences of primary and secondary prevention of gastrointestinal tumors. *Recent Results in Cancer Research, 142,* 163–192.

Goodwin, J. S., Hunt, W. C., Key, C. R., & Samet, J. M. (1987). The effect of marital status on stage, treatment, and survival of cancer patients. *Journal of the American Medical Association, 258,* 3125–3130.

Greer, S., Moorey, S., Baruch, J. D., Watson, M., Robertson, B. M., Mason, A., Rowden, L., Law, M. G., & Bliss, J. M. (1992). Adjuvant psychological therapy forpatients with cancer: A prospective randomized trial. *The British Medical Journal, 301,* 675–680.

Gregorio, D. I., Cummings, K. M., & Michalek, A. (1983). Delay, stage of disease and survival among white and black women with breast cancer. *American Journal of Public Health, 73,* 590–593.

Gregorio, D. I., Emrich, L. J., Graham, S., Marshall, J. R., & Nemoto, T. (1985). Dietary fat consumption and survival among women with breast cancer. *Journal of the National Cancer Institute, 75,* 37–41.

Grimes, D. A., & Economy, K. E. (1995). Primary prevention of gynecologic cancers. *American Journal of Obstetrics and Gynecology, 172* (pt. 1), 227–235.

Grossarth-Maticek, R., Schmidt, P., Vetter, H., & Arndt, S. (1984). Psychotherapy research in oncology. In A. Steptoe & A. Matthews (Eds.), *Health care and human behavior* (pp. 325–341). London: Academic Press.

Grunberg, N. E., Winders, S. E., & Wewers, M. E. (1991). Gender differences in tobacco use. *Health Psychology, 10,* 145–153.

Guide to clinical preventive services: Report of the US Preventive Services Task Force (2nd ed.). (1996). Baltimore: Williams & Wilkins.

Haenszel, W., & Kunhara, M. (1968). Studies of Japanese migrants: Mortality from cancer and other diseases among Japanese in the United States. *Journal of the National Cancer Institute, 40,* 43–68.

Havas, S., Heimendinger, J., Reynolds, K., Baranowski, T., Nicklas, T. A., Bishop, D., Buller, D., Sorensen, G., Beresford, S. A., Cowan, A., & Damron, D. (1994). 5-a-Day for better health: A new research initiative. *Journal of the American Dietetic Association, 94,* 32–36.

Havas, S., Heimendinger, J., Damron, D., Nicklas, T. A., Cowan, A., Beresford, S. A., Sorensen, G., Buller, D., Bishop, D., Baranowski, T., & Reynolds, K. (1995). 5-a-Day for better health—Nine community research projects to increase fruit and vegetable consumption. *Public Health Reports, 110,* 68–79.

Henderson, M. M., Kushi, L. H., Thompson, D. J., Gorbach, S. L., Clifford, C. K., Insull, W., Jr., Moskowitz, M., & Thompson, R.S . (1990). Feasibility of a randomized trial of a low-fat diet for the prevention of breast cancer: Dietary compliance in the Women's Health Trial Vanguard Study. *Preventive Medicine, 19,* 115–133.

Higginson, J. (1993). Environmental carcinogenesis. *Cancer, 72S,* 971–977.

Hill, H. A., & Austin, H. (1996). Nutrition and endometrial cancer. *Cancer Causes and Control, 7,* 19–32.

House, J. S., Landis, K. R., & Umberson, D. (1988). Social relationships and health. *Science, 241,* 540–544.

Hughes, J. R. (1993). Pharmacotherapy for smoking cessation: Unvalidated assumptions, anomalies, and suggestions for future research. *Journal of Consulting and Clinical Psychology, 62,* 751–760.

Hurwitz, S. (1988). The sun and sunscreen protection: Recommendations for children. *Journal of Dermatologic Surgery and Oncology, 14,* 657–660.

Kamb, M. L. (1995). Cervical cancer screening of women attending sexually transmitted disease clinics. *Clinical Infectious Diseases, 20* (Suppl. 1), S98–103.

Keesling, B., & Friedman, H. S. (1987). Psychosicial factors in sunbathing and sunscreen use. *Health Psychology, 6,* 477–493.

Klein, S., Kinney, J., Jeejeebhoy, K., Alpers, D., Hellerstein, M., Murray, M., & Twomey, P. (1997). Nutrition support in clinical practice: Review of published data and recommendations for future research direction. *American Journal of Clinical Nutrition, 66,* 683–706.

Kleinman, J., & Kopstein, A. (1981). Who is being screened for cervical cancer? *American Journal of Public Health, 71,* 73–76.

Kost, K., & Forrest, J. D. (1992). American women's sexual behavior and exposure to risk of sexually transmitted diseases. *Family Planning Perspectives, 24,* 244–254.

Koutsky, L. A., Holmes, K. K., Critchlow, C. W., Stevens, C. E., Paavonen, J., Beckman, A. M., DeRouen, T. A., Galloway, D. A., Vernon, D., & Kiviat, N. B. (1992). A cohort study of the risk of cervical intraepithelial neoplasia grade 2 or 3 in relation to papillomavirus infection. *New England Journal of Medicine, 327,* 1272–1278.

Lando, H.A. (1993). Formal quit smoking treatments. In C. T. Orleans & J. Slade (Eds.), *Nicotine addiction: Principles and management* (pp. 221–244). New York: Oxford University Press.

Landrigan, P.J. (1996). The prevention of occupational cancer. *CA: A Cancer Journal for Clinicians, 46,* 67–69.

Lerman, C., Rimer, B., & Glynn, T. (1997). Introduction: Priorities in behavioral research in cancer prevention and control. *Preventive Medicine, 26,* S3–S10.

Ley, C., Bauer, H. M., Reingold, A., Schiffman, M. H., Chambers, J. C., Tashiro, C. J., & Manos, M. M. (1991). Determinants of genital human papilloma virus infection in young women. *Journal of the National Cancer Institute, 83,* 997–1002.

Luepker, R. V., & Perry C. L. (1991). The Minnesota Heart Health Program—Education for youth and parents. *Annals of the New York Academy of Sciences, 623,* 314–321.

Luepker, R. V., Perry, C. L., McKinlay, S. M., Nader, P. R., Parcel, G. S., Stone, E. J., Webber, L. S., Elder, J. P., Feldman, H. A., Johnson, C. C., Kelder, S. H., & Wu, M. (1996). Outcomes of a field trial to improve children's dietary patterns and physical activity—The Child and Adolescent Trial for Cardiovascular Health (CATCH). *Journal of the American Medical Association, 275,* 768–776.

Lytle, L., & Achterberg, C. (1995). Changing the diet of america's children: What works and why? *Journal of Nutrition Education, 27,* 250–260.

Mandelblatt, J., Traxler, M., Lakin, P., Kanetsky, P, & Kao, R. (1993a). Targeting breast and cervical cancer screening to elderly poor black women: who will participate? The Harlem Study Team. *Preventive Medicine. 22,* 20–33.

Mandelblatt, J., Traxler, M., Lakin, P, Thomas, L., Chauhan, P, Matseoane, S, & Kanetsky, P. (1993b). A nurse practioner intervention to increase breast and cervical cancer screening for poor, elderly black women. The Harlem study team. *Journal of General Internal Medicine, 8,* 173–178.

Marks, R., & Hill, D. (1988). Behavioral change in adolescence: A major challenge for skin-cancer control in Australia. *Medical Journal of Australia, 149,* 514–515.

McGinnis, J. M., & Foege, W. H. (1993). Actual causes of death in the United States. *Journal of the American Medical Association, 270,* 2207–2212.

Miller, D. L., & Weinstock, M. A. (1994) Nonmelanoma skin cancer in the United States: Incidence. *Journal of the American Academy of Dermatology, 30,* 774–778.

Morrison, E. A., Ho, G. Y., Vermund, S. H, Goldberg, G. L., Kedish, A. S., Kelley, K. F., & Burk, R. D. (1991). Human papilloma virus infection and other risk factors for cervical neoplasia: A case–control study. *International Journal of Cancer, 49,* 6–13.

Muscat, J. E., Carmella, S. G., Akerhar, S., Scott, D., Hecht, S. S., & Richie, J. P. (1996a). Gender differences in the metabolism of the tobacco-specific nitrosamine 4-(methylnitrosamino)-1-(3-pyridyl)-1-butanone (NNK) (meeting abstract). *Proceedings of the Annual Meeting of the American Cancer Sociate for Cancer Research, 37,* A1720.

Muscat, J. E., Richie, J. P., Thompson, S., & Wynder, E. L. (1996b). Gender differences in smoking and risk for oral cancer. *Cancer Research, 56,* 5192–5197.

National Cancer Institute (NCI). (1986). Cancer control objectives for the nation: 1985–2000 (NIH Publication No. 86–2880, No. 2.) Washington, DC: US Government Printing Office.

National Research Council, Committee on Diet and Health. (1989). *Diet and health: Implications for reducing chronic disease risk.* Washington, DC: National Academy Press.

Nomura, A. M., Marchand, L. L., Kolonel, L. N., & Hankin, J. H. (1991). The effects of dietary fat on breast cancer survival among Caucasian and Japanese women in Hawaii. *Breast Cancer Research and Treatment, 18,* S135–S141.

Oliveria, S. A., Ellison, R. C., Moore, L. L., Gillman, M. W., Garrahie, E. J., & Singer, M. R. (1992). Parent–child relationships in nutrient intake: The Framingham Children's Study. *American Journal of Clinical Nutrition, 56,* 593–598.

Orleans, C. T. (1993). Treating nicotine dependence in medical settings: A stepped-care model. In C. T. Orleans & J. Slade (Eds.), *Nicotine addiction: Principles and management* (pp. 145–161) New York: Oxford University Press.

Orleans, C. T., Glynn, T. J., Manley, M. W., & Slade, J. (1993). Minimal contact quit smoking strategies for medical settings. In C. T. Orleans & J. Slade (Eds.), *Nicotine addiction: Principles and management* (pp. 181–220). New York: Oxford University Press.

Parcel, G. S., Simons-Morton, B., O'Hara, N. M., Baranowski, T., & Wilson, B. (1989). School promotion of healthful diet and physical activity: Impact on learning outcomes and self-reported behavior. *Health Education Quarterly, 16,* 181–199.

Patterson, B., & Block, G. (1991). Fruit and vegetable consumption: National survey data. In E. Bendich & C. Butterworth (Eds.), *Micronutrients in health and the prevention of disease* (pp. 409–436). New York: Marcel Dekker.

Peto, R. (1986). Influence of dose and duration of smoking on lung cancer rates. In D. G. Zaridze & R. Peto (Eds.), *Tobacco: A major international health hazard* (pp. 23–33). Lyon, France: International Agency for Research on Cancer.

Prentice, R. L., Thompson, D., Clifford, C., Gorbach, S., Goldin, B., & Byar, D. (1990). Dietary fat reduction and plasma estradiol concentration in healthy postmenopausal women. *Journal of the National Cancer Institute, 82*, 129–134.

Preston, D. S., & Stern, R. S. (1992). Nonmelanoma cancers of the skin. *New England Journal of Medicine, 327*, 1649–1662.

Reynolds, K. D., Racynski, J. M., Binkley, D., Franklin, F. A., Duvall, R C., Devane-Hart, K., Harrington, K. F., Caldwell, E., Jester, P., Bragg, C., & Fouad, M. (1997). Design of "High 5": A school-based study to promote fruit and vegetable consumption for cancer risk reduction. *Cancer Education, 12*, 89–94.

Rhodes, A. R., Weinstock, M. A., Fitzpatrick, T. B., Mihm, M. C. Jr, & Sober, A. J. (1987). Risk factors for cutaneous melanoma: A practical method of recognizing predisposed individuals. *Journal of the American Medical Association, 258*, 3146–3154.

Richardson, J. L., Marks, G., Solis, J. M., Collins, L. M., Birba, L., & Hisserich, J. C. (1987). Frequency and adequacy of breast cancer screening among elderly Hispanic women. *Preventive Medicine, 16*, 761–774.

Rigel, D. S. (1997). Malignant melanoma: Incidence issues and their effect on diagnosis and treatment in the 1990s. *Mayo Clinic Proceedings, 72*, 367–371.

Rigel, D. S, Friedman, R. J., & Kopf, A. W. (1996). Lifetime risk for development of skin cancer in the US population: Current estimate is now 1 in 5 [editorial]. *Journal of the American Academy of Dermatology, 35*, 1012–1013.

Rose, D. P. (1996). The mechanistic rationale in support of dietary cancer prevention. *Preventive Medicine, 25*, 34–37.

Schiffman, M. H. (1992). Recent progess in defining the epidemiology of human papillomarvirus infection and cervical neoplasia. *Journal of the National Cancer Institute, 84*, 394–398.

Schiffman, M. H., Bauer, H. M., Hoover, R. N., Glass, A. G., Cadell, D. H., Rush, B. B., Scott, D. R., Sherman, M. E., Kumman, R. J., & Wacholder, S. (1993). Epidemiologic evidence showing that human papilloma virus infection causes most cervical intraepithelial neoplasia. *Journal of the National Cancer Institute, 85*, 958–964.

Schneider, A., Sawada, E., Gissmann, L., & Shah, K. (1987). Human papilloma viruses in women with a history of abnormal Papanicolaou smears and in their male partners. *Obstetrics and Gynecology, 69*, 554–562.

Schwartz, J. L. (1987). *Review and evaluation of smoking cessation methods—The United States and Canada, 1978–1985.* (NIH Publication No. 87–2940). Bethesda, MD: US Department of Health and Human Services.

Serra-Majem, L., LaVecchia, C., Ribas-Barba, L., Prieto-Ramos, F., Lucchini, F., Ramon, J.M., & Salleras, L. (1993). Changes in diet and mortality from selected cancers in southern Mediterranean countries, 1960–1989. *European Journal of Clinical Nutrition, 47* (Suppl. 1), S25–S34.

Spiegel, D. (1994). Health caring: Psychosocial support for patients with cancer, *Cancer, 74*, 1453–1457.

Spiegel, D., & Bloom, J. (1983). Group therapy and hypnosis reduce metastatic breast carcinoma pain. *Psychosomatic Medicine, 45*, 333–339.

Spiegel, D., Bloom, J. R., Kraemer, H. C., & Gottheil, E. (1989). Effect of psychosocial treatment on survival of patients with metastatic breast cancer. *Lancet, 2*, 888–891.

Stein, M., Miller, A. H., & Trestman, R. L. (1991). Depression, the immune system, and health and illness: Findings in search of meaning. *Archives of General Psychiatry, 48*, 171–177.

Steinmetz, K. A., & Potter, J. D. (1996). Vegetables, fruit, and cancer prevention: A review. *Journal of the American Dietetic Association, 96*, 1027–1039.

Stellman, J. M., & Stellman, S. D. (1996). Cancer and the workplace. *CA: A Cancer Journal for Clinicians, 46*, 70–92.

Sterling, T., Rosenbaum, W., & Weinkam, J. (1993). Income, race, and mortality. *Journal of the National Medical Association, 85*, 906–911.

Stern R. S., Weinstein, M. C., & Baker, S. G. (1986). Risk reduction for nonmelanoma skin cancer with childhood sunscreen use. *Archives of Dermatology, 122*, 537–545.

Taylor, C. R., & Sober, A. J. (1996). Sun exposure and skin disease. *Annual Review of Medicine, 47*, 181–191.

Trijsburg, R. W., van Knippenburg, F. C., & Rijpma, S. E. (1992). Effects of psychological treatment on cancer patients: A critical review. *Psychosomatic Medicine, 54*, 489–517.

U.S. Department of Agriculture (USDA) and U.S. Department of Health and Human Services (USDHHS). (1990). *Nutrition and your health: Dietary guidelines for Americans* (Home and Garden Bulletin No. 232). Washington, DC: US Government Printing Office.

US Department of Health and Human Services (USDHHS). (1985). *Report of the Secretary's Task Force on black and minority health* (Vol. I). Washington, DC: US Government Printing Office.

US Department of Health and Human Services (USDHHS). (1989). *Reducing the health consequences of smoking: 25 years of progress. A report of the Surgeon General.* (DHHS publication No. (CDC) 89-8411). Washington, DC: US Government Printing Office.

US Department of Health and Human Services (USDHHS). (1990). *The health benefits of smoking cessaiton. A report of the Surgeon General.* (DHHS Publication No. (CDC) 90-8416). Washington, DC: US Government Printing Office.

US Department of Health and Human Services (USDHHS). (1991). *Healthy People 2000: National health promotion and disease prevention objectives.* (DHHS Publication PHS 91-50212). Washington, DC: US Government Printing Office.

US Department of Health and Human Services (USDHHS). (1994a). *Preventing tobacco use among young people. A report of the Surgeon General.* (DHHS publication No (CDC) N 017-001-00491-0). Washington, DC: US Government Printing Office.

US Department of Health and Human Services (USDHHS). (1994b). *Seventh annual report on carcinogens.* (pp. 1–16). Rockville, MD: Technical Resources.

US Department of Health and Human Services (USDHHS). (1996). *Cancer rates and risks* (4th ed., pp. 94–102). Washington, DC: US Government Printing Office.

Vargas, P. A., & Alberts, D. S. (1991). Primary prevention of colorectal cancer through dietary modification. *Cancer, 70* (Suppl.), 1229–1235.

Vessey, M. P., & Gray, M. (1985). *Cancer risks and prevention.* Oxford: Oxford University Press.

Weinstock, M. A. (1993). Epidemiology of melanoma. In L. Nathanson (Ed.), *Current research and clinical management of melanoma* (pp. 29–56). Boston: Kluwer Academic.

Weinstock, M. A. (1997). Skin cancer I: Melanoma and nevi. In H. C. Williams & D. P. Strachan (Eds.), *The challenge of dermatoepidemiology* (pp. 191–207). Boca Raton, FL: CRC Press.

Weinstock, M. A., Colditz, G. A., Willett, W. C., Stampfer, M. J., Bronstein, B. R., Mihm, M. C., Jr, & Speizer, F. E. (1989). Nonfamilial cutaneous melanoma incidence in women associated with sun exposure before 20 years of age. *Pediatrics, 84,* 199–204.

Willett, W. C., & Hunter, D. J. (1994). Prospective studies of diet and breast cancer. *Cancer, 74* (Suppl.), 1085–1089.

Willett, W. C., Stampfer, M. J., Colditz, G. A., Rosner, B. A., Hennekens, C. H., & Speizer, F. E. (1987). Dietary fat and the risk of breast cancer. *New England Journal of Medicine, 316,* 22–28.

Williams, C. L. (1992). Intervention in childhood. In I. S. Ockene & J. K. Ockene (Eds.), *Prevention of coronary heart disease* (pp. 65–97). Boston: Little Brown.

Windsor, R. A., Kronnefeld, J. J., Cain, M. G., Cutter, G. R., Goodson, L. A., & Edwards, E. (1981). Increasing utilization of a rural cervical cancer detection program. *American Journal of Public Health, 71,* 641–643.

Wood, P. E., Milligan, I., Christ, D., & Liff, D. (1978). Group counseling for cancer patients in a community hospital. *Psychosomatics, 19,* 147–152.

Zang, E. A., & Wynder, E. L. (1996). Differences in lung cancer risk between men and women: Examination of the evidence. *Journal of the National Cancer Institute, 88,* 183–192.

Ziegler, R. G. (1991). Vegetables, fruits and carotenoids and the risk of cancer. *American Journal of Clinical Nutrition, 53,* 251S–259S.

CHAPTER 14

Intentional Injury

*Philip R. Fine, Matthew D. Rousculp, Andrea D. Tomasek,
and Wendy S. Horn*

Introduction

This chapter focuses on events resulting from purposeful acts involving the use of violent physical force, unlike "accidental" or unintentional injuries resulting from car crashes, falls, burns, poisonings, drownings, and so on. In intentional injuries, there is conscious intent to inflict injury or death. While many tend to think first of intentional injuries as the consequence of forceful acts involving two or more people, we must also consider suicide, a self-directed intentional injury.

Epidemiology

Intentional Injuries and Current Crime Statistics

According to the National Center for Health Statistics, 65 people die and more than 6000 are physically injured by acts of *interpersonal* violence on an average day in the United States (Harlow, 1989; National Center for Health Statistics, 1992). This translates to nearly 24,000 deaths and over 2 million nonfatal injuries each year. When suicide statistics are included, intentional injuries are estimated to account for approximately 50,000 annual deaths. It is worth noting that nonfatal assaults and unsuccessful suicide attempts are estimated to outnumber "successful" homicides and suicides by a ratio of more than 100 to 1 (National Center for Health Statistics, 1987; Rosenberg & Mercy, 1986; US Department of Justice, 1988). To appreciate the extent of the intentional injury problem in this country, it is helpful to consider intentional injury statistics within the overall context of crime data. While the numbers are impressive, overall crime statistics appear to be coming down, if only modestly. For example, according to the Federal Bureau of Investiga-

Philip R. Fine, Matthew D. Rousculp, Andrea D. Tomasek, and Wendy S. Horn • Injury Control Research Center, University of Alabama at Birmingham, Birmingham, Alabama 35294

Handbook of Health Promotion and Disease Prevention, edited by Raczynski and DiClemente.
Kluwer Academic/Plenum Publishers, New York, 1999.

tion (FBI), the 1995 crime index rate of 5,278 crimes per 100,000 persons at risk was 2% lower than that reported in 1994 (Federal Bureau of Investigation, 1996). Violent crimes, including aggravated assault, rape, and murder, reported to US law enforcement agencies during 1995 dropped below 1.8 million offenses. This resulted in the lowest violent crime rate, 685 violent crimes for every 100,000 persons at risk, since 1989. Nonetheless, aggravated assaults accounted for 61% of all violent crimes reported to law enforcement agencies in 1995 (Federal Bureau of Investigations, 1996).

In 1995, 33% of all violent, aggravated assaults were committed with blunt objects. Personal weapons such as hands, fists, and feet were used in another 26% of the violent, aggravated assaults, while knives or cutting instruments were used in yet another 18%. By comparison, firearms were only used in the remaining 23% of aggravated assaults (see Table 1). Moreover, closer inspection of firearm-related data shows the proportion of violent crimes committed with firearms remained stable between 1994 and 1995 (Federal Bureau of Investigations, 1996).

As reported by Mercy, Rosenberg, Powell, Broome, and Roper (1993), there is a disproportionate representation of persons between 12 and 24 years of age among the perpetrators and victims of violent acts:

> Arrest rates for homicide, rape, robbery and aggravated assault in the United States peak among older adolescents and young adults. During the 1980s more than 48,000 people were murdered by youths ages twelve to twenty-four. Interviews with assault victims indicate that offenders in this age range committed almost half of the estimated 6.4 million nonfatal crimes of violence in 1991. Adolescents and young adults also face an extraordinarily high risk of death and injury from violence. Homicide is the second leading cause of death for Americans ages fifteen to thirty-four and is the leading cause of death for young African-Americans. Homicide rates among young American men are vastly higher than in other Western industrialized nations. In addition, persons ages twelve to twenty-four face the highest risk of nonfatal assault of any age group in our society. The average age of both violent offenders and victims has been growing younger in recent years.

While they contain an element of hope, trends in recent statistics reveal a number of disturbing findings about violence in America. While the numbers are impressive, overall crime statistics appear to be coming down, if only modestly. For example, according to the FBI, the 1995 crime index rate of 5,278 crimes per 100,000 persons at risk was 2% lower than that reported in 1994. In 1995, there were approximately 1.1 million reports of aggravated assault. That figure reflects a drop of approximately 1% for the second consecutive year. However, while declining slightly, aggravated assault continues to account for the bulk—61%—of this country's violent crime problem. In fact, there were 418 victims of aggravated assault for every 100,000 persons at risk nationwide in 1995. While its magnitude is alarming, this was still the lowest aggravated assault rate since 1989 (Federal Bureau of Investigations, 1996).

Table 1. Aggravated Assaults by Method (USA–1995)

33%	Blunt objects
25%	Personal weapons (hands, fists, and feet)
23%	Firearms
18%	Knives and other cutting instruments

Murder: The Ultimate Interpersonal Injury

According to the FBI, approximately 21,600 persons were murdered in the United States in 1995. That number translates to a rate of 8 per 100,000 persons at risk. The 1995 FBI murder statistic is 7% lower than the 1994 figure and 13% lower than the 1991 figure. In 1995, as in virtually all previous years, 77% of murder victims were males, and 88% were 18 years of age or older. By race, 49% were African American and 48% were white. Clearly, a disproportionate number of murder victims are black, because African Americans constitute only 13% of the entire US population. Fifty-five percent of murder victims were slain by strangers or persons unknown. Among all female murder victims in 1995, 26% were slain by husbands or boyfriends, while 3% of the male victims were slain by wives or girlfriends. By circumstance, 28% of the murders resulted from arguments and 18% from felonious activities such as robbery, arson, and so forth. In approximately 7 out of 10 murders reported during 1995, firearms were the weapons used.

Violence against Women

According to the Family Violence Prevention Fund, two thirds of all physical attacks on women are committed by someone they know, often a husband or boyfriend. In 1995, this translated to almost 4 million American women being physically abused by intimate male partners. If these estimates are correct, it means that every 9 seconds a woman in this country is physically injured by a domestic male companion and that women are more often victims of domestic violence than they are victims of burglary, mugging, or other physical crimes combined. Moreover, recent statistics suggest that as many as 42% of women who are murdered are killed by their intimate male partners.

Also, according to the Family Violence Prevention Fund, more than one in three Americans have witnessed an incident of domestic violence resulting in physical injury to a female. The same source claims that nearly 9 out of 10 Americans say that women being beaten is a serious problem facing many families, with concern cutting across race, gender, and age categories. According to the same survey, 81% of Americans believe something can be done to reduce domestic violence in this country.

Recently, the Milwaukee Women's Center broadened the definition of domestic violence to include physical abuse by intimate partners of the same or opposite sex. Additional terms, aimed at broadening the definition further, are coming into common usage. For example, partner violence is sometimes used to encompass all aspects of violence involving intimate partners—physical, sexual, and emotional. Additionally, "family and intimate violence" has been used to encompass partner violence, child abuse, elder abuse, dating violence, children affected by witnessing family violence, and other violence and abuse involving family and intimates (US Department of Health and Human Services, 1996).

Rape and Sexual Assault

In 1995, just over 97,000 forcible rapes were reported to law enforcement agencies across the country. This was the lowest reported total since 1989, and it was 5% lower than the number reported in 1994. However, in the FBI's Uniform Crime Reporting Program, the victims of forcible rape are always female and, while the 1995 rate was slightly lower than in the previous year, it is commonly acknowledged that an enormous number of rapes go unreported. The rate of forcible rape reported for 1995 was 72 per 100,000 females at risk (Federal Bureau of Investigations, 1996). In recent years, the definitional borders of rape have been extended to include subcategories defined by the intersection of forced sexual intercourse and the specific relationship between the victim and the rapist. For example, whereas in the past we spoke only of "rape," today we use qualifiers like *"acquaintance" rape, "date" rape, "marital rape,"* and *"stranger" rape.* Whether these distinctions are important from a prevention standpoint is unknown, although it could be argued that specific interventions are easier to conceptualize than are generic interventions. For example, an intervention targeting the prevention of date rape on a college campus would seem easier to institute and evaluate than would an intervention targeting the prevention of stranger rape.

Nonetheless, from an injury prevention perspective, there must be a distinction between victimization as a crime and victimization resulting in injury. As described by the National Committee for Injury Prevention and Control, the law may differentiate between forced genital rape as rape and forced oral copulation as merely sexual assault. Regretfully, this technical distinction does not consider nor convey the degree of physical, psychological, or emotional injury sustained by the victim, which in virtually all cases is equally devastating irrespective of the specific details of the physical act(s) involved (National Committee for Injury Prevention and Control, 1989). Finally, it should be remembered that more than 99% of assaults on women do not result in their death but rather in physical and psychological injuries. Exacerbating this finding are studies showing that such injuries increase the survivor's risk of subsequent suicide, alcoholism, drug addiction, depression, and other behavioral disorders including child abuse (Mercy *et al.*, 1993).

Violence against Children

In 1995, the National Center on Child Abuse and Neglect (NCCAN) reported that the number of children who were maltreated/abused increased from approximately 800,000 in 1990 to just over 1 million in 1993 (US Department of Health and Human Services, 1995). Over 47% of the cases fell into the "neglect" category. Physical abuse was documented in 24% of the children. Child sexual abuse ranged from a high of 16.0% in 1990 to a low of 13.8% in 1993. Other and unknown forms of maltreatment/abuse were reported in 12.6% of the children. Emotional maltreatment was reported in approximately 5.5% of the children. For the most part, distinctions between the categories seem irrelevant, since all these acts are heinous and because the victims are essentially incapable of protecting themselves or in most instances of even making their plight known (US Department of Health and Human Services, 1995).

According to the NCCAN, most abused children are between 2 and 5 years of age (25.4%). Children between 6 and 9 years of age are abused next most often (22.8%), followed by children between 10 and 13 years of age (19.4%). Children between 14 and 17 years of age make up approximately 14.7% of those who are violently abused, while children who are 1 year of age or less are violently abused about 13.4% of the time (US Department of Health and Human Services, 1995). Between 1990 and 1993, slightly more female than male children (52% and 45.6%, respectively) were victims of abuse. The percentages correspond very closely to the overall proportion of females and males in the general population, according to 1990 census figures (US Department of Health and Human Services, 1995). On average, 54.4% of the abused children in 1995 were white compared to 25.6% who were African American. When statistical population corrections are made [in the 1990 census, African Americans constituted only 12.1% of the US population (Bennett, 1996)], the incidence of violent child abuse is demonstrated to be significantly higher among African Americans than whites.

Violence against the Elderly

The problem of elder abuse and neglect first received attention in the early 1980s when reports appeared in mass media publications and on national television (Pillemer & Frankel, 1991). Despite this publicity, the National Committee for Injury Prevention and Control acknowledged that as late as 1989, there had been no major studies on the prevalence of elder abuse. Rather, most of what was known was based on data derived from small samples of older people and surveys of social workers and other professionals who worked with the elderly (National Committee for Injury Prevention and Control, 1989, pp. 233–242). However, as long ago as 1985, the House Select Committee on Aging estimated that each year more than 1 million older adults are physically, financially, and emotionally abused by their relatives (US House of Representatives, Select Committee on Aging, 1985).

One of the major difficulties associated with studying elder abuse or attempting to estimate its incidence and prevalence has been the lack of concise, widely adopted definitions. Phillips (1983) defined elder abuse using the dimensions of physical abuse and neglect, emotional abuse, neglect and deprivation, sexual exploitation and assault, verbal assault, medical neglect, material abuse, neglect of environment, and violation of rights. Others have suggested the categories of passive and active neglect, physical abuse, and verbal abuse (Bristow & Collins, 1989). Accordingly, Pillemer and Finkelhor (1989) focused on physical abuse, psychological abuse, and neglect.

As is often the case in public-health-related issues, prevalence estimates vary. Clark (1984) projected that as many as 10% of persons over 65 years of age experienced some form of maltreatment at the hands of others. The House Select Committee on Aging report concluded that as many as 4% of the elderly may have experienced moderate to severe abuse (Bristow & Collins, 1989). Extrapolating from studies conducted in Illinois, Ohio, and Massachusetts, the prevalence of abused elderly persons is around 3% (Crous, Cobb, Harris, Kopecky, & Poertner, 1981; Lau & Kosberg, 1979; Pillemer & Finkelhor, 1988) or between 820,000 and 1,860,000 abused elderly persons in the United States in 1996 (National Center on Elder Abuse, 1996). It is important to emphasize that all existing elder abuse statistics are confined to domestic settings. Thus, there is little useful information about elder abuse in institutional settings (National Center on Elder Abuse, 1996). According to the National Center on Elder Abuse (NCEA), there was a 106% increase in reports of elder abuse between 1986 and 1994, although the organization acknowledges that since 1990 the rate of increase has been quite low. Nonetheless, there is general agreement that elder abuse is far less likely to be reported than child or spousal abuse because of differences in the public's level of awareness. Statistical data reflecting the incidence of the common types of domestic abuse (see Table 2) reveal that neglect or self-abuse occurred most frequently, followed by physical abuse, financial exploitation, emotional abuse, other types of abuse, unknown causes, and finally sexual abuse.

Table 2. Types of Domestic Elder Abuse and Their
Reported Frequency of Occurrence

Type	Percent
Neglect/self-abuse	58.5
Physical abuse	15.7
Financial exploitation	12.3
Emotional ebuse	7.3
Other types	5.1
Unknown	0.6
Sexual	0.5

Although statistics are incomplete, it appears that around two thirds of the elder abuse victims are females and there is a linear relationship between age and abuse; that is, persons 80 years of age and older comprise more than one third of the elder abuse victims, although they do not constitute one third of the elderly. Table 3 shows a breakdown of persons who abuse the elderly in domestic settings. Note that more than two thirds of abusers are family members, a figure remarkably comparable to the 70% of perpetrators who abuse children.

Violence against the Poor

Mercy *et al.* (1993) quote a variety of workers who reported consistent and compelling evidence that "poor people bear a disproportionate share of the public health burden of violence in our society." For example, homicide rates were consistently higher in metropolitan areas where poverty is most prevalent; and in 1991 in the United States, the risk of being a nonfatal, violent assault victim was three times greater for persons from families with incomes below $7,500 than for those with family incomes above $50,000 (Centerwall, 1984; Lowry, Hassig, Gunn, & Mathison, 1988; Muscat, 1988; US Department of Justice, 1988).

Suicide

If one accepts the premise that killing oneself is a bad thing, then suicide is a problem in the United States. In fact, according to the Centers for Disease Control (CDC) and the National Center for Health Statistics (NCHS), more people in this

Table 3. Abusers and Their Relationship to the Elderly

Abusers	Percent
Adult children	35.0
Other relatives	13.6
Spouse	13.4
Service provider	6.2
Grandchildren	5.9
Friend/neighbor	5.2
Sibling	2.9
All others	10.3
Unknown	7.4

country kill themselves than die from homicide in a given year. For example, in 1992, suicide claimed the lives of nearly 30,500 persons, for a rate of 11.1 suicides per 100,000 persons at risk, compared to 25,000 who were reported to have been homicide victims, for an overall homicide rate of 9.09 per 100,000 persons at risk (Harlow, 1989; National Center for Health Statistics, 1992). On an average day in the United States, 84 people die from suicide and an estimated 1900 adults make an unsuccessful suicide attempt. Until boys and girls are 9 years old, their suicide rates are identical; from 10 to 14, the boys' rate is twice as high as the girls' rate; from 15 to 19, four times as high; and from 20 to 24, six times as high (US Department of Health and Human Services, 1988). The risk for suicide among young people is greatest among young white males; however, from 1980 through 1992, suicide rates increased most rapidly among young black males. For African-American males aged 15 to 19, the rate increased 165.3% (Harlow, 1989; National Center for Health Statistics, 1992). According to the National Institute of Mental Health (NIMH), the most prevalent risk factors for teen suicide are: family history of suicide; mental illness or substance abuse disorder; history of family violence, including emotional, physical, or sexual abuse; separation or divorce; prior suicide attempts; firearms in the home; incarceration; and exposure to suicidal behavior of others, including family members and/or peers.

Suicide rates increase with age and are highest among Americans aged 65 years and older. The 10-year period of 1980 to 1990 was the first decade since the 1940s that the suicide rate for older residents rose instead of declined (Harlow, 1989; National Center for Health Statistics, 1992). Risk factors for suicide among older persons differ from those among the young. Older persons have a higher prevalence of alcohol abuse, depression, a greater use of highly lethal methods, and social isolation. They also make fewer attempts per completed suicide, have a higher male-to-female ratio than other groups, have often visited a health care provider before their suicide, and have more physical illnesses.

Overall, males are at least four times more likely to die from suicide than are females, but females are more likely to try to kill themselves than are their male counterparts (Harlow, 1989; National Center for Health Statistics, 1992). It is postulated that the completion statistic is due to the method of choice among males, which is predominantly firearms. For women, the most frequently employed method is pill ingestion, which renders them capable of being resuscitated if discovered in time. Moreover, among suicide attempters and completers who are in therapy, women tend to commit suicide early in treatment, whereas men wait until they conclude there is neither hope nor a way out (Harlow, 1989; National Center for Health Statistics, 1992).

In 1992, white males accounted for 73% of all suicides and for 81% of suicides among persons aged 65 years and older. From 1980 to 1992, the rate for men in this age group increased 10% (from 34.8 per 100,000 to 38.4). The rate for women was unchanged. Historically, white males and females account for almost 91% of all suicides; however, there is a noticeable and alarming increase in the frequency of suicide among African-American males and females. Moreover, suicide rates are higher than the national average for some groups of Asian and Native Americans (Harlow, 1989; National Center for Health Statistics, 1992).

Nearly 60% of all successful suicides in this country are committed with a firearm (Harlow, 1989; National Center for Health Statistics, 1992). Firearms were the most common method of suicide used by both men (74%) and women (31%). Among persons aged 15 to 19 years, firearm-related suicides accounted for 81% of the increase in the overall rate of suicide from 1980 to 1992 (National Institute of Mental Health Report, 1992). In fact, according to Kellerman and co-workers (1992), people living in a household where a firearm is kept are almost five times more likely to die by suicide than people who live in gun-free homes. However, in a subsequent study appearing in the March 1990 issue of the *American Journal of Psychiatry*, Rich, Young, Fowler, Wagner, and Black (1990) reported that all gun suicides, though statistically reduced in the 5 years following Canada's handgun restrictions that began in 1976, were substituted 100% by suicides using other methods, mostly jumping off bridges. Apparently, eliminating firearms may not eliminate suicide: It seems merely to shift the accomplishment of suicide to other means.

Certainly it will be true that people who own parachutes will die more frequently in falls from airplanes than people who do not, but does that mean that parachute ownership constitutes an increased risk factor for death by falling from an airplane? Logic tell us that the risk of dying as a result of falling from an airplane would be far greater by those people who fall from airplanes who do not have a parachute handy.

Cronkite observes that:

> . . . between 93 and 95% of suicides are suffering a psychiatric illness, most commonly depression, substance abuse associated with depression, or schizophrenia. . . . There is not a lot of [evidence] yet, but it appears that only 7 to 10% of attempters die by suicide and that attempters and completers are two distinct groups that overlap. One difference between the two groups is that the completers have a higher rate of substance abuse. Alcohol plus other substances like marijuana or coke increases the risk by ten times. It has been shown that depressives' risk is thirty to ninety times higher than the general population . . . 7 to 10% of those who attempt suicide end up killing themselves and 60 to 70% of those who talk about it to relatives or friends do it within six months. (Cronkite, 1994, pp. 116-117)

Violence in the United States

It has been postulated that the United States has a history, although not a tradition, of violence (Hofstadter & Wallace, 1971). Historians have compared the differences in violence between the United States and Europe: violence in Europe is marked by insurrectionary citizens versus the state; violence in the United States consists mostly of citizens versus citizens (Weiner & Zahn, 1989). Experts on the National Research Council's Panel on the Understanding and Control of Violent Behavior agreed that the United States is generally more violent than other countries. The panel's assertion was that homicide rates in the United States far exceed those in other industrialized nations. In addition, the United States has shown the highest prevalence among industrialized nations for serious sexual assaults and for all other assaults including threats of physical harm. However, the same panel resoundingly agreed that the United States was no more violent now than in the past (Reiss & Roth, 1993).

Although our society's past is deemed violent, it does not logically follow that we must repeat the past. Thus, in the search for constructive solutions, good science should act as a solid foundation. The goal for good science is to move from studies that concentrate entirely on correlates and predictors of violence to more appropriate studies that identify the actual causes and the pathways leading to violent actions (Buka & Earls, 1993). This direction in violence prevention is based on the notion that time and lives are not expendable luxuries, and therefore antiviolence interventions must be based on something more than only best intentions (National Committee for Injury Prevention and Control, 1989).

Summary

While traditional public policy responds to interpersonal violence by assigning responsibility to the criminal justice system, Rosenberg and Mercy (1991) have posited that violence is also a public health problem capable of being solved, at least in part, using the disease prevention model. Of course, adopting this approach requires accepting the premise that injuries resulting from violence are a public health problem. While there is not universal acceptance of the premise that violence is a public health problem (Mercy *et al.*, 1993), our conclusion that injuries resulting from violent acts are a public health problem hardly seems arguable.

Intentional injury and its analogous term, violence, have been defined as the use of physical force with the intent to inflict injury or death upon oneself or another (National Committee for Injury Prevention and Control, 1989). With so broad a definition, and considering the enormous financial and other costs to society from violence, a wide array of academic disciplines and professions have approached the challenge of violence prevention. It is generally acknowledged that a single approach to alleviating violence does not exist; therefore a multidisciplinary strategy is warranted (Earls, Cairns, & Mercy, 1993).

In Fig. 1, the Venn diagram depicts the overlapping perspectives of criminal justice, behavioral science, and public health with regard to violence. Criminal justice generally views violence as it relates to violations of the law. On the other hand, behavioral science views violence as variations of aggressive human behavior that can

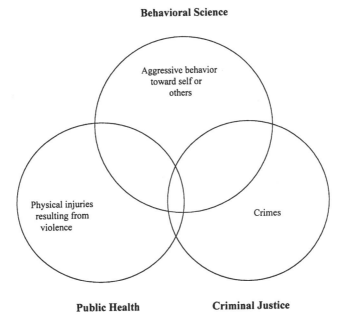

Figure 1. Overlapping perspectives of public health, criminal justice, and behavioral science. Adapted from National Committee for Injury Prevention and Control

harm individuals, their families, and their communities. Finally, public health views violent acts as precursors to physical injury and as such a detriment to health (National Committee for Injury Prevention and Control, 1989). Theoretically, each discipline's area of experience and viewpoints of violence would partially overlap. In practice, the clear distinctions between these disciplines begin to blur, resulting in larger areas of common perspectives (Moore, Prothrow-Stith, Guyer, & Spivak, 1994).

The Venn diagram presented does not provide a truly comprehensive representation of all the entities involved with violence prevention. Professionals such as police officers, social workers, judges, state public health professionals, probation officers, nurses, mental health professionals, teachers, and physicians are just a few examples of the groups involved in intentional injury control (National Committee for Injury Prevention and Control, 1989). Moreover, with the widely held belief that violence is a community problem, more and more individuals are taking a proactive stance and claiming a stake in violence prevention.

Theoretical Basis for Intervention

The National Research Council expressed frustration over the difficulty encountered when attempting to link fields of knowledge, such as criminology and public health, in a manner conducive to constructing a theoretical base on which to build violence intervention programs. The panel did acknowledge, however, that a significant "knowledge base exists regarding some aspects of violent events and behaviors and that certain areas of knowledge are expanding rapidly" (Reiss & Roth, 1993). In spite of lacking a theoretical base, the panel suggested that focusing on places where violence occurs holds promise for understanding, preventing, and controlling violence. One must consider risk factors related to both encounters and environments. For example, encounters brought about by threats and counterthreats, illegal drug sales, and armed robberies have a greater potential for generating violence than more mundane or ordinary encounters.

A better understanding of the interpersonal dynamics involved in these exchanges could lead to the development of violence intervention strategies to defuse high-risk encounters. Violent behavior results from a complex interplay of multiple factors throughout a lifetime, factors that include physical and emotional development, family influence, peers, and society (Earls, 1991). Behavioral interventions designed for a single stage of life are not necessarily effective over the long term. Earls *et al.* (1993) claim a significant problem in that the behavioral systems most readily changed through behavioral intervention programs are ironically also most vulnerable to rebound to their original state once the treatment is stopped or prior conditions are reestablished (i.e., reinstituted).

Interpersonal violence in the United States is concentrated among persons in the second decade of their life; yet, foundations for this type of violence are organized in childhood and activated in adolescence. Focusing on this "developmental" stage of life, behaviorists have found it useful in pointing to changes that are likely to be most effective. Like most other expressions of poor health, aggressive and violent behaviors are more readily prevented than they are ameliorated (Earls *et al.*, 1993).

Graphing the fatality rate from intrapersonal violence, one is struck by the bimodal distribution in different age cohorts. Deaths initially peak and then plateau in persons in their late 20s, and the fatality rate increases again in the elderly (Baker, O'Neill, Ginsburg, & Li, 1992). Although suicidology has grown in the past decade, the theoretical basis for suicide interventions has not truly evolved. There have been five categories postulated that form the foundation for all suicide prevention strategies (O'Carrol, Rosenberg, & Mercy, 1991): (1) improve the identification, referral, and treatment of persons at high risk of suicide; (2) focus on the underlying risk factors of suicide (i.e., clinical depression, alcohol and drug abuse); (3) educate the general population to decrease individual vulnerability to suicide; (4) provide or expand the accessibility of self-referral resources for suicidal persons; and (5) limit access to lethal means of suicide.

The Habits of Thought Model

This violence intervention model synthesizes empirical evidence regarding the development and control of aggression with a theoretical framework derived from social cognitive theory. The underlying premise is that benefits to individual children and communities can be achieved by intervening prior to the development of violence-promoting thought patterns, or by intervening before such thought patterns become ingrained and result in the development of violent lifestyle choices leading to increased morbidity and mortality. Slaby and Stringham (1994) refer to social experiences that increase exposure to and involvement with violent activity as "toxins for violence." These "toxins" include such things as: ". . . being victimized by violence, witnessing violence at home or in the community, viewing media violence, having ready access to firearms, becoming involved with alcohol and other drugs, experiencing verbal abuse, discrimination or coercion."

It is important to note that in and of themselves, these factors do not lead inevitably to violent behavior. It is rather the way in which individuals process these stimuli that seems to determine whether the individual affected by violence will turn to either violent or nonviolent behaviors. Slaby and Stringham (1994) explain that "much like a healthy functioning immune system, an individual's habits of thought are capable of neutralizing or counteracting the impact of social experiences that act as toxins for violence."

Skills, beliefs, and cognitive styles all play a role in processing social experiences and in responding to those experiences. Skills influence the ways in which we think about solving social difficulties. Beliefs provide structure for how we view the role or the appropriateness of violence in addressing these difficulties. Impulsive or reflective cognitive styles also influence the ways in which we interpret social problems. Not surprisingly, individuals who are reflective and "coolheaded" are more likely to think of multiple solutions to a particular problem and to consider the consequences of each solution, and as a result they are at lower risk for resorting to violent behavior. The contrary is also true. Individuals at high risk for violent behavior are generally less likely to weigh alternative courses of action, may harbor unrealistic beliefs regarding violence, and are more likely to respond impulsively in volatile situations.

The crux of the Slaby and Stringham (1994) model is that an individual's habits of thought are learned and therefore can be unlearned or modified through direct intervention. Through preventive intervention, individuals can be taught to consider nonviolent alternatives when resolving conflict, as well as to defuse or avoid situations likely to expose self or others to violence.

Community-as-Client Model

This model for public health nursing (Fig. 2) is multifaceted, holistic, and applicable to violence interventions. The main objectives of the model are to address community responses to stressors and to prevent actual or potential rifts in community equilibrium. The basic structure of the community consists of the people who reside within it as well as their cultural and religious beliefs, value systems, laws, and mores. Subsystems within the community, such as education, recreation, and safety, interact dynamically with the community members and contribute to what is termed the community's "normal line of defense." The normal line of defense represents the health status achieved by the community over time and is characterized by health-related events such as infant mortality rates and immunization rates. Gang-related violence and domestic violence also can be viewed as indicators of a community's well-being or lack thereof.

A buffer zone or "flexible line of defense" surrounds the community's normal line of defense and represents a dynamic level of health stemming from temporary responses to community stressors. Responses included under this heading can be as varied as neighborhood mobilization after a natural disaster to implementing a violence intervention program for elementary school children. In addition, methods for coping with stress and problem-solving skills play an important role in the viability of the community's lines of defense and bolster its lines of resistance. These are mechanisms unique to the community to ward off the effects of stressors. Neighborhood Watch programs and peer mediation programs can be seen as examples of lines of resistance.

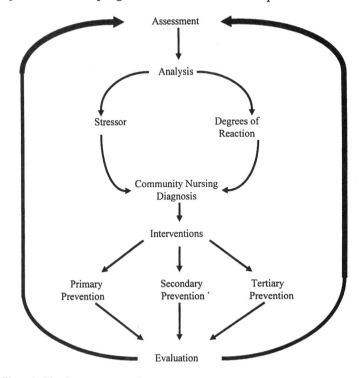

Figure 2. The Community-as-Client Model. Adapted from Anderson *et al.* (1986).

"Degree of reaction" is the term used to denote the amount of disruption that results after an assault by stressors upon a community's lines of defense. This may be reflected in crime statistics and unemployment figures, among other measures. The community nursing diagnosis is based on an assessment of a particular community's normal and flexible lines of defense, stressors, lines of resistance, and degree of reaction. The community diagnosis then shapes the development and implementation of interventions. Measuring a community's degree of reaction can provide important insight in relation to reinforcing lines of defense. A variety of approaches to intervening are possible, including eliminating or curtailing a stressor, or improving the community's ability to withstand a stressor by strengthening its flexible lines of defense (Anderson, McFarlane, & Helton, 1986).

Preventing Youth Violence

As part of the 1994 Violent Crime Control and Law Enforcement Act, the US Congress created the President's Crime Prevention Council. The findings of the council were integrated into a publication titled *Preventing Crime and Promoting Responsibility: 50 Programs That Help Communities Help Their Youth*. Although the strategies suggested by the council may not qualify as a "model" in the strictest sense of the term, their recommendations provide a practical and concrete approach to designing crime and violence intervention programs for our nation's youth. The essence of the strategies is described below.

Address All Levels of the Problem

Community-based prevention endeavors should be comprehensive in scope and ultimately should strive to increase responsible behavior among youth, rather than simply discourage criminal behavior. A well-designed program provides opportunities and incentives for reducing youth criminal behavior during all phases or levels of prevention, which the council describes as the following: (1) early prevention—reinforcing understanding and respect for the dangers of crime and crime-related behaviors and promoting and rewarding responsible behavior; (2) intervention—intervening with risk-involved individuals before serious crimes are committed; (3) suppression—punishing individuals in a consistent and appropriate manner for criminal behavior; and (4) reintegration—providing positive alternatives to individuals who are under the control of the juvenile justice system to discourage their future involvement in crime and crime-related behaviors (President's Crime Prevention Council, 1995).

Be Inclusive

To maximize efficacy, community-based crime prevention programs must be cooperatively developed and implemented by a spectrum of individuals and organizations with a vested interest in solving the problem at hand. Forging ties between community residents, law enforcement officials, and service providers has been shown to be of critical importance in the success of crime prevention programs.

Build On What Is Known

A variety of approaches and strategies are required, as well as a knowledge of the target population. Some programs have been shown to be more helpful than others in addressing specific societal problems or reaching specific populations. Program planners would be well advised to research what has already been tried as they move from establishing general goals to devising specific intervention components.

Assess What Is Being Done

It is easy to lose sight of long-term goals once program implementation is under way. It is therefore of great importance to evaluate continuously goals and strategies to determine whether programs are effective and sufficient to meet a specific challenge or if additional interventions might be necessary. Setting specific goals also aids policymakers and can help garner public support for local crime prevention endeavors.

Target Efforts and Tailor Strategies

Very few communities have the luxury of unlimited resources at their fingertips. It is therefore incumbent upon program developers to decide which group will constitute the intervention target population. If an intervention is not sufficiently focused, even the most modest of goals may be difficult to achieve. The council recommends thinking of interventions in terms of which segment of the youth population will be reached: general, vulnerable, risk-involved, delinquent, or serious, violent, and chronic. Strategies found to be highly effective with one group may prove less than effective with another group. For example, conflict resolution classes or peer mediation groups may work beautifully for lower-risk youth but may become fraught with difficulty when working with high-risk youth.

Members of the President's Crime Prevention Council emphasize that the greatest weakness of many prevention programs is that they are short-lived and fragmented attempts to intercede (President's Crime Prevention Council, 1995).

Intentional Injury: Violence Interventions

The crux of the violence intervention challenge has been summed up nicely by Dr. David Satcher and his colleagues: "We must recognize that violence prevention, like a healthy diet, requires diversity of input. There is no single simple solution. The monotonous application of limited strategies, even effective strategies, like eating only apples, will be insufficient" (Satcher, Powell, Mercy, & Rosenberg, 1996, p. v.). Violence does not occur in a vacuum, but rather emanates from a complex, tangled web of personal and social factors that must be addressed. The National Committee for Injury Prevention and Control (1989) recommends an interdisciplinary approach incorporating elements of public health, criminal justice, and behavioral science. Public health professionals contribute methods and knowledge from the related area of injury control, and behavioral scientists treat aggressive human behavior as harmful to individuals, families, and communities. From the field of criminal justice, violence must be handled as criminal and in violation of the law. All three disciplines offer vital components for effective programs to prevent violence. Summarized below are some of the programs that have been developed to address intentional injury.

Intentional Injury Prevention Programs for Youth

Safe Streets Now!

When arson began to seem like a reasonable stratagem for closing down a neighborhood drug house, a single mother in Berkeley, California, was struck by a novel idea. Rather than rely on the police to arrest drug dealers, Molly Wetzel and 18 of her neighbors sued the landlord of the drug house in small claims court for allowing his property to be used for purposes that "prevented the enjoyment of life and property." The suit was precipitated by the robbery of Wetzel's children at gunpoint, a rash of burglaries in the vicinity, and the gunfire that erupted in the area with alarming regularity. The band of neighbors won their case, each was awarded $2,000, and the drug house was shut down. This triumph led Wetzel to begin Safe Streets Now!, a national, nonprofit organization that supports citizens who utilize small claims courts to address community blight. Since 1992, the grassroots organization has closed 800 drug houses in several states and has won over $1 million in California court settlements (Lappe, 1995).

Crisis Intervention Network (CIN)

In response to increasing gang-related violence in "the city of brotherly love," a municipal agency emerged in 1975 with the purpose of dispatching negotiation teams among gangs in Philadelphia. By 1979, the organization had metamorphosed into a multifaceted, nonprofit social service agency. In addition to their original mission, CIN teams respond to tips of impending violence left by callers on a 24-hour hotline and also monitor community functions such as street festivals and block parties that lend themselves to gang activity and violence. Through an innovative arrangement with probation departments, CIN members are assigned to work with adolescents and young adults who are on probation or parole after conviction of gang-related activities. The benefits of this violence intervention strategy are twofold: it allows CIN members to stay abreast of gang activity and encourages parolees to seek nonviolent resolution of disputes. One of the negotiation teams specializes in defusing racial and ethnic conflicts.

The CIN is involved in a variety of programs designed to help youth resist the lifestyle of violence. Workshops are hosted in local schools, churches, and community centers to foster self-esteem, leadership skills, and career interests in high-risk youth. Youth offenders who would otherwise face incarceration attend day treatment programs coordinated by CIN and the city's family court. The CIN also serves as a referral center for the Philadelphia Private Industry Council's employment training programs, administers summer employment and athletic programs, and champions job readiness training programs.

The CIN claims that it has played an integral role in the decline of gang-related homicide in Philadelphia, which has plummeted from a high of 32 in 1974 to an annual average of 2.18 between 1975 and 1987. Similar programs have been organized in other major US cities such as Los Angeles, Chicago, and Miami (Crisis Intervention Network, 1987; National Committee for Injury Prevention and Control, 1989).

Mad Dads

In 1990, a small group of African-American fathers in Omaha, Nebraska, began patrolling the streets of their neighborhoods. As self-appointed street parents, they were in search of drug dealers and community youth who might be using drugs in an effort to curb violence and a host of other ills associated with drug abuse. According to Frank May, a program development coordinator, Mad Dads endeavor to address the underlying problems that lead people to use drugs. Mad Dads are out en masse on Friday and Saturday evenings, clad in distinctive black and green T-shirts and caps. They go to the places where kids hang out and engage them in dialogue. The organization now has 40 chapters in 12 states across the country.

Bill Patten, the coordinator of substance abuse prevention in Ocala–Marion County, Florida, believes firmly in the positive impact of Mad Dads. Patten explains that in 1990, there were 16 young people killed in one single neighborhood. That was the year Mad Dads began their crusade. Several years after organizing, the same neighborhood experienced only one homicide in the course of a year. Bill Patten summarizes the crux of grass roots violence intervention programs in the following manner: "Mad Dads taught us that ours was not a black or white problem but a community problem. The only way to help a community is for the community to help itself—one house, one block at a time" (Lappe, 1995, pp. 1–2).

PeaceBuilders

PeaceBuilders is a violence prevention program for elementary schoolchildren (K–5) that endeavors to change the school climate in a positive manner and to promote prosocial behavior among students and staff. The main objective of this comprehensive program consists of instilling in children the following five principles: (1) praise people, (2) avoid putdowns, (3) seek wise people as advisors and friends, (4) notice and correct hurts we cause, and (5) right wrongs. PeaceBuilders' activities are deliberately woven into the school's everyday routine to make them a way of life, rather than an isolated exercise without meaningful application. This "way of life" strategy reflects the educational, psychological, and criminology research on which the program is based and is designed to be echoed and reinforced at home, in the community, and in the mass media. In many respects, PeaceBuilders appears to be the embodiment of the African proverb, "it takes a village to raise a child." PeaceBuilders recognizes that violent behavior neither evolves nor flourishes in a vacuum, but rather in a broad social context of harmful or protective factors including neighborhoods, communities, and media. For this reason, the program includes four components: (1) parent education, (2) family marketing, (3) collateral training (for community volunteers), and (4) mass media tie-ins.

The intervention structure of PeaceBuilders entails nine broad behavior change techniques: (1) common language for "community norms," (2) story and live models for positive behavior, (3) environmental cues to signal desired behaviors, (4) role-plays to increase range of responses, (5) rehearsals of positive solutions after negative events, (6) group and individual rewards to strengthen positive behavior, (7) threat reduction to reduce reactivity, (8) self- and peer-monitoring for positive behavior, and (9) generalization promotion to increase maintenance of change across time, places, and people. One of the findings is that "changing the behavior of one child may involve changing the behavior of 10 or more other people" (Embry *et al.*, 1996).

A consortium of the Pima County (AZ) Community Services Department, the University of Arizona, and the Tucson-based company Heartsprings, Inc., is currently conducting a formal evaluation of 10 schools considered to be "at risk." The Embry *et al.* (1996) reported that the program had gained momentum and spread to 55 other schools in the community, mainly as a result of word-of-mouth support from teachers and parents.

Operation Night Light

An innovative crime prevention program in Boston has achieved impressive results in reducing the incidence of homicide among young adults. Like other cities, Boston experienced escalating youth violence. The program is based on pragmatic, inexpensive strategies combining benevolent social programs with aggressive police enforcement. Operation Night Light grew out of a friendship between a Boston police detective active with the Youth Violence Strike Force and a probation officer. At the scene of a youth homicide where both men happened to be present, it became apparent that the youth hovering around the crime scene were much less reluctant to speak with the parole officer than with the police officer. Youth offenders who receive court-ordered curfews are now paid evening visits by teams of parole officers and police officers. Young probationers in violation of their curfews are written up and face possible arrest. In addition to curfew enforcement visits, the Boston Police Department has worked with area churches and businesses over the last few years to develop job programs and recreation opportunities for young offenders. Since the initiation of the Night Light program in 1993, the number of probation violators who have been jailed has tripled, and the rate of curfew compliance among young probationers has jumped from 15% to 70%. The homicide rate for individuals under 24 years of age reportedly dropped more than 70% during 1996, while the number of juveniles arrested for assault with guns declined 81% since 1993 ("Boston finds recipe," 1997).

Drug Abuse Resistance Education (DARE)

The Department of Justice and the Department of the Interior are sponsors of the DARE curriculum, which was developed by the Los Angeles Unified School district. Specially trained uniformed police officers deliver the program to approximately 5,000,000 students annually in all 50 states, and the program even operates internationally. DARE represents a collaborative endeavor between education and law enforcement to provide accurate information, coping, and decision-making skills and positive alternatives to substance abuse. The curriculum is designed to teach students that maturity entails resisting peer pressure, making decisions on one's own, and learning to cope with life's difficulties in positive ways. Components of DARE include curricula for junior high schools, senior high schools, parenting programs, and afterschool activity programs (President's Crime Prevention Council, 1995).

Although DARE appears to promote cordial school–police relations, little hard evidence is available to support the program as an effective means for curbing substance abuse. In a review of the literature that included 17 published and unpublished reports of program evaluation, drug use among schools implementing DARE and drug use among control schools was found to be roughly equivalent. Several longitudinal studies detected neither short- nor long-term benefits from this program, which nonetheless continues to enjoy widespread political and community support, as well as tremendous financial support (Ennett, Ringwalt, & Flewelling, 1993). In fiscal year 1995, the federal government earmarked $1.75 million for DARE implementation, which did not include financial support contributed by community organizations. Plans are currently under way by program developers to revise the DARE curriculum, although more dramatic steps (including well-designed, outcome-based evaluations) may be necessary to revitalize the program and contribute to effective drug abuse prevention among the nation's youth (DiClemente, Hansen, & Ponton, 1996).

Youth Suicide Prevention

In response to increasing incidence rates of suicide and attempted suicide among adolescents and young adults over the past five decades, the CDC's (1992) National Center for Injury Prevention and Control published *Youth Suicide Prevention Programs: A Resource Guide*. This guidebook describes theories and evidence in support of the efficacy of myriad suicide prevention strategies, and it identifies current model programs that incorporate these strategies. Intended for use as a community tool for developing or enhancing existing prevention programs, the report summarizes eight strategies: (1) school gatekeeper training, (2) community gatekeeper training, (3) general suicide education, (4) screening programs, (5) peer support programs, (6) crisis centers and hotlines, (7) restriction of access to lethal means, and (8) intervention after a suicide (CDC, 1992).

Findings described in the CDC's (1994) *Morbidity and Mortality Weekly* with regard to the *Resource Guide* include the observation that most suicide prevention programs target adolescents in high school, while very few include young adults (individuals up to 25 years of age). Perhaps the relative ease of access to adolescents in high school plays an important role in this phenomenon. It was also determined that links between suicide prevention programs and existing community mental health resources frequently are inadequate. Certainly, this is an important hurdle to overcome if programs are to succeed. The lack of evaluation research is the single greatest obstacle to improving current suicide prevention programs for adolescents and young adults. Without evidence to support the potential of programs effectively to reduce suicidal behavior, it is difficult to recommend one particular strategy over another for any given population. In light of this, a multifaceted approach to suicide prevention is currently recommended (CDC, 1994).

Preventing Violence against Women

Seizing the opportunity to address the complex problem of domestic violence is particularly important in health care settings. In one study, partner abuse was found to result in three times more injuries to women than automobile crashes and is the most widely committed but least reported form of violence. One fourth of women in the United States (12 million) will be abused by a current or former partner at some point during their lifetime; phrased another way, 3 to 4 million women are physically abused each year (National Woman Abuse Prevention Project, n.d.). In light of the fact that battered women come into contact with health professionals more often than with police officers, judges, or domestic violence service providers, it is particularly critical that health care providers receive training that will enable them to recognize the signs of domestic violence.

Studies indicate that failure to identify partner abuse is the primary problem with the health care system's response to adult victims of domestic violence. One study, for example, indicated that 40% of women treated in the emergency room showed signs of abuse, although only 4% were actually identified as such (New York State Office for the Prevention of Domestic Violence, 1994). In addition, battered women are likely to see physicians frequently for increasingly severe injuries as a result of the cyclic, escalating nature of domestic violence over time (Stark & Flitcraft, 1979). With proper training, health care providers could become important allies in campaigns to combat domestic violence.

The National Committee for Injury Prevention and Control (1989) suggests that domestic violence intervention protocols must incorporate the following elements to be effective: (1) the identification of suggestive injury and complaint patterns, (2) a review of the medical history, (3) a confidential interview with the woman when battering is suspected, (4) a lethality assessment with battered women, (5) validation of the battered woman's experience, (6) presentation of options for safety and referrals to other services, and (7) the counseling the victim to resist blaming herself.

Health Care Provider Education and Activism

To achieve integration of routine screening for partner abuse during the intake process at local departments of public health, the state of Illinois has implemented a computer-based client management and tracking system called Cornerstone. An abuse assessment question is included on the intake screen; if abuse is indicated, follow-up questions on an additional screen help service providers acquire more information specifically about the abuse (Illinois Department of Public Health, 1996).

Safe at Home

The Milwaukee Women's Center spearheaded a comprehensive campaign to reduce violence against women. The first phase of Safe at Home entails a public awareness project in which all 550 buses of the Milwaukee (Wisconsin) Transit Company display interior placards. In 1996, Safe at Home became one of five community-based, intervention evaluation projects to be funded by the National Center for Injury Prevention and Control. Along with the public awareness campaign, Safe at Home will evaluate three treatment models for working with batterers, provide training for health care professionals, and provide violence prevention education in city schools and the community. The treatment approaches for working with abusive partners will be evaluated individually against their own programmatic goals, rather than evaluated and compared across groups. Curricula are being developed to provide training for groups as diverse as staff in probation and parole offices, emergency department staff in hospitals affiliated with the Aurora Health Care System, and staff from various social service agencies. Referring to the prevention programs, Terri Strodthoff, Project Manager for Safe at Home, observed that most of the men who come to these sessions don't want to be there—they feel pushed into it. ... We hope to help them realize that preventing domestic violence is their responsibility and to give them tools to make a change. So we'll track changes in attitude, as well as changes in behavior. (US Department of Health and Human Services, 1996, p.14)

Lexington Rape Crisis Center

In 1985, the Lexington (Kentucky) Rape Crisis Center was praised as an exemplary program for rape crisis intervention by the National Institute of Mental Health. The center is a private, nonprofit organization providing 24-hour crisis line services, counseling, legal and medical advocacy, as well as companion services for adult survivors of sexual assault and their families. The center is also involved with developing programs to help detect and prevent child sexual abuse. Antirape activities fall into three categories of prevention. Tertiary prevention entails providing services to victims of rape, sexual assault, incest, and child sexual abuse with the objective of assisting the survivor and preventing additional trauma. Secondary prevention is geared toward raising awareness about the scope and extent of the problem and increasing sensitivity and knowledge related to treatment and service delivery as well as providing knowledge and skills to reduce the risk and fear of sexual assault. Finally, primary prevention involves changing societal attitudes and dispelling myths about rape (Lexington Rape Crisis Center, n.d.).

Summary

In closing, let us return to Satcher's analogy of designing violence intervention programs in the same way that we would approach implementing a well-balanced diet: "Although currently we lack the knowledge to construct a violence prevention model with the precision of the nutrition pyramid, we can suggest the components most likely to be important" (Satcher *et al.*, 1996, p. v). Multidisciplinary efforts among public health, criminal justice, and behavioral science professionals hold promise, as do efforts at the community grassroots level. Intervention programs designed to reduce risk factors that develop at family, peer, community, and societal levels need to be developed and implemented. We agree with Dr. Satcher, who emphasizes that all age groups must be addressed and that empirical evidence must guide decisions or, in the absence of such evidence, it must be sought: "In sum, the approach to violence prevention must be diverse and scientific. We need to avoid unitary approaches, draw from and develop a range of workable interventions and mobilize new partnerships representing diverse sectors of our population" (Satcher *et al.*, 1996, p. vi).

References

Anderson, E., McFarlane, J., & Helton, A. (1986). Community-as-client: A model for practice. *Nursing Outlook, 34*, (5), 220–224.

Baker, S. P., O'Neill, B., Ginsburg, M. J., & Li, G. (1992). *The Injury Fact Book, 2nd ed.* New York: Oxford University Press.

Bennett, C. E. (1996). United States Department of Commerce. Economic and Statistics Administration. Bureau of the Census.

Boston finds recipe to cut shootings among young. (Sunday, January 26, 1997). *The Birmingham News*, p. 5A.

Bristow, E., & Collins, J. B. (1989). Family mediated abuse of noninstitutionalized frail elderly men and women living in British Columbia. *Journal of Elder Abuse and Neglect, 1,* 45–64.

Buka, S., & Earls, F. (Winter, 1993). Early detriment of delinquency and violence. *Health Affairs, 12(4),* 46–64.

Centers for Disease Control (CDC). (1992). *Youth suicide prevention programs: A resource guide.* Atlanta, GA: US Department of Health and Human Services, Public Health Service, CDC.

Center for Disease Control (CDC). (1994). Programs for the prevention of Suicide Among Adolescents and Young Adults. *Morbidity and Mortality Weekly Report, 43,* 1–7.

Centerwall, B. S. (1984). Race, socioeconomic status and domestic homicide, Atlanta, 1971–1972. *American Journal of Public Health, 74,* 813–815.

Clark, C. B. (1984). Geriatric abuse: Out of the closet. *Journal of the Tennessee Medical Association, 77,* 470–471.

Crisis Intervention Network. (1987). *Crisis Intervention Network Report, 1975–1987: New approach to youth violence.* Philadelphia: Author.

Cronkite, K. (1994). *On the edge of darkness.* New York: Dell.

Crous, J. S., Cobb, D. C., Harris, B. B., Kopecky, F. J., & Poertner, J. (1981). *Abuse and neglect of the elderly in Illinois: Incidence and characteristics, legislation and policy recommendations.* Chicago: Illinois Department of Aging.

DiClemente, R. J., Hansen, W. B., & Ponton, L. E. (Eds.). (1996). *Handbook of adolescent health risk behavior.* New York: Plenum Press.

Earls, F. (1991). A development to understanding and controlling violence. In H. E. Fitzgerald. (Ed.), *Theory and research in behavioral pediatrics* (vol 5, pp. 61–88). New York: Plenum Press.

Earls, F., Cairns, R., & Mercy, J. (1993). The control of violence and the promotion of nonviolence in adolescents. In S. Millstein, A. Petersen, & E. Nightengale. (Eds.), *Adolescent health promotion* (pp. 285–304). New York: Oxford University Press.

Embry, D. D., Flannery, D. J., Vazsonyi, A.T., Powell, K. E., & Atha, H. (1996). PeaceBuilders: A theoretically driven school-based model for early violence prevention. In *Youth violence prevention: Descriptions and baseline data from 13 evaluation projects,* published as a supplement to the *American Journal of Preventive Medicine, 12,* (5), 91–100.

Ennett, S. T., Ringwalt, C., & Flewelling, R. .L. (1993). *How effective is project D.A.R.E.? A review and assessment of D.A.R.E. evaluations.* San Diego: University of California.

Federal Bureau of Investigation. (1996). *Highlights from crime in the United States, 1995.* Washington, DC: US Government Printing Office.

Harlow, C. W. (1989). *Injuries from crime: Bureau of justice statistics special report,* Pub. No. NCJ-116811. Washington, DC: US Department of Justice, Bureau of Justice Statistics.

Hofstadter, R., & Wallace, M. (1971). *American violence: A documentary history.* New York: Vintage Books.

Illinois Department of Public Health. (1996). *Partner abuse in Illinois: Knowing the facts and breaking the cycle.* Report to the General Assembly.

Kellerman, A. L., Rivara, F. P., Somes, G., Reay, D. T., Francisco, J., Banton, J. G., Prodzinski, J., Fligner, C., & Hackman, B. B. (1992). Suicide in the home in relation to gun ownership. *New England Journal of Medicine, 327,* (7), 467–472.

Lappe, F. M. (September, 1995). The drug war at home—Citizens' success in the streets. *The American News Service,* 1–2.

Lau, E. E., & Kosberg, J. I. (September–October, 1979). Abuse of the elderly by informal care providers. *Aging,* 10–15.

Lowry, P. W., Hassig, S. E., Gunn, R. A., & Mathison, J. B. (1988). Homicide victims in New Orleans: Recent trends. *American Journal of Epidemiology, 128,* 1130–1136.

Mercy, J. A., Rosenberg, M. L., Powell, K. E., Broome, C. V., & Roper, W. L. (1993). Public health policy for preventing violence. *Health Affairs, 12,* (4), 7–29.

Moore, M., Prothrow-Stith, D., Guyer, B., & Spivak, H. (1994). Violence and intentional injuries: Criminal justice and public health perspectives on an urgent national problem. In A. Reiss & J. Roth (Eds.), *Understanding and preventing violence: vol. 4—Consequences and control* (pp. 167–216). Washington, DC: National Academy Press.

Muscat, J. E. (1988). Characteristics of childhood homicide in Ohio, 1974–1984. *American Journal of Public Health, 78,* 822–824.

National Center for Health Statistics (1987). *Advance report of final mortality statistics, 1987.* Hyattsville, MD: National Center for Health Statistics. DHHS Publication Number (PHS)89-1120 (Monthly Vital Statistics Report; vol 38, No. 5 supplement).

National Center for Health Statistics (1992). National Vital Statistics System; US Department of Justice. *Criminal victimization in the United States, 1991*, Pub. No. NCJ-139563. (Washington, DC: US Department of Justice, Office of Justice Programs, Bureau of Justice Statistics.

National Center on Elder Abuse. (1996). *Elder abuse: Questions and answers. An Information guide for professionals and concerned citizens*, 6th ed. Washington, DC: American Public Welfare Association.

National Committee for Injury Prevention and Control (1989). *Injury prevention: Meeting the challenge*. Supplement to the *American Journal of Preventive Medicine, 5*(3), 192–203. New York: Oxford University Press.

National Institute of Mental Health (1992). *Suicide facts*. (National Institute of Mental Health Report). Washington, DC: Author.

New York State Office for the Prevention of Domestic Violence. (Spring 1994). Domestic violence—A public health issue. *OPDV Bulletin*, 3.

O'Carrol, P. W., Rosenberg, M. L., & Mercy, J. (1991). Suicide. In M. L. Rosenberg & M. Fenley (Eds). *Violence in America: Public health approach* (pp. 184–196). New York: Oxford University Press.

Phillips, L. R. (1983). Abuse and neglect of the frail elderly at home: An exploration of theoretical relationships. *Journal of Advanced Nursing, 8*, 379–392.

Pillemer, K., & Finkelhor, D. (1989). Causes of elderly abuse: Caregiver stress versus problem relatives. *American Journal of Orthopsychiatry, 59*, 179–187.

Pillemer, K., & Finkelhor, D. (1988). The prevalence of elder abuse: A random sample survey. *Gerontologist, 28*, (1), 51–57.

Pillemer, K., & Frankel, S. (1991). Domestic violence against the elderly. In M. L. Rosenberg & M. Fenley (Eds.), *Violence in America: A public health approach* (p. 158), New York: Oxford University Press.

The President's Crime Prevention Council. (1995). *Preventing crime and promoting responsibility: 50 programs that help communities help their youth*. Washington, DC: US Government Printing Office.

Reiss, A. J., & Roth, J. (1993). *Understanding and preventing violence* (pp. 1–27). Washington, DC: National Academy Press.

Rich, C. L., Young, J. G., Fowler, R. C., Wagner, J., & Black, N. A. (1990). Guns and suicide: Possible effects of some specific legislation. *American Journal of Psychiatry, 147* (3), 342–346.

Rosenberg, M. L., & Mercy, J. (1986). Homicide: Epidemiologic analysis at the national level. *Bulletin of the New York Academy of Medicine, 62*(5), 376–394.

Rosenberg, M. L., & Mercy, J. A. (1991). Introduction. In Rosenberg & Fenley (Eds.), *Violence in America: A public health approach* (pp. 3–4). New York: Oxford: Oxford University Press.

Satcher, D., Powell, K. E., Mercy, J. A., & Rosenberg, M. L. (1996). Opening commentary: Violence prevention is as American as apple pie. In *Youth violence prevention: Descriptions and baseline data from 13 evaluation projects*. Supplement to the *American Journal of Preventive Medicine, 12*(5), p. v.

Slaby, R. G., & Stringham, P. (1994). Prevention of peer and community violence: The pediatrician's role. *Pediatrics, 94* (4), 608–616.

Stark, E., & Flitcraft, A. (1979). Medicine and patriarchal violence: The social construction of a private event. *International Journal of Health Services, 9*, 461–493.

US Department of Health and Human Services. (1996, Spring/Summer). Public Health Service. Centers for Disease Control and Prevention. Family and Intimate Violence: Milwaukee Mobilizes Resources to Keep Women "Safe at Home." *Injury Control Update*.

US Department of Health and Human Services. National Center for Health Statistics. (1991). *Vital statistics of the United States*, (Vol. 2, Part A, "Mortality," p. 51, tables 1–9, "Death rates for 72 selected causes by 5-year age groups, race, and sex: US 1988). Washington, DC: Government Printing Office.

US Department of Health and Human Services. National Center on Child Abuse and Neglect. (1995, April). National Child Abuse and Neglect Data System, Working Paper 2, 1991 Summary Data Component, May, 1993; Child Maltreatment—1992, May, 1994; and Child Maltreatment—1993. (Internet reference)

US Department of Justice. (1991). *Criminal victimization in the United States* (National Crime Victimization Survey). Washington, DC: Author.

US Department of Justice, Bureau of Justice Statistics. (1988). *Criminal victimization in the United States, 1986: A national crime survey report*. Washington, DC: Bureau of Justice Statistics, US Department of Justice (NCJ-111456).

US House of Representatives, Select Committee on Aging, Subcommittee on Health and Long-Term Care. (1985). *Elder abuse: A national disgrace*. (Committee Publication No. 99–502). Washington, DC: Government Printing Office.

Weiner, N., & Zahn, M. (1989). Violence arrests in the city: The Philadelphia story 1857–1980. In T. Gurr (ed.) *Violence in America: The history of crime* (pp. 102–121). Newbury Park, CA: Sage.

CHAPTER *15*

Unintentional Injury

Philip R. Fine, Andrea D. Tomasek, Wendy S. Horn, and Matthew D. Rousculp

Introduction and Background

In the mid-1980s, the National Research Council described injury as ". . . the principal public health problem in America today" (National Academy of Science, 1985, p. v). Now, more than a decade later, injuries retain this auspicious distinction. Although some argue that acquired immunodeficiency syndrome (AIDS) is a greater public health threat than injury, an objective comparison of morbidity and mortality statistics, risk factors, and lifetime costs demonstrates that, while AIDS clearly deserves much concern and attention, its public health significance pales by comparison to that of injury. For example, during a 1992 presidential debate, then-Arkansas Governor Bill Clinton (1992) stated: "AIDS has (already) killed 150,000 people and 1.25 million are HIV-positive . . . that is, at risk" (Clinton, 1992). Although now-President Clinton did not specify his exact time frame, a review of AIDS-related mortality suggests the period in question was between 1982 and 1992, give or take a year. However, when AIDS and injury statistics were compared, injuries were found to claim as many lives in each and every year as AIDS during the entire decade. Moreover, unlike AIDS, everyone is and will always be at risk of being injured. Finally, while an eventual vaccine is likely for AIDS, there will never be a vaccine capable of immunizing against the many injuries and potential sequelae facing all age groups (see Table 1).

Injuries are physical (i.e., tissue) damage resulting from a transfer of energy or physical damage resulting from the absence of elements or conditions needed to sustain life, such as oxygen or heat. The energy transfer may be acute (i.e., sudden and of very short duration), such as that which occurs in an automobile crash, or the period during which the energy transfer occurs may be protracted, as in the case of carbon monoxide poisoning where death typically occurs after several hours of

Philip R. Fine, Andrea D. Tomasek, Wendy S. Horn, and Matthew D. Rousculp • Injury Control Research Center, University of Alabama at Birmingham, Birmingham, Alabama 35294.

Handbook of Health Promotion and Disease Prevention, edited by Raczynski and DiClemente. Kluwer Academic/Plenum Publishers, New York, 1999.

Table 1. Ten Leading Causes of Death by Age Group—1994[a]

					Age groups						
RA	<1	1–4	5–9	10–14	15–24	25–34	35–44	45–54	55–64	65+	Total
1 RA	Congenital anomalies	Unintentional injuries	Unintentional injuries	Unintentional injuries	Unintentional injuries	Unintentional injuries	HIV	Malignant neoplasms	Malignant neoplasms	Heart disease	Heart disease
2	Short gestation	Congenital anomalies	Malignant neoplasms	Malignant neoplasms	Homicide	HIV	Malignant neoplasms	Heart disease	Heart disease	Malignant neoplasms	Malignant neoplasms
3	SIDS	Malignant neoplasms	Congenital anomalies	Homicide	Suicide	Homicide	Unintentional injuries	Unintentional injuries	Bronchitis Emphysema Asthma	Cerebro-vascular	Cerebro-vascular
4	Respiratory distress syndrome	Homicide	Homicide	Suicide	Malignant neoplasms	Suicide	Heart disease	HIV	Cerebrovascular	Bronchitis Emphysema Asthma	Bronchitis Emphysema Asthma
5	Maternal complications	Heart disease	Heart disease	Heart disease	Heart disease	Malignant neoplasms	Suicide	Cerebro-vascular	Diabetes	Pneumonia and influenza	Unintentional injuries
6	Placenta cord membranes	HIV	HIV	Congenital anomalies	HIV	Heart disease	Homicide	Liver disease	Unintentional injuries	Diabetes	Pneumonia and influenza
7	Unintentional injuries	Pneumonia and influenza	Pneumonia and influenza	Bronchitis Emphysema Asthma	Congenital anomalies	Cerebro-vascular	Liver disease	Suicide	Liver disease	Unintentional injuries	Diabetes
8	Perinatal infections	Perinatal period	Benign neoplasms	HIV	Bronchitis Emphysema Asthma	Liver disease	Cerebro-vascular	Diabetes	Pneumonia and influenza	Nephritis	HIV
9	Pneumonia and influenza	Septicemia	Bronchitis Emphysema Asthma	Benign neoplasms	Pneumonia and influenza	Diabetes	Diabetes	Bronchitis Emphysema Asthma	Suicide	Alzheimer's disease	Suicide
10	Intrauterine hypoxia	Benign neoplasms	Anemias	2 Tied	Cerebro-vascular	Pneumonia and influenza	Pneumonia and influenza	Pneumonia and influenza	HIV	Septicemia	Liver disease

[a] Adapted from the Centers for Disease Control and Prevention, National Center for Injury Prevention and Control's web page. (http://www.cdc.gov/ncipc/pub-res/map.htm)

exposure. Injuries are divisible into two major categories: unintentional and intentional. Unintentional injuries account for approximately two thirds of all injury-related deaths that occur each year and consist of those events commonly referred to as "accidents." These include motor vehicle crashes, falls, fires and burns, poisonings, and drownings. Intentional injuries are those resulting from acts of violence, accounting for the remaining one third of the injury-related deaths. Intentional injuries are subdivided further into the categories of interpersonal and intrapersonal violence. The several components of these two subcategories will be elaborated in this chapter.

Injuries are not accidents. This recently adopted axiom and fundamental distinction between phenomena is critical because accidents, by definition, are unforeseen, unplanned, and unexpected events. In the case of "an accident," the implication is that there was no fault or misconduct on the part of those injured and that which occurred could not have been predicted nor prevented. However, since injuries can be studied in much the same way as infectious and chronic diseases using epidemiological principles and techniques, we have learned that unlike "accidents," injuries are predictable and, to a measurable extent, preventable.

Injury control consists of three distinct but related phases. The first phase, primary prevention, focuses on the ultimate goal of injury control workers and includes the sum total of efforts intended to prevent the occurrence of an event with injury-producing potential. Anti–drunk-driving legislation and its associated enforcement is an example of primary prevention and is intended to keep a motor vehicle crash caused by intoxicated driver from ever occurring. The second phase encompasses the sum total of efforts intended to reduce the severity of injuries when they do occur, since it is not possible to prevent the occurrence of all injury-producing events. Examples of secondary interventions include automobile seat belts and helmets for bicycle and motorcycle operators. The third phase, acute care and rehabilitation, encompasses the sum total of efforts used to preserve life and restore functional capacity after an injury has occurred. Activities such as highly organized, well-trained emergency medical service systems, spinal cord injury care systems, traumatic brain injury care systems, burn centers, poison centers, and rehabilitation centers generally constitute that which the injury control community includes under the rubric of tertiary prevention.

By far, primary prevention is the most cost-effective form of injury control, but in many respects it is also the most abstract and elusive for two reasons. First, it is difficult to measure precisely that which does not happen, especially in the absence of historically accurate surveillance data. Second, cause–effect relationships are notoriously difficult to prove, especially when attempting to ascribe change to something as complex as human behavior. For example, while tough, new anti–drunk-driving laws have been adopted by state legislatures across the country, it cannot be proven, with any measure of certainty, that such laws result directly in a significant reduction in motor vehicle crash mortality statistics. Clearly, a variety of other factors must be considered, such as improved roadway characteristics, vehicle design that is inherently safer today than in the past, a documented reduction in per capita alcohol consumption, and the like. Nonetheless, by its very nature, primary prevention has the potential to be the most cost-effective component of the injury control continuum. Certainly, the least expensive head injury is the one that does not occur.

Epidemiology

Overall, injuries—unintentional and intentional—are the leading cause of death for persons up to 45 years of age. They are the fourth-leading cause of death when all age groups are combined and impact the lives of one in three Americans each year. As the leading killer of children, injuries have been characterized as the last major plague of the young. Approximately 150,000 injury-related deaths were estimated to have occurred each year during the past several decades; about two thirds or 100,000 annual injury-related deaths fall into the unintentional injury category, about half of which, in any given year, result from motor vehicle crashes.

Unintentional Injury Mortality

According to the National Safety Council, the number of annual unintentional injury deaths peaked at 116,385 in 1969. Interestingly, the number of reported motor vehicle-related deaths peaked at 56,278 some 3 years later, in 1972. The cyclic decline in motor vehicle-related mortality after that time appears to reflect an association with the Arab oil embargo, the 55 mile per hour national speed limit of the early 1970s, and the economic recessions of the early and late 1980s (National Safety Council, 1996). However, as with any public health problem, it is important to consider rates rather than relying solely on total numbers to fully appreciate the magnitude of the phenomenon. According to current data, unintentional injury deaths, increased from 91,600 in 1993 to 92,200 in 1994. Motor vehicle death rates also increased in 1994 for the second consecutive year (Graham, 1993). However, over the past quarter century, there has been an overall decline in the number of unintentional injury-related deaths, with a non–motor vehicle death linear trend that appears to be less influenced by economic cycles than for motor vehicle-related deaths (National Safety Council, 1996).

Unintentional Injury Morbidity

Typically, the magnitude of the unintentional injury problem is expressed by citing the number of deaths or the mortality rate resulting from a specific category or cause. However, the extent of the injury problem cannot begin to be appreciated without considering the staggering number of injury-producing events that do not result in a person being killed, but rather being injured badly enough to be rendered temporarily or permanently disabled. The figures are breathtaking: National Safety Council data suggest that each hour of the day throughout the year there are approximately 2,120 disabling injuries (National Safety Council, 1996), translating to over 50,000 disabling injuries per day, nearly 360,000 disabling injuries per week, or approximately 18.6 million disabling injuries annually.

Injury Costs

The economic impact of injuries is estimated by calculating direct costs (the expense associated with medical treatment and rehabilitation) and indirect costs (the projected value of lost earnings and opportunities resulting from short- and long-term disability and/or premature death). Various methods have been used to estimate the lifetime cost of injury (Rice et al., 1989; National Safety Council, 1996). For example, for the 57 million persons injured in 1985, total lifetime costs have been estimated at $157.6 billion dollars, out of which $44.8 billion are estimated to be direct expenses for physicians services, hospital and nursing home care, drugs, and related medical and rehabilitation services (Rice *et al.*, 1989). Mortality costs or losses resulting from premature injury fatalities amounted to $47.9 billion. Finally, the value of lost productivity (morbidity) due to injuries occurring in 1985 was estimated to be $64.9 billion. By 1988, the total lifetime cost of injury estimate had increased approximately 14% to $180 billion (Rice *et al.*, 1989). The National Safety Council extensively revised previous cost-estimating procedures to include new components, the adoption of new benchmarks, and the inclusion of a new discount rate (National Safety Council, 1996), resulting in estimated total costs of unintentional injury in 1994 to be $440.9 billion dollars, an amount that included fatal and nonfatal unintentional injuries together with employer costs, vehicle damage costs, property-related fire losses, wage and productivity losses, medical expenses and administrative expenses (National Safety Council, 1996).

Despite the difference in projected estimates, two conclusions seem inescapable: First, injuries impose a multibillion dollar burden on the economy each year. Second, debate over the relative merits of different techniques for projecting total lifetime costs of injuries is best suited for another forum, because the difference between the two does not significantly lessen the impact of the more conservative figure on our economy or on society as a whole.

Epidemiology of the Major Unintentional Injury Categories

Motor Vehicles

Since 1900, motor vehicle crashes have killed 2.8 million people in the United States (Committee on the National Agenda, 1992). Crashes remain the leading cause of death in this country for persons between 1 and 34 years of age and are the source for more deaths of people between 1 and 75 years of age than any other injury-producing event (Graham, 1993; Baker, O'Neill, Ginsburg, & Guohau, 1992). For persons between 5 and 29 years of age, more than 20% of deaths from all causes (including non–injury-related deaths) are motor vehicle-related, and crashes account for more than 40% of all deaths for persons in their late teens. Crashes are responsible for over 500,000 hospitalizations, with another approximately 5 million injuries not requiring hospitalization each year, and are the major cause of catastrophic spinal cord injuries (60%) and account for between 30 and 60% of all traumatic brain injuries. The National Safety Council estimated the overall costs associated with motor vehicle crashes in 1994 to be approximately $176.5 billion (National Safety Council, 1996).

Falls

Falls are the second-leading cause of unintentional injury-related deaths (Baker *et al.*, 1992). Although falls happen in all age groups, older persons are more vulnerable, and hence more likely to die from falls than any other segment of our population, accounting for more than 10,000 deaths annually among older Americans (United States Public Health Service, 1991). Moreover, these mortality data are probably much higher than suggested, since death certificates may report only the primary cause of death and may miss cases in which, for example, the primary cause of death might be listed as pneumonia but the injured senior citizen may have been bedfast as the result of an earlier fall (Committee on the National Agenda, 1992). Falls are the most common cause of injuries and of trauma-related hospital admissions (Baker *et al.*, 1992), the source of virtually all fractures among the elderly (Fife & Barancik, 1985), and the second- or third-leading cause of brain and spinal cord injury, accounting for approximately 20% of all reported neurotrauma in a given year. Each year, 1 person in 20 is treated in a hospital emergency department because of a fall. Falls in younger age groups account for far fewer deaths but for an enormous amount of nonfatal injury, accounting for only 328 deaths in 1985 among persons up to 19 years of age but nearly 123,000 hospital admissions and over 3.6 million emergency department visits (Gallagher *et al.*, 1982; Guyer & Ellers, 1990; National Committee for Injury Prevention and Control, 1989; Spiegel & Lindaman, 1977). In 1985, total lifetime costs associated with falls was estimated to be in excess of $37 billion, with nearly $10 billion attributable to falls for people over age 65.

Fires and Burns

Deaths resulting from fires and burns occur most often among the very young, the elderly, and in minority populations (Committee on the National Agenda, 1992). The high death rates among children and the elderly appear to be associated with their difficulty in escaping from a residential fire. Some relationship between economic status and fire-related mortality also appears to exist, with house fire death rates being almost five times as high in areas of low per capita income. In recent years, fires and burns have been responsible for approximately 5000 deaths annually (Baker *et al.*, 1992). Residential fires account for about 75% of all fire and burn deaths, with smoke inhalation and resulting carbon monoxide poisoning responsible for two thirds of these deaths (Committee on the National Agenda, 1992). Fires and burns are responsible for nearly 1.5 million injuries annually, and of these, approximately 54,000 require hospitalization (Baker *et al.*, 1992). Burns from sources other than house fires are associated with extensive morbidity; for example, scalds caused 29% of all burn-related hospital admissions in a New York State study (Baker *et al.*, 1992; Committee on the National Agenda, 1992). The estimated lifetime costs for fire and burn-related injuries occurring in 1985 were $3.8 billion, out of which an estimated $920 million were direct costs, $1.5 billion were morbidity-related costs, and $1.4 were mortality related costs (Rice *et al.*, 1989).

Poisonings

Approximately 13,000 poison-related deaths occur each year in the United States. While commonly perceived to be a childhood problem, data reveal that more than 99% of fatal poisonings occur among adults, with almost half attributable to suicide (a self-inflicted intentional injury that is discussed at greater length in Chapter 14). In 1989, less than 5% of all poison-related deaths were reported to poison centers because in such cases death often occurs without help ever having been sought (Baker *et al.*, 1992; Committee on the National Agenda, 1992). While the number of unintentional poisoning deaths in the United States is comparatively modest (i.e., 6500 +), nearly 250,000 persons are admitted to hospitals each year for treatment of poisoning. Between 80,000 and 90,000 poisonings involve children less than 5 years of age, and of these approximately 20,000 require hospitalization. A documented 60% of all calls to poison centers involve children who are less than 5, although this age group constitutes less than one half of 1% of all fatal poisonings (Baker *et al.*, 1992; Committee on the National Agenda, 1992). Including suicides and suicide attempts, poisonings accounted for only 3% of the total injuries in 1985, but were estimated to account for $8.5 billion or 5% of the total lifetime cost of injury.

Drownings

Drowning is defined as a death resulting from suffocation within 24 hours of submersion in water. Between 4000 and 5000 persons are estimated to drown each year in the United States, placing drowning as the third most common cause of unintentional injury-related death for all age groups combined and second for persons between 5 and 44 years of age, excluding deaths resulting from floods or other disasters (Baker *et al.*, 1992; Committee on the National Agenda, 1992). The overall drowning death rate is highest between ages 1 and 18, with persons between 15 and 24 years of age known to be at exceptionally high risk. Drowning is broken down into two major categories: drownings not associated with the use of boats or other watercraft account for approximately 84% of all drownings; those that involve boats primarily used for recreational purposes account for the remaining 16%, although boat-related drownings are often inappropriately classified as water transport deaths and excluded from overall drowning statistics (Baker *et al.*, 1992). For drownings not associated with boats, the rate is highest for children who are 1 to 2 years of age (Baker *et al.*, 1992). The male-to-female ratio is approximately 14 to 1 for drowning related to boats and about 5 to 1 for non–boat-related drownings. Drowning rates are highest among Native Americans and lowest among Asians and whites. For all age groups combined, the drowning rate for African Americans is almost twice that for whites. However, among children between 1 and 4 years of age, the rate among whites is almost twice that for African Americans. There is an inverse relationship between drowning rates and per capita income, which helps to explain why these rates are highest among residents of rural areas, especially among African Americans (Baker *et al.*, 1992). There are many reported cases of permanent disability that result from near-drowning, which is defined as survival beyond 24 hours after suffocation from submersion in water. In fact, it has been estimated that for every 10 children who drown, 36 survive but require a hospital admission and another 140 require emergency medical treatment (Committee on the National Agenda, 1992). On average, drownings and near-drownings account for $2.5 billion in lifetime cost of injury, and per-person costs of near drownings are $65,000 in 1985 dollars, compared with an average fatality cost of $362,000 (Rice *et al.*, 1989).

Firearms

Unintentional fatalities involving firearms account for less than 2% of all unintentional injury deaths and less than 5% of total firearm-related mortality [Baker *et al.*, 1992; Centers for Disease Control (CDC), 1992; Fingerhut, 1993]. While minuscule when compared to unintentional deaths from other causes, the figures defy the popular notion that we are in the midst of an epidemic of firearm-related deaths. The reason for this seeming disparity is that firearm-related mortality are often based on combining all four types of gun-related deaths—homicides, suicides (both of which are obviously intentional) with "accidents" (unintentional) and with deaths involving guns resulting from undetermined motivation—while keeping multiple types of other "causes" separated (Blackman, 1994). There is substantial disagreement on the number of nonfatal gunshot wounds that occur annually. For example, a position paper on firearm injuries appearing in the *Proceedings of the Third National Injury Control Conference* states: ". . . in recent years, more than 65,000 injuries requiring hospitalization and an additional 236,000 less severe injuries have occurred annually from firearms" (Committee on the National Agenda, 1992, p. 291). These figures, when combined, yield an estimated 301,000 nonfatal firearm-related injuries. Using Rice and MacKenzies' (Rice, *et al.*, 1989) own data, there were 236,000 nonfatal firearm-related injuries, not 301,000 injuries. The point to be made is dual. First, while raw numbers are certainly important indices of magnitude, meaningful interpretations of numeric differences—for any and all injuries as well as for other diseases—are only possible if rates are compared. Second, it is essential to separate scientific fact from political agendas, no matter how well-intentioned the latter (Cole, 1995).

Firearm injuries, both unintentional and intentional, were estimated to cost the nation about $14.4 billion dollars in 1985 (Rice *et al.*, 1989) and about $20.4 billion in 1993, out of which approximately $1.4 billion or 6.8% was estimated to go for actual medical care of gunshot wound victims annually (Max & Rice 1993). Other estimates suggest that the actual medical costs of treating gunshot wounds is $4 billion (Chafee, 1992; Mercy & Houk, 1993). These estimates may vary according to the economic models employed. With regard to associated lifetime costs, firearms ($14.4 billion) rank a distant third behind injuries resulting from motor vehicle crashes ($49 billion) and falls ($37 billion). While injuries from firearms account for only one half of 1% of total injuries, they account for 9% of the total lifetime costs (Martin, Hunt, & Hulley, 1988).

Summary

According to the US Department of Health and Human Services, the unintentional injury death rate declined by approximately 14% between 1987 and 1994. Yet, unintentional injuries continue to be the leading cause of death among children and young adults aged 1 to 34 years. As public health and medical advancements through the early part of this century improved survival from infectious diseases, people began living long enough to die from other causes, specifically those related to heart, cancer, stroke, and injuries. Heart disease, cancer, and stroke affect mostly middle-aged and older persons, so it is not surprising nor alarming, when viewed in perspective, that unintentional injuries are the leading cause of death for persons between 1 and 34 years of age. The challenge is to reduce the incidence of injuries to minimal levels by identifying and dealing with realistic risk factors in an organized and systematic way based on rigorously conducted research findings. A decline in hospitalizations for nonfatal unintentional injuries was noted in 1993, when there were 699 hospitalizations per 100,000 persons, falling below the Healthy People 2000 goal of 754 [Department of Health and Human Services (DHHS), 1996]. Although declining hospital admissions with health care delivery system changes may account for some of this reduction in nonfatal unintentional injuries, it is likely that injury control initiatives contributed to the year 2000 hospital admission goal being achieved years in advance of the target date.

An analysis of specific causes of unintentional injury shows decreases in mortality rates in almost every category. Motor vehicle death rates have declined significantly between 1987 and 1994, likely resulting from a variety of National Highway

Traffic Safety Administration (NHTSA)-driven interventions (e.g., seat belts, child restraint systems, motor cycle helmets, vigorous anti-drunk-driving initiatives) in combination with dramatically improved vehicular safety standards as well as highway design standards resulting from NHTSA's regulatory authority (CDC, 1992; National Safety Council, 1996; Haddon, 1980b; Shinar, 1993). Mortality rates from falls and fall-related injuries have declined from 2.7 to 2.5 per 100,000, but hospitalizations for hip fractures increased alarmingly from 714 to 841 per 100,000 persons 65 years of age and older. Thus, falls remain a real health hazard for older persons (DHHS, 1996). Drowning-related mortality rates have declined from 2.1 to 1.7; however, drownings remain the third-leading cause of death for children between 1 and 4 years of age as well as an important cause of death for persons who are intoxicated. The poisoning-related mortality rate has dropped dramatically from 87 per 100,000 to 49 per 100,000 in the 7-year period between 1987 and 1994, likely in part due to a substantial change in the poison reporting process used by poison control centers (DHHS, 1996).

Theoretical Models

Measures to prevent injuries or to lessen the severity of their consequences have been used since ancient times (Haddon, 1980a). Today, the rapidly expanding field of injury control has become a complex mixture of disciplines as diverse as medicine, engineering, sociology, psychology, epidemiology, health education, health promotion, political science, and criminal justice (National Committee for Injury Prevention and Control, 1989). Biomechanics, a subspecialty within engineering, is generally regarded as the "basic" science of injury control (Committee on the National Agenda, 1992; National Academy of Science, 1985).

Nonetheless, while biomechanics is regarded as the basic science of this new discipline, it has been recommended that injury control employ fundamental public health doctrine in its general approach (National Academy of Science, 1985; National Committee for Injury Prevention and Control, 1989; Teutsch, 1992). Thus, the National Center for Injury Prevention and Control, one of the freestanding centers constituting the federal CDC, recommends a four-step approach to injury prevention that reflects this more generic public health doctrine (see Fig. 1) (National Center for Injury Prevention and Control, 1996). The first step in the public health approach addresses surveillance, defining the nature and extent of the problem. Surveillance is considered by many to be the very foundation of injury control because of the need for accurate data that enable injury control workers to establish the incidence, severity, and in some cases even the costs associated with a specific injury or injury category. The second step is to identify the risk factors for a particular type of injury through using analytical techniques that enable scientists to identify groups of individuals at increased risk for injury. It is important during this step to identify both the factors leading to the injury-producing event as well as those factors that increase the likelihood of a more severe injury. The third step is to develop an intervention to prevent injury through one or more interventions intended to: (1) prevent the injury from occurring, (2) prevent exacerbation of the injury, or (3) reduce the potential long-term sequelae or disability often associated with more severe injuries. One of the most important components of any intervention is a well-designed evaluation component capable of measuring the intended outcome. The final step is actual implementation of the intervention at a community level; a goal we recommend should be pursued only

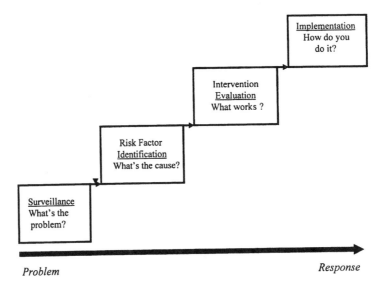

Figure 1. Public health's four step scientific approach to preventing injury and disease. Adapted from National Center for Injury Prevention and Control (1996).

after the intervention's efficacy has been proven in a small-scale, pilot project. Each step of this strategy reflects a logical progression toward the development of a successful injury control program. The strategy's organization is deliberate and sequential, with each component building on the previous one.

Health Behavior Models

In the remainder of this chapter we focus on the theoretical foundation of behavioral change as historically utilized in injury control. Like infectious and chronic disease control (McLeroy *et al.*, 1993), there is no single psychological or social behavioral change theory that is adequate for developing truly effective, comprehensive injury control programs. In part, the reason for this is that injury control is problem focused. This means that injuries are not solely the fault of the victims, but rather are the result of numerous factors. As such, strategies intended to modify behavior must address the behavior of all variables in the injury control equation: individuals, manufacturers, legislators, and regulators (National Committee for Injury Prevention and Control, 1989, pp. 4–18). The models presented herein will exhibit a gradual progression from the basic foundation conceived by Dr. William Haddon to a recently constructed model that incorporates the basic "injury control" philosophy with the current thinking in health behavior.

"Active" and "passive" are terms applied to injury control interventions that describe the role of the individual. Interventions that require cooperation from individuals to confer protection from an injury are defined as active countermeasures. On the other hand, interventions requiring little or no individual action are defined as passive (automatic) countermeasures (Haddon, 1980a). A prime example of each intervention is in passenger restraint systems used in modern motor vehicles. The nonautomatic seatbelt is an active countermeasure, requiring the passenger to buckle up for protection.

The airbag is a passive countermeasure because it does not require the person being protected to do anything. Passive countermeasures will never be unilaterally effective without addressing the psychological–behavioral components of injury-producing events. In fact, Roberts, Fanunik, and Layfield (1987) conclude that for an intervention to be effective, acceptable, and implementable, it will have to be active and individually oriented. This strengthens the premise that the number of cases is limited in which passive countermeasures alone will be sufficient to reduce the risk of injury (Roberts 1987).

The Haddon Matrix

William Haddon, Jr., generally acknowledged as the father of injury control, constructed an aid to resource allocation, strategy identification, and planning paradigm that came to be known as the Haddon matrix (Haddon, 1968, 1972, 1980b). In its simplest form, Haddon's matrix has two dimensions. The first dimension divides an injury producing event into three separate temporal stages: "preevent," "event," and "postevent" or in the case of a motor vehicle-related injury, "precrash," "crash," and "postcrash." These stages correlate with the classic public health notion of primary, secondary, and tertiary prevention, as can be seen in Table 2.

The second dimension of the matrix is divided into three factors that evolved from a classic, epidemiological model. The theory about injury occurrence is based on the premise that like other diseases, injuries only occur when certain factors are present. Gordon (1949) gave examples of how injuries can be characterized by point epidemics, seasonal variations, long-term trends, and geographic and socioeconomic factors. Gordon's descriptive studies on injuries parallel those of infectious disease used in constructing the host–agent–environment model (H-A-E model) (Haddon, 1980a). The H-A-E model is based on the epidemiological triad used in identifying intervention points. In this model, the host is the individual in which a disease process or an injury occurs. The agent is an environmental entity whose excess or relative absence is necessary for the particular disease or injury to occur (e.g., energy or lack of an essential component such as oxygen or heat). The agent is brought into contact with the host through a vehicle or vector (e.g., a motor vehicle, a knife, a gun, etc.).

Table 2. Summary of Correspondence of Haddon's Stages with Classic Public Health Notion of Primary, Secondary, and Tertiary Prevention

	Levels of prevention	
	Classic	Haddon
Primary	Focus during stage of subclinical disease. (Reduce incidence.)	Prevent the event from occurring. This can be accomplished by controlling the hazard. (Eradicate event or reduce the frequency of its occurrence.)
Secondary	Focus during stage of susceptibility. (Reduce complications.)	Prevent the impairment from progressing to a disability. This can be accomplished by minimizing the energy transfer through the modification of the environment, the agent, or the host.
Tertiary	Focus during stage of clinical disease. Prevent long-term disability.	Minimize the dependency that might otherwise ensue. Accomplished by organizing and applying the treatment and rehabilitation resources of the community.

The environment is composed of many factors that affect both the exposure of potential hosts to agents and the ability of the host to maintain a high level of resistance to the agent. The environment can be divided into physical or social components.

Consider a hypothetical case involving a head-on crash between two motor vehicles in a rural area. One of the drivers is drunk, has been convicted repeatedly of driving under the influence of alcohol (DUI), and is not wearing a seatbelt on this rainy evening. In this situation, some of the factors that could lead to injury and thus be identified using the Haddon matrix are summarized in Table 3.

Haddon also developed what he termed "10 logically based strategies" for reducing damage from injury-producing events (Haddon, 1970; Waller, 1987). Though Haddon's initial strategy was to be injury specific, his countermeasures can be used to reduce damage (to either animate or inanimate objects) from all forms of agents. Since being introduced, it has become a basic tool that can be helpful in public health and throughout other professions (McLeroy, et al., 1993). Countermeasures were defined according to phases (Haddon, 1970; Waller, 1987). During the preinjury phase (primary prevention), the three countermeasures consisted of: (1) prevent the creation of the hazard in the first place; (2) reduce the amount of hazard brought into being; and (3) prevent the release of the hazard that already exists. During the injury phase (secondary prevention), the five countermeasures consisted of: (1) modify the rate or spatial distribution of release of the hazard from its source; (2) separate, in time or space, the hazard and that which is to be protected; (3) separate the hazard and that which is to be protected by interposition of a material barrier; (4) modify relevant basic qualities of the hazard; and (5) make what is to be protected more resistant to damage from the hazard. The two countermeasures associated with the postinjury phase (tertiary phase) include: (1) begin to counter the damage already done by the environmental hazard; and (2) stabilize, repair, and rehabilitate the object of the damage. To prevent an injury, only one countermeasure may be needed. However, implementing more than one countermeasure may be prudent (Waller, 1987). As mentioned, these countermeasure strategies are not injury control specific. Rather, they are useful strategy organizers for all health-oriented prevention interventions. In fact, one of Haddon's classic examples using this strategy focused on prevention of unplanned pregnancies (Haddon, 1970).

Table 3. Haddon's Matrix as Applied to Example of Drunk Driving

	Factors		
Phases	Host	Agent (vehicle)	Environment physical / psychosocial
Preevent	I	II	III
Event	IV	V	VI
Postevent	VII	VIII	IX

[a] Variables that play a role in the outcome of injuries in example of driving under the influence of alcohol:

I	Alcohol impairment	VIa	Physical: Slippery roadway
II	Speed of travel	VIb	Psychosocial: Society's attitude about seat belt use
IIIa	Physical: Nondivided highway	VII	Age of the injured persons
IIIb	Psychosocial: Laws sentencing of DUI	VIII	Integrity of auto fuel system
IV	Not wearing seat belts	IXa	Physical: Effectiveness of emergency communication system
V	Design of auto's interior and how it changes during a crash	IXb	Psychosocial: Availability of medical insurance

The Haddon countermeasures focus primarily on changing or controlling the agent and the environment, but less so in relation to the host. This should not be construed as diminishing the importance of the role of the individual in controlling injuries, but rather represents a shift in injury control thinking from "blaming the victim" to the inclusion of other factors in the prevention of injury (McLeroy et al., 1993). The modern view of injury control does not eliminate personal responsibility, but it does assign greater weight to other factors. Additionally, Haddon's model represents a complete menu, but does not offer direct guidance as to which options should be given the highest priority or which countermeasure or mixture of countermeasures will produce the greatest return in terms of cost-benefits (Haddon, 1970; Waller, 1987).

Precede–Proceed Model

The precede–proceed model, developed for widespread use in general health promotion and disease prevention (Green & Kreuter, 1991), is often employed in the field of injury control (Gielen, 1992; Macrina, Macrina, Horvath, Gallaspy, & Fine, 1996; McLeroy et al., 1993; National Committee for Injury Prevention and Control, 1989). The overriding principle of this planning model centers on the notion that the most enduring health behavior change is voluntary. A systematic planning process was developed to empower individuals with understanding, motivation, and skills needed to become active in community affairs so as to improve their quality of life (Glanz & Rimer, 1995). The precede–proceed model consists of nine phases that can be grouped into diagnostic, implementation and evaluation categories. The application of behavioral theory occurs primarily in the behavioral and environmental diagnosis, educational and organizational diagnosis, and administrative and policy diagnosis (Glanz & Rimer, 1995). More specifically, it is within the educational and organizational diagnosis phase that this model addresses the factors that shape behavioral actions and environmental factors. In this phase, the primary study of interest is shaped by predisposing, reinforcing, and enabling factors (Green & Kreuter, 1991). In the precede–proceed model, *predisposing factors* provide the motivation, or reason, behind a behavior; this includes relevant knowledge, attitude, and cultural beliefs. *Enabling factors* make it possible for a motivation to be realized; this includes the availability and accessibility of personal resources, supportive policies, and community services. *Reinforcing factors* come into play after a behavior has begun and provide continuing rewards or incentives; this includes social support, praise, reassurance, and symptom relief (Glanz & Rimer, 1995; Green & Kreuter, 1991).

One example of an injury control intervention using the precede–proceed model is a program initiated to increase the documentation of the Glasgow Coma Score (GCS) of trauma patients in hospital emergency departments (see Fig. 2) (Macrina et al., 1996). The GCS is a clinical tool used to measure a patient's neurological status by assessing orientation, eye opening, and limb movement. In addition to being a clinical tool, research has determined that the GCS is a predictor of survivor outcome after traumatic brain injury and found that the GCS score is a tool used by physicians in their decision to refer patients to rehabilitation (Wrigley, Yoels, Webb, & Fine, 1994). In spite of the proven utility and relative simplicity, the GSC's use has been less than optimal. Therefore, Macrina et al. implemented an educational program to increase the use and documentation of the GCS by emergency department nurses. Education alone was not enough to produce change; however, GCS education combined with changes in hospital policy resulted in greater assessment by emergency department staff (Macrina et al., 1996).

Integrative Planning Network

A unique planning model integrating the Haddon matrix, Haddon countermeasures, and the precede–proceed model into a four-step plan for injury control interventions has been devised by Dr. Andrea Gielen (Gielen, 1992). Step 1, epidemiological diagnosis, involves problem diagnosis via descriptive epidemiological analysis, addressing variables such as mortality and morbidity data, characteristics of the individuals at greater risk of being injured (e.g., sex, age, ethnicity, and other injury-specific risk factors), and different data that are specific to the injury-producing hazard. Step 2, environmental and behavioral diagnosis, involves access to the nonbehavioral and behavioral determinants associated with the specific injury-producing incident. Referring to the H-A-E model, the nonbehavioral component includes the environment and the agent and the behavioral component refers to host factors. Step 3, influencing factors diagnosis, consists of accepting that multiple factors exist that determine whether an injury-producing event will occur, and if such an event does occur, determining which factors determine severity of injury among both the behavioral and nonbehavioral determinants. To organize various factors, Gielen suggests using predisposing, enabling, and reinforcing factors from the precede–proceed model. Finally, Step 4, intervention planning, involves examining the distribution of individuals affected, and the determining factors that are attributed to the particular injury of interest are identified. Specific interventions can be linked using known information addressing the predisposing, enabling, and reinforcing factors for behavioral and nonbehavioral determinants.

Interventions can be divided into three separate categories: (1) education–behavior change, (2) engineering–technology, and (3) legislation–enforcement (see Fig. 3). The

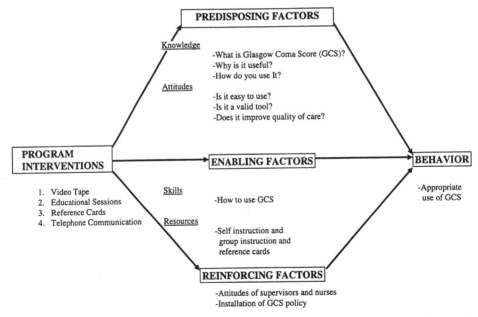

Figure 2. Adaptation of the precede–proceed model used for an educational intervention to increase the use the Glasgow Coma Scale by emergency department nurses. From Macrina *et al.* (1996).

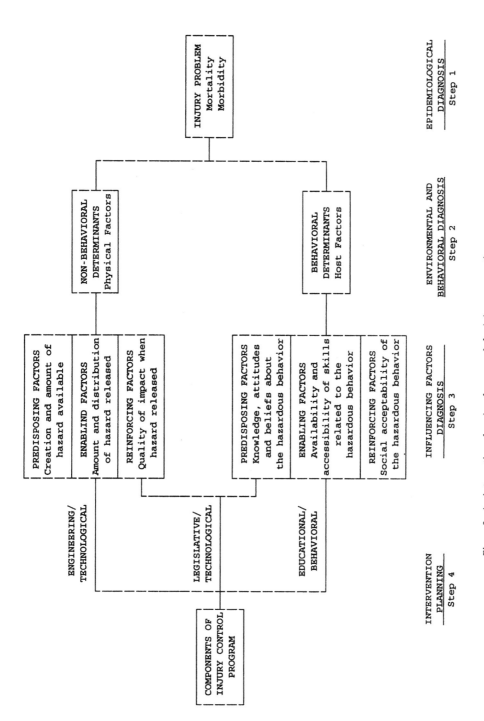

Figure 3. An integrative planning framework for injury prevention programs.

education–behavior change category addresses behavioral determinant factors. Gielen (1992) recognized that educational strategies are often employed in informing and persuading decision makers such as legislators and manufacturers, but within this framework, the education–behavior change category refers to interventions addressing change in behavior of the individuals at risk. As for the second and third categories, engineering–technology interventions generally address factors associated with nonbehavioral determinants, while legislation–enforcement interventions may address either behavioral or nonbehavioral determinants. In the schematic of Gielen's model, it may appear that equal weight is given to each of the plausible intervention categories, although that is not really the intention. In fact, Gielen adheres to the injury control principle that passive systems that do not require any action on the part of the individual are generally more effective.

Unintentional Injury: The Interventions

As discussed earlier in this chapter, designing an effective intervention often requires a well-choreographed balancing act. Proposed curtailment of personal liberty must be carefully scrutinized and weighed against the expected benefit to society as a whole. For example, passive strategies (e.g., automatic seat belts) are likely to be more efficacious than those requiring radical behavioral changes; however, alienation of the public also may become an unwanted side effect. On the other hand, attempting to coax a target population into long-term behavior modification is also fraught with difficulty and may not be realistic, or may run the risk of appearing to "blame the victim" or place an inordinate burden of responsibility for injury prevention on the individual. Gielen (1992) has examined the tension between those in the field of injury prevention who endorse circumventing the role of individual behavior through the provision of automatic or passive protection and those who support attempting to change the behavior of the individual. Ideally, the two approaches can complement one another and provide a stronger framework for effective intervention than either approach by itself (Gielen, 1992). Another facet of this controversy entails designing interventions that successfully meld educational, legal, and engineering components. As one might expect, striking a balance can be challenging at best and an exercise in frustration at worst.

Primary Prevention

Primary prevention entails successful avoidance or prevention of a disease or injury (Pickett & Hanlon, 1990). Familiar examples include improving highway design (Finkelstein & Smolkin, 1987), requiring child-resistant caps on many drugs and medications (CDC, 1985; Clarke & Walton, 1979; Walton, 1982), and requiring children's sleepwear to be constructed of flame-retardant fabric (McLoughlin et al., 1977). Described below are several injury prevention programs and examples that illustrate combinations of educational, legal, and engineering strategies in the prevention of unintentional injuries.

Children Can't Fly

In response to a high incidence rate of children falling from windows of high-rise apartment buildings, the New York City Department of Health launched a pilot program in 1972 known as Children Can't Fly. This program illustrates the potential effectiveness of injury prevention programs combining environmental, behavioral, and regulatory components. Intervention strategies included free distribution (and in some cases installation) of window guards, mass media campaigns, community outreach activities, education about the hazards of unguarded windows for at-risk families, and follow-up visits to families of fall victims to provide referrals and window guards and to collect demographic and sociological data. A 35% decline in childhood mortality related to falls from heights was documented between 1973 and 1975. In 1976, the New York City health code was amended to include a requirement that landlords provide window guards in apartment buildings inhabited by children under 10 years of age, and the educational interventions were revised to reflect this new mandate. Property owners were advised regarding compliance with the regulation and families with children under 10 years of age were informed about their right to window guard installation. This third component of the intervention culminated in an overall reduction of 50% in childhood mortality stemming from falls from high-rise apartments (Spiegel & Lindaman, 1977).

LifeSavers: A Residential Fire Injury Prevention Project

In November 1986, burn injuries resulting in hospitalization or death became a reportable condition in the state of Oklahoma. During 32 months of data collection, Oklahoma City had the highest rate of residential fire-related injuries among cities reporting greater than 10 injuries, accounting for 66 injuries and 34 deaths. Two thirds of the injuries were concentrated in the southern region of the city, which included predominately nonwhite, nonblack ethnic minorities with lower median household incomes and lower housing condition ratings when compared to the rest of the city. In an effort to combat this phenomenon, the Oklahoma State Department of Health developed the Oklahoma Injury Prevention Project in conjunction with the Oklahoma City Fire Department and a variety of other organizations.

The objective of the intervention was to assess the efficacy of a large-scale smoke alarm giveaway (10,000 alarms) in reducing morbidity and mortality stemming from residential fires in south Oklahoma City. Four methods of participant solicitation were evaluated as well as two methods of smoke alarm distribution and installation. Distribution strategies included either: (1) canvassing neighborhoods with a fire truck, sounding its alarm, and announcing over a loudspeaker system that volunteers were distributing free smoke alarms curbside, (2) mailing flyers to all residents informing them of a free smoke alarm distribution program, (3) posting the flyers in public places, or (4) placing flyers in residential doors. The canvassing method proved by far the most efficacious, with approximately 80% of the homes in need within the targeted area receiving alarms. Final analysis indicated that between May 1, 1990 (when the intervention began) and April 30, 1994 (48 month follow-up), there was a 73% decrease in the rate of injury compared to a 30% increase in the remainder of Oklahoma City. Furthermore, preliminary cost-benefit analysis suggests an impressive ratio of 1:20 or a savings of $20 for every $1 invested (Injury Update, 1995).

Queens Boulevard Pedestrian Safety Project

One of the most celebrated endeavors in the prevention of pedestrian injuries among the elderly took place in New York City in 1985. Based on police reports from 1982 to 1984, the Traffic Safety Unit of the New York City Police Department plotted severe and fatal pedestrian injuries on a spot map of the city. The spot map, a classic tool in epidemiological outbreak investigations, revealed that 39 severe and fatal injuries occurred along a 2 ½-mile stretch of Queens Boulevard. Upon scrutiny, 75% of those injured and 85% of those killed were found to be over the age of 65. In the city as a whole, only 30% of pedestrian fatalities were among this age group. A thorough investigation determined that: (1) Queens Boulevard is very wide, requiring pedestrians to cross distances of 150 feet; (2) the boulevard is heavily trafficked; (3) the 30 mile per hour speed limit is often exceeded; (4) the "WALK" signs allowed only 35 seconds for pedestrian crossing, although elderly individuals required an average of 50 seconds to cross the boulevard; (5) vision loss among the elderly contributed to confusion regarding the direction from which traffic was approaching, as well as making it difficult to read the signs; and (6) indistinct boundaries between the curb and street often contributed to the elderly stepping off the curb and into the path of oncoming vehicles.

The Traffic Safety Unit incorporated the following key elements: (1) increased police enforcement of the speed limit and installation of oversized speed limit signs at frequent intervals; (2) placement of additional "WALK/DON'T WALK" signs on medians and resetting signs to allow greater time for crossing; (3) painting large arrows on the pavement near crosswalks to indicate from which direction traffic would be approaching; (4) painting median island edges to provide a visible distinction between the curb and the street; and (5) launching a consciousness-raising campaign for senior citizens in the vicinity regarding pedestrian injuries. A comparison of the injury data for Queens Boulevard 30 months after program implementation and 5 years prior to implementation demonstrated a 60% reduction in the rate of fatal and severe injuries (National Committee for Injury Prevention and Control, 1989).

The Injury Prevention Program (TIPP)

Initially developed by the American Academy of Pediatrics in 1983, TIPP was expanded in 1988 to include age-specific topics tailored for newborns through children 12 years of age. The educational program provides pediatricians with a systematic method for counseling parents regarding the adoption of behaviors likely to prevent the occurrence of injuries. The Academy developed a schedule of recommended counseling topics for each preventive health visit, complete with safety sheets to distribute to parents and safety surveys to assist the health care provider in pinpointing individual counseling needs of each family (American Academy of Pediatrics, n.d.). A cost-benefit analysis of TIPP demonstrated that every dollar spent on TIPP counseling targeting children from ages 0 to 4 years yielded a return of nearly $13 saved in injury costs (Miller & Galbraith, 1995).

Safe Moves

Safe Moves was founded in 1983 by Pat Hines, world-class bicycle racer, in response to the death of a friend in a bicycle crash while training for the 1984 Olympic trials. The primary objective of Safe Moves is to achieve a reduction in traffic-related fatalities through educational programs designed to reduce the vulnerability of child pedestrians and bicyclists in their communities. Safe Moves targets all preschools, elementary schools, and middle schools in the city and county of Los Angeles. Through various partnerships, the nonprofit organization brings interactive workshops, traffic safety rodeos, parent training seminars, and community outreach programs to approximately 1 million children and families each year. Evaluation data reveal benefits from the program. By evaluating school attendance and health records, a 34% decrease in bicycle- and pedestrian-related injuries and deaths in the city and county of Los Angeles were documented (Safe Moves, 1994; US Department of Transportation, 1996).

Louisiana's Car Seat Loaner Program

The state of Louisiana implemented an innovative approach to documenting that correct usage of child car seats and education of parents play a vital role in saving young lives. A statewide survey revealed that only about 18% of children in Louisiana were restrained in car seats or by seat belts, prompting the Office of Public Health to launch a car seat loaner program at local health departments in three southeastern Louisiana parishes in 1990. In addition to loaning the car seats, health educators accompanied parents to the family car to demonstrate correct installation and use of the seats in the car. Out of 26 car seats known to have been involved in collisions between 1990 and 1993, 24 car seats were returned and police information was obtained regarding 23 of the incidents. Out of the 23 crashes for which information was available, 17 resulted in hospitalization or death of at least one unrestrained adult occupant; however, none of the crashes resulted in the serious injury or death of an infant or small child (Child Car Safety Seats, 1996).

Harlem Hospital Injury Prevention Program

A study conducted in 1984 by the Pediatric Trauma Service of Harlem Hospital Center and the Columbia University School of Public Health documented that a high percentage of local children were sustaining serious injuries, many requiring hospitalization. Further research indicated that this phenomenon was the result of dangerous and filthy playground areas that prompted children to play in the street, leading to increased vehicle–pedestrian crashes and bicycle collisions. The Harlem Hospital injury prevention team came into being with assistance from hospital staff, community leaders, community-based organizations, and parent associations, among other groups. Playgrounds were renovated and new playgrounds were built, transportation injury prevention programs were sponsored, and the hospital implemented a car seat loaner program and a low-cost bike helmet distribution program. These efforts resulted in a 55% reduction in hospital injury admissions of Harlem children under 17 years of age and culminated in the organization receiving the 1996 Secretary of Transportation's Community Partnership Award (US Department of Transportation, 1996).

Drivers' Education

Occasionally, the development and implementation of injury control programs appear so rational and prudent that evaluation falls by the wayside. Driver's education is a rather surprising example of this phenomenon. One would think that if lack of driving skill or driver error plays a significant role in motor vehicle crashes, then bolstering those skills through training should lead to a reduction in crashes. However, driver education training in high schools does not appear to reduce the number of crashes per mile driven, but rather increased the number of licensed young drivers. Ultimately, this development led to an increased risk of motor vehicle crashes among this cohort as a result of increased numbers of young drivers on the road (Shaoul, 1975). Teenagers who attended high schools that had discontinued drivers' education programs were also found to be involved in fewer crashes than their counterparts attending schools that retained the programs (Robertson, 1980). The Third National Injury Control Conference concluded that raising the minimum age of licensure may reduce the risk of crashes stemming from driver immaturity (USDHHS, 1991). It seems logical that the next phase in the evolution of educating teenaged drivers would combine an older age at the time of licensure with tactics from traditional driver's education programs.

Drownproofing

Another injury prevention strategy that has generated considerable controversy is organized swimming and "drownproofing" lessons for infants and young children. Some experts believe that rather than guarding against unintentional immersion, prematurely exposing children to training may increase a child's risk of drowning as a result of increasing exposure to the water, decreasing fear of the child near water, and encouraging a false sense of security among parents (National Committee for Injury Prevention and Control, 1989). For this reason, the American Academy of Pediatrics does not endorse swimming instruction for children under 5 years of age (Committee on Accident and Poison Prevention, 1987). The efficacy of swimming pool barriers, on the other hand, has been documented in several studies of childhood pool drownings, preventing 70% of the fatalities in one study (Baxter, n.d.). Although swimming lessons are certainly worthwhile for older children, this is clearly a case in which a technological injury countermeasure (i.e., pool enclosures) is more effective than an educational intervention by itself.

Tap Water Burn Prevention

In 1983, Washington state approved legislation requiring new water heaters to be preset at 120° F (49° C) as a means of reducing the incidence of scald injuries (Erdmann *et al.*, 1991). Compared to an average of 5.5 hospital admissions per year as a result of scalding during the 1970s, an average of 2.4 people per year were admitted from 1979 to 1988. Compared to the 1970s, total body surface area burned, grafting, scarring, length of hospital stay, and mortality were also all reduced. Among admitted patients, however, the likelihood of scald burns as a result of abuse was found to be 1.6 times greater at the time of follow-up (1988) than between 1969 and 1976, possibly suggesting a greater awareness of the manifestations of abusive tap water scalds.

Researchers in Kentucky designed a prospective study to evaluate the impact of care-giver education and antiscald device installation on the incidence of pediatric scald burns. Data from the Kosair Children's Hospital Trauma Registry were analyzed to determine the zip code area at greatest risk. Overall admissions to the Kosair Children's Hospital Burn Unit as a result of scald injuries declined the year following implementation of the project. During the year prior to the intervention (1989), 48% of 31 admitted scald victims were from the targeted zip code area, compared to 32% of 37 admitted scald victims during 1991 (Fallat & Rengers, 1993).

Secondary Prevention

According to the National Center for Injury Prevention and Control, secondary prevention curtails the progression of an injury or disease from an impairment to a disability (Pickett & Hanlon, 1990). In cases where an impairment has already occurred, disability may be prevented or minimized through early intervention. Often this entails acute care or emergency care, during which time is of the essence; prehospital care, stabilization in the emergency department, and surgical intervention in the operating room must all be provided within the first critical postinsult "Golden Hour" (Pre-Hospital Trauma Life Support Committee of the National Association of Emergency Medical Technicians in Cooperation with the Committee on Trauma of the American College of Surgeons, 1994). Examples of secondary prevention interventions include the development of regional poison control centers (Thompson *et al.*, 1983) with 24-hour hotlines (National Committee for Injury Prevention and Control, 1989), use of the Glasgow Coma Scale in the management of traumatic brain injury (Macrina *et al.*, 1996), and the use of helicopters as a component of well-developed trauma systems (Baxt & Moody, 1983). The use of bicycle helmets and the installation of seat belts and air bags in automobiles also fall under the rubric of secondary prevention. Refinements in patient treatment strategies comprise another facet of secondary prevention. For example, Dr. Michael Rosner has determined that using cerebral perfusion pressure management techniques in patients with traumatic brain injuries results in outcomes superior to those achieved using traditional techniques based on management of intracranial pressure (Rosner, Rosner, & Johnson, 1995).

Bicycle Helmet Campaigns

The Seattle Children's Helmet Campaign and the Howard County Helmet Legislation Campaign in Maryland are both examples of multifaceted, successful injury control interventions. Effectiveness of the Seattle campaign (launched in 1986) is largely attributed to clear objectives and strategically directed interventions on the part of project coordinators, while success of the Howard County campaign (legislation passed in 1990) resulted from a synergistic convergence of multiple factors.

Activism in Seattle

Project coordinators at the Harborview Injury Prevention and Research Center (HIPRC) in Seattle, Washington decided to restrict the scope of their helmet campaign to three clearly defined objectives: (1) to convince parents that riding bicycles without helmets is hazardous; (2) to lower the price of helmets to more affordable levels; and

(3) to overcome the reluctance of children to wear helmets. Although 8- to 16-year-olds sustain the greatest numbers of bicycle-related head injuries, elementary schoolchildren were selected as the target group (i.e., attempting to alter the behavior of teenagers was deemed overly ambitious). Educational messages designed to raise parental awareness regarding the importance of helmet use emanated from a variety of sources: physician offices, hospitals, health departments, events such as trade shows for parents, and most importantly, mass media public service announcements (newspapers, television, and radio). Lowering the price of bicycle helmets became a reality when Mountain Safety Research created a subsidiary to mass-produce and market helmets under a new label. Overcoming the "nerd factor" required a bit of creativity. Prominent sports figures were recruited from the Seattle Seahawks, Seattle Mariners, and the University of Washington Huskies to promote helmet use as a standard component of any bicyclist's uniform, just as they are for baseball batters and football players. An observational survey conducted in September 1989, indicated that the helmet use rate among Seattle schoolchildren had risen to 23% from a baseline of 5%. During the course of the study, Portland, Oregon, served as a control community. As of September 1988, the helmet use rate had increased to only 3% from a baseline of 1% (Bergman *et al.*, 1990; Rivara *et al.*, 1994).

Education and Legislation in Howard County

Howard County, Maryland, was the first area in the country to mandate the use of helmets for bicyclists under 16 years of age. Introduction of the legislation fortuitously coincided with a national helmet promotion campaign designed by the American Academy of Pediatrics. The kickoff for the campaign was a highly visible event at a local elementary school that received a great deal of publicity from both local newspapers and television stations. Reports from legislators suggest that the testimonies of health professionals and students during the hearing were particularly persuasive, as well as the following factors: (1) epidemiological surveillance helped focus national attention on the issue; (2) a specific, feasible strategy for preventing bicycle-related head injuries had been identified; (3) bicycle safety programs at the local level had been endorsed and promoted by highly regarded organizations such as the American Academy of Pediatrics and the Johns Hopkins University School of Hygiene and Public Health; (4) through educational and legislative approaches, highly motivated students and teachers organized a local movement to reduce head injuries stemming from bicycling; (5) highlighting of the issue by the media; and (6) the concerted efforts of a local councilman in introducing the helmet bill. Multifaceted efforts are indispensable to the passage of new public health legislation (Cote *et al.*, 1992; Scheidt, Wilson, & Stern, 1992).

Tertiary Prevention

Arresting the progression of a disability to a state of dependency is the role of tertiary prevention (Pickett & Hanlon, 1990). Expedient medical care followed by rehabilitation can prevent some of the dependencies associated with traumatic injuries such as spinal cord injuries. Patients who are confined to wheelchairs can help prevent pressure sores, as well as muscle atrophy in their upper bodies by doing simple wheelchair push-ups. Other examples of pressure sore prevention include proper bed, positioning and frequent turning, protective devices that prevent the heel from touching the patient's bed, and the use of special, pressure-relieving wheelchair cushions (Stover, DeLisa, & Whiteneck, 1995). In some cases, rehabilitation professionals have played indispensable roles in primary prevention activities. During the mid-1970s in Seattle, Washington, for example, physicians at the University of Washington Spinal Cord Injury Center noticed an increase in the frequency of adolescents with broken necks, leading to a successful campaign to remove trampolines, the source of the injuries, from schools (National Committee for Injury Prevention and Control, 1989).

Summary

Unintentional injuries result in nearly 100,000 deaths and millions of nonfatal injuries each year. Unintentional injuries are the leading cause of death in the United States for people aged 1 to 44. The leading causes of death from unintentional injuries are motor vehicle crashes, fires, burns, falls, drownings, and poisonings. Unintentional injury statistics are sobering. For example, according to the National Center for Injury Prevention and Control (1989) and other reliable sources, motor vehicle crases are the leading cause of death in the United States for people aged 1 to 34; for every injury death, there are approximately 19 hospitalizations, 233 emergency department visits, and 450 office-based physician visits; motor vehicle crashes claimed the lives of approximately 5,800 teenagers and 2,600 children between the ages of birth and 12 years in 1994; drowning is the second-leading cause of death due to unintentional injuries among children and young adults; each year about 60,000—nearly 165 people each day—are hospitalized for burns; among people over age 65, falls account for about 7,400 deaths each year; alcohol is involved in many injuries, including 40% of all deaths due to motor vehicle crashes and about 40% of deaths in residential fires; and, each year, over 600,000 people are treated in hospital emergency departments and over 800 die from bicycle injuries. Because of their diverse etiology, the very nature of injury control necessitates a multidisciplinary approach to problem solving. As a consequence, professionals representing a constellation of disciplines as well as individuals potentially affected by the injury problem should participate in defining the problems and planning solutions (Gielen, 1992).

References

American Academy of Pediatrics. (1994). TIPP: The Injury Prevention Program, A Guide to Safety Counseling in Office Practice. Elk Grove Village, Illinois: Author.

Baker, S. P., O'Neill, B., Ginsburg, M. J., & Guohau, L. (1992). *The injury fact book*, 2nd ed. New York: Oxford University Press.

Baxt, W. G., & Moody, P. (1983). The impact of a Rotorcraft aeromedical emergency care service on trauma mortality. *Journal of the American Medical Association, 249* (22), 3047–3051.

Baxter, L. (n.d.). 1986–1987 Consumer product safety commission study of child drownings. In D. Brill, S. Micik, & J. Yuwilwe (Eds.), *Childhood drownings: Current issues and strategies for prevention* (pp. 37–44). Orange, CA: California Drowning Prevention Network, North County Health Service. Orange County Trauma Society.

Bergman, A. B., Rivara, F. P., Richards, D. D., & Rogers, L. W. (1990). The Seattle Children's Bicycle Helmet Campaign. *American Journal of Diseases of Children, 144,* 727–731.

Blackman, P. H. (1994, March). *The federal factoid factory on firearms and violence: A review of CDC research and politics*. A paper presented at the annual meeting of the Academy of Criminal Justice Sciences, Chicago, Illinois.

Centers for Disease Control (CDC). (1985). Update: Childhood poisonings—United States. *Morbidity and Mortality Weekly Report, 34* (9), 26–27.

Centers for Disease Control (CDC). (1992). Unintentional firearm-related fatalities among children and teenagers—United States, 1982–1988. *Morbidity and Mortality Weekly Report, 41*, 442–445.

Chaffee, Senator John. (October 1, 1992). Testimony before the Senate Committee on the Judiciary on Children Carrying Weapons.

Child car safety seats: Imaginative Louisiana program links education and evaluation. (Spring/Summer, 1996). In *Injury Control Update*, 8–9.

Clarke, A., & Walton, W. W. (1979). Effect of safety packaging on aspirin ingestion by children. *Pediatrics, 63*, 687–693.

Clinton, Governor William Jefferson. (October 11, 1992). First presidential debate (video). Washington University, St. Louis, MO.

Cole, P. (1995). *The Moral Bases for Public Health Interventions Journal: Epidermiology, 6*(1), 78–83.

Committee on Accident and Poison Prevention. (1987). *Injury control for children and youth*. Elk Grove Village, IL: American Academy of Pediatrics.

Committee on the National Agenda. (1992). *Position papers from the Third National Injury Control Conference*. Atlanta, GA: Centers for Disease Control.

Cote, T. R., Sacks, J. J., Lambert-Huber, D. A., Lambert-Huber, D. A., Dannenberg, A. L., Kresnow, M. J., Lipsitz, C. M., & Schmidt, E. R. (1992). Bicycle helmet use among Maryland children: Effect of legislation and education. *Pediatrics, 89* (6), 1216–1220.

Department of Health and Human Services. (1996). *Healthy people 2000 progress review. Unintentional injury*. Washington, DC: United States Public Health Service.

Erdmann, T. C., Feldman, K. W., Rivara, F. P., Heinbach, D. M., & Wall, H. A. (1991). Tap water burn prevention: The effect of legislation. *Pediatrics, 88* (3), 572–577.

Fallat, M. E., & Rengers, S. J. (1993). The effect of education and safety devices on scald burn prevention. *The Journal of Trauma, 34*,(4), 560–564.

Fife, D., & Barancik, J. I. (1985). Northeastern Ohio Trauma Study III: Incidence of fractures. *Annals of Emergency Medicine, 14*, 244–248.

Fingerhut, L. A. (1993). *Firearm mortality among children, youth, and young adults 1–34 years of age, trends and current status: United States, 1985–1990*. Advance data from Vital and Health Statistics. No. 231. Washington, DC: US Government Printing Office.

Finkelstein, M., & Smolkin, H. (1987). Feasibility of roadway countermeasures to reduce alcohol-related crashes (a joint NHTSA/FHWA review paper), unpublished manuscript. Washington, DC: NHTSA, FHWA.

Gallagher, S. S., Guyer, B., Kotelchuck, M., Bass, J., Lovejoy, F. H., McLoughlin, E., & Mehta, K. (1982). A strategy for the reduction of childhood injuries in Massachusetts: SCIPP. *New England Journal of Medicine, 307*, 1015–1019.

Gielen, A. C. (1992). Health education and injury control: Integrating approaches. *Health Education Quarterly, 19* (2), 203–218.

Glanz, K., & Rimer, B. (1995). *Theory at a glance: A guide for health promotion practice*. (NIH Pub. No. 95-3896). Bethesda, Maryland: National Cancer Institute.

Gordon, J. (1949). The epidemiology of accidents. *American Journal of Public Health, 39*, 504–515.

Graham, J. D. (1993). Injuries from traffic crashes: Meeting the challenge. *Annual Review of Public Health, 14*, 515–543.

Green, L., & Kreuter, M. (1991). *Health education planning: An educational and environmental approach*. 2nd ed. Mountain View, CA: Mayfield Publishing.

Guyer, B., & Ellers, B. (1990) Childhood injuries in the United States: Mortality, morbidity and cost. *American Journal of Diseases of Children, 144*, 649–652.

Haddon, W. (1968). The changing approach to the epidemiology, prevention, and amelioration of trauma: The transition to approaches etiologically rather than descriptively based. *American Journal of Public Health, 58*, 1431–1438.

Haddon W. (1970). On the escape of tigers: An ecological note. *American Journal of Public Health, 60*, 2229–2234.

Haddon, W. (1972). A logical framework for categorizing highway safety phenomena and activity. *Journal of Trauma, 12*, 193–207.

Haddon, W. (1980a). The basic strategies for reducing damage from hazards of all kinds. *Hazard Prevention, 16* (11), 8–12.

Haddon, W. (1980b). Options for the prevention of motor vehicle crash injury. *Israel Journal of Medical Sciences, 16,* 45–68.

Injury Control Update. A report to Oklahoma injury surveillance participants. (October 23, 1995). Life-Savers, A residential fire injury prevention project update: 48 month follow-up. Atlanta, Georgia: NCIPC/CDC.

Macrina, D., Macrina, N., Horvath, C., Gallaspy, J., & Fine, P. (1996). An educational intervention to increase use of the Glasgow Coma Scale by emergency department personnel. *International Journal of Nursing, 2,* 7–12.

Martin, M. J., Hunt, T. K., & Hulley, S. B. (1988). The cost of hospitalization for firearm injuries. *Journal of the American Medical Association, 260,* 3048–3050.

Max, W., & Rice, D. P. (1993). Shooting in the dark: Estimating the cost of firearm injuries. *Health Affairs, 12(4),* 171–185.

McLeroy, K., Steckler, A., Simons-Morton, B., Goodman, R., Gottlieb, N., & Burdine, J. (1993). Social science theory in health education: Time for a new model? *Health Education Research, 8* (3), 305–312.

McLoughlin, E., Clarke, N., Stahl, K., & Crawford, J. D. (1977). One pediatric burn unit's experience with sleepwear-related injuries. *Pediatrics, 60,* 405–409.

Mercy, J. A., & Houk, V. N. (1993). The public health impact of firearm injuries. *American Journal of Preventive Medicine, 9* (3), 8–11.

Miller, T. R., & Galbraith, M. (1995). Injury prevention counseling by pediatricians: A benefit-cost comparison. *Pediatrics, 96* (1), 1–4.

National Academy of Science. (1985). *Injury in America.* Washington, DC: National Academy Press.

National Center for Injury Prevention and Control. (1996). *1996 fact book.* Atlanta, GA: Centers for Disease Control.

National Committee for Injury Prevention and Control. (1989). Injury prevention: Meeting the challenge. *American Journal of Preventive Medicine, 5* (3) (Suppl.).

National Safety Council. (1996). *Accident facts 1995 edition.* Itasca, IL: Author.

Pickett, G., & Hanlon, J. (1990). *Public health administration and practice,* 9th ed., St. Louis, Missouri: Times Mirror/Mosby College Publishing.

Pre-Hospital Trauma Life Support Committee of the National Association of Emergency Medical Technicians in Cooperation with the Committee on Trauma of the American College of Surgeons. (1994). *PHTLS: Basic and advanced pre-hospital trauma life support,* 3rd ed. St. Louis, MO: Mosby-Year Book.

Rice, D. P., MacKenzie, E. J., Jones, A. S., Kaufman, S. R., deLissovoy, G. V., Max, W., McLoughlin, E., Miller, T. R., Robertson, L. S., Salkever, D. S., Smith, G. S., & Red, I. V. S. W. (1989). *Cost of injury in the United States: A report to Congress 1989.* San Francisco, CA: Institute for Health and Aging, University of California and Injury Prevention Center, The Johns Hopkins University.

Rivara, F. P., Thompson, D. C., Thompson, R. S. (1994). The Seattle Children's Bicycle Helmet Campaign: Changes in helmet use and head injury admissions. *Pediatrics, 93* (4), 567–569.

Roberts, M., Fanunik, D., & Layfield, D. (1987). Behavioral Approaches to prevention of childhood injuries. *Journal of Social Issues, 43* (2), 105–118.

Robertson, L. S. (1980). Crash involvement of teenaged drivers when driver education is eliminated from high school. *American Journal of Public Health, 70,* 599–603.

Rosner, M., Rosner, S., & Johnson, A. (1995). Cerebral perfusion pressure: Management protocol and clinical results. *Journal of Neurosurgery, 83,* 949–961.

Safe Moves. (1994, October). A guide to traffic safety (brochure). Marina Del Ray, CA: US Department of Transportation.

Scheidt, P. C., Wilson, M. H., & Stern, M. S. (1992). Bicycle helmet law for children: A case study of activism in injury control. *Pediatrics, 89* (6), 1248–1250.

Shaoul, J. (1975). *The use of accidents and traffic offenses as criteria for evaluating courses in driver education.* Salford, England: University of Salford.

Shinar, D. (1993). Demographic and socioeconomic correlates of safety belt use. *Accident Analysis and Prevention, 25,* 745–755.

Spiegel, C. N., & Lindaman, F. C. (1977). Children can't fly: A program to prevent childhood morbidity and mortality from window falls. *American Journal of Public Health, 67,* 1143–1147.

Stover, S. L., DeLisa, J. A., & Whiteneck, G. G. (1995). *Spinal cord injury, clinical outcomes from the model systems.* Gaithersburg, MD: Aspen Publishers.

Teutsch, S. A. (1992). Framework for assessing the effectiveness of disease and injury prevention. *Morbidity and Mortality Weekly Report, 41*, 1–12.

Thompson, D. F., Trammel, H. L., Robertson, N. J., & Reigart, J. R. (1983). Evaluation of regional and non-regional poison centers. *New England Journal of Medicine, 308*, 191–194.

US Department of Health and Human Services (USDHHS). (1991). *Injury control: Position papers from the Third National Injury Control Conference, "Setting the National Agenda for Injury Control in the 1990's."* Pub. no. 1992-634-666. Washington, DC: US Government Printing Office.

US Department of Transportation. (1996). 1996 Secretary of Transportation's community partnership award program (bulletin). Washington, DC: US Government Printing Office.

United States Public Health Service. (1991). *Healthy people 2000: National health promotion and disease prevention objectives: Full report with commentary.* (DHHS Publication No. (PHS) 91-50212.) Washington, DC: US Government Printing Office.

Waller, J. (1987). Injury: Conceptual shifts and preventive implications. *Annual Reveiw of Public Health, 8*, 21–49.

Walton, W. (1982). An evaluation of the Poison Prevention Packaging Act. *Pediatrics, 69*, 363–370.

Wrigley, M., Yoels, W., Webb, C., & Fine, P. (1994). Social and physical factors in the referral of people with traumatic brain injuries to rehabilitation. *Archives of Physical Medicine and Rehabilitation, 75*, 149–155.

CHAPTER 16

Pulmonary Disorders

Connie L. Kohler, Susan L. Davies, Anne Turner-Henson, and William C. Bailey

Introduction

Pulmonary and respiratory disorders are among the most prevalent of chronic diseases in this country, affecting both children and adults and costing millions a year in health care dollars. The pulmonary disorders referred to in this chapter include asthma, chronic bronchitis, and emphysema. These three disorders are sometimes referred to as a group as chronic obstructive pulmonary disorders (COPD), although asthma is usually considered as a distinct pulmonary disorder, because it does not always involve obstruction. COPD is the fourth-leading cause of death and the second-leading cause of disability in this country (Murray & Nadel, 1988; Singh *et al.*, 1994). Prevalence estimates for COPD range from 5 to 10% of the adult population (Bang, 1993; NCHS, 1985). Asthma is another very common lung disease estimated to affect 5 to 10% of the population in North America. A recent study estimated the direct costs of asthma in the United States at $6.2 billion per year and the indirect costs at $1 billion per year due to reduced productivity related to absenteeism (Weiss, Gergen, & Hodgson, 1992).

Asthma during childhood has a profound impact on the growth and development of children and on their families. The most common of all chronic childhood conditions, asthma affects approximately 5 million children in the United States (Friday & Fireman, 1988). The overall prevalence of asthma is greater in blacks compared to whites, with greater frequencies seen in males and children living in poverty and inner cities (Taylor & Newacheck, 1992). Asthma morbidity accounts for approximately 20% of all hospital admissions (NCHS, 1986). When children with asthma miss school, their parents often miss work. This reduced parental productivity contributes to the impact of asthma on the family budget and on the indirect costs of

Connie L. Kohler and Susan L. Davies • Department of Health Behavior, School of Public Health, UAB Center for Health Promotion, University of Alabama at Birmingham, Birmingham, Alabama 35294. *Anne Turner-Henson* • School of Nursing, UAB Center for Health Promotion, University of Alabama at Birmingham, Birmingham, Alabama 35294. *William C. Bailey* • Department of Pulmonary and Critical Care, School of Medicine, University of Alabama at Birmingham, Birmingham, Alabama 35294.

Handbook of Health Promotion and Disease Prevention, edited by Raczynski and DiClemente. Kluwer Academic/Plenum Publishers, New York, 1999.

asthma (Taggart & Fulwood, 1993). Pediatric asthma is the leading cause of school absenteeism and ranks first among childhood chronic conditions in limiting activities of daily living (Newacheck, Budetti, & Halfon, 1986). African-American children experience significantly greater restrictions in daily activity, significantly fewer contacts with primary care services, increased frequency of emergency department utilization and hospitalization, and more severe functional disability (Sly, 1989; Taylor & Newacheck, 1992).

Persons affected by chronic lung diseases can retard their disease progression, greatly reduce their disability, and improve their quality of life by taking an active role in managing their disease. Research with chronically ill patients has shown that exercising influence over their treatment regimens contributes to positive mood and functioning (Bandura, 1997). The National Asthma Education and Prevention Program (NAEPP) expert panel on the management of asthma concluded in its guidelines that patient education is one of four critical components of asthma treatment, along with diagnosis, treatment, and environmental measures (NAEPP, 1991, 1997). This chapter will outline the major tasks involved in "self-management" of pulmonary disorders and describe self-management interventions including their theoretical underpinnings. In addition, this chapter will cover objectives of self-management interventions for adults and children with chronic pulmonary problems, their content, and the settings and formats for delivery of such programs.

Objectives of Self-Management Programs

Theoretical Foundations of Self-Regulation and Self-Management

A number of theories have been useful in developing and promoting the self-management of chronic disease. Theories of empowerment and self-regulation have been recommended among others (Clark, Evans, Zimmerman, Levinson, & Mellins, 1994; Leventhal, Zimmerman & Gutmann, 1984). The theory of empowerment asserts that individuals who have a sense of ownership or control over decisions that impact their health will be more successful in managing their condition (Green & Frankish, 1994). Theories of self-regulation include the processes of self-observation, self-judgment, and self-reaction, which can influence patients to use more strategies to control their symptoms, leading to a reduction in excessive health care utilization (Clark et al., 1994).

While any number of theories of disease and human behavior may be compatible with the concept of involving patients in the daily management of their chronic disease (Bruhn, 1983), there are a limited number of theories that provide a useful foundation for developing and evaluating programs to teach and promote self-management. One that has been used successfully is social cognitive theory, especially as outlined by Bandura (1977). Self-management programs developed within the framework of social cognitive theory address a triad of interrelated factors including environmental factors, such as the triggers of an asthma attack and the social support patients receive; cognitive factors, such as knowledge and self-confidence to manage illness episodes; and behavioral factors, such as physical activity and medication compliance. Further, such programs incorporate modeling techniques, self-monitoring, reinforcement, and observational learning of skills through guided mastery practice and informative feedback (Bandura, 1986, 1997).

The Objectives of Pulmonary Disease Self-Management

Generally, self-management of chronic disease is aimed toward the alleviation of symptoms, maintenance of functioning, and self-regulative skills (Bandura, 1997). For pulmonary disorders the primary objectives are to manage episodes of illness or symptoms such as asthma attacks, to manage interpersonal relationships central to reducing disruption of daily life, and to use self-regulation to prevent illness episodes (Clark, Gotsch & Rosenstock, 1993; Wilson, 1993). Specific tasks within these categories may differ for adults and children and for the specific type of pulmonary disorder (i.e., asthma, emphysema, or chronic bronchitis). Management of illness episodes includes resting (and staying calm in the face of an attack), taking medications as prescribed, using predetermined criteria to call a health care provider, and following other instructions outlined by the provider (Clark & Starr-Schneidkraut, 1994).

Because pulmonary disorders can limit activity, they may cause disruption of daily life. Strategies that enable the patient to manage interpersonal relationships can reduce disruption; these skills include effective communication and negotiation strategies within the family, with health care personnel, at school and the workplace, and related to leisure pursuits (Clark & Starr-Schneidkraut, 1994) and skills in locating helpful community resources (Holman & Lorig, 1992). Self-regulation to control illness involves following treatment regimens and avoiding health threats. This means performing such activities as proximal goal setting (i.e., setting small, achievable goals), using self-applied incentives or rewards, self-monitoring and interpreting changes in health status, and using coping and/or problem-solving skills (Holman & Lorig, 1992; Abrams, Emmons, & Linnan, 1997). For pulmonary disorders this entails recognizing early signs of problems and acting on those signs to prevent an infection or attack, using a peak flowmeter to anticipate problems related to a change in breathing, identifying and controlling the behavioral and environmental factors that trigger breathing problems, and taking prescribed medications correctly and on schedule (Clark & Starr-Schneidkraut, 1993).

Interventions to promote patient self-management not only should provide guidance for achieving the above objectives, but also should include a goal of increasing the patient's and family's perceived self-efficacy for doing so. It is a distrust in their own ability to manage breathing difficulties that causes people to lead constricted lives (Wigal, Creer, & Kotses, 1991; Bandura, 1997). In fact, perceived self-efficacy to manage chronic disease appears to have a stronger influence on functioning than either the degree of physical impairment (Baron, Dutil, Berkson, Lander, & Becker, 1987) or the actual use of coping skills (Bandura, 1997). In a study to evaluate interventions to increase exercise in patients with progressive pulmonary function loss, Kaplan, Atkins, and Reinsch (1984) found that higher perceived efficacy correlated with better adherence to prescribed exercise, improved lung function, an increased capacity for physical exertion, and an increased sense of well-being. In a study of the correlates of health status in patients with COPD (Kohler *et al.*, 1994), patients' scores on a quality of well-being measure were a function of their perceived self-efficacy in addition to their actual pulmonary function. The investigators concluded that the effects of pulmonary function on patients' quality of well-being were mediated by self-efficacy. Similiarly, a study by Katz, Yelin, Smith, and Blanc (1997) found that perceived control of asthma was negatively associated with adverse asthma outcomes. Thus, research suggests that patient-centered interventions that focus on perceived self-efficacy or perceived control can improve asthma outcomes.

Self-Management Interventions

Interventions should include behavioral components related to the objectives of self-management programs along with strategies to enhance perceived self-efficacy across all behaviors. The NAEPP panel (1991, 1997) emphasized the importance of information (e.g., how bronchodilator medicines work), skills training (e.g., using a medication inhaler correctly, controlling triggers), and self-confidence development (i.e., self-efficacy) as crucial elements in helping patients manage their condition. Other important elements include increasing cognitive skills, fostering positive attitudes, increasing adherence, and helping develop effective social support.

The following sections describe typical elements of pulmonary disease self-management interventions.

Self-Monitoring Activities

Self-monitoring provides patients with data to increase self-control of their symptoms and disease progress. Self-monitoring includes observing and recording of factors related to a behavioral problem, such as physiological processes, environmental stimuli, cognitive processes, and behaviors (Tobin, Reynolds, Holroyd, & Creer, 1986). Forms of self-monitoring useful in pulmonary disease self-management include monitoring signs and symptoms, monitoring peak expiratory flow rate (a measure of lung capacity), keeping medication diaries, and using logs to record episodes of symptoms along with their precipitating events.

The value of self-monitoring is that by observing and recording disease-related factors and situations in which they occur, patients can identify cause-and-effect relationships between these factors and the occurrence of symptoms, infections, or missed medication doses. Armed with this knowledge, they can then determine appropriate responses to these factors and develop cues to prompt the responses (Tobin et al., 1986). For example, if patients use diaries to observe and record their medication-taking behaviors and link these behaviors to the their disease status, they will be able to: (1) analyze the situations (such as, "left inhaler in other purse or trousers"); and (2) come up with means of improving their own adherence (such as, "attach inhaler to car keys, which rarely fail to get transferred to other purses, trousers"). A device called a peak flowmeter is a simple tool to measure the force with which individuals can exhale air. By monitoring peak expiratory flow rate with a peak flowmeter, patients can link missed medication doses, as well as certain activities, with a drop in their peak flow rate and learn to avoid these activities as necessary.

Parents and children need to be educated to recognize the patterns of symptoms that indicate that the child's asthma is out of control and that additional treatments are needed. An asthma education plan for children should include daily symptom monitoring and a crisis management plan for attacks. Daily peak flow monitoring, while recommended in adult asthma care, is not a realistic goal for young children. Therefore, parents should be taught to assess asthma symptoms such as increased coughing, wheezing, shortness of breath, or irritability.

The association of self-monitoring strategies with improvements in health status has been supported empirically (Clark *et al.*,1994; Kotses *et al.*, 1995; Madsen *et al.*, 1993). For example, Kotses *et al.* (1995), developed an intervention based on the self-monitoring of symptoms, medications taken, peak expiratory flow rates, and asthma attack precipitants. The investigators reasoned that keeping track of these factors gave patients information that signaled them to begin using strategies to help control their asthma attack. This training led to improved symptoms and fewer physician visits and to fewer attacks over time.

Strategies Targeting Environmental Factors

According to social cognitive theory (Bandura, 1986; Tobin *et al.*, 1986) and other self-regulation theories (e.g., Leventhal *et al.*, 1984), environmental factors are reciprocal determinants of behavioral factors, and so changes in the environment affect changes in behavior and vice versa. This notion is especially pertinent to self-management of pulmonary disorders, in which environmental irritants can precipitate severe breathing problems. For example, every case of asthma has unique triggers (i.e., factors that "trigger" an attack), and treatment measures taken without concurrent environmental control are less effective (NAEPP, 1991). The most recent report (NAEPP, 1997) lists those things patients with asthma should avoid: exposure to allergens, exposure to environmental tobacco smoke, exertion when levels of air pollution are high, and certain foods and medications to which they may be sensitive.

Asthma management interventions for children need to be directed toward reducing exposure to environmental triggers in children with asthma. Children have unique physical and developmental characteristics that place them at greater risk for exposure to certain types of environmental agents. Triggers and environmental factors such as respiratory infections, cigarette smoke, dust mites, cockroach allergens, air pollution, pets, and outdoor seasonal allergens are the leading causes of acute asthma exacerbations, and control of such triggers is an essential component in pediatric asthma management. Passive smoke exposure continues to be the most potent trigger in childhood asthma. Exposure to high ambient air pollution is another environmental trigger for children with asthma. Children, particularly school-age children, are at greater risk for ozone exposure because they are physically active outdoors in the afternoon, a time when ozone levels are at their highest (Bates, 1995a). Ozone exposure is a prime suspect in asthma because it provokes airway inflammation and may increase the effects of allergens (e.g., dust mites, pollens, etc.) by increasing lung permeability (Bates, 1995b).

A self-management program developed by Bailey and colleagues (1990) suggests three behavioral options for dealing with asthma triggers: (1) avoid the trigger entirely (e.g., avoid contact with animals, have housecleaning done by someone else); (2) limit exposure to the trigger if complete avoidance is not possible (e.g., leave the room if someone starts smoking or is wearing strong perfume); and (3) take an extra dose of bronchodilator medication before trigger exposure if neither of the first two options is possible.

Another important environmental factor is the pulmonary patient's social support. An environment that includes supportive others to provide encouragement for and assistance in self-management is extremely important. This is one reason why improving social and communication skills is considered to be one of the three main objectives of asthma self-management programs (Clark *et al.*, 1993). Patient treatment and activity affects other family members and the behavior of family members likewise has a direct impact on patients. As with the physical environment, patient behaviors can improve the social environment. Educating the family and others who play a significant role in the patient's life can help to create an environment conducive to favorable patient outcomes, especially in relation to adherence, positive attitude, and managing and coping with symptoms (NAEPP, 1991). Interventions that include support groups for both patients and "support" persons provide an effective context in which the person without disease can learn about special needs and concerns of pulmonary patients and see supportive behaviors modeled by others (Bailey *et al.*, 1990). Also, a focus on developing an open and trusting relationship with health care staff is an intervention strategy that can improve the social environment.

Finally, given that cigarette smoke plays a crucial role in the development and progression of pulmonary diseases and is a key factor in the initiation of respiratory attacks in both adults and children, smoking cessation is an extremely important aspect of pulmonary disease self-management. Attention should be given to assist patients and parents who smoke or smokers who live in close proximity to persons with pulmonary disorders in successfully quitting smoking (see Chapter 8, this volume).

Development of Medication Skills

Many pulmonary medications are delivered by a metered dose inhaler (MDI), through which patients inhale a spray of medicine. For children with asthma, inhaled medications can be administered through a metered dose inhaler or through a nebulizer. While nebulizers are generally used for children less than 8 years of age, MDIs with spacers can be used with the older school-age child. For both delivery systems, there are certain techniques to get the optimal dose of medicine into the patient's lungs. This requires careful training and periodic assessment of the patient's technique. Incorrect technique in using MDIs and nebulizers can compromise the effectiveness of the medication regimen (Interiano & Guntapalli, 1993; Wilson *et al.*, 1993). While pharmaceutical companies have addressed this problem by developing devices that are easier to use, even these require careful instruction when first introduced to the patient. Pulmonary disease self-management programs may include an inhaler use instruction component. Following social cognitive theory tenets, this often entails correct MDI use demonstrated by a nurse or patient educator and followed by supervised practice by the patient (using placebo inhalers). Patients' techniques then may be periodically assessed to ensure that errors are caught and corrected. This approach has resulted in a decrease in errors by patients with pulmonary disease (Greene *et al.*, 1994).

Adherence to medication regimens is a well-documented problem for individuals with chronic disease, and pulmonary disease is no exception. Reported rates of adherence with pulmonary medication range from 6 to 70% (Dekker, Dieleman, Kaptein, & Mulder, 1993; Rand & Wise, 1994). Patients report a number of reasons for not taking medicine as prescribed, only one of which is forgetting. Other reasons include inability to get the medicine (e.g., due to lack of transportation or money or forgetting to order refills in a timely manner); disbelief in the need for the medicine (e.g., due to denial of the disease, or wrongly concluding that the medicine is no longer needed when symptoms go away); disbelief in the efficacy of the medicine to treat the illness; social pressures to avoid being continuously "on medication"; misunderstanding of the regimen (especially, but not only, by those who have less education or low literacy skills); and medication side effects (Greene *et al.*, 1994; Hindi-Alexander & Thromm, 1987; Rand & Wise, 1994). Pulmonary patients are at particular risk for nonadherence, because medication regimens are long in duration, include multiple medications with varying dosing schedules, and are to be continued over periods of symptom remission (Rand & Wise, 1994).

Self-management interventions often include strategies to increase medication adherence. One such strategy is self-monitoring, as described earlier. Keeping a written record of medication use can help patients identify times and situations in which taking medicine is a problem. Strategies to minimize forgetting include reminders, such as pill dispensers marked with the days of the week or setting computer or wristwatch alarms, and pairing medication taking with other routine daily activities, such as toothbrushing. Providing education regarding the physiology of the disease and how medications work to relieve symptoms can increase the likelihood of proper medication use. But even with full understanding of the importance of and benefit from medications, nonadherence can exist if side effects are present from pulmonary medications (Busse, Maisiak, & Young, 1994). To counteract nonadherence due to side effects, patients may be counseled to report side effects to the health care provider so adjustments to the regimen can be made. Often patients do not realize there are alternatives and simply stop taking the medicine because they cannot tolerate the side effects. Strategies to address other reasons for nonadherence are counseling on sources of financial aid for medication and on the need for medications even when asymptomatic, using color-coded medication containers and easy-to-read instructions for what to take when, and simplifying the dosing schedule whenever possible (e.g, some medications come in forms that need to be taken only once a day).

Self-Efficacy Enhancing Strategies

Self-management interventions should include strategies to enhance patients' perceived self-efficacy for the skills described above. Promoting mastery of skills is the most powerful method to enhance perceptions of efficacy, but self-efficacy perceptions can also be learned vicariously (Bandura, 1997). In combination, these two sources of efficacy beliefs can be applied by modeling the skills to be learned followed by guided mastery practice. For example, asthma patients may be asked to monitor their peak expiratory flow rate on a regular basis. Peak expiratory flow rate is a measure of the amount of air a person can exhale and a drop in this rate signals airway narrowing. Patients may have low levels of efficacy for getting themselves to measure their peak flow rate on a regular basis. To increase their self-efficacy, patients can be introduced to peers who have overcome the difficulties of regular monitoring and can "model" the process by relating their own strategies to the patient. This vicarious learning gives the patient the sense that since others can manage the process, they too are likely to be able to manage. Patients may then be asked to set small, achievable goals, such as measuring peak flow one weekday morning and one weekend morning. Success at attaining a small goal may be followed by an increase in perceived self-efficacy and an increased willingness to try a more demanding monitoring schedule. Strategies of modeling and proximal goal setting can be used to increase self-efficacy for doing most of the tasks outlined in the self-management of chronic disease.

Important Considerations for Children with Asthma

Health promotion and disease prevention in children with asthma are of great importance. Chronic conditions in childhood have been found to be associated with excess morbidity in the short term and with a poor perception of health in adulthood (Power & Peckham, 1990). Long-term health risks for children with asthma appear to track into adulthood, and these risks are enhanced by a sedentary lifestyle. The establishment of a regular program of physical activity could improve cardiorespiratory fitness, muscular strength, muscular endurance, and flexibility. For children with asthma, a positive attitude toward physical activity may be associated with greater exercise involvement (Brook, Stein, & Alkalay, 1994). Children with asthma are often excluded from physical activity, in both organized sports and vigorous free play (Verma & Hyde, 1976; Strunk, Rubin, Kelly, Sherman, & Fukuhura, 1988; Taylor & Newacheck, 1992). This exclusion may be due to parents, physicians, physical education teachers, or even their own reluctance to provoke an attack of exercise-induced asthma. Physical fitness programs for asthmatic children have been successful in improving physical fitness parameters and vital capacity (Orenstein, Reed, Grogan & Crawford, 1985), while decreasing school absences and improving sociability, self-assertion, and peer acceptance (Szentagothai, Gyene, Szocaska, & Osvath, 1987).

Developing a partnership between the family and the health care team should be at the foundation of any comprehensive asthma management plan, with parents playing an essential role in pediatric asthma management. To date, interventions to improve adherence in pediatric populations have focused primarily on education and case management strategies, rather than on behavioral outcomes. However, studies done in high-risk populations for asthma morbidity have demonstrated that knowledge alone is insufficient to affect behavioral change and appropriate health care utilization. Hence, interventions that provide skills for behavioral change while providing "essential" asthma knowledge can be more effective in improving asthma outcomes in this population.

Settings and Formats for Self-Management Interventions

Self-management interventions are delivered in a variety of settings and formats. Settings include hospitals, clinics, outside agencies such as the American Lung Association or local community facilities such as the public library, and even the telephone. Formats include large- and small-group instruction and support, one-to-one instruction and counseling, self-help or self-instructional materials (written, video, and computer-based), and combinations of these.

Intervention Settings

Clark et al. (1993) identified the settings for large-scale evaluations of asthma education programs. Most took place primarily in the outpatient clinic setting. Other settings were schools (for programs aimed at children and parents) and a voluntary health organization. Self-management education may be delivered in less traditional settings such as neighbor-to-neighbor interactions (Huss *et al.*, 1994) and community centers (Fisher *et al.*, 1994) and over the telephone. Nontraditional venues are employed to reach people who may not utilize the clinic on a regular basis, including those who may not even be aware they have pulmonary disease.

Intervention Formats

In a recent study of the effectiveness of individual teaching compared with small-group teaching in a clinic-based asthma education program, the investigators concluded that both small-group education and individual education were associated with improved self-management practices, but that the group program was easier to administer, better received by patients and educators, and more cost-effective (Wilson *et al.*, 1993). Kotses and colleagues (1995) identified three format components related to the effectiveness of their self-management intervention: presentation of material by a highly credible individual, a small-group setting, and the inclusion of written material.

Research on other intervention formats such as videos, manuals, or computer-based instruction in pulmonary disease is scarce (Bailey *et al.*, 1992). Print materials are a common format for communicating about self-management of pulmonary disorders. The American Lung Association publishes a variety of materials designed to teach patients about lung disease. The advantages of print materials are that they can be widely distributed and used by patients according to their own needs and learning styles. The disadvantages include the lack of social support and professional feedback featured in person-to-person programs. Other forms of self-help materials include audiotapes, videotapes, and computer software, all of which are often available from pharmaceutical companies. Increasingly, computer-based interventions are being developed for chronic disease self-management. This type of intervention can increase patient knowledge and reduce the amount of clinic staff time used on education and can be highly motivating (Tomita *et al.*, 1995).

Although asthma directly affects only from 5 to 10% of the general population, recent efforts to employ the community in addressing this health problem have been promising, especially in inner-city neighborhoods where asthma prevalence may be elevated. In St. Louis, a neighborhood asthma coalition was formed to raise awareness of asthma and support for people with asthma. Among their strategies was to disseminate a simple four-point message about asthma through ongoing community activities (Fisher *et al.*, 1996). In Baltimore, neighborhood community health workers were trained to work with asthma patients, going on home visits to teach asthmatic children and their families in basic asthma self-management (Butz *et al.*, 1994).

In an effort to curtail the significant increase in asthma-related morbidity and mortality among inner-city children, a number of asthma education programs have been developed using various instructional methods (e.g., group classes, individualized instruction, pamphlets, computer-assisted learning tools, videotapes, etc.) The National Cooperative Inner-City Asthma Study (Butz *et al.*, 1994; Crain *et al.*, 1994) sponsored by the National Institutes of Health from 1991 to1996 used an asthma counselor to work with each family to identify and help solve problems in the four key areas: access to medical care, adherence to treatment regimens, control of environmental triggers, and adoption of behavioral strategies to manage asthma. A 1-year follow-up of these subjects indicated a significant improvement in asthma outcome measures. However, whether this intensive and expensive intervention will result in sustained behavioral change remains to be determined.

Effectiveness of Self-Management Interventions

While self-management programs may vary in content and format, most include the fundamental skills needed for prevention and control of respiratory exacerbations. But while most programs show success in increasing self-management knowledge and skills, significant progress has not been evidenced for more meaningful outcome measures. The fact that asthma-related morbidity and mortality has risen significantly in recent years (Hanania, David-Wang, Kesten, & Chapman, 1997) suggests that self-management practices are not being implemented despite widespread education to improve asthma outcomes. Findings by Kolbe, Vamos, James, Elkind, and Garrett (1996) suggest there is a gap between knowledge about treatment and actual practice. Other research (Bernard-Bonnin, Stachenko, Bonin, Charette, & Rousseau, 1995) has shown that asthma education programs improve knowledge but do not reduce morbidity. In addition, the relationship between self-management teaching and asthma morbidity is confounded by multiple factors, such as environmental conditions, that are not directly amenable to change by education (Bernard-Bonnin et al., 1995). Not surprisingly, engagement in self-management practices is highly associated with the severity of asthma symptoms. Lahdensuo and colleagues (1996) found that patients with mild symptoms had a compliance rate of only 29%, while patients with severe symptoms were 100% compliant. Studies evaluating the effectiveness of self-management programs indicate that in order to reach maximal impact, patient education needs to be relevant, realistic, and repeated (Kolbe et al., 1996). As noted earlier, studies evaluating the effectiveness of community-based interventions have had positive results, but much more work needs to be done in this area.

Kolbe and colleagues (1996) found that patients who had received considerable self-management education were unsuccessful in applying the knowledge to appropriately manage their condition. They evaluated patients using hypothetical situations in which breathing difficulties arose to assess practical knowledge of asthma self-management. Also alarming, their findings indicate the poorest responses were to scenarios that depicted an attack of slow-onset (over several days), where half the subjects responded that they would not call for emergency assistance even in what was clearly a potentially life-threatening situation. This same study found that peak flowmeter use was a greatly underutilized strategy in attack prevention and control. The majority of subjects indicated that they would not perform peak flow monitoring even during asthma exacerbations. This is consistent with Garrett and colleagues (1994), who found that only 8% of patients who had peak flowmeters used them at the early stages of an attack and 26% rarely or never used their peak flowmeter. These findings clearly indicate that before asthma management decisions are based on measures of peak flow, an accurate assessment of each patient's knowledge, attitudes, and actual use of this device must be made. Moreover, before practitioners assume that self-management education will lead to better attack prevention and control, further research is needed to understand why a gap exists between cognitive understanding and the decision to put such knowledge into action at the appropriate time. Such investigations will be essential in bringing about significant reductions in asthma-related morbidity and mortality.

Conclusions

Chronic diseases and their management represent a significant area of study in health behavior. As the populations of developed countries age, the prevalence of chronic disease and its associated costs will increase. In addition, with an ever-more polluted environment, asthma and other respiratory problems are increasing in all age groups. A challenge for health promotion professionals is to apply behavioral theory and empirically evaluated interventions to the problem of involving those with pulmonary disease in their own disease management. Based on available evidence, successful self-management will lead to improved health status, better quality of life, and lower health care costs.

References

Abrams, D. B., Emmons, K. M., & Linnan, L. A. (1997). Health behavior and health education, the past, present and future. In K. Glanz, F. M. Lewis, & B. K. Rimer (Eds.), *Health behavior and health education* (2nd ed., pp. 453–478). San Francisco: Jossey Bass.

Bailey, W. C., Richards, J. M., Brooks, C. M., Soong, S. J., Windsor, R. A., & Manzella, B. A. (1990). A randomized trial to improve self-management practices of adults with asthma. *Archives of Internal Medicine, 150,* 1664–1668.

Bailey, W. C., Clark, N. M., Gotsch, A. R., Lemen, R. J., O'Connor, G. T., & Rosenstock, I. M. (1992). Asthma prevention. *Chest, 102,* 216s–231s.

Bandura, A. (1977). Self-efficacy: Toward a unifying theory of behavior change. *Psychology Review, 84,* 191–215.

Bandura, A. (1986). *Social foundations of thought and action.* Englewood Cliffs, NJ: Prentice Hall.

Bandura, A. (1997). *Self-efficacy: The exercise of control.* New York: W. H. Freeman.

Bang, K. M. (1993). Prevalence of chronic obstructive pulmonary disease in blacks. *Journal of the National Medical Association, 85,* 51–55.

Baron, M., Dutil, E., Berkson, L., Lander, P., & Becker, R. (1987). Hand function in the elderly. Relation to osteoarthritis. *Journal of Rheumatology, 14,* 815–819.

Bates, D. V. (1995a). Observations on asthma. *Environmental Health Perspectives, 103,* 243–247.

Bates, D. V. (1995b). The effects of air pollution on children. *Environmental Health Perspectives, 103,* 49–53.

Bernard-Bonnin, A. C., Stachenko, S., Bonin, D., Charette, C., & Rousseau, E. (1995). Self-management teaching programs and morbidity of pediatric asthma: a meta-analysis. *Journal of Allergy and Clinical Immunology, 95,* 34–41.

Brook, U., Stein, D., & Alkalay, Y. (1994). The attitude of asthmatic and nonasthmatic adolescents toward gymnastic lessons at school. *Journal of Asthma, 31,* 171–175.

Bruhn, J. G. (1983). Then application of theory in childhood asthma self-help programs. *Journal of Allergy and Clinical Immunology, 72,* 561–577.

Busse, W. W., Maisiak, R, & Young , K. R. (1994). Treatment regimen and side effects of treatment measures. *American Journal of Respiratory Critical Care Medicine, 149,* S44–S50.

Butz, A. M., Malveaux, F. J., Eggleston, P., Thompson, L., Schneider, S., Weeks, K., Huss, K., Murigande, C., & Rand, C. S. (1994). Use of community health workers with inner city children who have asthma. *Clinical Pediatrics, 33,* 135–141.

Clark, N. M., & Starr-Schneidkraut, N. J. (1994). Management of asthma by patients and families. *American Journal of Respiratory Critical Care Medicine, 149,* S54–S66.

Clark, N. M., Gotsch, A., Rosenstock, I. R. (1993). Patient, professional, and public education on behavioral aspects of asthma: A review of strategies for change and needed research. *Journal of Asthma, 30,* 241–255.

Clark, N. M, Evans, D., Zimmerman, B. J., Levinson, M. J., & Mellins, R. B. (1994). Patient and family management of asthma. Theory based techniques for the clinician. *Journal of Asthma, 31*, 427–435.

Crain, E. F., Weiss, K. B., Bijur, P. E., Hersh, M., Westbrook, L., & Stein, R. E. (1994). An estimate of the prevalence of asthma and wheezing among inner city children. *Pediatrics, 94*, 356–362.

Dekker, F. W., Dieleman, F. E., Kaptein, A. A., Mulder, J. D. (1993). Compliance with pulmonary medication in general practice. *European Respiratory Journal, 6*, 886–890.

Fisher, E. B., Jr., Sussman, L. K., Arfken, C., Harrison, D., Munro, J., Sykes, R. K., Sylvia, S., & Strunk, R. C. (1994). Targeting high risk groups. Neighborhood organization for pediatric asthma management in the neighborhood asthma coalition. *Chest, 106* (Suppl.) 248s–259s.

Fisher, E. B., Jr., Strunk, R. C., Sussman, L. K., Arfken, C., Sykes, R. K. Munro, J. M. Haywood, S., Harrison, D., & Bascom, S. (1996). Acceptability and feasibility of a community approach to asthma management: The Neighborhood Asthma Coalition (NAC). *Journal of Asthma, 33*, 367–383.

Friday, G. A., & Fireman, P. (1988). Morbidity and mortality of asthma. *Pediatric Clinics of North America, 35*, 1149–1152.

Green, L. W., & Frankish, C. J. (1994). Theories and principles of health education applied to asthma. *Chest, 106*, 5–9.

Greene, P. G., Kohler, C. L., Baker, A., Richards, J. M., Jr., Jackson, J. R., & Bailey, W. C. (1994). Nonadherence to medication regimens: Factors associated with medication overutilization in the treatment of chronic obstructive pulmonary disease. In *Proceedings of the 28th Annual Association of Behavioral Therapy Conference* (p. 128). New York: Association for the Advancement of Behavioral Therapy.

Hanania, N. A., David-Wang, A., Kesten, S., and Chapman, K. R. (1997). Factors associated with emergency department dependence of patients with asthma. *Chest, 111*, 290–295.

Hindi-Alexander, M. C. & Thromm, J. (1987). Compliance or noncompliance: That's the question. *American Journal of Health Promotion, 1*, 5–11.

Holman, H., & Lorig, K. (1992). Perceived self-efficacy in self-management of chronic disease. In R. Schwarzer (Ed.), *Self-efficacy: Thought control of action* (pp. 305–323). Washington, DC: Hemisphere.

Huss, K., Rand, C. S., Butz, A. M., Eggleston, P. A., Murigande, C., Thompson, L. C., Schneider, S., Weeks, K., & Malveaux, F. J. (1994). Home environmental risk factors in urban minority asthmatic children. *Annals of Allergy, 72*, 173–177.

Interiano, B., & Guntapalli, K. (1993). Metered dose inhalers: Do health care providers know what to teach? *Archives of Internal Medicine, 153*, 81–85.

Kaplan, R. M., Atkins, C. J., & Reinsch, S. (1984). Specific efficacy expectations mediate exercise compliance in patients with COPD. *Health Psychology, 3*, 223–242.

Katz, P. P., Yelin, E. H., Smith, S., & Blanc, P. D. (1997). *American Journal of Respiratory Critical Care Medicine, 155*, 577–582.

Kohler, C. L., Greene, P. G., Baker, A., Richards, J. M., Jr., Jackson, J. R., & Bailey, W. C. (1994). A social–cognitive model of chronic obstructive pulmonary disease: Implications for patient evaluation and treatment. *Proceedings of the 28th Annual AABT Convention* (p. 128). New York Association for the Advancement of Behavioral Therapy.

Kolbe, J., Vamos, M., James, F., Elkind, G., & Garrett, J. (1996). Assessment of practical knowledge of self-management of acute asthma. *Chest, 109*, 86–90.

Kotses, H., Bernstein, L., Bernstein, D. I., Reynolds, R. V. C., Korbee, L., Wigal, J. K., Ganson, E., Stout, C., & Creer, T. L. (1995) A self-management program for adult asthma. Part I: Development and evaluation. *Journal of Allergy and Clinical Immunology, 95*, 529–540.

Lahdensuo, A., Haahtela, T., Herrala, J., Kava, T., Kiviranta, K., Kuusisto, P., Peramaki, E., Poussa, T., Saarelainen, S., & Svahn, T. (1996). Randomised comparison of guided self-management and traditional treatment of asthma over one year. *British Medical Journal, 312*, 748–752.

Leventhal, H., Zimmerman, R., & Gutmann, M. (1984). Compliance: A self-regulation perspective. In D. Gentry (Ed.), *Handbook of behavioral medicine* (pp. 369–423). New York: Guilford Press.

Madsen, J., Sallis, J. F., Rupp, J. W., Senn, K. L., Patterson, T. L., Atkins, C. J., & Nader, P. B. (1993). Relationship between self-monitoring of diet and exercise change and subsequent risk factor changes in children and adults. *Patient Education and Counseling, 21*, 61–69.

Murray, J. F., & Nadel, J. A. (1988). *Textbook of respiratory medicine.* Philadelphia: W.B. Saunders.

National Asthma Education Program Expert Panel (NAEPP). (1991). *Guidelines for the diagnosis and management of asthma.* Bethesda, Maryland: National Institute of Health.

National Asthma Education Program Expert Panel. (1997). *Expert panel report 2. Guidelines for the diagnosis and management of asthma.* Bethesda, Maryland: National Institutes of Health.

National Center for Health Statistics (NCHS). (1985). *Current estimates from the national health interview survey.* Washington, DC: Govternment Printing Office.

National Center for Health Statistics (NCHS). (1986). *Advance data from vital and health statistics.* National Ambulatory Medical Care Survey. (DHHS Publication No. PHS 87-2350). Washington, DC: Government Printing Office.

Newacheck, P. W., Budetti, P. P., & Halfon, N. (1986). Trends in activity-limiting chronic conditions among children. *American Journal of Public Health, 76,* 178–184.

Orenstein, D. M., Reed, M. E., Grogan, F. T. Jr & Crawford, L. V. (1985). Exercise conditioning in children with asthma. *Journal of Pediatrics,* 556–560.

Power, C., & Peckham C. (1990). Childhood morbidity and adulthood ill health. *Journal of Epidemiology and Community Health, 44,* 69–74.

Rand, C. S., & Wise, R. A. (1994). Measuring adherence to asthma medication regimens. *American Journal of Respiratory Critical Care Medicine, 149,* S69–S76.

Singh, G. K., Matthews, T. J., Clarke, S. C., Yannicos, T., & Smith, B. L. (1994) Annual summary of births, marriages, divorces and deaths: United States, 1994. *Monthly vital statistics report, 43.* Hyattsville, MD: National Center for Health Statistics.

Sly, R. M. (1989). Mortality from asthma. *Journal of Allergy and Clinical Immunology, 84,* 421–434.

Strunk, R. C., Rubin, D., Kelly, L., Sherman, B., & Fukuhura, J. (1988). Determination of fitness in children with asthma. Use of standardized tests for functional endurance, body fat composition, flexibility, and abdominal strength. *American Journal of Diseases in Children, 142,* 940–944.

Szentagothai, K., Gyene, I., Szocska, M., & Osvath, P. (1987). Physical exercise program for children with bronchial asthma. *Pediatric Pulmonology, 3,* 166–172.

Taggart, V. S., & Fulwood, R. (1993). Youth health report card: Asthma. *Preventive Medicine, 22,* 579–584.

Taylor, W. R., & Newacheck, P. W. (1992). Impact of childhood asthma on health. *Pediatrics, 90,* 657–662.

Tobin, D. L., Reynolds, R. V. C., Holroyd, K. A., & Creer, T. L. (1986). Self-Management and social learning theory. In K. A. Holroyd & T. L. Creer (Eds.), *Self-management of chronic disease* (pp. 29–55). Orlando, FL: Academic Press.

Tomita, M., Takabayashi, K., Honda, M., Yamakazi, S., Suszuki, T., Tomoika, N., Nishimoto, M., Nakano, M., Satoh, Y., & Noriji, M. (1995). Computer assisted instruction on multi-media environment for patients. *Medinfo, 8* (2), 1192–1197.

Verma, S., & Hyde, J. S. (1976). Physical education programs and exercise-induced asthma. *Clinical Pediatrics, 15,* 697–705.

Weiss, K. B., Gergen, P. F., & Hodgson, T. A. (1992). An economic evaluation of asthma in the United States. *New England Journal of Medicine, 326,* 862–866.

Wigal, J. K., Creer, T. L., & Kotses, H. (1991). The COPD self-efficacy scale. *Chest, 99,* 1193–1196.

Wilson, S. R. (1993). Patient and physician behavior models related to asthma care. *Medical Care, 31,* MS49–MS60.

Wilson, S. R., Scamagas, P., German, D. F., Hughes, G. W., Lulla, S., Coss, S., Chardon, L., Thomas, R. G., Starr-Schneidkraut, N., Stancavage, F. B., & Arsham, G. M. (1993). A controlled trial of two forms of self-management education for adults with asthma. *American Journal of Medicine, 94,* 564–576.

CHAPTER 17

Behavioral and Social Dimensions of Pain in Rheumatic Disease

Laurence A. Bradley

Introduction

A large number of behavioral and social factors may influence the health status of patients with rheumatic disease (Bradley, 1997). Although investigators have focused primarily on these factors among patients with rheumatoid arthritis (RA), behavioral and social variables are important in all rheumatic conditions and disorders of the musculoskeletal system.

One of the most important dimensions of health status in patients with rheumatic disease is pain (Bradley, 1996b). Indeed, it has been found that pain is more important than physical or psychological disability in explaining medication use among patients with RA (Kazis, Meenan, & Anderson, 1983). Pain is also a significant predictor of patient and physician assessments of patients' general health status and their future levels of pain and disability (Kazis *et al.*, 1983). Although important advances have been made in the medical management of rheumatic disease, patients rarely experience complete pain relief in response to their pharmacological and physical treatment regimens (Bradley, 1996b). Given that patients' perceptions of pain and pain behaviors are more strongly associated with behavioral and social variables than with measures of rheumatic disease activity (e.g., joint counts), it should not be surprising that pharmacological and physical therapies often do not provide optimal reductions in pain (Bradley, 1994a).

The primary purposes of this chapter are to: (1) review the relationships that have been established between behavioral and social factors and pain among individuals with three common rheumatic disorders: RA, osteoarthritis (OA), and fibromyalgia (FM); and (2) examine the behavioral treatments that have been shown to help these individuals manage their pain. Before addressing these issues, however, the chapter will present information on the prevalence, pathogenesis, and medical

Laurence A. Bradley • Division of Clinical Immunology and Rheumatology, Department of Medicine, University of Alabama at Birmingham, Birmingham, Alabama 35294.

Handbook of Health Promotion and Disease Prevention, edited by Raczynski and DiClemente. Kluwer Academic/Plenum Publishers, New York, 1999.

treatment of these three disorders. Attention also will be devoted to the social and economic consequences of rheumatic disease.

Review of Three Major Rheumatic Diseases

Rheumatic disease poses great challenges to individual patients and their family members as well as to society. The pain, fatigue, and progressive damage to soft tissues and joints associated with most rheumatic disorders may produce highly negative effects on the daily lives of patients and their relatives. Thus, patients may experience impairments in their activities of daily life that may include personal care tasks (e.g., grooming, toileting), household tasks (e.g., housework, paying bills), and discretionary activities (e.g., hobbies) (Mitchell, Burkhauser, & Pincus, 1988; Schned & Reinertsen, 1997). Diminished functional ability affects patients' interactions with spouses, children, and other family members and also may produce highly negative economic impacts (Callahan, 1996). For example, it has been found that men with RA report half the earnings of men without arthritis, while women with the same disease report one fourth of the earnings of women with no arthritis (Mitchell *et al.*, 1988). Similarly, 10% of patients with OA report reduced work hours and 13.7% take early retirement; only 1.7% of cohort members without arthritis report working fewer hours and 3.4% retire early (Gabriel, Crowson, & O'Fallon, 1995). With respect to persons with FM, it has been found that 25% report that they have received disability payments, including 15% who have received Social Security Disability (Bennett, 1996). The total cost to our society of all forms of arthritis has been estimated to be 64.8 billion in 1992 dollars (Schned & Reinertsen, 1997). As the mean age of our citizens continues to increase, it is expected that these costs will increase dramatically over time. We now will examine the epidemiology and pathogenesis of the three rheumatic disorders noted above.

Rheumatoid Arthritis

Rheumatoid arthritis is a systemic, inflammatory disease that is found in 0.5 to 1% of the population across many cultures (Pincus, 1996). However, the prevalence is about 2.5 times higher in women than in men. This disease is characterized by an acute inflammatory response, with symmetric polyarticular joint pain and swelling, morning stiffness, and fatigue. For most persons, RA is a progressive illness in which the inflammatory activity produces irreversible joint damage. However, the course of the disease, the amount of joint damage, as well as the severity of pain are quite variable among individuals with RA. There is no cure for RA, although some individuals experience spontaneous remissions of their disease.

There appears to be a genetic predisposition for RA, in that it tends to cluster in families and there is a high concordance of disease in monozygotic twins (Winchester, 1994). It has been estimated that a first-degree relative of an RA patient has a 16-fold increased risk of developing the disease compared to members of the general population.

The etiology of the initial events that evoke the inflammatory response underlying RA is not known. Indeed, it may well be that different exogenous (e.g., viral infection) and endogenous factors [e.g., perturbations of the hypothalamic–pituitary–adrenal (HPA) axis] can precipitate inflammation in the synovial tissue lining of the joint. In persons with RA, this inflammatory response does not remit. The continued production of cytokines and other mediators of the inflammatory response produces a hypercellular pannus that leads to destruction of the cartilage and other structural components of the joint (Pincus, 1996).

The course of RA is quite variable across individuals. However, most patients do show a progressive course with severe declines in functional ability that are independent of age (Pincus, 1996). In addition, patients with RA tend to die at an earlier age than expected for persons of similar ages and sex in the general population.

Medical therapies for RA include nonsteroidal anti-inflammatory drugs (NSAIDS) (e.g., naproxen), corticosteroids (e.g., prednisone), and "disease-modifying" antirheumatic drugs (DMARDS) (e.g., methotrexate). It is well recognized that education as well as physical and occupational therapy and joint protection strategies are also essential for optimal disease management, especially among patients with severe disease and poor prognostic features (Paget, 1997). For some individuals, joint replacement surgery may be needed to reduce pain and increase functional ability.

Osteoarthritis

Osteoarthritis is the most common of the joint diseases and is the second-most common cause of long-term disability among adults in the United States (Stein, Griffin, & Brandt, 1996: Fife, 1997). The prevalence of OA varies among different nationalities. However, over one half of all persons over age 65 show radiographic evidence of OA in the knees. Nevertheless, OA is not considered to be a normal feature of aging. Fewer than one half of persons in their 70s with radiographic evidence of OA experience pain or functional disability (Bagge, Bjelle, Eden, & Svanborg, 1991). Indeed, several variables other than age are involved in OA. For example, women, especially those over the age of 55, are more likely to suffer OA than are men of the same age. In addition, occupations that produce repetitive trauma to joints tend to predispose persons to develop OA in those joints. Obesity also tends to be associated with OA of the knees. Finally, heredity may play a role in the development of OA in some persons, especially those with inflammatory OA of the hand (Fife, 1997).

The etiology of OA is not completely understood. The initiating event is usually identified as a mechanical stress that leads to altered metabolism of chondrocytes, the production of proteolytic enzymes, and disruption of matrix properties (Fife, 1997; Stein et al., 1996). Multiple microfractures may result, leading to gradual loss of the articular cartilage. As the cartilage is lost, "bone-on-bone" contact occurs in the joint, which results in more rapid deterioration in joint movement and function, greater stress on and damage to the joint, and release of damaging degradative enzymes within the joint. Thus, OA becomes a self-perpetuating process that produces pain, stiffness, and functional disability.

As is the case with RA, there is no cure for OA. Thus, treatment usually consists of pharmacological therapy, in conjunction with patient education, physical and occupational therapy, joint protection devices, range-of-motion exercises, and weight loss. In addition, there are orthopedic surgical interventions available for patients who do not respond adequately to pharmacologic therapies and who experience moderate to high levels of pain and functional impairment.

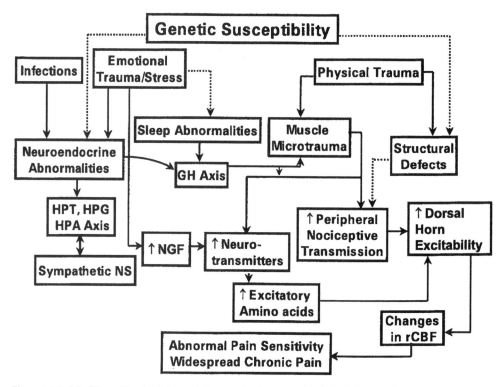

Figure 1. Model of the pathophysiology of abnormal pain perception in FM. Genetic factors, as well as several precipitating events (i.e., physical trauma, emotional trauma or stress, and infections) may contribute to abnormalities in the neuroendocrine axes, sleep, muscle tissue, or spinal structures. Muscle and structural abonormalities may directly lead to hyperexcitability of dorsal horn spinal neurons through increased nociceptive transmission from the periphery to the dorsal horn and through central release of neuropeptide transmitters such as substance P, dynorphin, and calcitonin gene-related peptide as well as by activation of neurons at *N*-methyl-D-aspartate (NMDA) receptor sites by excitatory amino acids. Similarly, neuroendocrine axis and sleep abnormalities may indirectly lead to hyperexcitability of dorsal horn spinal neurons through their disruptive effects on growth hormone (GH) secretion and their stimulation of nerve growth factor (NGF) production. The increased excitability of the dorsal horn spinal neurons produces a barrage of nociceptive input to the brain which eventually alters the functional activity, as measured by regional cerebral blood flow (rCBF), of brain structures that process the sensory–discriminative and affective–motivational dimensions of pain. That is, there appears to be decreased activity in structures that modulate nociceptive input and increased activity in structures that process the affective–motivational dimensions of pain (Bradley *et al.*, 1998). The endpoint of this process is abnormal pain thresholds and widespread, persistent pain. In this model, solid lines between variables indicate relationships for which there is reliable empirical evidence; dotted lines indicate relationships for which there is only preliminary evidence.

Fibromyalgia

Fibromyalgia is a disorder characterized by widespread pain and exquisite tenderness at multiple anatomic sites (Bradley & Alarcón, 1997). Other symptoms include fatigue, disturbed sleep, and irritable bowel. The prevalence of FM is 2% in population studies across cultures; however, approximately 90% of persons with FM are women. The etiopathogenesis of FM is unknown, but several biological abnormalities have been identified in patients with this syndrome. These include alpha electroencephalogram (EEG) intrusion during non–rapid eye movement (REM) sleep, abnormal function of the HPA axis, development of collagen cuffs around nerve terminals, metabolic abnormalities in muscle tissue, elevated cerebrospinal fluid levels of substance P, and inhibited functional activity of two brain structures—the thalamus and caudate nucleus—during resting conditions. Only recently, however, have investigators attempted to develop models of the pathogenesis of FM that incorporate all these biological abnormalities (Bradley & Alarcón, 1997). For example, Weigent, Bradley, Blalock, and Alarcón (1998) recently proposed a model that posits that among individuals with a genetic predisposition for the development of FM, one or more precipitating events (e.g., physical injury, emotional distress) may alter neuroendocrine function or produce muscle microtraumas (Fig. 1). These events, in turn, can produce prolonged transmission of nociceptive input from the periphery to the dorsal horns of the spinal cord. This input eventually produces hyperexcitability of the dorsal horn spinal neurons, which leads to high levels of nociceptive transmission from the spinal cord to the brain. The process of central sensitization thus described alters the function of brain structures involved in pain processing, such as the thalamus, and produces the persistent pain and low pain thresholds characteristic of FM.

There are no well-accepted treatment protocols for FM. Most physicians employ regimens consisting of antidepressant medications and exercise instruction. Indeed, several randomized controlled trials have shown that cardiovascular training exercise, amitriptyline, cyclobenzoprine, and combinations of medications (e.g., fluoxetine and amitriptyline) are superior to placebo in reducing pain (Bradley & Alarcón, 1997). However, none of the interventions thus described may have a great impact on the abnormalities in nociceptive transmission that may be responsible for the major symptoms of FM.

Behavioral and Social Factors that Influence Pain in the Rheumatic Diseases

Depression and Anxiety

Depression and anxiety are negative psychological states that frequently are found in patients with rheumatic disease. For example, the frequency with which depression and anxiety disorders are diagnosed among RA patients ranges from 14 to 42% (Blalock et al., 1989; Frank et al., 1988; Ahles et al., 1991). Similarly, the frequency of lifetime diagnoses of major depression and anxiety disorders in patients with FM ranges from 26 to 71% (Hudson et al., 1985, 1992; Aaron et al., 1996). Clinically significant levels of depression are found in 14 to 23% of patients with OA (Dexter & Brandt, 1994); little is known, however, regarding the frequency of anxiety disorders in these patients. Although there are large differences in the frequency of depression and anxiety among patients with rheumatic disease, all the frequency rates reported in the literature are substantially greater than the population base rates for these psychological disorders (Frank & Hagglund, 1996).

Depression and anxiety are associated with several other health status variables in patients with rheumatic disease. For example, patients with RA who experience depression report significantly higher levels of pain, greater number of painful joints, and poorer functional ability and they spend significantly more days in bed than patients who are not depressed (Katz & Yelin, 1993). Depression also is associated with higher levels of pain and functional disability in patients with OA and FM (Summers, Haley, Reveille, & Alarcón, 1988; Bradley & Alarcón, 1997). Moreover, psychological distress is associated with high levels of medical service use among patients with RA. For example, it was found that over a 5-year period, RA patients with elevated scores on a geriatric depression scale reported a significantly greater number of physician visits and hospitalizations related to their disease than patients whose depression scores were within normal limits (Katz & Yelin, 1993). This is a particularly important finding when one considers that in 1992 terms, $62 billion, or 1% of the gross national product, were spent on direct costs of medical care for patients with arthritis and related musculoskeletal conditions. Thus, early identification and treatment of psychological distress might contribute to a reduction in patients' medical costs.

Some effort has been devoted to identifying the predictors of depression and anxiety in patients with RA. There is evidence that measures of disease activity, such as the number of tender or painful joints, are associated with anxiety and depression (Parker et al., 1991, 1992). However, both cross-sectional and longitudinal studies have shown that pain severity, age, neuroticism, lack of satisfaction with current lifestyle, and degree of functional impairment are better predictors of psychological distress than are joint counts and other disease activity measures (Frank et al., 1988; Hawley & Wolfe, 1988; Affleck et al., 1992a).

Several studies of patients with FM also have examined the role of depression and anxiety in health care seeking. For example, a cross-sectional investigation revealed that the frequency of lifetime psychiatric diagnoses assessed by a computerized form of the Diagnostic Interview Schedule (Robins, Helzer, Croughan, & Ratcliff, 1981) reliably differentiated three groups of individuals from one another: (1) patients with FM recruited from a university-based rheumatology clinic; (2) volunteer community residents with FM who had not sought treatment for their pain during a 10-year period prior to the study (i.e., nonpatients); and (3) healthy community residents without FM (Aaron et al., 1996). The mean number of lifetime psychiatric diagnoses among the FM patients was nearly three times greater than those of both the nonpatients and the controls. Moreover, major depression and anxiety disorders were found most frequently among the FM patients. There were no differences in psychiatric morbidity between the nonpatients and the healthy controls. Thus, lifetime history of psychiatric disorders appears to be an important determinant of health-care-seeking behavior among persons with FM.

This conclusion received additional support in a 2 ½-year longitudinal study of the nonpatients. That is, it was found that only 25% of the nonpatients obtained medical treatment for their pain during the 2 ½-year follow-up study (Aaron et al., 1997c). Although several measures of stress (e.g., working more than one job) and prescription medication use at baseline predicted the receipt of medical care for pain during follow-up, the best predictor of medical treatment was the baseline number of lifetime psychiatric diagnoses. Indeed, the mean baseline number of lifetime psychiatric diagnoses among the nonpatients who obtained medical care during the follow-up was nearly identical to that of the FM patients assessed in the initial cross-sectional study.

Psychosocial factors also are associated with frequency of health-care-seeking behavior among established patients with FM. For example, rheumatology clinic patients with FM who report that psychological trauma preceded or coincided with the onset of their pain more frequently obtain medical consultations and report significantly higher levels of functional disability than FM patients without trauma (Aaron *et al.*, 1997b). One form of psychological trauma that has received particular attention from investigators is sexual and/or physical abuse. It has been found that between 53 and 67% of rheumatology clinic patients with FM report one or more incidents of sexual or physical abuse during childhood or adulthood (Alexander *et al.*, 1998). Patients with histories of abuse, relative to nonabused patients, have significantly higher levels of psychiatric morbidity and report significantly higher levels of pain and functional disability as well as significantly greater frequencies of physician visits for medical problems other than FM. Abused patients also report using a significantly greater number of medications for pain than nonabused patients. In contrast, the frequency of abuse among nonpatients with FM does not differ from that established for the general population (approximately 30%). Thus, it appears that abuse may predispose individuals for the development of psychiatric illness and thus indirectly contribute to high usage of the health care system for FM.

Stress

Rheumatological disorders produce numerous stressors, in addition to psychological distress, that may influence pain. These stressors include activity limitations and functional impairments in the home and workplace as well as financial hardships produced by loss of income and high health care costs (Felts & Yelin, 1989; Liang *et al.*, 1984a; Yelin, 1992; Pincus, Mitchell, & Burkhauser, 1989; Clarke *et al.*, 1993). Another important source of stress is change in patients' social relationships and in their appearance. It has been found, for example, that between 43 and 52% of patients with RA report dysfunction in the areas of social interaction, communication with others, and emotional behavior (Deyo *et al.*, 1982). In addition, two independent studies have reported that about 60% of patients with RA experience at least one major psychosocial change related to family functioning such as increased arguments with spouses, changes in the health of family members, and sexual dysfunction (Liang *et al.*, 1984b; Yelin *et al.*, 1979).

Most of the research concerning stress and pain has been performed with patients with RA. It has been found that these patients frequently report that stress tends to precede flareups in disease activity (Affleck *et al.*, 1987). Indeed, there is evidence that the HPA axis and other neural structures involved in stress responses are also involved in the inflammatory process in RA (Chikanza *et al.*, 1992). For example, patients with RA are characterized by relatively low levels of cortisol and low corticosteroid receptor densities on peripheral blood mononuclear cells (Neeck, Federlin, Graef, Rusch, & Schmidt, 1990; Morand, Jefferies, Dixey, Mitra, & Goulding, 1994). These cortisol abnormalities may indicate dysregulation of the immune system–HPA axis relationship with impaired down-regulation of inflammatory responses by the HPA axis. Abnormal function of the HPA axis also may be involved in abnormal pain perception among patients with FM through its effects on production of nerve growth factor and on the function of brain limbic system structures involved in pain processing (Crofford *et al.*, 1994; Weigent *et al.*, 1998). Finally, there is some evidence that daily stressors and mood are both involved in immune system responses and pain among patients with RA. That is, it has been shown that daily stresses are associated with mood disturbances, which, in turn, are related to decreases in soluble interleukin-2 receptor levels and increases in joint pain (Harrington *et al.*, 1993). In addition, interpersonal stress is associated with elevated immune markers among patients with RA as well as subsequent increases in disease activity (Zautra *et al.*, 1997).

Sleep Disturbance

High frequencies of sleep disturbances have been documented in patients with a variety of rheumatological disorders including RA and OA (Wegener, 1996). However, sleep disturbance is most consistently found among patients with FM. These patients frequently show a specific anomaly characterized by intrusion of alpha waves during non-REM delta (i.e., slow wave) sleep (Moldofsky, 1986). This "alpha–delta" sleep anomaly is associated with local tenderness, pain, and stiffness in patients with FM. It also has been demonstrated in healthy persons that noise-induced disruption of non-REM delta sleep directly leads to the appearance of the alpha–delta sleep anomaly as well as to onset of musculoskeletal pain and negative mood changes (Moldofsky & Scarisbrick, 1976). A return to undisturbed sleep in these healthy persons is followed by normalized sleep physiology and alleviation of symptoms. However, patients with FM who display the alpha–delta sleep anomaly do not report greater symptom severity than those without the anomaly. Moreover, the anomaly does not respond to a nightly regimen of low-dosage amitriptyline (Carette, Oakson, Guimont, & Steriade, 1995). Thus, disturbed sleep plays a role in symptom production and amplification in FM, but the precise physiological mechanism underlying the relationship has not yet been identified.

Beliefs and Coping Strategies

There is consistent evidence that patients' beliefs about their abilities to control or influence their symptoms are associated with pain. Two beliefs that have been studied extensively in patients with rheumatic diseases are *learned helplessness* and *self-efficacy*. These beliefs also may influence patients' abilities to effectively use various coping strategies to reduce or adapt to their pain and other symptoms.

Learned Helplessness

This is a phenomenon characterized by emotional, motivational, and cognitive deficits in adaptive coping with stressful situations. The deficits are produced by the belief that no viable solutions are available to eliminate or reduce the source of stress (Garber & Seligman, 1980). It has been hypothesized that learned helplessness may underlie a portion of the psychological distress and pain experienced by patients with RA and other rheumatological disorders (Bradley, 1985). That is, many patients may develop the belief that their diseases are beyond their effective control because they tend to be characterized by causes that are not well understood, chronic and unpredictable courses, and variable responses to medical treatments. These patients tend to perceive that, regardless of their actions, they will not be able to substantially reduce the pain or other symptoms associated with their conditions. This perception of uncontrollability may cause patients to experience depression and anxiety (i.e., emotional deficits), which in turn may lead to increased pain and reduced attempts to either engage in activities of daily living (i.e., motivational deficits) or to develop new means of adapting to their pain, disabilities, and distress (i.e., cognitive deficits).

These deficits may be particularly profound and resistant to change among patients who view the consequences of their conditions as relatively stable over time and global in nature (i.e., adversely affecting numerous vocational, recreational, social, and marital or sexual activities).

The importance of helplessness beliefs in adaptation to rheumatic disease has been demonstrated in many studies (Bradley, 1994a, 1999b). For example, high levels of helplessness are associated with high levels of pain, depression, and functional disability among patients with RA both at baseline and over follow-up periods of up to 3 years (Smith, Peck, & Ward, 1990; Lorish, Abraham, Austin, Bradley, & Alcarón, 1991). These studies initially led many health professionals to believe that the perception of control over pain and other symptoms (low helplessness) is desirable for patients with rheumatological illnesses. Subsequently, however, it was found that RA patients who believe they can control their symptoms tend to suffer psychological distress in response to flares in disease activity and pain unless they are able to cognitively restructure their pain experiences (Tennen *et al.*, 1992). An example of cognitive restructuring would be the adoption of the belief that one's pain has allowed one to better appreciate the preciousness of life. Thus, psychologists and other health professionals currently tend to focus on enhancing both perceptions of control and coping with flare-induced losses of control among their patients with rheumatic disease (Keefe & Van Horn, 1993).

Self-Efficacy

This construct is closely related to belief in one's level of symptom control or helplessness. However, in contrast to perceptions of loss of control over symptoms, self-efficacy (SE) represents a belief that one can perform specific behaviors to achieve specific health-related goals. Thus, whereas loss of control as manifested in learned helplessness tends to represent a relatively consistent belief regarding a wide array of symptoms, an individual may vary with respect to SE beliefs concerning different behaviors. An individual with RA, for example, may have high SE for pacing her daily activities to reduce pain and fatigue, but she also may have low SE for performing water-based exercise to improve physical function (Lorig *et al.*, 1989).

The importance of SE is that it tends to predict pain and other dimensions of health status if individuals believe that the relevant behaviors will lead to improved health status (Bradley, 1994a). Indeed, it has been reported that high SE for pain is correlated with low frequencies of observable displays of pain behavior among patients with RA and FM even after controlling for demographic factors and disease activity (Buescher *et al.*, 1991; Buckelew *et al.*, 1994). Given these findings, current behavioral interventions for patients with rheumatic disease are designed to foster the development of high levels of SE for pain control through rehearsal of adaptive behaviors in the home, social, and work environments. Many of these adaptive behaviors may be considered as coping strategies.

Coping Strategies

Coping is defined as behaviors that are performed to manage environmental and internal demands (i.e., stressors and conflicts among them) that tax or exceed a person's resources (Bradley, 1994a). The coping process consists of several stages.

These are (1) appraisal of the threat associated with a particular stressor; (2) performing the adaptive behaviors or coping strategies that may control the effects of the stressor; and (3) evaluating the outcomes produced by these behaviors and, if necessary, performing alternative coping responses. It should be noted that coping strategies may be categorized as either direct action or palliative strategies (Burish & Bradley, 1983). Direct action strategies consist of behaviors that contribute to the removal of the stressor, whereas palliative strategies are responses that diminish the negative impact of the stressor. For example, a patient with RA who experiences a flare-up in disease activity may seek treatment from her physician (direct action) and use relaxation or other cognitive distracters (palliative) to better control the impact of pain associated with the flare.

Numerous studies have been performed on the coping responses of patients with rheumatic disease. Three instruments have been used to evaluate coping among patients with these illnesses. These are the Ways of Coping scale (Lazarus & Folkman, 1984), Coping Strategies Questionnaire (Rosenstiel & Keefe, 1983), and the Vanderbilt Pain Management Inventory (Brown & Nicassio, 1987). Despite the differences among these instruments, there has been remarkable consistency in the findings reported across investigations and across disorders. For example, it has been shown repeatedly that passive coping strategies, such as catastrophizing (e.g., believing that if medication is not effective, no other coping strategy will effectively control pain and other symptoms) and escapist fantasies (e.g., hoping that pain will get better someday) are correlated with high levels of pain (Brown & Nicassio, 1987; Martin *et al.*, 1996) and psychological distress (Martin *et al.*, 1996; Keefe *et al.*, 1989) in patients with RA, OA, and FM. In addition, it recently has been found that catastrophizing among FM patients moderates the relationships between morning levels of pain intensity and evening levels of pain intensity, functional impairment, and fatigue severity (Aaron *et al.*, 1997a). That is, FM patients who produce relatively high scores on the Coping Strategies Questionnaire measure of catastrophizing report stronger relationships between morning pain intensity and evening levels of pain, impairment, and fatigue than do patients who produce relatively low catastrophizing scores. However, catastrophizing does not moderate the relationships between morning pain levels and evening levels of depression, anxiety, and hassles. In contrast to the findings reported above, psychological adjustment and relatively low levels of pain tend to be associated with strategies such as attempts to derive personal meaning from the illness experience, seeking information about arthritis, focusing on positive thoughts during pain episodes, and infrequent use of catastrophizing (e.g., Affleck *et al.*, 1992b).

Cognitive–Behavioral Pain Management Interventions for Patients with Rheumatic Disease

Given the relationships that have been documented between pain and patients' beliefs and coping strategies, several cognitive–behavioral therapy (CBT) interventions have been developed to alter patients' perceptions of control, SE beliefs, as well as their coping strategies and thereby improve pain and other health status variables. All these interventions tend to share similar treatment components. These include education, training in relaxation and other coping skills, rehearsal of these newly learned skills in patients' home and work environments, and relapse prevention. Each component included in CBT interventions is described below. A detailed manual for the use of CBT for patients with RA has been presented by Bradley (1996a).

Education

The primary purposes of the educational component are to present a credible rationale for the treatment intervention, to elicit the active collaboration of patients and spouses or other caregivers with the therapist, and to help patients and spouses begin to alter negative perceptions regarding their abilities to manage the pain and other consequences of their disease. During this phase of treatment, it is especially important to encourage the patients and spouses to adopt the belief that they can learn the skills necessary to cope better with the patients' pain and other illness-related problems. This frequently may be accomplished through (1) discussions of the relationships among perceptions of helplessness or low self-efficacy, negative behavior (e.g., low adherence with medication regimes), and poor health status; and (2) demonstrations of the power of behavioral interventions such as relaxation or controlled breathing to enhance control of these symptoms. In a behavioral intervention study performed with RA patients, the educational component comprised the first two treatment sessions. The therapists initiated the education by discussing with the patients and their spouses the learned helplessness construct and the relationships between perceptions of helplessness and pain, depression, and functional disability (Bradley *et al.*, 1987). Once the patients and spouses acknowledged the importance of those relationships in their experiences, the therapists described the major components of the behavioral intervention to them and explained how the components of the intervention were designed to help the patients maintain better control of their pain, psychological reactions, and health-related behaviors. This was followed by a brief demonstration with the patients of the power of relaxation and deep breathing to temporarily reduce perceptions of stress and pain.

Coping Skills Training; Cognitive and Behavioral Rehearsal

The purpose of the coping skills training component is to help patients and spouses engage actively in the process of learning new behaviors and cognitions that will help them better manage pain and other disease-related problems. The purpose of the rehearsal component is to help patients and spouses practice and consolidate new pain management behaviors and cognitions and to apply these effectively in their home and work environments.

The Bradley *et al.* (1987) intervention study featured 11 sessions of training in and rehearsal of three major coping skills. These skills were (1) progressive muscle relaxation training with relaxation imagery and deep breathing; (2) thermal biofeedback aimed at increasing skin temperature at joints affected by RA; and (3) behavioral goal setting by patients and spouses, with reinforcements provided by the spouses and other family members following patients' displays of adaptive coping. For example, patients and spouses who reported fatigue as a problem frequently identified spending more time together in leisure activities as a behavioral goal. Therefore, these couples usually agreed to written daily time schedules for patients' activity and rest periods in an attempt to reduce patients' illness behaviors and to create more opportunities for shared leisure activities. The rewards for following these time schedules often included verbal self-reinforcement, as well as allowing the patients to choose the leisure activities they desired.

Relapse Prevention

The purpose of this component is to help patients retain their newly learned coping skills and to avoid increases in pain or other unpleasant symptoms following treatment. It has been suggested that relapses among patients with rheumatic disease tend to occur when patients' symptoms begin to increase in intensity and their perceptions of symptoms control are diminished (Keefe & Van Horn, 1993). Indeed, these circumstances can be expected to occur relatively often, given the unpredictable courses of most of the rheumatic diseases. At these times, patients are likely to experience psychological distress, show reduced or maladaptive strategies for coping with their symptoms, and thus experience a relapse in pain, emotional distress, and functional ability. Relapse prevention training, then, is designed to help patients respond effectively to potential relapse situations. Specifically, training includes (1) identification of high-risk situations that are likely to tax patients' coping resources; (2) identification of the early signs of relapse, such as increases in pain or depression; (3) rehearsal of cognitive and behavioral skills for coping with these early relapse signs; and (4) provision of self-rewards for effective performance of coping responses to potential relapse (Keefe & Van Horn, 1993).

The Bradley *et al.* (1987) intervention study devoted the final two sessions of the treatment protocol to relapse prevention. During these sessions, patients and their spouses discussed their beliefs and feelings regarding new problems they might encounter after the termination of the treatment intervention. These problems often were associated with possible increases in disease activity or disability with advancing age. Therefore, the therapists asked the patients and spouses to describe possible goals, behavioral strategies, and rewards for coping with their anticipated problems. The therapists also frequently encouraged them to use their newly learned skills to cope with problems unrelated to RA that they might confront in the future. It should be noted that 1-year follow-up analyses indicated that this relapse prevention component produced a sustained reduction in health care services use but failed to maintain improvement in pain behavior (Young, Bradley, & Turner, 1995). Findings such as these have led Keefe and Van Horn (1993) to suggest that relapse prevention training should be introduced early in treatment and repeated throughout the protocol.

Outcomes Produced by Cognitive–Behavioral Interventions

Cognitive–behavioral and other psychosocial interventions have been evaluated in patients with rheumatic disease in over 100 published studies. Overall, it has been shown that these interventions produce a mean reduction of 16% in patients' reports of pain relative to customary medical management (Mullen *et al.*, 1987). However, they generally have not produced substantial reductions in patients' functional disabilities. Only a small number of the studies have examined the effects of treatment on health care utilization or related costs. Nevertheless, the findings that have been reported are positive. The following discussion will review the outcomes produced by the major, well-controlled studies published to date on the effects of CBT and similar interventions on pain and other dimensions of health status among patients with RA, OA, and FM.

Rheumatoid Arthritis

Bradley and colleagues (1987) performed one of the first studies of the effects of behavioral interventions on the pain behavior of patients with RA. The components of this intervention, which were described in preceding section, primarily emphasized training in progressive muscle relaxation, thermal biofeedback, and behavioral goal setting. It was found that, relative to a credible attention placebo (i.e., social support group meetings) and no adjunct treatment conditions, the intervention produced significant reductions in patients' displays of pain behavior (e.g., guarded movement during walking) and the number of painful or tender joints identified during physical examination. The change in the joint count is quite important, as this is one of the best markers for assessing disease activity in patients with RA. Indeed, the joint count reduction produced by this relaxation-based therapy has been replicated by several other investigators (e.g., O'Leary et al., 1988). Moreover, during a 1-year follow-up period, patients who received the intervention reported significantly lower usage of outpatient health care services (13% reduction in RA clinic visits) and incurred lower medical service costs (17% reduction in RA clinic charges) than patients in the other two study conditions (Young et al., 1995). The former patient group also reported significantly lower levels of pain intensity and depression than patients who received no adjunct treatment. However, posttreatment reductions in pain behavior and joint counts produced by the behavioral intervention were not maintained at 1-year follow-up.

Unpublished post hoc analyses of the data from this study suggested that treatment gains on all variables, including pain behavior and joint counts, were best maintained at follow-up by patients who reported good adherence with at least two of the major treatment components (i.e., relaxation, biofeedback, behavioral goal setting). Similar observations by other investigators have led to increased interest in improving relapse prevention among large numbers of patients who participate in behavioral treatment protocols. Indeed, a recent study of a stress management intervention that incorporated the relapse prevention procedures advocated by Keefe and Van Horn (1993) showed that, relative to attention placebo and no adjunct treatment conditions, stress management produced significant improvements in RA patients' pain ratings, reports of helplessness, and coping strategy usage that persisted for 15 months following treatment (Parker et al., 1995).

Osteoarthritis

Two investigations have examined the effects of a coping skills training intervention on patients with OA of the knee (Keefe et al., 1990a, b). This training program, relative to arthritis education and no adjunct treatment, produced significant reductions in patients' ratings of pain and psychological disability that generally were maintained at 6 month follow-up. The coping skills intervention also produced significant improvements in patients' reports of physical disability from posttreatment to follow-up.

The Arthritis Self-Management Program (ASMP) is a standardized intervention that is designed to enhance patients' perceptions of SE for pain, disability, and other arthritis symptoms. It has been evaluated primarily with large groups of patients with OA and RA. The most recent study of the effectiveness of the ASMP with these patients showed that it produced significant increases in SE for pain and other symptoms as well as significant reductions in pain ratings and arthritis-related physician visits that persisted up to 4 years after treatment (Lorig, Mazonson, & Holman, 1993).

Provision of behavioral counseling by telephone represents a new, inexpensive method for improving patients' health status. The first of these interventions, developed for patients with OA, reviewed educational information, medications, and clinical problems identified by the patients. Moreover, it taught them strategies for increasing their involvement in their encounters with their physicians (Weinberger, Tierney, Cowper, Katz, & Booher, 1993). The intervention produced significant reductions in patients' reports of pain and functional ability and did not substantially increase their health care costs.

Recently, telephone-based counseling interventions have been tested with patients with RA and systemic lupus erythematosus (Maisiak, Austin, West, & Heck, 1996). However, the results produced by these interventions have not been uniformly positive. It remains to be determined, then, whether the promising initial results of telephone-based counseling can be consistently reproduced in OA patients as well as in patients with other rheumatic diseases.

Fibromyalgia

Bradley (1989) first suggested that CBT interventions might prove to be beneficial for patients with FM. Since then, several investigators have produced studies of the outcomes produced by CBT interventions with FM patients. Most of these investigators have reported that CBT interventions produce significant reductions in patients' ratings of pain, other clinical symptoms, and functional disability as well as in pain behavior and pain thresholds at the tender points (Bennett *et al.*, 1991; Bennett, Burckhardt, Clark, O'Reilly, & Wiens, 1996; Goldenberg *et al.*, 1994; Nielson, Walker, & McCain, 1992; White & Nielson, 1995). However, none of these investigators employed attention placebo comparison groups to control for the nonspecific effects of prolonged or frequent contact with concerned health professionals. Thus, it is not possible to attribute the treatment gains to the interventions, although it is promising that two studies found that patient improvements in observed pain behavior, reports of functional ability, and the tender point count were maintained for periods ranging from 6 to 30 months after treatment termination (Bennett *et al.*, 1996; White & Nielson, 1995).

Three groups of investigators have performed controlled studies of behavioral treatments for patients with FM. Each group examined the effects of cognitive–behavioral interventions, which included electromyographic (EMG) biofeedback and/or relaxation training as well as training in coping strategies (Vlaeyen *et al.*, 1997; Buckelew *et al.*, 1998; Nicassio *et al.*, 1997). Vlaeyen and colleagues (1997) and Nicassio *et al.* (1997) reported that patients who received CBT interventions did not show greater improvements on any measure of pain or health status than patients who received education-based, attention placebo intervention. It should be noted, however, that Vlaeyen *et al.* (1997) reported there was poor compliance among the CBT patients with home practice of the pain control and coping skills; this intervention, then, may have failed to produce change because many patients did not attempt to fully learn these skills or to incorporate their use in their home and work environments. In contrast, the results reported by Nicassio *et al.* (1997) indicated that the CBT and attention placebo conditions both produced significant improvements for patients on several outcome measures. Therefore, it appears that the negative findings produced by this study may have been due to the unanticipated development of a powerful educational intervention. Indeed, Carette and colleagues (1995) have shown that placebo interventions may produce strong, positive effects on FM patients' symptom reports in pharamacological intervention studies.

Unlike the investigators above, Buckelew and colleagues (1998) compared the effects of brief CBT intervention, exercise training, and a combination of the two treatments with an education based, attention placebo condition. At 2-year follow-up, all of the active treatments had produced significant improvements in a tender point index relative to the attention placebo condition. Only exercise training and the combination of exercise and behavior therapy produced significant improvements in physical activity relative to attention placebo. There were no other group differences on any measure of pain or health status. However, the investigators suggested that the effects of the behavioral and exercise interventions may have been enhanced if the treatments had not been limited to only six training sessions.

In summary, well-controlled studies of the effects of CBT interventions for patients with FM have produced modest effects compared to those produced by similar interventions for patients with RA and OA. It should be emphasized, however, that the potential power of CBT has not been adequately assessed with FM patients due to difficulties with patient compliance, development of powerful attention placebo interventions, and the use of training periods that were much shorter than those used for patients with RA (6 vs. 15) (Buckelew *et al.*, 1998; Bradley *et al.*, 1987). These methodological problems must be resolved before the value of CBT interventions for patients with FM may be accurately assessed.

Future Directions

An important issue that has not been adequately addressed to date involves the mechanisms that might underlie the positive effects produced by CBT on pain among patients with rheumatic disease. Most CBT interventions are designed to reduce perceptions of helplessness or impaired self-efficacy and thereby lead to improved pain control. However, some investigators have produced evidence consistent with this theoretical model (Lorig *et al.*, 1993), while others have reported that CBT produces significant improvements in symptoms but has little effect on perceived symptom control (e.g., Bradley *et al.*, 1987). To date, there have been no attempts to determine whether improvements in health status produced by CBT might also be mediated by changes in physiological variables. Among patients with RA and FM, for example, it would be useful to know whether CBT alters physiological markers of the HPA axis function, such as cortisol levels, which typically are depressed in these patients.

Investigators recently have become interested in documenting abnormal functional brain activity, as measured by regional cerebral blood flow, in patients with chronic pain using neuroimaging methods such as positron emission tomography and single photon emission computed tomography (Mountz, Bradley, & Alarcón, 1998). Several investigations have found evidence of decreased functional activity in the thalamus among patients with advanced cancer pain (DiPiero *et al.*, 1991) and neuropathic pain (e.g., Iadarola *et al.*, 1995). One study has documented low levels of functional activity in both the thalamus and caudate nucleus among patients with FM (Mountz *et al.*, 1995). This finding recently was replicated by a group of investigators in Australia (Kwiatek, Barnden, Rowe, & Pile, 1997). Mountz and colleagues (1995, 1998) have speculated that diminished functional activity in these brain structures may reflect impaired capacity to inhibit transmission of sensory information from ascending spinal afferents to the cortex or other brain structures. Therefore, some investigators have begun to examine whether pharamacological and surgical interventions produce changes in functional brain activity that may mediate changes in pain perception (e.g., Di Piero *et al.*, 1991). Neuroimaging eventually may help us better understand the changes in brain function produced by interventions such as relaxation training that might mediate changes in patients' reports of pain.

Summary and Conclusions

This chapter has shown there are strong relationships between psychosocial factors and pain in patients with rheumatic disease. Factors that tend to increase pain include the presence of depression and anxiety, stress, sleep disturbances, and maladaptive pain beliefs or coping strategies. In contrast, relatively adaptive pain beliefs, such as perceived self-efficacy, tend to be associated with lower levels of pain. These findings have led investigators to devote considerable effort to studying the effects of CBT interventions on pain and other symptoms among patients with RA, OA, and FM.

The CBT intervention studies have shown consistently that these treatments produce significant reductions in ratings of pain and psychological distress among patients with RA and OA. The small number of well-controlled intervention studies performed with FM patients generally have not produced positive results. However, resolution of methodological problems in this area of the behavioral intervention literature may produce improved outcomes for FM patients.

It is anticipated that four issues will receive greater attention from investigators during the next 5 years. First, greater emphasis will be devoted to the prevention of relapse among patients following CBT treatment. Second, increased efforts will be made to document treatment-related reductions in health care use and other costs of chronic pain in addition to changes in patients' reports of symptoms. Third, special attention will be devoted to the development and evaluation of low-cost interventions, such as telephone-based counseling or self-help therapies, that may reduce the health care costs incurred by patients. Finally, it is expected that investigators will devote particular attention to treatment-related alterations in physiological variables that may mediate changes in patients' perceptions of pain.

ACKNOWLEDGMENTS. Supported by National Institute of Arthritis, Musculoskeletal and Skin Diseases grants 1RO1-AR-43136-04 and PO-AR-20164, National Center for Research Resources grant 5-MO1-00032, and grants from the American Fibromyalgia Syndrome Association and the Arthritis Foundation.

References

Aaron, L. A., Bradley, L. A., Alarcón, G. S., Alberts, K. R., Martin, M. Y., & Sotolongo, A. (1997a). Catastrophizing is a specific moderator of daily pain and health status in patients with fibromyalgia (FMS). *Arthritis and Rheumatism 40*, S129.

Aaron, L. A., Bradley, L. A., Alarcón, G. S., Alexander, R. W., Alexander, M. T., Martin, M. Y., Alberts, K. R. (1996). Psychiatric diagnoses are related to health care seeking behavior rather than illness in fibromyalgia. *Arthritis and Rheumatism, 39*, 436–445.

Aaron, L. A., Bradley, L. A., Alarcón, G. S., Triana-Alexander, M., Alexander, R. W., Martin, M. Y., Alberts, K. R. (1997b). Perceived physical and emotional trauma as precipitating events in fibromyalgia: Associations with health care seeking and disability status but not pain severity. *Arthritis and Rheumatism, 40*, 453–460.

Aaron, L. A., Bradley, L. A., Alexander, M. T., Alexander, R. W., Alberts, K. R., Martin, M. Y., & Alarcón, G. S. (1997c). Work stress, psychiatric history, and medication usage predict initial use of medical treatment for fibromyalgia symptoms: A prospective analysis. In T. S. Jensen, J. A. Turner, & Z. Weisenfeld-Hallin (Eds.), *Proceedings of the VIIIth World Congress on Pain, Progress in Pain Research and Management* (Vol. 5, 683–691). Seattle: IASP Press.

Affleck, G., Tennen, H., Pfeiffer. C., & Higgins, P. (1987). Appraisals of control and predictability in adapting to a chronic disease. *Journal of Personality and Social Psychology, 53*, 273–279.

Affleck, G., Tennen, H., Urrows, S., & Higgins, P. (1992a). Neuroticism and the pain–mood relation in rheumatoid arthritis: Insights from a prospective daily study. *Journal of Consulting and Clinical Psychology, 60*, 119–126.

Affleck, G., Urrows, S., Tennen, H. & Higgins, P. (1992b). Daily coping with pain from rheumatoid arthritis: Patterns and correlates. *Pain, 51*, 221–230.

Ahles, T. A., Khan, S., Yunus, M. B., Spiegel, D. A., & Masi, A. T. (1991). Psychiatric status of patients with primary fibromyalgia, patients with rheumatoid arthritis, and subjects without pain: A blind comparison of DSM-III diagnoses. *American Journal of Psychiatry, 148*, 1721–1726.

Alexander, R. W., Bradley, L. A., Alarcón, G. S., Triana-Alexander, M., Aaron, L. A., Alberts, K. R., Martin, M. Y., & Stewart, K. E. (1998). Sexual and physical abuse is associated with outpatient health care utilization and pain medication usage in women with fibromyalgia. *Arthritis Care and Research, 11*, 102–115.

Bagge, E., Bjelle, A., Eden, S., & Svanborg, A. (1991). Osteoarthritis in the elderly: Clinical and radiographic findings in 79–85 year olds. *Annals of Rheumatic Disease, 50*, 535–539.

Bennett, R. M. (1996). Fibromyalgia and the disability dilemma: A new era in understanding a complex, multidimensional pain syndrome. *Arthritis and Rheumatism, 39*, 1627–1634.

Bennett, R. M., Campbell, S., Burckhardt, C., Clark, S., O'Reilly, C., & Weins, A. (1991). Balanced approach provides small but significant gains. A multidiscplinary approach to fibromyalgia management. *Journal of Musculoskeletal Medicine, 8*, 21–32.

Blalock, S. J., DeVellis, R. F., Brown, G. K., & Wallston, K. A. (1989). Validity of the Center for Epidemiologic Studies Depression scale in arthritis populations. *Arthritis and Rheumatism, 32*, 991–997.

Bradley, L. A. (1985). Psychological aspects of arthritis. *Bulletin on the Rheumatic Diseases, 35*, 1–12.

Bradley, L. A. (1989). Cognitive–behavioral therapy for primary fibromyalgia. *Journal of Rheumatology, 16*, 131–136.

Bradley, L. A. (1994a). Psychological dimensions of rheumatoid arthritis. In F. Wolfe, & T. Pincus (eds.), *Rheumatoid arthritis: Critical issues in etiology, assessment, prognosis, and therapy* (pp. 273–295). New York: Marcel Dekker.

Bradley, L.A. (1994b). Behavioral interventions for managing chronic pain. *Bulletin on the Rheumatic Diseases 43:* 2–5.

Bradley, L. A.. (1996a). Cognitive–behavioral therapy for chronic pain. In R. J. Gatchel, D. C. Turk, (Eds) *Psychological approaches to pain management: A practitioner's handbook* (pp. 131–147). New York: Guilford Press.

Bradley, L. A. (1996b). Pain. In S. T. Wegener, B. L. Belza, & E. P. Gall (eds.), *Clinical care in the rheumatic diseases* (pp. 111–115). Atlanta: American College of Rheumatology.

Bradley, L. A. (1997). Psychosocial factors. In J. H. Klippel, C. M. Weyand, & R. L. Wortmann, (eds.), *Primer on the rheumatic diseases* (11th ed., pp. 413–415). Atlanta: The Arthritis Foundation.

Bradley, L. A., & Alarcón, G. S. (1997). Fibromyalgia. In W. J. Koopman (ed.), *Arthritis and allied conditions* (13th ed., pp. 1619–1640). New York: Lippincott.

Bradley, L. A., Young, L. D., Anderson, K. O., Turner, R. A., Agudelo, C. A., McDaniel, L. K., Pisko, E. J., Semble, E. L., & Morgan, T. M. (1987). Effects of psychological therapy on pain behavior of rheumatoid arthritis patients: Treatment outcome and six-month follow-up. *Arthritis and Rheumatism, 30*, 1105–1114.

Bradley, L. A., Alarcón, G. S., Mountz, J. M., Sotolongo, A., Alberts, K. R., Liu, H-G, Kersh, B. C., Domino, M. L., DeWaal, D. (1998). Acute pain produces abnormal regional cerebral blood flow (rCBF) inthe antierior cingulate (AC) cortex in patients with fibromyalgia (FM). *Arthritis and Rheumatism 41*, S353 (abstract).

Brown, G. K., Nicassio, P. M. (1987). Development of a questionnaire for the assessment of active and passive coping strategies in chronic pain patients. *Pain, 31*, 53–64.

Buckelew, S. P., Parker, J. C., Keefe, F. J., Deuser, W. E., Crews, T. M., Conway, R., Kay, D. R., & Hewett, J. E. (1994). Self-efficacy and pain behavior among subjects with fibromyalgia. *Pain, 59*, 377–384.

Buckelew, S. P., Conway, R., Parker, J., Deuser, W. E., Jennings, J., Read, J., Witty, T. E., Hewett, J. E., Minor, M., Johnsen, J. C., Van Maler, L., McIntosh, M. J., Nigh, M., & Kay, P. R. (1998). Biofeedback/relaxation training and exercise interventions for fibromyalgia: a prospective trial. *Arthritis Care and Research, 11*, 196–209.

Buescher, K. L., Johnston, J. A., Parker, J. C., Smarr, K. L., Buckelew, S. P., Anderson, S. K., & Walker, S. E. (1991). Relationship of self-efficacy to pain behavior. *Journal of Rheumatology, 18*, 968–972.

Burish, T. G., & Bradley, L. A. (1983). Coping with chronic disease: Definitions and issues. In T. G. Burish, L. A. Bradley (Eds.), *Coping with chronic disease: Research and applications* (pp. 3–12). New York: Academic Press.

Callahan, L. F. (1996). Impact of rheumatic disease on society. In S. T. Wegner, B. L. Belza, & E. P. Gall (Eds.), *Clinical care in the rheumatic diseases* (pp. 209–213). Atlanta: American College of Rheumatology.

Carette, S., Oakson, G., Guimont, C., & Steriade, M. (1995). Sleep electroencephalography and the clinical response to amitriptyline in patients with fibromyalgia. *Arthritis and Rheumatism, 38*, 1211–1217.

Chikanza, I. C., Petrou, P, Kingsley, G., Chrousos, G., & Panaji, G. S. (1992). Defective hypothalamic response to immune and inflammatory stimuli in patients with rheumatoid arthritis. *Arthritis and Rheumatism, 35*, 1281–1288.

Clarke, A. E., Esdaile, J. M., Bloch, D. A., Lacaille, D., Danoff, D. S., & Fries, J. F. (1993). A Canadian study of the total medical costs for patients with systemic lupus erythematosus and the predictors of costs. *Arthritis and Rheumatism, 36*, 1548–1559.

Crofford, L. F., Pillemer, S. R., Kalogeras, K. T., Cash, J. M., Michelson, D., Kling, M. A., Sternberg, E. M., Gold, P. W., Chrousos, G. P., & Wilder, R. L. (1994). Hypothalamic–pituitary–adrenal axis perturbations in patients with fibromyalgia. *Arthritis and Rheumatism, 37*, 1583–1592.

Dexter, P., & Brandt, K. (1994). Distribution and predictors of depressive symptoms in osteoarthritis. *Journal of Rheumatology, 21*, 279–286.

Deyo, R. A., Inui, T. S., Leininger, J., & Overman, S. (1982). Physical and psychosocial function in rheumatoid arthritis: Clinical use of a self-administered health status instrument. *Archives of Internal Medicine, 142*, 879–882.

Di Piero, V., Jones, A. K. P. Iannotti, F., Powell, M., Perani, D., Lenzio, G. L., & Frackowiak, R. J. J. (1991). Chronic pain: A PET study of the central effects of percutaneous high cervical cordotomy. *Pain, 46*, 9–12.

Felts, W., & Yelin, E. H. (1989). The economic impact of the rheumatic diseases in the United States. *Journal of Rheumatology, 16*, 867–884.

Fife, R. S. (1997). Osterarthritis. Epidemiology, pathology, and pathogenesis. In J. H. Klippel, C. M. Weyand, & R. L. Wortmann (Eds.), *Primer on the rheumatic diseases* (11th ed., pp. 216–218). Atlanta: The Arthritis Foundation.

Frank, R. G., & Hagglund, K. J. (1996). Mood disorders. In S. T. Wegener, B. L. Belza, & E. P. Gall (Eds.) *Clinical care in the rheumatic diseases* (pp. 125–130). Atlanta: American College of Rheumatology.

Frank, R. G., Beck, N. C., Parker, J. C., Kashami, J. H., Eliott, T. R., Haw, A. E., Smith, E., Allwood, C., Brownlee-Duffeck, M., & Kay, D. R. (1998). Depression in rheumatoid arthritis. *Journal of Rheumatology, 15*, 920–929.

Gabriel, S. E., Crowson, C. S., O'Fallon, W. M., Brodeur, C., Smith, S., & Schmid, C. H. (1995). Cost of osteoarthritis estimates from a geographically defined population. *Journal of Rheumatology, 22*(Suppl. 43), 23–25.

Garber, J., & Seligman, M. E. P. (Eds.). (1980). *Human helplessness: Theory and applications.* New York: Academic Press.

Goldenberg, D. L., Kaplan, K. H., Nadeau, M. G., Tennen, H., Higgins, P., Zautha, A., & Hoffman, S. (1994). A controlled study of a stress-reduction, cognitive–behavioral treatment program in fibromyalgia. *Journal of Musculoskeletal Pain, 2*, 53–66.

Harringon, L., Affleck, G., & Urrows, S. (1993). Temporal covariation of soluble interleukin-2 receptor levels, daily stress, and disease activity in rheumatoid arthritis. *Arthritis and Rheumatism, 36*, 199–203.

Hawley, D. J., & Wolfe, J. (1988). Anxiety and depression in patients with rheumatoid arthritis: A prospective study of patients. *Journal of Rheumatology, 15,* 932–941.

Hudson, J. I., Hudson, M. S., Pliner, L. F., Goldenberg, D. L., & Pope, H. G. (1985). Fibromyalgia and major affective disorder: A controlled phenomenology and family history study. *American Journal of Psychiatry, 142,* 441–446.

Hudson, J. I., Goldenberg, D. L., Pope, H. G., Keck, P. E., & Schlesinger, L. (1992). Comorbidity of fibromyalgia with medical and psychiatric disorders. *American Journal of Medicine, 92,* 363–367.

Iadarola, M. J., Max, M. B., Berman, K. F., Byas-Smith, M. G., Coghill, R. C., Gracely, R. H., & Bennett, G. J., (1995). Unilateral decrease in thalamic activity observed with positron emission tomography in patients with chronic neuropathic pain. *Pain, 63,* 55–64.

Katz, P. P., & Yelin, E. H. (1993). Prevalence and correlates of depressive symptoms among persons with rheumatoid arthritis. *Journal of Rheumatology, 20,* 790–796.

Kazis, L. E., Meenan, R. F., & Anderson, J. J. (1983). Pain in the rheumatic diseases: investigation of a key health status component. *Arthritis and Rheumatism, 26,* 1017–1022.

Keefe, F. J., & Van Horn, Y. (1993). Cognitive–behavioral treatment of rheumatoid arthritis pain: Maintaining treatment gains. *Arthritis Care and Research, 6,* 213–222.

Keefe, F. J., Brown, G. K., Wallston, K. A., & Caldwell, D. S. (1989). Coping with rheumatoid arthritis pain: catastrophizing as a maladaptive strategy. *Pain, 37,* 51–56.

Keefe, F. J., Caldwell, D. S., & Williams, D. A., Gil, K. M., Mitchell, D., Robertson, C., Martinez, S., Nunley, J., Beckham, J. C., Crisson, J.E., & Helms, M. (1900a). Pain coping skills training in the management of osteoarthritic knee pain: A comparative study. *Behavior Therapy, 21,* 49–62.

Keefe, F. J., Caldwell, D. S., Williams, D. A., Gil, K. M., Mitchell, D., Robertson, C., Martinez, S., Nunley, J., Beckham, J. C., Crisson, J. E., & Helms, M. (1990b). Pain coping skills training in the management of osteoarthritic knee pain: II. Follow-up results. *Behavior Therapy, 21,* 435–447.

Koopman, W. J., (Ed.). (1997). *Arthritis and allied conditions* (13th ed.). New York: Lippincott.

Kwiatek, R., Barnden, L., Rowe, C., & Pile K. (1997). Pontine tegmental regional cerebral blood flow (rCBF) is reduced in fibromyalgia. *Arthritis and Rheumatism, 40,* S43.

Lazarus, R. S., & Folkman, S. (1984). *Stress, appriasal, and coping.* New York: Springer.

Liang, M. H., Larson, M,, Thompson, M., Eaten, H. M., McNamara, E., Katz, R., & Taylor, J. (1984a). Costs and outcomes in rheumatoid arthritis and osteoarthritis. *Arthritis and Rheumatism, 27,* 522–529.

Liang, M. H., Rogers, M., Larson, M., Eaton, H. M., Murawski, B. J., Taylor, J. E., Swofford, J., & Shur, P. H. (1984b). The psychosocial impact of systemic lupus erythematosus and rheumatoid arthritis. *Arthritis and Rheumatism, 27,* 13–19.

Lorig, K., Chastain, R. L., Ung, E., Shoor, S., & Holman, H. R. (1989). Development and evaluation of a scale to measure perceived self-efficacy in people with arthritis. *Arthritis and Rheumatism, 32,* 37–44.

Lorig, K. R., Mazonson, P. D., & Holman, H. R. (1993). Evidence suggesting that health education for self-management in patients with chronic arthritis has sustained health benefits while reducing health care costs. *Arthritis and Rheumatism, 36,* 439–446.

Lorish, C. D., Abraham, N., Austin, J., Bradley, L. A., & Alarcón, G. S. (1991). Disease and psychosocial factors related to physical functioning in rheumatoid arthritis patients. *Journal of Rheumatology, 18,* 1150–1157.

Maisiak, R., Austin, J. S., West, S. G., & Heck, L. (1996). The effect of person-centered counseling on the psychological status of persons with systemic lupus erythematosus or rheumatoid arthritis: A randomized controlled trial. *Arthritis Care and Research, 9,* 60–66.

Martin, M. Y., Bradley, L. A., Alexander, R. W., Alarcón, G. S., Triana-Alexander, M., Aaron, L. A., & Alberts, K. R. (1996). Coping strategies predict disability in fibromyalgia. *Pain, 68,* 45–53.

Mitchell, J. M., Burkhauser, R. V., & Pincus, T. (1998) The importance of age, education, and comorbidity in the substantial earning losses of individuals with symmetric polyarthritis. *Arthritis and Rheumatism, 31,* 348–357.

Moldofsky, H. (1992). Sleep and musculoskeletal pain. *American Journal of Medicine, 81*(Suppl. 3A), 85–89.

Moldofsky, H., & Scarisbrick, P. (1976). Induction of neurasthenic musculoskeletal pain syndrome by selective sleep stage deprivation. *Psychosomatic Medicine, 38,* 35–44.

Morand, E. F., Jefferiss, C. M., Dixey, J., Mitra, D., & Goulding, N. J. (1994). Impaired glucocorticoid induction of monomuclear leudocyte lipocortin-1 in rheumatoid arthritis. *Arthritis and Rheumatism, 37,* 207–211.

Mountz, J. M., Bradley, L. A., Modell, J. G., Alexander, R. W., Triana-Alexander, M., Aaron, L. A., Stewart, K. E., Alarcón, G. S., & Mountz, J. D. (1995). Fibromyalgia in women: Abnormalities of regional cerebral blood flow in the thalamus and the caudate nucleus are associated with low pain threshold levels. *Arthritis and Rheumatism, 38,* 926–938.

Mountz, J. M., Bradley, L. A., & Alarcón, G. S. (1998). Abnormal functional activity of the central nervous system in fibromyalgia syndrome. *American Journal of the Medical Sciences, 315,* 385–396.

Mullen, P. D., Laville, E., Biddle, A. K., & Lorig, K. (1987). Efficacy of psycho-educational interventions on pain, depression, and disability with arthritis adults: A meta-analysis. *Journal of Rheumatology, 14,* 33–39.

Neeck, G., Federlin, K., Graef, V., Rusch, D., & Schmidt, K. L. (1990). Adrenal secretion of cortisol in patients with rheumatoid arthritis. *Journal of Rheumatology, 17,* 24–29.

Nicassio, P. M., Radojevic, V., Weisman, M. H., Schuman, C., Kim, J. Schoenfeld-Smith, T., & Kral, T. (1997). A comparison of behavioral and educational interventions with fibromyalgia. *Journal of Rheumatology, 24,* 2000–2007.

Nielson, W., Walker, G., & McCain, G. A. (1992). Cognitive–behavioral treatment of fibromyalgia syndrome: Preliminary findings. *Journal of Rheumatology, 19,* 98–103.

O'Leary, A., Shoor, S., Lorig, K., & Holman, H. R. (1988). A cognitive–behavioral treatment for rheumatoid arthritis. *Health Psychology, 7,* 527–544.

Paget, S. A. (1997). Rheumatoid arthritis. C. Treatment. In J. H. Klippel, C. M. Weyand, R. L. Wortmann, (Eds.), *Primer on the rheumatic diseases* (11th ed., pp. 168–174). Atlanta: The Arthritis Foundation.

Parker, J., Smarr, K., Anderson, S., Hewett, J., Walker, S., Bridges, A., & Caldwell, W. (1992). Relationship of changes in helplessness and depression to disease activity in rheumatoid arthritis. *Journal of Rheumatology, 19,* 1901–1905.

Parker, J. C., Smarr, K. L., Walker, S. E., Haggland, K. J., Andersen, S. K., Hewett, J. E., Bridges, A. J., & Caldwell, C. W. (1991). Biopsychosocial parameters of disease activity in rheumatoid arthritis: a prospective study of 400 patients. *Arthritis Care and Research, 4,* 73–80.

Parker, J. C., Smarr, K. L., & Buckelew, S. P., (1995). Effects of stress management on clinical outcomes in rheumatoid arthritis. *Arthritis and Rheumatism, 38,* 1807–1818.

Pincus. T. (1996) Rheumatoid arthritis. In S. T. Wegener, B. L. Belza, & E. P. Gall (Eds.), *Clinical care in the rheumatic diseases* (pp. 147–155). Atlanta: American College of Rheumatology.

Pincus, T., Mitchell, J., & Burkhauser, R. V. (1989). Substantial work disability and earnings losses in individuals less than age 65 with osteoarthritis: Comparisons with rheumatoid arthritis. *Journal of Clinical Epidemiology, 42,* 449–457.

Robins, L. N., Helzer, J. E., Croughan, J., & Ratcliff, K. S. (1981). National Institute of Mental Health Diagnostic Interview Schedule. *Archives of General Psychiatry, 38,* 381–389.

Rosenstiel, A. K., & Keefe, F. J. (1983). The use of coping strategies in chronic low back pain patients: Relationship to patient characteristics and current adjustment. *Pain, 17,* 33–44.

Schned, E. S., & Reinertsen, J. L. (1997). The social and economic comsequences of rheumatic disease. In J. H. Klippel, C. M. Weyand, & R. L. Wortmann (Eds.), *Primer on the rheumatic diseases* (11th ed., pp. 6–9). Atlanta: The Arthritis Foundation.

Smith, T. W., Peck, J. R., & Ward, J. R. (1990). Helplessness and depression in rheumatoid arthritis. *Health Psychology, 9,* 377–389.

Stein, C. M., Griffin, M. R., & Brandt, K. D. (1996). Osteoarthritis. In S. T. Wegener, B. L. Belza, & E. P. Gall (Eds.), *Clinical care in the rheumatic diseases* (pp. 177–182). Atlanta: American College of Rheumatology.

Summers, M. N., Haley, W. E., Reveille, J. D., & Alarcón, G. S. (1988). Radiographic assessment and psychologic variables as predictors of pain and functional impairment in osteoarthritis of the knee or hip. *Arthritis and Rheumatism, 31,* 204–209.

Tennen, H., Affleck, G., Urrows, S., Higgins, P., & Mendolan, R. (1992). Perceiving control, construing benefits, and daily processes in rheumatoid arthritis. *Canadian Journal of Behavioral Science, 24,* 186–203.

Vlaeyen, J. W. S., Teeken-Gruben, N. J. G., Goosens, M. E. J. B., Rutten-van Molken, M. P. M. H., Pelt, R. A. G. B., van Eek, H., & Heuts, P. H. T. G. (1997). Cognitive-educational treatment of fibromyalgia: A randomized clinical trial. I. Clinical effects. *Journal of Rheumatology, 23,* 1237–1245.

Wegener, S. T. (1996). Sleep disturbance. In S. T. Wegener, B. L. Belza, & E. P. & Gall EP (Eds.), *Clinical care in the rheumatic diseases* (pp. 121–124). Atlanta: American College of Rheumatology.

Weigent, D. A., Bradley, L. A., Blalock, J. E., & Alarcón, G. S. (1998). Current concepts in the pathophysiology of abnormal pain perception in fibromyalgia. *American Journal of the Medical Sciences, 315,* 405–412.

Weinberger, M., Tierney, W. M., Cowper, P. A., Katz, B. P., & Booher, P. A. (1993). Cost-effectiveness of increased telephone contact for patients with osteoarthritis: A randomized controlled trial. *Arthritis and Rheumatism, 36,* 243–246.

White, K. P., & Nielson, W. R. (1995). Cognitive–behavioral treatment of fibromyalgia syndrome: A follow-up assessment. *Journal of Rheumatology, 22,* 717–721.

Winchester, R. (1994). The molecular basis of susceptibility to rheumatoid arthritis. *Advances in Immunology, 56,* 389–466.

Yelin, E. (1992). Arthritis: The cumulative impact of a common chronic condition. *Arthritis and Rheumatism, 35,* 489–497.

Yelin, E., Feshbach, D. M., Meenan, R. F., & Epstein, W. (1979). Social problems, services, and policy for persons with chronic disease: The case of rheumatoid arthritis. *Social Science and Medicine, 13,* 13–20.

Young, L. D., Bradley, L. A., & Turner, R. A. (1995). Decreases in health care resource utilization in patients with rheumatoid arthritis following a cognitive–behavioral intervention. *Biofeedback and Self-Regulation, 20,* 259–268.

Zautra, A. J., Hoffman, J., Potter, P., Matt, K. S., Yocum, D., & Castro, L. (1997). Examination of changes in interpersonal stress as a factor in disease exacerbations among women with rheumatoid arthritis. *Annals of Behavioral Medicine, 19,* 279–286.

CHAPTER 18

Prevention of HIV/AIDS

Ralph J. DiClemente, Gina M. Wingood, Sten H. Vermund, and Katharine E. Stewart

Introduction

The human immunodeficiency virus (HIV) epidemic is a biomedical phenomenon given the viral etiology of the acquired immunodeficiency syndrome (AIDS). However, the HIV epidemic is equally, if not more so, a psychosocial and cultural phenomenon. It is not only the virus per se, but an individual's behavior, more specifically, the lack of appropriate health-promoting behavior that propels the epidemic (DiClemente & Peterson, 1994a). Moreover, much of the behavior associated with HIV exposure is of an interpersonal nature resulting from intimate sexual interaction; and, precisely because HIV infection links sexuality with disease, it is inextricably a psychosocial and cultural phenomenon.

Recently, there have been remarkable advances in the treatment of HIV/AIDS (Deeks, Smith, Holodniy, & Kahn, 1997). However, the persistence of other sexually transmitted diseases (STDs) as a major public health problem suggests that the presence of an effective medical treatment alone is not sufficient to control the HIV epidemic (Yankauer, 1986, 1994; Eng & Butler, 1997). Therefore, we must rely not only on our burgeoning and increasingly effective pharmacological armamentarium to control HIV disease, but we must reduce the prevalence of risk behaviors that result in exposure and infection.

This chapter provides an overview, albeit brief, of HIV prevention research as it relates to four populations: adolescents, women, men who have sex with men, and injection drug users (IDUs). Recognizing that there are many ways in which the information in this chapter could have been categorized and presented, we have

Ralph J. DiClemente and Gina M. Wingood • Department of Behavioral Sciences and Health Education, Rollins School of Public Health, Emory University, and Emory/Atlanta Center for AIDS Research, Atlanta, Georgia 30322.   *Sten H. Vermund* • Department of Epidemiology, School of Public Health, UAB Center for AIDS Research, University of Alabama at Birmingham, Birmingham, Alabama 35294.   *Katharine E. Stewart* • Departments of Psychology and Medicine, UAB Center for AIDS Research and UAB Center for Health Promotion, University of Alabama at Birmingham, Birmingham, Alabama 35294.

Handbook of Health Promotion and Disease Prevention, edited by Raczynski and DiClemente.
Kluwer Academic/Plenum Publishers, New York, 1999.

elected to follow a conventional approach that provides population-specific information. We recognize, however, that there is some inconsistency with respect to using this taxonomic strategy. In reality, individuals can be members of multiple categories, for example, gay adolescents. However, the advantages of consistency with the research literature outweigh many of the disadvantages that may arise from inevitable oversimplifications when complex individuals are categorized within groups.

To facilitate an understanding of the prevention research, we initially describe the epidemiology of HIV including temporal changes. Then, we present population-specific epidemiology and discuss primary interventions designed to reduce the risk of HIV infection. To further illustrate the components of effective interventions, we highlight key interventions in greater depth. Finally, we identify a core of programmatic features and constructs that are associated with effective behavior change interventions.

Adolescents

Epidemiology

Adolescents have been identified as a population at increased risk for HIV infection (Select Committee on Children, Youth, and Families, 1992; Office of National AIDS Policy, 1996; National Institutes of Health, 1997). Currently, however, there are no representative population-based studies for estimating HIV seroprevalence among adolescents. The absence of population-based data limits assessing the magnitude of risk for adolescents and reduces the capability to monitor changes in infection rates over time. Much of the HIV seroprevalence data are derived from selected segments of the adolescent population such as studies of applicants for military service or active duty military personnel. Other studies have focused on disadvantaged youth receiving training in the Job Corps, homeless youth, adolescents seeking treatment in STD clinics, and adolescents seeking medical care. HIV seroprevalence data from a variety of adolescent surveys indicate that African-American adolescents have, with few exceptions, markedly higher seroprevalence rates (DiClemente, 1992, 1996; D'Angelo & DiClemente, 1996; Bowler, Sheon, D'Angelo, & Vermund, 1992).

While trend data are limited, recent findings from the continuing HIV serosurvey of Job Corps training program applicants have identified marked changes in infection rates between 1988 and 1992 with African-American female applicants experiencing a twofold increase in seroprevalence rates, from 3.2 per 1000 to 6.6 per 1000. In 1992, African-American females had seroprevalence rates that exceeded not only rates for white and Hispanic women, but also exceeded HIV seroprevalence rates for African-American males (Conway et al., 1993). Overall, the findings suggest that African Americans, particularly females, are at greatest risk for HIV infection.

Prevention Interventions with Adolescents

Sexual abstinence is clearly the most effective strategy for prevention of HIV infection. However, a substantial proportion of adolescents (Anderson et al., 1990; DiClemente, 1990; Hein, 1992; Kann et al., 1991) do not adopt this preventive practice.

Indeed, the expectation that sexually active adolescents will adopt routinely sexual abstinence as an HIV prevention strategy may be unrealistic. For sexually active adolescents, appropriate and consistent use of latex condoms represents the most effective strategy for preventing transmission of HIV (Cates & Stone, 1992), although condom efficacy as a risk-reduction strategy is dependent on appropriate and consistent use (Hein, 1993; Roper, Peterson, & Curran, 1993). High-risk sex among adolescents is not random, uncontrollable, or inevitable. Many factors—individual (intrapersonal), social (interpersonal), environment, and societal—contribute to the propensity to engage in HIV-related sexual risk taking (Sweat & Denison, 1995). More importantly, many of these factors are modifiable.

Behavior change interventions have attempted to reduce or eliminate adolescents' HIV-related risk behaviors. While modifying adolescents' sexual behavior has been a formidable challenge, there are accumulating data suggesting that increasing adolescents' condom use is an achievable goal, as summarized below. Adolescents are not a homogeneous population, but rather a mosaic of subgroups, each with differing subcultural values and norms. Thus, the prevention interventions described below, while broadly applicable for changing adolescents' sexual risk behaviors, should be tailored to the needs of specific adolescent subgroups to be maximally effective.

To facilitate a description of prevention interventions, we have elected to provide site-specific analyses and describe in some detail a few successful interventions that may be useful for others engaged in health-promotion activities. Thus, the following section will be divided into intervention studies conducted in schools, community settings, and clinics.

School-Based HIV Prevention Programs

Schools, primarily in response to the growing threat of HIV, are implementing prevention programs in many districts in the United States as the primary strategy for educating adolescents about STDs and HIV (Kenney, Guardado, & Brown, 1989; Britton, de Mauro, & Gambrell, 1992). Initially, programs focused on enhancing adolescents' knowledge of HIV, particularly the identified routes of disease transmission. These programs were based on the explicit assumption that increased knowledge of HIV would result in reductions in risk behavior. Unfortunately, this is not necessarily the case. Many of the limited program evaluations indicate no significant behavior changes, although most increased knowledge about HIV disease and, to a lesser degree, modification of attitudes. Unfortunately, many of these program evaluations did not or could not measure sexual risk behavior, and thus there is no evidence of effectiveness in modifying behaviors that increase adolescents' risk for HIV in the United States (Kirby & DiClemente, 1994).

Recently, a school-based HIV prevention program has demonstrated efficacy in reducing adolescents' sexual risk behaviors (Walter & Vaughan, 1993). Based on a 3-month follow-up, the findings indicate that the intervention was most effective in increasing knowledge, changing adolescents' beliefs, enhancing self-efficacy, and, most importantly, in reducing high-risk sexual behaviors. Adolescents in the intervention group reported a lower frequency of sexual intercourse with high-risk partners, decreased number of sex partners, and an increase in consistent condom use relative to their peers in the control group.

There are a number of key elements that contribute to the intervention's success. The prevention curriculum is based on established psychological models of behavior change. Moreover, the investigators were able to target key psychosocial constructs that directly effect adolescents' decision making and sexual risk taking based on a needs assessment and recent empirical data. In particular, the prevention curriculum emphasized risk information, self-efficacy and sexual negotiation skills, beliefs about perceived susceptibility, barriers and benefits to engaging in preventive behaviors, and perceptions of the acceptability and norms for involvement in preventive behaviors. Finally, teacher in-service was provided to familiarize teachers with the curriculum.

In another report, Main and colleagues (1994) developed a 15-session skills-based HIV prevention curriculum implemented by trained teachers. Results indicate that students receiving the intervention exhibited greater knowledge about HIV and greater intent to engage in safer sex practices than students in the comparison schools. Among sexually active students at the 6-month follow-up assessment, intervention group students reported fewer sexual partners within the 2 months prior to assessment ($P = 0.046$), greater frequency of condom use ($P = 0.048$), and greater intentions to engage in sexual intercourse less frequently ($P = 0.017$) and to use condoms when having sexual intercourse ($P = 0.039$). This intervention, however, neither delayed the onset nor decreased the frequency of sexual intercourse or the frequency of alcohol and other drug use before sex.

Many of the elements identified in the above studies and other effective school-based interventions have been summarized in a review by Kirby and DiClemente (1994). These critical elements include: (1) using social learning theories as a foundation for program development (e.g., social learning theory, cognitive behavioral theory, social influence theory), (2) maintaining a narrow focus on reducing sexual risk-taking behaviors, (3) using active learning methods of instruction, (4) including activities that address the social and/or media influences and pressures to have sex, (5) focusing on and reinforcing clear and appropriate values against unprotected sex (i.e., postponing sex, avoiding unprotected intercourse, avoiding high risk partners), and (6) providing modeling and practice of communication or negotiation skills. Furthermore, to maximize program effectiveness, HIV prevention programs also must be tailored to be developmentally appropriate and culturally relevant. Clearly, the studies reviewed may provide the impetus for the development of a new generation of school-based HIV prevention programs: those that are theoretically based, empirically driven, emphasize social competency skills acquisition, and are systematically evaluated. Although some findings are encouraging, the modest effect sizes observed suggest that other innovative and effective strategies are urgently needed (DiClemente, 1993).

Community-Based HIV-Prevention Programs

Schools offer a great deal of promise for developing and implementing adolescent HIV prevention interventions. However, the impact of schools as agents of change, promoting the adoption and/or maintenance of HIV-preventive behaviors, should not be exaggerated. Schools alone will not achieve maximal effectiveness if adolescents live in environments that counteract newly acquired HIV-prevention knowledge and skills. There is ample evidence, for instance, that adolescents who do not attend school are at disproportionately greater risk for HIV infection (CDC, 1994).

Thus, community-based HIV prevention interventions may be better able to access this hard-to-reach adolescent population.

Studies conducted with non–school-based adolescent populations indicate that increasing health-promoting behavior change is possible when skills training is incorporated into prevention curricula. A study by Jemmott, Jemmott, and Fong (1992) tested the effectiveness of a sexual risk reduction intervention for African-American male adolescents. Adolescents in the HIV risk reduction condition received a 5-hour intervention involving videotapes, games, and exercises aimed at increasing AIDS-related knowledge, weakening problematic beliefs and attitudes toward HIV risk-associated sexual behavior, and increasing skills at negotiating safer sex. Adolescents randomly assigned to the control condition also received a 5-hour intervention. Structurally similar to the HIV risk reduction intervention, the program involved culturally and developmentally appropriate videotapes, exercises, and games, but the topic was career opportunities rather than HIV risk reduction.

The results revealed that adolescents who received the HIV risk reduction intervention subsequently had greater AIDS knowledge, less favorable attitudes toward risky sexual behavior, and reduced intentions for such behavior compared with adolescents in the control condition. At 3-month follow-up, adolescents in the HIV risk reduction condition reported less risky sexual behavior in the 3 months postintervention than did those in the control condition. Specifically, these adolescent males reported having coitus less frequently and with fewer women and using condoms more consistently during coitus. Fewer reported engaging in heterosexual anal intercourse. In summarizing their community-based research, Jemmott and Jemmott (1994) emphasized the need for further methodologically rigorous research design that incorporates social psychological theory in the selection of variables to be assessed and in guiding the development of the behavior change intervention.

Similarly, St. Lawrence and colleagues (1995) randomly assigned African-American adolescents to an educational program or a social cognitive–behavioral skills intervention in which health educators provided training in correct condom use, sexual assertion, refusal, self-management, problem-solving strategies, and risk recognition. Six- and 12-month follow-up showed that the behavioral skills training participants reported a greater percentage of condom-protected intercourse and were more skillful at handling high-risk sexual situations than control participants.

In another community-based prevention program, Rotheram-Borus and associates (Rotheram-Borus, Koopman, Haignere, & Davies, 1991; Rotheram-Borus, Feldman, Rosario, & Dunne, 1994) developed and evaluated sexual risk reduction programs for high-risk runaway and homeless adolescents. Runaways participating in the risk reduction program were exposed to a multiple-session intervention administered by skilled trainers. The program addressed the following: general knowledge about HIV/AIDS, coping skills, access to health care and other resources, and individual barriers to use of safer sex practices. General HIV knowledge was addressed by having adolescents participate in video and art workshops and review commercial AIDS/HIV commercial videos. Coping skills training addressed runaways' unrealistic expectations regarding emotional and behavioral responses in high-risk situations. Additional medical and mental health care and other resources were made available to address specific individual health concerns. Individual barriers to adopting and maintaining safer sex practices were reviewed in private counseling sessions. Participants in the nonintervention condition were exposed to individual counseling from staff, but this counseling did not specifically address HIV prevention. Condoms were available and staff members were trained to discuss condom use.

Runaways in the risk reduction program demonstrated a significant and marked increase in consistent condom use and less frequently reported engaging in a high-risk pattern of HIV-associated behaviors over 6 months. A high-risk pattern of sexual behavior was defined as consistent condom use occurring in fewer than 50% of sexual encounters, 10 or more sexual encounters, and/or three or more sexual partners in the 6-month interval. A greater proportion of adolescents (22%) in the control group reported this high-risk pattern of sexual behavior compared to those adolescents (9%) who received between 10 and 14 intervention sessions and those (0%) who received 15 or more intervention sessions. Reports of consistent condom use increased from about 32% of runaways at initiation of the project to 62% 6 months after receiving more than 15 intervention sessions. A 2-year follow-up of the same sample continued to show significant reductions in risk acts among those who received the intervention. While highly encouraging, the intensity (> 15 sessions) of the needed intervention limits applicability to all settings.

Finally, Stanton and colleagues (1996) recently reported a study involving 383 low-income African-American youth (ages 9 to 15) randomly assigned in preexisting friendship groups to one of two 8-week interventions. The HIV prevention intervention focused on decision-making and risk-reducing skills. Knowledge regarding HIV, birth control, and human development were also provided. Two annual booster sessions (consisting of didactic sessions and community projects) were completed 15 and 27 months after the eight-session intervention series. Youths in the control condition attended weekly sessions at which a factual movie was shown. However, only the intervention group youths received these facts in the context of decision-making and skills training based on social cognitive theory.

Six months following the intervention, condom use rates were one third higher among sexually active intervention youth (from 59 to 85%) than among control youth (from 65 to 61%, $P < 0.05$). At 12 months, differences in condom use rates were no longer statistically significant between intervention and control group youth. However, following an annual "booster" sessions, rates of condom use at 18 months were again one third higher among intervention youth ($P < 0.05$). In addition, several other HIV risk behaviors expectations and feelings were less common among intervention youth compared to control youth.

Clinic-Based HIV Prevention Programs

While school- and community-based prevention efforts are undoubtedly important in disseminating HIV prevention information, another critical but underutilized access point for educating adolescents about HIV is during the provision of health care. Physicians, in particular pediatricians, adolescent medicine specialists, family practitioners, internists, and gynecologists, are most likely to be engaged in treating adolescents during the time of their onset of sexual and drug behaviors. Thus, clinical interactions between the pediatrician and adolescent patient become an opportunity to assess sexual and drug risk behaviors, evaluate the adolescent's physical and psychological maturation, and provide developmentally appropriate HIV prevention information (DiClemente & Brown, 1994). Little work has been done to examine the comparative successes of nurse practitioners or physician assistant-based care for adolescents.

In one report, the effects of physician's assessment of adolescents' risk behaviors and counseling about HIV risks and prevention were evaluated in an inner-city hospital-based adolescent clinic (Mansfield, Conroy, Emans, & Woods, 1993). Adolescents seeking care were randomly assigned to one of two groups: a standard care group in which physicians interviewed adolescents about high-risk behaviors related to HIV disease and an counseling group in which physicians provided discussion of HIV risks and prevention. At follow-up approximately 2 months after baseline assessments and randomization, 25% of patients reported less sexual activity; 32% and 18%, respectively, of the standard care and counseling group reported less sexual activity. Consistent use of condoms also significantly increased among adolescents in both groups (standard care, $P = 0.03$; counseling $P = 0.02$). Use of condoms at last intercourse increased in the counseling group from 37% to 42% ($P = 0.03$). Another adolescent clinic-based intervention implemented a peer educator risk reduction program targeting multiethnic females 12–19 years of age (Slap, Plotkin, Khalid, Michelman, & Forke, 1991). This study used a single group pretest–posttest research design to evaluate an intervention that consisted of a single counseling session of HIV education and condom skills administered by peer educators using observational learning techniques (i.e., videos and brochures). At follow-up, 2–6 weeks after baseline assessment, adolescents' demonstrated increased HIV knowledge ($P < 0.05$), decreased adolescents' frequency of sexual intercourse ($P < 0.05$) and decreased the frequency of times adolescents reported "never using condoms" during sexual intercourse from 22% at baseline to 11% at follow-up ($P < 0.05$).

Overall, the findings from school, community, and clinic-based studies suggest that behavior change, while difficult, is attainable. Significant reductions in adolescents' risk behaviors over a brief and less often extended follow-up period have been reported. Thus, while much remains to be learned, these findings are promising and suggest key intervention constructs that may enhance the efficacy of prevention interventions.

Women

Epidemiology

Women represent the population that has experienced the most rapid growth in AIDS cases since the inception of the AIDS epidemic (Centers for Disease Control and Prevention, 1990b). For example, in 1997, of the 60,161 persons older than 13 years of age diagnosed with AIDS, 22% were women, nearly threefold greater than the proportion of women diagnosed with AIDS in 1985. AIDS cases attributable to heterosexual transmission are increasing faster than any other exposure category. From 1983 to 1994, AIDS cases attributed to heterosexual contact in women increased from 15% to 38% (Chu & Whortley, 1995). Given the sharp increase in heterosexually transmitted HIV among women, prevention approaches in this population represent an understudied theme. While epidemiological data are informative with respect to quantifying the prevalence of AIDS/HIV in women, they provide limited insight into the influence of pervasive cultural, gender-specific, and psychosocial factors that are the determinants of sexual behavior. Thus, identifying the psychosocial, relational, and gender-related factors associated with a couple's failure to use condoms during sexual intercourse may be useful for developing more efficacious HIV prevention interventions for women.

Psychosocial Correlates of HIV-Related Sexual Risk Taking in Women

Socioeconomic status (SES) is an important correlate of behavior that affects health, access to health services, the risk of disease, the risk of an adverse outcome once disease occurs, and mortality (Adler, Boyce, Chesney, Folkman, & Syme, 1993; Pappas, Queen, Hadden, & Fisher, 1993). Economic factors play an important role in enhancing women's risk of infection. One study reported that women having lower income levels were less likely to use condoms (Peterson *et al.*, 1992b). Similarly, another study noted that compared to employed women, women who were welfare (AFDC) recipients (Wingood & DiClemente, 1998) were less likely to use condoms. In addition to socioeconomic factor, there are numerous beliefs associated with HIV-related sexual risk taking. These include believing that condoms have a negative impact on sexual enjoyment (Catania *et al.*, 1992; Peterson *et al.*, 1992b), feeling that using condoms is embarrassing (Peterson *et al.*, 1992b), perceiving oneself to be at risk for HIV (Sikkema *et al.*, 1995), perceiving that your partner will think you are unfaithful if you ask them to use a condom (Wingood & DiClemente, 1998) and having a negative attitude toward sex (Harlow, Quina, Morokoff, Rose, & Grimley, 1993).

Self-efficacy is the confidence in one's ability to effect change in a specific practice (Bandura, 1986). Self-efficacy regarding sexual communication/negotiation is the confidence a women has in bargaining for safer sex in light of the social cost of such negotiations (Worth, 1990; Wingood, Hunter, & DiClemente, 1993). Women's inability to negotiate condom use is one of the strongest correlates of never having used a condom (Peterson *et al.*, 1992b; Wingood & DiClemente, 1998; Catania *et al.*, 1992; Harlow *et al.*, 1993). Additionally, a number of studies have reported that women with low levels of self-efficacy for using condoms (Peterson *et al.*, 1992) and women who are less confident in their ability to avoid HIV (Harlow *et al.*, 1993) are also more likely to engage in HIV-related sexual risk taking.

At the core of partner-related influences exacerbating women's HIV risk are the power inequities that exist between the sexes. Power inequalities in heterosexual relationships are evident in social norms dictating monogamy for women and not for men, men having control over condom use, and violence directed toward women as well as the threats of such victimization. Several studies have demonstrated that monogamous women, women who have one sexual partner are four times less likely, and women who have a partner who is resistant toward using condoms (Wingood & DiClemente, 1998) are nearly three times less likely to use condoms (Catania *et al.*, 1992; Wingood & DiClemente, 1998). Other partner-related factors associated with HIV sexual risk taking include having a physically abusive partner (Wingood & DiClemente, 1997), having a sexually abusive partner (Zierler, 1997) and fearing partner victimization (Harlow *et al.*, 1993). In addition, if one or both partners wishes to conceive, the desire for pregnancy may undermine conscientious use of condoms (Adler & Tschann, 1993).

As the development of an effective therapeutic treatment or prophylactic vaccine may not be available in the foreseeable future, reducing the risk of HIV infection among sexually active women requires the adoption of preventive strategies that effectively inhibit viral transmission. (Wingood & DiClemente, 1996). Thus, identifying HIV-related socioeconomic factors, beliefs, skills, and partner-related influences is crucial for designing and implementing efficacious HIV prevention interventions for women.

Effective HIV Behavioral Interventions for Women

Behavioral interventions based on theories of health behavior, designed to reduce HIV-related sexual risk practices are critical for preventing further acceleration of HIV among women. While behavioral interventions have been developed for a number of at-risk populations (DiClemente & Peterson, 1994b), unfortunately programs developed specifically for women have lagged behind those developed for other populations (Choi & Coates, 1994; Coates, 1990; Wingood & DiClemente, 1996). We briefly review, several HIV prevention interventions that have been tailored to women.

El-Bassel and Schilling (1992) conducted an HIV prevention intervention for females 21 to 42 years of age, the majority of whom where either African-American or Hispanic, recruited from a methadone maintenance program in Bronx, New York. Women were randomly assigned to either a skills-based intervention condition (n = 48) or an information-only control condition (n = 43). Participants randomized to the peer-led skills-based intervention condition received training in AIDS education, proper condom use, assertiveness and communication skills, as well as identifying personal barriers to implementing safer sex practices. The theoretical framework guiding the intervention was social cognitive theory. The study reported a significant increase in the mean frequency of condom use 15 months postintervention ($P < 0.01$).

Hobfoll, Jackson, Lavin, Britton, and Shepherd (1994) conducted an HIV sexual risk reduction intervention for single pregnant women 16 to 29 years of age, the majority of whom where either African American or Caucasian, recruited from three inner-city obstetric clinics in Akron, Ohio. Women were randomly assigned to one of three conditions: a four-session AIDS prevention condition (n = 68), a health promotion comparison condition (n = 77), or a control condition (n = 61). Participants randomized to the four-session peer-led AIDS prevention condition received AIDS education, assertiveness skills, negotiation skills, planning skills, skills in cleaning drug works, and relapse prevention. Peer leaders utilized role playing to refine participants' sense of mastery, positive expectations of success, problem-solving skills, and sense of vulnerability. The theoretical models underlying the intervention were the social cognitive theory and conservation of resources theory (COR). The COR theory posits that an intervention must increase both a woman's personal and social resources in order to combat her increased threat of AIDS. The COR theory further suggests that target groups must see the intervention as both adding new resources and building on current strengths. Participants randomized to the intervention demonstrated favorable changes in mean scores on a composite measure of spermicide and condom use over a 6-month period compared to the no-intervention control conditions (χ^2 = 2.44; $P < 0.05$).

Kelly and colleagues (1994) conducted an HIV sexual risk-reduction intervention among women 18 to 40 years of age recruited from a primary health care clinic in Milwaukee, Wisconsin. The majority of women were African American with multiple male sexual partners who had a diagnosis of a sexually transmitted infection or had sex with a high-risk male partner. Participants were randomized to either a five-session peer-led HIV/AIDS intervention condition (n = 100) or a comparison condition

($n = 87$). Women randomized to the intervention condition received five sessions that emphasized AIDS education, attitudinal and social factors affecting safer sex, proper condom use skills, identifying personal triggers such as involvement in coercive or power imbalanced sexual relationships, and peer support elements (e.g., endorsing the norm that men can be denied sex unless condoms are used). As in the other theoretically based interventions, social cognitive theory was used to guide intervention development. Women randomized to the intervention condition demonstrated increased frequency of condom use from 26% at baseline to 56% of all intercourse occasions in the 3-months postintervention assessment ($P < 0.001$). The comparison group showed little change in condom use at follow-up assessment.

DiClemente and Wingood (1995) conducted an HIV sexual risk reduction intervention among African-American women 18–29 years of age recruited from the Bayview Hunter's Point neighborhood in San Francisco, California. Participants were randomized to either a five-session peer-led HIV/AIDS intervention condition ($n = 53$), an HIV education-only condition ($n = 35$), or a delayed HIV education control condition ($n = 40$). Women randomized to the five-session peer-led HIV/AIDS intervention received five sessions that emphasized ethnic and gender pride, HIV risk reduction information, sexual self-control, sexual assertiveness and communication skills, proper condom use skills, and developing relationship norms supportive of consistent condom use. The theoretical frameworks guiding intervention development were the social cognitive theory and theory of gender and power. The theory of gender and power posits that difficulties arise in following safer sex practices because self-protection often is swayed by feelings of intimacy, abusive partners, economic factors, and norms supporting women's passive behavior within sexual relationships. The theory of gender and power addresses the influence of these larger social structures that can compromise the sexual health of women (Connell, 1987). Women randomized to the intervention condition, compared to the delayed HIV education control condition, demonstrated increased consistent condom use (adjusted odds ratio = 2.1, 95% CI 1.03-4.15; $P = 0.04$). No statistically significant differences in condom use were observed between the HIV education-only condition relative to the delayed HIV education control condition.

In general, HIV interventions that are guided by social psychological theories, in particular, social cognitive theory, provide skills training in condom use and sexual communication and emphasize social support for behavior change are more effective at promoting the adoption and maintenance of condom use (Bandura, 1994; Moore, Harrison, & Doll, 1994). In addition to the application of a theoretical framework, these interventions have several other programmatic and methodological characteristics that may facilitate program efficacy. Many effective interventions emphasize gender-related influences, such as stressors facing women, gender-based power imbalances within the relationship, and sexual assertiveness. While HIV preventive skills are clearly important, unsafe sexual behavior often is not only the result of a deficit of knowledge, motivation, or skills, but also has meaning within a women's personal relationships and sociocultural context. Furthermore, many effective interventions are peer led. Peer educators may be a more credible source of information, communicate in a language that is more likely to be understood, and serve as positive role models to dispel the normative misconception that most women are engaging in high-risk behaviors. This is especially important in high-risk social environments where many women may perceive the community norm as supporting risky behavior rather than HIV preventive behavior. Finally, most effective interventions were multiple-session programs. Interventions in which women received 8 to 10 hours of HIV prevention education and skills training were more effective at enhancing and maintaining condom use than single session interventions. Given that results depend on self-report, prevention research that can study HIV seroconversion outcomes (Allen *et al.*, 1991) or that minimize the likelihood of responses that are incorrect, that is, overreported safe behavior, (Turner *et al.*, 1998) are needed.

Men Who Have Sex with Men

Epidemiology

AIDS was initially described in a cohort of homosexual men in Los Angeles in 1981 (CDC, 1981). Since then, homosexual and bisexual men, or men who have sex with men (MSMs), have typically been thought to comprise the majority of those affected by the HIV epidemic. Indeed, MSMs comprise 49% of the total AIDS cases reported to the Centers for Disease Control and Prevention (CDC) since 1981 (CDC, 1998). However, MSMs comprised only 35% of AIDS cases in 1997. This reflects the fact that the HIV epidemic is shifting slightly away from MSMs, and affecting injection drug users and heterosexual populations more than in the past.

It would be a mistake, however, to conclude that the AIDS epidemic is ending for MSMs. While Coates (1990) has characterized the extent of the behavior changes made by urban gay men as one of public health's most dramatic successes, the epidemic continues to spread rapidly in some subsections of the gay male population. For example, younger MSMs may be at higher risk than older men (Hays, Kegeles, & Coates, 1990). Among men aged 20 to 24, MSMs comprise 63% of HIV cases (CDC, 1995). In addition, minority MSMs (Peterson *et al.*, 1992a) and MSMs in small cities (Kelly, 1994) tend to report higher levels of risky behavior and display increasing rates of HIV seroprevalence. Thus, these subgroups of the larger MSM population continue to be in particular need of prevention interventions.

Several authors (Hays & Peterson, 1994; Kelly *et al.*, 1995) have identified other demographic and psychological characteristics associated with increased risk taking. These include high risk-taking behavior in the past, lower self-efficacy, lower educational levels, use of alcohol or drugs, less integration into a gay community, stronger beliefs that peers do not support preventive behaviors, and stronger beliefs that high-risk sexual activities are more enjoyable than low-risk activities. Careful examination of this list reveals important parallels to a well-recognized theory of behavior change—social learning theory (Bandura, 1986, 1994).

Knowledge about the need for change, perceived self-efficacy, social support for behavior change, and a belief that such changes are desirable in one's community are all components of successful behavior modification, according to social learning theory. Interventions implemented both at the individual (Kelly, St. Lawrence, Hood, & Brasfield, 1989; Leviton *et al.*, 1990; Roffman *et al.*, 1997) and community (Kegeles, Hays, & Coates, 1996) levels have incorporated this model, generally with considerable success. Overall, interventions that have either explicitly followed social learning principles or implicitly included these principles have demonstrated more consistent successes than those focusing on education or on counseling and testing alone (Kalichman, Carey, & Johnson, 1996).

Prevention Interventions with MSMs

Individual and Small-Group Interventions

Interventions at this level focus typically on provision of information about HIV transmission, counseling about risky behaviors, and training in preventive behaviors, such as condom use. Many of these interventions have been evaluated; however, many have also suffered from a lack of theoretical underpinning, a lack of control samples, or reliance on attitude or knowledge change rather than behavior change as outcome variables.

On the individual level, the CDC Community Demonstration Project (CDC, 1992) focused not only on provision of information, but also on skills training about correct condom use with persons referred from community organizations, clinics, and other word-of-mouth advertising. Participants (all MSMs) reduced their frequency of unprotected anal intercourse and increased their condom use; however, no control group was employed in this study. Given the explosion of information regarding safer sexual behaviors during the late 1980s and early 1990s, the lack of a control group makes it difficult to determine whether these changes reflect the intervention or an overall increase in community awareness. Another important shortcoming inherent in the individual approach is the lack of opportunity for social norms, supports, and pressures to exert their considerable influence during the intervention. For this reason, as well as for cost-effectiveness reasons, small-group interventions have been more thoroughly investigated.

In small-group meetings, participants can observe peers espousing desired attitudes regarding sexual risk reduction and can receive positive feedback about their personal ability to implement such changes from members of their own community. These combine to enhance a sense of self-efficacy for the desired behavior, a critical component in the social learning model (Bandura, 1994). Many small-group interventions have also employed "peer educators," members of the target community trained to implement the group sessions, to further enhance these social modeling and normative effects.

Kelly *et al.* (1989) based a 12-session group intervention with MSMs on social learning theory and cognitive–behavioral theory and compared their results to wait-listed controls. The sessions included information about HIV transmission and risk, identification of cognitive or behavioral risk triggers (e.g., alcohol use) and ways to manage these triggers, role-playing of assertive sexual behaviors (e.g., negotiating condom use), and formation of a sense of community solidarity. This intervention program reduced frequencies of unprotected anal intercourse in the intervention group to near zero and increased condom use from 23% to 75%.

This team achieved similar results when they replicated their study using only a seven-session intervention (Kelly, St. Lawrence, Betts, Brasfield, & Hood, 1990). Of particular note is the ethnic composition of this replication study's sample: nearly 20% of the sample were minority men, permitting greater generalizability of findings compared to most other contemporaneous interventions with MSMs.

Another randomized, controlled trial (Leviton *et al.*, 1990) compared lectures on HIV risk reduction to lectures that were combined with skills training, again using role-playing and feedback exercises with MSMs. The groups receiving the combination intervention not only reported significantly safer behaviors, such as increased condom use and decreased unprotected anal intercourse, but maintained these changes at 6- and 12-month follow-ups. For example, condom use in the combination group was 36% at pretrial, rising to 80% at the 12-month follow-up, significantly higher than rates for the lecture-alone group. Attitudinal changes about the importance of high- versus low-risk activities were also maintained at follow-up. This use of a knowledge-enhancing control group effectively demonstrates the limited effects that knowledge alone may have on modifying behavior; specific skills training and social support for such behaviors appear critical to the behavior change process.

A unique intervention that attempts to provide social support and peer norms about low-risk activities to individuals who may otherwise be isolated from receiving such messages is the use of telephone conference calls (Roffman *et al.*, 1991, 1997). This intervention uses the conference call technology to provide information and some skills training while advancing a social norm about reducing high-risk activities. Participants in these small groups have consistently been more likely to identify as bisexual, to be more secretive about their sexual orientation, and to feel strongly that their sexual orientation needed to remain hidden. They also reported similar rates of high-risk behavior as other groups of MSMs.

After the conference call interventions and at a 1-month follow-up, participants reported increased low-risk activity and decreased high-risk activity and also perceived their social norms as more affirming of preventive behaviors. Thus, innovative or creative interventions may be effective in addressing the needs of MSMs who often are not participants in studies that enroll volunteers; in fact, this "hidden" group is a subpopulation of MSMs that may be at particular risk of HIV (Hays & Peterson, 1994).

Community Interventions

Community-level interventions seek to change the behavior and attitudinal norms on a wider basis than individual and small-group interventions. This approach is particularly powerful in the area of HIV prevention, and particularly so with MSMs, because of the often well-defined social networks already in existence in this population (Kelly, 1994). In both large and small cities there are often bars, community organizations, and residential neighborhoods where MSMs tend to meet and socialize. This provides a critical test of the social learning theory model, since changes in social norms, combined with skills training, should lead to particularly noticeable changes in behavior within communities.

Honnen and Kleinke (1990) demonstrated that simply raising awareness within the community can potentially decrease risk taking. When signs were posted in three gay men's bars about the rate of HIV in the community and the efficacy of condoms in reducing the spread of HIV, the numbers of condoms taken by bar patrons was nearly 50% higher than when the signs were not present. Although the number of condoms taken is not an absolute measure of safer sexual behavior, this study is relatively unique for its reliance on a measure of risk taking not based on self-report. Objective indicators of behavior change may include STD or HIV seroincidence, actual condom use, or other verifiable markers. These are likely to be subject to minimal bias from recall or from the giving of responses perceived to be socially desirable, which is a problem with self-reported data.

More elaborate community interventions have specifically focused on addressing the social components of behavior change. Kelly and colleagues (1992) utilized Rogers' (1983) theory of social diffusion, which argues that attitudes and behavior change often move through social networks from "opinion leaders," or popular community members, to others. This team identified several opinion leaders in bars where MSMs met and socialized and trained these men to actively discuss and espouse safer sex messages and reduction of risky behaviors. The focus was primarily on the leaders' initiating conversations about their own changes in behavior and attitudes, as well as modeling acceptance and approval of low-risk activities.

The intervention proved successful at both 3- and 6-month follow-ups, with 25 to 30% reductions in self-reported unprotected anal intercourse, increases in condom use, and decreases in number of sexual partners. Control comparisons in another city showed no changes. This intervention is particularly noteworthy because it focused on MSMs in cities that were relatively small. Such populations are in particular need of such large-scale change, since MSMs in small cities have been shown in general to have higher rates of high-risk activity than that of MSMs in HIV epicenters where prevention interventions have been ongoing.

Focusing on another population that may benefit from wide-scale normative changes, Kegeles *et al.* (1996) developed an intervention specifically for younger MSMs. Called the M-Powerment Project, this intervention focused not only HIV prevention, but the often unique social needs of younger MSMs, who may not have as well-defined social networks. Thus, part of the project was focused on helping young men create such networks, through social activities (dances, group meetings, "movie nights," etc.) and informal networking, before implementing HIV risk-reduction messages. Risk reduction was accomplished through peer outreach, similar to the Kelly *et al.* (1992) study described above, as well as more formal small-group meetings and a communitywide publicity campaign targeted to young men.

The M-Powerment Project resulted in considerable decreases in unprotected anal intercourse among the young MSM population and also significantly changed attitudes about the favorability of lower-risk versus higher-risk activities. Further analyses (described in Hays & Peterson, 1994) demonstrated that the use of various modes of interventions (e.g., dances and large informal social gatherings where theatrical productions espousing safer sex were performed, informal peer interactions, and small-group workshops) may be particularly useful. Men who engaged in high rates of high-risk behavior typically declined to participate in small-group activities, but they did report behavior changes after informal interactions or social gatherings where salutary social norms were evident.

Most interventions targeted at MSMs have focused on primarily white, relatively well-educated men who self-identify as gay and volunteer to participate in intervention studies. While they have repeatedly demonstrated the effectiveness of various interventions, particularly those that are based on the social learning model, these studies must be followed by well-designed interventions with other subgroups of the MSM population who may be at particular risk. These groups include minority MSMs, MSMs who do not identify as gay, less well-educated men, and rural MSMs. Studies with such groups can provide additional evidence of the generalizability of the social cognitive and other models.

In addition, leaders in this field have called for a standard of outcome measurement, such as frequency of unprotected anal intercourse, to allow easier comparisons between studies and for outcomes that are not self-report in nature, such as condom purchase rates or STD rates (Kelly, 1994), to control for some of the social desirability effects and recall errors inherent in self-report data. Finally, Kalichman *et al.* (1996) make a strong argument in favor of interventions based on theoretical models, particularly social learning theory. Since most studies that have demonstrated desirable behavior changes that are maintained over time incorporate most or all of the components of this model, continued adherence to the model while adapting it for specific populations is most likely to yield positive results.

Injection Drug Users

Epidemiology

Injection drug users (IDUs) account for a substantial proportion of HIV cases in the United States. In 1995, injection drug use was the principal risk factor in 26% of new AIDS diagnoses (CDC, 1995). Another 5% of cases were due to unprotected sex with an IDU. In women, injection drug use is the single-most common cause of HIV infection; over 50% of new cases of HIV were IDU-related (CDC, 1995).

Traditionally in this country, intravenous drug use has been approached with either a legal or medical model. That is, IDUs have typically been "handled" by either arrest and conviction, or by either compulsory or voluntary enrollment in addiction treatment programs that emphasize total abstinence from drug use as the primary goal. However, these approaches may miss a substantial proportion of IDUs, including those who do not wish to seek treatment, those who have sought treatment but have been unable to find treatment available, and those who evade arrest successfully (Watters & Guydish, 1994).

Another approach to reducing the spread of HIV infection in IDUs is the harm reduction model, which emphasizes safer injection and sex practices, such as avoiding sharing of equipment and use of bleach to clean syringes and condoms during sex. This has typically been the primary approach of the majority of interventions with this population, particularly those that are community based. However, it is important to note that this approach conflicts substantially with many treatment centers' goals to decrease and eliminate drug use (Sorensen, Costantini, & London, 1989). This conflict may make implementation of interventions somewhat difficult in clinic settings without appropriate communication between clinic and public health workers. Community leaders and politicians commonly confuse risk reduction with "permissiveness," failing to appreciate the HIV-related benefits and the "bridge" function to definitive drug treatment services.

Prevention Interventions with IDUs

Individual and Clinic-Level Interventions

Most individual-level interventions have been conducted within clinic settings. Their findings are generalizable only to the in-treatment subpopulation of IDUs.

However, a variety of different approaches have been implemented and have been successful, from the drug treatment itself to education, skills training, and small-group interventions.

Drug treatment, specifically methadone maintenance treatment, repeatedly has been shown to decrease IDU (Ball, Lange, Myers, & Friedman, 1988; Yancovitz *et al.*, 1991) and rates of HIV seroconversion (Moss *et al.*, 1994; Williams *et al.*, 1990). However, since relapse rates in drug treatment programs are fairly high (Ball & Ross, 1991), it is unclear whether these reductions in injection drug use and seroconversion can be maintained over time without additional behavioral modification, both of IDU and high-risk sexual activities.

Although there has been some concern that testing for HIV in the clinic context might be distressing to patients, most investigations have found that testing tends to be perceived as beneficial by most patients even though they may experience some anxiety (Casadonte, Des Jarlais, Friedman, & Rostrosen, 1990). Testing for HIV affords another intervention opportunity. Farley, Cartter, Wassell, and Hadler (1992) reviewed methadone maintenance patient records and found decreased levels of IDU among those patients who received HIV testing and counseling compared to those who did not, and also found HIV testing did not lead to an increased rate of discontinuing drug treatment. However, Calsyn, Saxon, Freeman, and Whittaker (1992) found no significant differences in behavior change among patients in treatment who were randomly assigned to AIDS education, education plus testing, or wait-list control groups, even though the patients reduced their high-risk behavior overall.

Several interventions have attempted to incorporate the social learning model into their interventions, primarily by designing small-group interventions that included skills training in either lower-risk injection behavior or sexual behavior. McCusker, Stoddard, Zapka, and Lewis (1993) found that IDUs who participated in group sessions reported increased self-efficacy for desired behaviors and reported reduced frequency of injection at a 6-month follow-up, when compared to patients who were in educational programs alone. A similar group intervention (Des Jarlais, Casriel, Friedman, & Rosenblum, 1992) resulted in a reduction in the number of patients who converted from snorting to injecting heroin.

However, other group-based interventions have not been as effective in changing behavior. In a primarily education-based group intervention, Colon, Robles, Freeman, and Matos (1993) found no differences between their intervention and control groups in injection behaviors, despite knowledge changes. Similarly, Sorensen *et al.* (1994) obtained knowledge and attitude changes with a combination education and skills-training group approach, but again found no behavior changes. This may be due partially to the interventions not targeting those issues believed to be critical in social learning theory, especially modeling by credible peers and establishing self-efficacy for desired behaviors. In addition, Sorensen *et al.* (1994) point out that IDUs may require more potent interventions than some of the briefer programs, primarily because they may be attempting to learn fairly complex behaviors (such as "works" syringe cleaning) as well as multiple risk reduction behaviors (drug use avoidance and safer sexual behaviors) simultaneously.

Reviewing several studies of small-group interventions, Roehrich, Wall, and Sorensen (1994) conclude that small groups are effective in reducing IDU overall. However, they make several suggestions for improving their effectiveness, including "booster" sessions to reinforce learning, peer-led interventions, and interventions targeted at the specific needs of women and minorities. These suggestions correspond to similar findings in the MSM population, and point again to the social learning model, with its emphases on peer instruction, targeted interventions to subpopulations, and intensive training and reinforcement, as the standard for program development.

Community-Level Interventions: Needle Exchange Programs

To attempt to reach IDUs who either cannot or do not wish to enter treatment programs, various community approaches to reducing risky behavior, particularly sharing of syringes, have been developed. Perhaps none is so controversial in the United States as needle exchange programs. In needle exchange, IDUs may obtain sterile needles and syringes in exchange for new ones at no cost from community health workers. Rather than reusing old syringes or borrowing a used syringe from another IDU, the recipient can use a sterile needle and syringe. The primary concern about needle exchange programs has been whether they encourage or increase the rate of injection drug use. Guydish *et al.* (1993) evaluated this question and found no evidence that the programs increase injection among IDUs or increase the rate of conversion from noninjecting users to injecting users. A comprehensive review by the Institute of Medicine (1995) came to the same conclusion.

Needle exchange programs have been successful in reducing the sharing of injection equipment among IDUs. Hagan, DesJarlais, Purchase, Reid, and Friedman (1991a) demonstrated a decrease in self-reported sharing of syringes in an exchange program in Tacoma. Following up on these self-reported data, the same team (1991b) found that participants in the exchange program had lower HIV seroprevalence rates than the nonexchangers. Kaplan and Heimer (1992) implemented an exchange and tracking program by numbering syringes given to IDU; they were thus able to determine if syringes were taken and returned by different individuals (implying sharing had taken place). They estimated a one third reduction in new cases of HIV during the exchange program period using molecular HIV diagnosis of residual blood in needle bevels and mathematical models.

While needle exchange programs reduce HIV incidence, they do not eliminate syringe sharing behaviors and they do not address other important concerns, such as sexual transmission of HIV and access to drug treatment for those who desire it. As Watters and Guydish (1994) point out, needle exchange programs are likely to be successful only in communities with broad support for such programs from political and community-based groups, and are likely to remain a fairly controversial intervention strategy in the United States. The best programs, as in New Haven, offer needle exchange as one component of more comprehensive treatment and HIV prevention social services.

Community-Level Interventions: Street Outreach Programs

Needle exchange is but one type of community intervention with IDUs. Street outreach programs that provide education, skills training, and encouragement for the social norm of safer injecting behavior and drug-free lifestyles are also a focus of prevention efforts. Watters *et al.* (1990) developed a community health outreach plan that sent workers to areas where IDUs gathered throughout San Francisco. The workers provided education regarding the need to refrain from sharing equipment, to use bleach to clean used syringes, and to use condoms during sexual activity. Over the course of more than a year, several follow-ups revealed significant increases in self-reported bleach and condom use and decreases in syringe sharing.

Stephens, Feucht, and Roman (1991) obtained similar success in their community outreach program, with reductions from 67% to 24% in the proportion of IDU who shared syringes, a change that was maintained at a 3-month follow-up. Other larger-scale studies of several cities have found an overall positive effect of outreach programs (CDC, 1990a). Watters and Guydish (1994) point out that these successful programs generally have been losing funding over the past several years due to political opposition.

Of note is the relative lack of theoretical focus in many of the community interventions for IDU. Although many interventions incorporate elements of various models, as a group they do not focus on components that have been found to be critical in other populations (i.e., MSMs). Additional research needs to evaluate whether incorporation of these elements, such as peer modeling, self-efficacy building, and practice of acquired skills, increases the adoption of health-promoting behavior changes within this population.

Like interventions targeted at MSMs, interventions focusing on IDUs have demonstrated successes in behavior changes toward less risky activities. Small-group interventions appear particularly effective with this population, perhaps because these interventions have been more intensive in their education and skills-building components.

Interventions focused on IDUs who are not in treatment, female and minority IDUs, and young IDUs all could benefit from further development. Theory-based programs that emphasize skills training and peer encouragement and feedback need to be studied, as well as those that address the particularly complex set of psychosocial needs and forces that affect the various IDU subpopulations.

Of course, standardized outcome measurement and assessments that do not rely on self-report are needed. However, as Watters and Guydish (1994) point out, relying on HIV seroprevalence or other biological markers as outcome measures also has statistical problems, particularly in areas where the base rate of infection is high. Continued creative and well-developed research that addresses these concerns is particularly important as the epidemic continues to spread among IDUs, particularly their female sex partners.

Core Components Associated with Reducing Sexual Risk Behaviors: A Synthesis

There are several key theoretical and implementation features that appear to be associated with changing sexual risk behavior. Foremost, programs need to be tailored to meet the specific needs of different populations. "Tailoring" would include assuring that the intervention was culturally sensitive, developmentally appropriate, gender-relevant, and risk-relevant (Wingood & DiClemente, 1992, 1998).

Second, using a theoretical model on which to base the intervention, one that addresses the interplay between cognition, attitudes, beliefs, behaviors, and environmental influences, improves the likelihood of program efficacy. Sexual behavior, in particular, takes place within a social–cultural context. Effective program development depends on an understanding of the contextual nature of behavior, the factors that promote the adoption of preventive behaviors, and those countervailing influences that reinforce risk taking behavior. One model that has demonstrated utility as a foundation for developing sexual risk reduction interventions is social cognitive theory (Bandura, 1994). The cornerstones of this model include the provision of timely and accurate information, developing and mastering social competency skills through observational learning techniques (e.g., social modeling) and active learning techniques (e.g., role playing, preferably a series of graded-intensity high-risk situations), enhancing self-efficacy to communicate assertively and effectively with sex partners, and developing a supportive peer network to reinforce the maintenance of safer sex behaviors. Many of the effective prevention interventions reviewed earlier were based on this model.

Another key component is maintaining a narrow focus on reducing sexual risk-taking behaviors. Thus, each sexual risk behavior targeted for change, whether it is enhancing condom use, reducing the number of sexual partners, or even postponing sexual intercourse, should be clearly specified with appropriate strategies designed to address them directly. Far too often prevention programs have targeted a broad spectrum of risk behaviors for change without including behavior-specific change strategies in the program. An example will help to illustrate this key concept. Designing a prevention intervention to enhance adolescents' self-efficacy to reduce their number of sexual partners is an important and appropriate endpoint. However, the behavior-specific strategies and techniques used to enhance their self-efficacy may not succeed in increasing self-efficacy to assert that sex partners use condoms. Programs designed to reduce the number of sex partners and increase condom use are addressing two important but qualitatively different risk behaviors. To be maximally effective, each risk behavior, the underlying psychosocial factors that reinforce these behaviors, and the strategies and skills needed to achieve behavior change must be addressed adequately in synergistic, mutually reinforcing ways.

Finally, there are specific psychosocial constructs that have been identified as associated with condom use. Interventions tailored to emphasize these constructs are more likely to be effective in modifying adolescents' behaviors. Key constructs include: (1) providing specific skills training in sexual communication, negotiation, and assertiveness skills; (2) enhancing perceptions of peer norms as supporting abstinence and/or safer sex behavior; (3) enhancing self-efficacy to avoid high-risk situations and refuse high-risk sex; (4) increasing awareness of the effects of alcohol and drug use on their sexual behavior; and (5) providing condom use skills and increasing the availability of condoms where they are not readily accessible. Though we have identified core components of prevention interventions that have yielded promising results, given the magnitude of observed behavioral changes reported and the limited follow-up periods for evaluating the stability of treatment effects, new and innovative interventions remain a priority.

Conclusions

There is an overriding urgency to develop and implement social and behavioral interventions that motivate individuals to adopt and/or maintain HIV preventive practices. Without continued research designed to identify those constructs most closely associated with behavior change, for specific populations and subgroups within populations, interventions, though effective, cannot hope to achieve optimal efficacy. Much remains to be done. And, unfortunately, the HIV epidemic continues to exact a high toll in suffering and death. However, there are encouraging findings, across populations, suggesting that researchers are reaching closure on a set of constructs predictive of intervention-induced behavior change. Further refinements and innovations of program design and implementation, in concert with rigorous evaluation strategies, will pave the way for the advent of a new and more effective generation of HIV prevention interventions.

References

Adler, N. E., & Tschann, J. M. (1993). Conscious and preconscious motivation for pregnancy among female adolescents. In A. Lawson & D. L. Rhode (Eds.), *The politics of pregnancy: Adolescent sexuality and public policy* (pp. 144–158). New Haven, CT: Yale University Press.

Adler, N. E., Boyce, T., Chesney, M. A., Folkman, S., & Syme, L. (1993). Socioeconomic inequalities in health, no easy solution. *Journal of the American Medical Association, 269,* 3140–3145.

Allen, S., Lindan, C., Serufilir, A., Van de Perrre, P., Rundle, A. C., Nsengumuremyi, F., Carael, M., Schwalbe, J., & Hulley, S. (1991). Human immunodeficiency virus infection in urban Rwanda. Demographic and behavioral correlates in representative sample of childbearing women. *Journal of the American Medical Association, 266,* 1657–1663.

Anderson, J. E., Kann, L, Holtzman, D., Arday, S., Truman, B., & Kolbe, L. (1990). HIV/AIDS knowledge and sexual behavior among high school students. *Family Planning Perspectives, 22,* 252–255.

Ball, J. C., & Ross, A. (1991). *The effectiveness of methadone treatment.* New York: Springer-Verlag.

Ball, J. C., Lange, W. R., Myers, C. P., & Friedman, S. R. (1988). Reducing the risk of AIDS through methadone maintenance treatment. *Journal of Health and Social Behavior, 29*(3), 214–226.

Bandura, A. (1986). *Social foundations of thought and action: A social cognitive theory.* Englewood Cliffs, NJ: Prentice Hall.

Bandura, A. (1994). Social cognitive theory and exercise of control over HIV infection. In R. J. DiClemente & J. L. Peterson (Eds.), *Preventing AIDS: Theories and methods of behavioral interventions* (pp. 25–60). New York: Plenum Press.

Bowler, S., Sheon, A. R., D'Angelo, L. J., & Vermund, S. H. (1992). HIV and AIDS among adolescents in the United States: Increasing risk in the 1990s. *Journal of Adolescence, 15,* 345–371.

Britton, P. O., de Mauro, D., & Gambrell, A. E. (1992). HIV/AIDS education. *SIECUS Report, 21,* 1–8.

Calsyn, D. A., Saxon, A. J., Freeman, Jr., G., & Whittaker, S. (1992). Ineffectiveness of AIDS education and HIV antibody testing in reducing high-risk behaviors among injection drug users. *American Journal of Public Health, 82*(4), 573–574.

Casadonte, P. P., Des Jarlais, D. C., Friedman, S. R., & Rostrosen, J. P. (1990). Psychological and behavioral impact among intravenous drug users of learning HIV test results. *International Journal of the Addictions, 25,* 409–426.

Catania, J. A., Coates, T. J., Kegeles, S., Fullilove, M. T., Peterson, J., Marin, B., Siegel, D., & Hulley, S. (1992). Condom use in multi-ethnic neighborhoods of San Francisco: the population-based AMEN (AIDS in multi-ethnic neighborhoods) study. *American Journal of Public Health, 82,* 284–287.

Cates, W., & Stone, K. M. (1992). Family planning, sexually transmitted diseases and contraceptive choice: A literature update—part I. *Family Planning Perspectives, 24,* 75–84.

Centers for Disease Control and Prevention (CDC). (1981). Kaposi's sarcoma and *Pneumocystis pneumonia* among homosexual men—New York City and California. *Morbidity and Mortality Weekly Report, 30*(25), 305–308.

Centers for Disease Control and Prevention (CDC) (1990a). Update: Reducing HIV transmission in intravenous drug users not in treatment—United States. *Morbidity and Mortality Weekly Report, 39,* 529–538.

Centers for Disease Control and Prevention. (CDC) (1990b). AIDS in women—United States. *Mortality and Morbidity Weekly Report, 39,* 845–846.

Centers for Disease Control and Prevention (CDC). (1992). AIDS community demonstration projects: Implementation of volunteer networks for HIV-prevention programs—selected sites, 1991–1992. *Morbidity and Mortality Weekly Report, 41*(46), 868–869, 875–876.

Centers for Disease Control and Prevention (CDC). (1994). Health risk behaviors among adolescents who do and do not attend school—United States, 1992. *Morbidity and Mortality Weekly Report, 43,* 129–132.

Centers for Disease Control and Prevention (CDC). (1995). *HIV/AIDS surveillance report, 7*(2), 7–35.

Centers for Disease Control and Prevention (CDC). (1998). *HIV/AIDS surveillance report, 10*(1), 5–27.

Choi, K. H., & Coates, T. J. (1994). Prevention of HIV infection. *AIDS, 8,* 1371–1389.

Chu, S. Y., Wortley, P. M. (1995). Epidemiology of HIV/AIDS in women. In H. Minkoff, J. A. DeHovitz, & A. Duerr (Eds.), *HIV infection in women* (pp. 1–12). New York: Raven Press.

Coates, T. J. (1990). Strategies for modifying sexual behavior for primary and secondary prevention of HIV disease. *Journal of Consulting and Clinical Psychology, 58,* 57–69.

Colon, H. M., Robles, R. R., Freeman, D., & Matos, T. (1993). Effects of a risk-reduction education program among injection drug users in Puerto Rico. *Puerto Rico Health Sciences Journal, 12*(1), 27–34.

Connell, R. W. (1987). *Gender and power.* Stanford CA: Stanford University Press.

Conway, G. A., Epstein, M. R., Hayman, C. R., Miller, C. A., Wendell, D. A., Gwinn, M., Karon, J. M., and Peterson, L. R. (1993). Trends in HIV prevalence among disadvantaged youth: Survey results from a national job training program 1988 through 1992. *Journal of the American Medical Association, 269,* 2887–2889.

D'Angelo, L., & DiClemente, R. J. (1996). Sexually transmitted diseases and human immunodeficiency virus infection among adolescents. In R. J. DiClemente, W. Hansen, & L. E. Ponton (Eds.), *Handbook of adolescent risk behavior* (pp. 333–368). New York: Plenum Press.

Deeks, S. G., Smith, M., Holodniy, M., & Kahn, J. O. (1997). HIV-1 protease inhibitors. *Journal of the American Medical Association, 277,* 145–153.

Des Jarlais, D. C., Casriel, C., Friedman, S. R., & Rosenblum, A. (1992). AIDS and the transition to illicit drug injection: Results of a randomized trial prevention program. *British Journal of Addiction, 87*(3), 493–498.

DiClemente, R. J. (1990). The emergence of adolescents as a risk group for human immunodeficiency virus infection. *Journal of Adolescent Research, 5,* 7–17.

DiClemente, R. J. (1992). Epidemiology of AIDS, HIV seroprevalence and HIV incidence among adolescents. *Journal of School Health, 62,* 325–330.

DiClemente, R. J. (1993). Preventing HIV/AIDS among adolescents: Schools as agents of change. *Journal of the American Medical Association, 270,* 760–762.

DiClemente, R. J. (1996). Adolescents at-risk for acquired immune deficiency syndrome: Epidemiology of AIDS, HIV prevalence and HIV incidence. In S. Oskamp & S. Thompson (Eds.), *Understanding and preventing HIV risk behavior* (pp. 13–30). Newbury Park, CA: Sage.

DiClemente, R. J. (1997). Looking forward: Future directions for prevention of HIV among adolescents. In L. Sherr (Ed.), *AIDS and adolescents* (pp. 189–199). Reading, Berkshire, United Kingdom: Harwood Academic Publishers.

DiClemente, R. J., & Brown, L. K. (1994). Expanding the pediatrician's role in HIV prevention for adolescents. *Clinical Pediatrics, 32,* 1–6.

DiClemente, R. J., & Peterson, J. (1994a). Changing HIV/AIDS risk behaviors: The role of behavioral interventions. In R. J. DiClemente & J. Peterson (Eds.), *Preventing AIDS: Theories and methods of behavioral interventions* (pp. 1–4). New York: Plenum Press.

DiClemente, R. J., & Peterson, J. (Eds.). (1994b). *Preventing AIDS: Theories and methods of behavioral interventions.* New York: Plenum Press.

DiClemente, R. J., & Wingood, G. M. (1995). A randomized controlled trial of a community-based HIV sexual risk reduction intervention for young adult African-American females. *Journal of the American Medical Association, 274,* 1271–1276.

El-Bassel, N., & Schilling, R. F. (1992). 15-month follow-up of women methadone patients taught skills to reduce heterosexual HIV transmission. *Public Health Reports, 107,* 500–504.

Eng, T. R., & Butler, W. T. (1997). *The hidden epidemic. Confronting sexually transmitted diseases.* Washington, DC: National Academy Press.

Farley, T. A., Cartter, M. L., Wassell, J. T., & Hadler, J. L. (1992). Predictors of outcome in methadone programs: Effect of HIV counseling and testing. *AIDS, 6,* 115–121.

Guydish, J., Bucardo, J., Young, M., Woods, W., Grinstead, O., & Clark, W. (1993). Evaluating needle exchange: Are there negative effects? *AIDS, 7*(6) 871–876.

Hagan, H., Des Jarlais, D. C., Purchase, D., Reid, T., & Friedman, S. R. (1991a). The Tacoma syringe exchange. *Journal of Addictive Diseases, 10,* 81–88.

Hagan, H., Des Jarlais, D. C., Purchase, D., Reid, T., & Friedman, S. R. (1991b). Lower HIV seroprevalence, declining HBV and safer injection in relation to the Tacoma syringe exchange. Poster presented at the VII International Conference on AIDS, Florence (Abstract W.C.3291).

Harlow, L. L., Quina, K., Morokoff, P. J., Rose, J. S., & Grimley, D. M. (1993). HIV risk in women: A multi-faceted model. *Journal of Applied Biobehavioral Research, 1,* 3–38.

Hays, R. B., & Peterson, J. L. (1994). HIV prevention for gay and bisexual men in metropolitan cities. In R. J. DiClemente & J. L. Peterson (Eds.), *Preventing AIDS: Theories and methods of behavioral intervention* (pp. 267–296). New York: Plenum Press.

Hays, R. B., Kegeles, S. M., & Coates, T. J. (1990). High HIV risk taking among younger gay men. *AIDS, 4,* 901–907.

Hein, K. (1992). Adolescents at risk for HIV infection. In R. J. DiClemente (Ed.), *Adolescents and AIDS: A generation in jeopardy* (pp. 3–16). Newbury Park, CA: Sage.

Hein, K. (1993). "Getting real" about HIV in adolescents. *American Journal of Public Health, 83,* 492–494.

Hobfoll, S. E., Jackson, A. P., Lavin, J., Britton, P. J., & Shepherd, J. B. (1994). Reducing inner-city women's AIDS risk activities: A study of single, pregnant women. *Health Psychology, 13,* 3979–403.

Honnen, T. J., & Kleinke, C. L. (1990). Prompting bar patrons with signs to take free condoms. *Journal of Applied Behavior Analysis, 23*(2), 215–217.

Institute of Medicine. (1995). *Preventing HIV transmission: The role of sterile needles and bleach.* Washington, DC: National Academy Press.

Jemmott, J. B., & Jemmott, L. S. (1994). Interventions for adolescents in community settings. In R. J. DiClemente & J. Peterson (Eds.), *Preventing AIDS: Theories and methods of behavioral interventions* (pp. 141–174). New York: Plenum Press.

Jemmott, J. B., Jemmott, L. S., & Fong, G. T. (1992). Reductions in HIV risk-associated sexual behaviors among black male adolescents: Effects of an AIDS prevention intervention. *American Journal of Public Health, 82,* 372–377.

Kalichman, S. C., Carey, M. P., & Johnson, B. T. (1996). Prevention of sexually transmitted HIV infection: A meta-analytic review of the behavioral outcome literature. *Annals of Behavioral Medicine, 18*(1) 6–15.

Kann, L., Anderson, J. E., Holtzman, D., Ross, J., Truman, B. I., Collins, J., & Kolbe, L. J. (1991). HIV-related knowledge, beliefs, and behaviors among high school students in the United States: Results from a national survey. *Journal of School Health, 61,* 397–401.

Kaplan, E. H., & Heimer, R. (1992). HIV prevalence among intravenous drug users: Model-based estimates from New Haven's legal needle exchange. *Journal of Acquired Immune Deficiency Syndromes, 5,* 163–169.

Kegeles, S. M., Hays, R. B., & Coates, T. J. (1996). The Mpowerment Project: A community-level HIV prevention intervention for young gay men. *American Journal of Public Health, 86*(8), 1129–1136.

Kelly, J. A. (1994). HIV prevention among gay and bisexual men in small cities. In R.J. DiClemente & J. Peterson (Eds.), *Preventing AIDS: Theories and methods of behavioral interventions* (pp. 297–318). New York: Plenum Press.

Kelly, J. A., & Murphy, D. A. (1992). Psychological interventions with AIDS and HIV: Prevention and treatment. *Journal of Consulting and Clinical Psychology, 60*(4), 576–585.

Kelly, J. A., St. Lawrence, J. S., Hood, H. V., & Brasfield, T. L. (1989). Behavioral intervention to reduce AIDS risk activities. *Journal of Consulting and Clinical Psychology, 57,* 60–67.

Kelly, J. A., St. Lawrence, J. S., Betts, R., Brasfield, T. L., & Hood, H. V. (1990). A skills training group intervention to assist persons in reducing risk behaviors for HIV infection. *AIDS Education and Prevention, 2,* 24–35.

Kelly, J. A., St. Lawrence, J. S., Stevenson, L. Y., Hauth, A. C., Kalichman, S. C., Diaz, Y. E., Brasfield, T. L., Koob, J. J., & Morgan, M. G. (1992). Community AIDS/HIV risk reduction: The effects of endorsements by popular people in three cities. *American Journal of Public Health, 82,* 1483–1489.

Kelly, J. A., Murphy, D. A., Washington, C. D., Wilson, T. S., Koob, J. J., Davis, D. R., Ledezma, G., & Davantes, B. (1994). The effects of HIV/AIDS intervention groups for high-risk women in urban clinics. *American Journal of Public Health, 84,* 1918–1922.

Kelly, J. A., Sikkema, K. J., Winett, R. A., Solomon, L. J., Roffman, R. A., Heckman, T. G., Stevenson, L. Y., Perry, M. J., Norman, A. D., & Desiderato, L. J. (1995). Factors predicting continued high-risk behavior among gay men in small cities: psychological, behavioral, and demographic characteristics related to unsafe sex. *Journal of Consulting and Clinical Psychology, 63*(1), 101–107.

Kenney, A. M., Guardado, S., & Brown, L (1989). Sex education and AIDS education in the schools: What states and large school districts are doing. *Family Planning Perspectives, 21*(2), 56–64.

Kirby, D., & DiClemente, R. J. (1994). School-based interventions to prevent unprotected sex and HIV among adolescents. In R. J. DiClemente & J. Peterson (Eds.), *Preventing AIDS: Theories and methods of behavioral interventions* (pp. 117–139). New York: Plenum Press.

Leviton, L. C., Valdiserri, R. O., Lyter, D. W., Callahan, C. M., Kingsley, L. A., Huggins, J., & Rinaldo, C. R. (1990). Preventing HIV infection in gay and bisexual men: Experimental evaluation of attitude change from two risk reduction interventions. *AIDS Education and Prevention, 2*(2), 95–108.

Main, D. S., Iverson, D. C., McGloin, J., Banspach, S. W., Collins, J. L., Rugg, D. L., & Kolbe, L. J., (1994). Preventing HIV infection among adolescents: Evaluation of a school-based education program. *Preventive Medicine, 23,* 409–417.

Mansfield, C. J., Conroy, M. E., Emans, S. J., & Woods, E. R. (1993). A pilot study of AIDS education and counseling of high-risk adolescents in an office setting. *Journal of Adolescent Health, 14,* 115–119.

McCusker, J., Stoddard, A. M., Zapka, J. G., & Lewis, B. F. (1993). Behavioral outcomes of AIDS educational interventions for drug users in short-term treatment. *American Journal of Public Health, 83*(10), 1463–1466.

Moore, J. S., Harrison, J. S., & Doll, L. S. (1994). Interventions for sexually active, heterosexual women in the United States. In R. J. DiClemente & J. L. Peterson (Eds.), *Preventing AIDS: Theories and methods of behavioral interventions* (pp. 243–266). New York: Plenum Press.

Moss, A. R., Vranizan, K., Gorter, R., Bacchetti, P., Watters, J., & Osmond, D. (1994). HIV seroconversion in intravenous drug users in San Francisco, 1985–1990. *AIDS, 8*(2), 223–231.

National Institutes of Health (1997). *NIH consensus development conference on interventions to prevent HIV risk behaviors.* Washington, DC: Government Printing Office.

Office of National AIDS Policy (1996). *Youth and HIV/AIDS: An American agenda.* Washington DC: Government Printing Office.

Pappas, G., Queen, S., Hadden, W., & Fisher, G. (1993). The increasing disparity in mortality rates between socioeconomic groups in the United States, 1960 and 1986. *New England Journal of Medicine, 329,* 103–109.

Peterson, J. L., Grinstead, O. A., Golden, E., Catania, J. A., Kegeles, S., & Coates, T. J. (1992b). Correlates of HIV risk behaviors in black and white San Francisco heterosexuals: The population-based AIDS in multiethnic neighborhoods (AMEN) study. *Ethnicity and Disease, 2,* 361–370.

Roehrich, L., Wall, T. L., & Sorensen, J. L. (1994). Behavioral interventions for in-treatment drug users. In R. J. DiClemente & J. L. Peterson (Eds.), *Preventing AIDS: Theories and methods of behavioral intervention* (pp. 189–208). New York: Plenum Press.

Roffman, R. A., Beadnell, B. A., Stern, M., Gordon, J. R., Downey, L., & Siever, M. (1991, August). *Phone counseling in reducing barriers to AIDS prevention.* Paper presented to the Annual Meeting of the American Psychological Association, San Francisco.

Roffman, R. A., Picciano, J. F., Ryan, R., Beadnell, B., Fisher, D., Downey, L., & Kalichman, S. C. (1997). HIV-prevention group counseling delivered by telephone: An efficacy trial with gay and bisexual men. *AIDS and Behavior, 1,* 137–154.

Rogers, E. M. (1983). *Diffusion of innovations.* New York: Free Press.

Roper, W. L., Peterson, H. B., & Curran, J. W. (1993). Commentary: Condoms and HIV/STD prevention—Clarifying the message. *American Journal of Public Health, 83,* 501–503.

Rotheram-Borus, M. J., Koopman, C., Haignere, C., & Davies, M. (1991). Reducing HIV sexual risk behaviors among runaway adolescents. *Journal of the American Medical Association, 266,* 1237–1241.

Rotheram-Borus, M. J., Feldman, J., Rosario, M., & Dunne, E. (1994). Preventing HIV among runaways: Victims and victimization. In R. J. DiClemente & J. Peterson (Eds.), *Preventing AIDS: Theories and methods of behavioral interventions* (pp. 175–188). New York: Plenum Press.

Select Committee on Children, Youth, and Families. (1992). *A decade of denial: Teens and AIDS in America.* Washington, DC: Government Printing Office.

Sikkema, K. J., Heckman, T. G., Kelly, J. A., Anderson, E. S., Winett, R. A., Solomon, L. J., Wagstaff, D. A., Roffman, R. A., Perry, M. J., Cargill, V., Crumble, D. A., Fuqua, R. W., Norman, A. D., & Mercer, M. B. (1995). HIV risk behaviors among women living in low-income, inner-city housing developments. *American Journal of Public Health, 86,* 1123–1128.

Slap, G. B., Plotkin, S. L., Khalid, N., Michelman, D. F., & Forke, C. M. (1991). A human immunodeficiency virus peer education program for adolescent females. *Journal of Adolescent Health, 12,* 434–442.

Sorensen, J. L., Costantini, M. F., & London, J. A. (1989). Coping with AIDS: Strategies for patients and staff in drug abuse treatment programs. *Journal of Psychoactive Drugs, 21,* 435–440.

Sorenson, J. L., Loudon, J. Heitzmann, C., Gibson, D. R., Morales, E. S., Dumentet, R., & Acree, M. (1994). Psychoeducational group approach: HIV risk reduction in drug users. *AIDS Education and Prevention, 6*(2), 95–112.

Stanton, B. F., Xiaoming, L., Ricardo, I., Galbraith, J., Feigelman, S., & Kaljee, L. (1996). A randomized, controlled effectiveness trial of an AIDS prevention program for low-income African-American youths. *Archives of Pediatrics and Adolescent Medicine, 150,* 363–372.

Stephens, R. C., Feucht, T. E., & Roman, S. W. (1991). Effects of an intervention program on AIDS-related drug and needle behavior among intravenous drug users. *American Journal of Public Health, 81*(5), 568–571.

St. Lawrence, J. S., Brasfield, T. L., Jefferson, K. W., Alleyne, E., O'Bannon, R. E., & Shirley, A. (1995). Cognitive–behavioral intervention to reduce African-American adolescents' risk for HIV infection. *Journal of Consulting and Clinical Psychology, 63,* 221–237.

Sweat, M. D., & Denison, J. A. (1995). Reducing HIV incidence in developing countries with structural and environmental interventions. *AIDS, 9* (Suppl. A), S251–S257.

Turner, C. F., Ku, L., Rogers, S. M., Lindberg, L. D., Pleck, J. H., & Sonenstein, F. L. (1998). Adolescent sexual behavior, drug use, and violence: Increased reporting with computer survey technology. *Science, 280,* 867–873.

Walter, H. J., & Vaughan, R. D. (1993). AIDS risk reduction among multiethnic urban high school students. *Journal of the American Medical Association, 270,* 725–730.

Watters, J. K., & Guydish, J. (1994). HIV/AIDS prevention for drug users in natural settings. In R. J. DiClemente & J. L. Peterson (Eds.), *Preventing AIDS: Theories and methods of behavioral intervention* (pp. 209–225). New York: Plenum Press.

Watters, J. K., Downing, M., Case, P., Lorvick, J., Cheng, Y-T., & Fergusson, B. (1990). AIDS prevention for intravenous drug users in the community: Street-based education and risk behavior. *American Journal of Community Psychology, 18,* 587–596.

Williams, A., Vranizan, D., Gorter, R., Brodie, B., Meakin, R., & Moss, A. (1990, June). *Methadone maintenance, HIV serostatus and race in injection drug users (IDU) in San Francisco, CA.* Poster presented at the VI International Conference on AIDS, San Francisco, California.

Wingood, G. M. & DiClemente, R. J. (1992). Cultural, gender and psychosocial influences on HIV-related behavior of African-American female adolescents: Implications for the development of tailored prevention programs. *Ethnicity and Disease, 2,* 381–388.

Wingood, G. M., & DiClemente, R. J. (1996). HIV sexual risk reduction interventions for women: A review. *American Journal of Preventive Medicine, 12*(3), 209–217.

Wingood, G. M., & DiClemente, R. J. (1997). Consequences of having a physically abusive partner on condom use and sexual negotiation of young adult African-American women. *American Journal of Public Health, 87,* 1016–1018.

Wingood, G. M. & DiClemente, R. J. (1998). Relationship characteristics associated with noncondom use among young adult African-American women. *American Journal of Community Psychology, 26,* 29–53.

Wingood, G. M., Hunter, D., & DiClemente, R. J. (1993). A pilot study of sexual communication and negotiation among young African-American women: Implications for HIV prevention. *Journal of Black Psychology, 19,* 190–203.

Worth, D. (1990). Sexual decision making and AIDS: Why condom promotion among vulnerable women is likely to fail. *Studies in Family Planning, 20,* 297–307.

Yancovitz, S. R., Des Jarlais, D. C., Peyser, N. P., Drew, E., Friedman, P., Trigg, H. L., & Robinson, J. W. (1991). A randomized trial of an interim methadone maintenance clinic. *American Journal of Public Health, 81*(9), 1185–1191.

Yankauer, A. (1986). The persistence of public health problems: SF, STD and AIDS. *American Journal of Public Health, 76,* 494–495.

Yankauer, A. (1994). Sexually transmitted diseases: A neglected public health priority. *American Journal of Public Health, 84,* 1894–1897.

Zierler, S., Witbeck, B., & Mayer, K. (1996). Sexual violence against women living with or at risk for HIV infection. *American Journal of Preventive Medicine, 12,* 304–310.

PART *VI*

Intervention Channels

CHAPTER 19

Schools as a Setting for Health Promotion and Disease Prevention

Kim D. Reynolds, Mary Ann Pass, Melissa Galvin,
Scott D. Winnail, Kathleen F. Harrington,
and Ralph J. DiClemente

Introduction

Three areas of school-based health promotion and disease prevention will be described in this chapter, including school-based intervention research, comprehensive school health programs, and school-based health clinics. School-based intervention research is the process of developing and evaluating interventions that are delivered in the schools and designed to modify a specific set of health behaviors. Comprehensive school health programs involve the implementation of eight objectives for school health education. These objectives impact health education curricula, as well as school health policy, staff wellness, and staff training for health education. School-based health clinics involve the delivery of health services and prevention activities directly to children through clinics in the schools.

Each area is unique and involves a separate set of goals, problems, and logistic considerations. However, the three areas are also complementary and can work together to enhance health promotion and disease prevention efforts in the schools. In this chapter, we will describe school-based intervention research, comprehensive school health programs, and school-based health clinics and outline the ways in which they promote health and prevent disease among youth. In our view, carefully

Kim D. Reynolds • Center for Behavioral Studies, AMC Cancer Research Center, Lakewood, Colorado 80214. *Mary Ann Pass* • Department of Maternal and Child Health, School of Public Health, University of Alabama at Birmingham, Birmingham, Alabama 35294. *Melissa Galvin and Kathleen F. Harrington* • Department of Health Behavior, School of Public Health, University of Alabama at Birmingham, Birmingham, Alabama 35294. *Scott D. Winnail* • Department of Human Studies, School of Education, University of Alabama at Birmingham, Birmingham, Alabama 35294. *Ralph J. DiClemente* • Department of Behavioral Sciences and Health Education, Rollins School of Public Health, Emory University, and Emory/Atlanta Center for AIDS Research, Atlanta, Georgia 30322.

Handbook of Health Promotion and Disease Prevention, edited by Raczynski and DiClemente. Kluwer Academic/Plenum Publishers, New York, 1999.

orchestrated prevention efforts in each area will maximize the health promoter's ability to reduce disease risk among youth and adolescents. In this chapter, we cannot fully describe the methods used in each area of school health promotion. However, we will note some important issues to consider when working in each area and will guide the reader to additional sources of information.

School-Based Intervention Research

School-based intervention research involves the development, implementation, and testing of interventions in the schools. These interventions often focus on a single set of health behaviors (eating behaviors), or on a specific health threat [e.g., human immunodeficiency virus (HIV)]. Over time, the development and testing of interventions in the schools provides a set of strategies with known ability to alter behavior and reduce disease risk. In this section, we will (1) describe the rationale for school-based intervention research, (2) describe several intervention approaches used, and (3) describe several technical issues that the school-based health promoter should consider in developing a high quality school-based intervention effort.

Rationale for School-Based Intervention Research

Today's youth experience a number of infectious and chronic diseases, exhibit risk factors for disease, and often fail to engage in behaviors that are shown to be protective from disease. Four major causes account for 72% of the mortality in youth and young adults, aged 5 to 24, including motor vehicle crashes, other unintentional injuries, homicide, and suicide (National Center for Health Statistics, 1996; Kann et al., 1996). The health behavior of youth may contribute to these causes of mortality. For example, 21.7% of adolescents rarely or never use seat belts (Sells & Blum, 1996), 43.8% of motorcycle riders rarely or never use helmets, 15.4% of adolescents have driven after using alcohol in the past year, 38.8% rode with someone who had been drinking alcohol in the past year, 38.7% of adolescents reported being in a physical fight in the past 12 months, and 9.8% reported carrying a weapon on school property (Kann et al., 1996). Adolescents in the United States experience high rates of pregnancy, with approximately 1,000,000 pregnancies among adolescents each year (National Center for Health Statistics, 1995). More than half (51.6%) of adolescents reported having at least one drink of alcohol in the past 30 days (Kann et al., 1996), current cigarette use is estimated to be 34.8%, and frequent cigarette use is 16.1% (Office on Smoking and Health, 1996; Kann et al., 1996). Marijuana was used at least once in the past 30 days by 25.3% of adolescents (Kann et al., 1996) and the 30-day prevalence of illicit drug use among high school seniors has been estimated at 18% (Sells & Blum, 1996). Estimates indicate that only 6.8 to 27.7% of children eat five or more fruits and vegetables per day as recommended, that children and adolescents consume greater than the recommended 30% of calories from fat (Kann et al., 1996; Basch, Zybert, & Shea 1994; Krebs-Smith et al., 1996; Berenson et al., 1991) and that levels of obesity are higher than optimal (Enrst & Oberzanek, 1994). Physical activity occurs less frequently and with less intensity than recommended (Kann et al., 1996; Sallis & McKenzie, 1991; U.S. Department of Health and Human Services, 1991). Sexual behavior occurs in youth, with 37.9% of adolescents estimated to have had sexual intercourse in the previous 3 months and 17.8% reporting four or more lifetime partners

(Kann *et al.*, 1996). Since risk factors, high-risk behavior, and low protective behavior are present in youth, there is a compelling need to intervene to address these factors.

Substantial evidence, particularly from research in heart disease epidemiology, indicates that risk factors and risk behaviors present in youth carry over, or "track," into later childhood and early adulthood (Nicklas, Webber, Johnson, Srinivasan, & Berenson, 1995; Perry, Kelder, & Klepp, 1994; Webber, Srinivasan, Wattigney, & Berenson, 1991; Berenson *et al.*, 1991; Porkka, Viikari, & Akerblom, 1991; Clarke, Schrott, Leaverton, Connor, & Lauer, 1978). Longitudinal evidence supporting the tracking of behaviors in youth is somewhat limited, particularly for the transition from youth into adulthood. However, several studies have identified the tracking of smoking behavior (Kelder, Perry, Klepp, & Lytle, 1994; Esobedo, Marcus, Hotzma, & Giovino, 1993; Taioli & Wynder, 1991), physical activity (Kelder *et al.*, 1994), and dietary behavior (Kelder *et al.*, 1994; Stein, Shea, Basch, Contento & Zybert, 1991). Since risk factors and protective behaviors may track throughout youth and into adulthood, it is important to intervene with youth to help formulate good health behavior. School-based interventions may help reduce risk behavior and form positive health behaviors that will last into adulthood, reducing disease risk for many years.

More than 95% of children ages 5 to 17 are enrolled in school, making schools an ideal setting to reach children and adolescents with health promotion and disease prevention programs (Kann *et al.*, 1995). Because a wide range of children and adolescents attend school, traditionally "hard-to-reach" groups can also receive health promotion and disease prevention programs through this setting (Kirby & DiClemente, 1994). In addition, regular attendance at school provides health promoters with repeated access to children and enables repeated exposure to intervention activities. Complex interventions can be developed that repeat key messages and build from activities that target knowledge and attitude change, to more intensive activities including behavioral skills building, goal setting, and self-monitoring. Repeated access to students also confers advantages for research and evaluation. In many cases, repeated access facilitates the completion of follow-up assessments, leading to higher completion rates.

The school setting provides opportunities for environmental change that can produce long-term behavior change well after the original intervention team has left the schools. School policies can be changed, teachers and other personnel can be trained, and changes in the physical environment can be made to support behavior change. Once made, the environmental changes support the positive health behavior of succeeding generations of students. Schools can also provide access to families with recruited children providing a link to their parents and siblings. This can multiply the efforts of the health promotion team by changing the parents and siblings behavior, reducing their disease risk as well as creating a home environment that is supportive of the change being produced in the recruited child.

All school-based interventions are not equally effective. School-based intervention research shows which interventions are effective, limiting the expenditure of scarce school district funds to programs that will have a positive effect on the health of children and adolescents.

Intervention Approaches

School-based intervention researchers have used three main components in the design of interventions, including a curriculum component, a parent involvement component, and an environmental component. Two or three of these components are often used together to produce the strongest possible intervention effect (Parcel *et al.*, 1987; Perry *et al.*, 1990). To provide a clear focus, this section will draw examples primarily from the school-based nutrition education literature.

Curriculum Component

This component involves the development of a health curriculum that is delivered in the classroom. When used alone, the curriculum approach has produced mixed results with some programs being effective (Schaalma *et al.*, 1996; Mitchell-DiCenso *et al.*, 1997; Rooney & Murray, 1996; Contento *et al.*, 1995). Several factors may influence the effectiveness of the curriculum approach including whether a program is theory-based (Flay, 1985; Lytle & Achterberg, 1995), the duration of the program (Connell, Turner, & Mason, 1985), the quality of training of personnel (Basen-Engquist *et al.*, 1994; Gingiss, 1992), the extent of formative evaluation, the pretesting used for the program, and the personnel who deliver the intervention.

The personnel who deliver an intervention are particularly critical in determining its success. The choice is typically between the use of existing classroom teachers or the use of staff hired by the intervention project to conduct education. The use of staff hired by the project may result in a program that is more fully delivered as designed (integrity), leading to higher dose and greater potential effectiveness (Rossi & Freeman, 1993). However, this comes at the cost of reduced generalizability of the program. Programs delivered by existing classroom teachers can be viewed as effectiveness trials (Flay, 1986). If positive results are obtained, we can have greater confidence that they will produce changes in behavior if delivered later in a standard classroom setting by classroom teachers. However, if null results are obtained, it is difficult to determine whether this was due to an ineffective program or to a failure to fully implement the program by the classroom teachers. When delivered by project staff, the school-based intervention study comes closer to satisfying the conditions for an efficacy trial (Flay, 1986). It provides a test of the intervention under the best conditions, providing a clear indication of whether the program will produce results when delivered as designed. The choice of approach depends on whether a researcher wishes to test the program as it was originally designed (efficacy trial) or as it works under real-world conditions (effectiveness trial). Some researchers prefer and/or advocate the conduct of efficacy trials first, to establish programs known to change behavior (Flay, 1986). This can be followed by effectiveness trials to establish the conditions under which the programs will work in the real world.

Parent Involvement Component

This component involves the delivery of intervention programs to parents and, occasionally, other family members, using a child recruited in the schools. This strategy is sometimes used in conjunction with a classroom intervention (Hopper, Gruber, Munoz, & Herb, 1992; Perry *et al.*, 1988; Luepker *et al.*, 1996); however, it has also been used as an independent intervention strategy with some success (Perry *et al.*, 1988, 1989). The parent involvement strategy provides support for psychosocial and behavior changes occurring for the child as a result of intervention activities received in the school, but it also provides an opportunity to reach family members and change their behavior as well. Although some studies have successfully conducted family interventions outside of the home (Nader *et al.*, 1989), most parents prefer to receive intervention materials at home (Perry, Crockett, & Pirie, 1987); studies that attempt to bring parents into the school after hours usually meet with low attendance rates.

Environmental Component

This component involves the modification of the physical, social, and policy environment of the school to produce or support behavior change in the children. Relatively few interventions have used only an environmental intervention component (Ellison, Capper, Goldberg, Witschi, & Stare, 1989); however, future work in this area may prove fruitful (Bowen, Kinne, & Orlandi, 1995). Environmental intervention activities are sometimes combined with classroom or family intervention activities as part of a larger intervention program. Mass media also has been used recently, in collaboration with intervention activities occurring in the schools, as an environmental intervention component. Several authors have evaluated this approach for the prevention of tobacco use among adolescents with mixed results (Flay *et al.*, 1995; Flynn *et al.*, 1992). One study showed greater reductions in cigarette consumption among children who received both school and media intervention components compared to children who only received intervention in the school (Flynn *et al.*, 1992).

Theories Used to Develop School-Based Interventions

Theory is an essential tool in the design and evaluation of school-based interventions. Theory provides the framework for the development of intervention components and their sequencing in the intervention. Theory can also guide a researcher in the selection of constructs to measure to assess the effectiveness of an intervention. The number of theories that can be applied to school-based interventions is large. Planning theories, such as Precede–Proceed, might be used to plan a programmatic school-based intervention effort (Bush *et al.*, 1989; Green & Kreuter, 1991). Psychologically based theories, such as social cognitive theory (SCT) (Bandura, 1986), the theory of planned behavior (Ajzen, 1991), or fear communication and attitude change theories (Stiff, 1994), can be used in the design of a specific intervention and its components. Finally, theories from specific research domains might have applicability to the intervention effort. For example, theories of media effectiveness might be used to assist in designing a school-based intervention with a media component (Flay *et al.*, 1995; Flynn *et al.*, 1992).

Social cognitive theory has been widely used to develop school-based intervention research efforts (Perry *et al.*, 1990; Reynolds *et al.*, 1998; Parcel, 1984), and it approaches being a theoretical paradigm for school-based intervention research (Parcel, 1984). SCT guides researchers to develop intervention components targeting person factors, environmental factors, and behavior factors that continuously influence one another in a process called *reciprocal determinism*. Within these three broad determinants of behavior (i.e., person factors, environmental factors, behavior factors), the theory delineates several components that have an effect on the variation of behavior. These components include environment, situation, behavioral capability, expectations, expectancies, reinforcement, perceived self-efficacy, outcome expectancies, observational learning, goal setting and self-monitoring, and emotional coping responses (Baranowski, Perry, & Parcel, 1997). The task of the school-based intervention researcher is to develop intervention activities that will influence each of these components, leading to changes in the behavior of the target children. For example, intervention activities should be designed that will produce skills for completing the target behavior (behavioral capability). If we are trying to teach adolescents not to ride with drivers who have been drinking, we might teach them how to find another ride, how to persuade the drunk driver not to drive, and how to maintain friendships when refusing to ride with a drunk driver. SCT also guides us in the selection of constructs to measure in the evaluation of the program. For example, SCT states that perceived self-efficacy is an important determinant of behavior. Thus, self-efficacy will be incorporated into the intervention and measured as a part of the evaluation of the intervention. In sum, SCT provides an outstanding theory from which to design a school-based intervention.

One example of the use of SCT in the design of an intervention and evaluation is presented here. In the High 5 study, an innovative school-based intervention was developed using SCT with the objective of increasing fruit and vegetable consumption in 4th-grade children according to the National Cancer Institute's 5-a-Day for Better Health guidelines (Reynolds *et al.*, 1998; National Cancer Institute, 1991). The intervention was designed using reciprocal determinism and was delivered to 14 of 28 schools randomly assigned to an immediate intervention condition. The intervention used a classroom component, a parent component, and an environmental/food service component to target the three elements of reciprocal determinism: person factors, environmental factors, behavior factors. The specific constructs within SCT (e.g., outcome expectancies, behavioral capability) were manipulated in the intervention to produce changes in psychosocial mediators and behavior. To limit the length of our description, we will focus on the classroom component of the intervention; however, SCT was also used to develop intervention activities within the parent and food service components. The 14-session classroom component included activities manipulating most of the constructs within SCT. For example, stories were read to increase the perceived positive consequences and reduce the perceived negative consequences of eating fruit and vegetables (perceived outcome expectancies) and the perceived ability to increase consumption of fruit and vegetables (perceived self-efficacy). Goal setting and self-monitoring of behavior were used by having students plan to eat five fruits and vegetables on one day during the week. Students then recorded their performance and were rewarded if they reached the target behavior, engaging the SCT construct of reinforcement. Behavioral skills were increased by having students learn and practice the preparation of their favorite fruits and vegetables, and to negotiate with parents to purchase their favorite fruit and vegetables. Perceived self-efficacy was enhanced through the modeling of target behaviors using role-playing and stories, structured success experience in eating five fruits and vegetables per day, and through persuasion.

Although we have highlighted SCT, numerous other theories can be used in school-based intervention research, as noted above. The use of new theories is encouraged and can help build the efficacy of school-based interventions by testing alternative intervention strategies (McBride *et al.*, 1995). The use of culturally (Baldwin *et al.*, 1996) and developmentally specific approaches (Garcia *et al.*, 1995; Osborne, Kistner, & Helgemo, 1993) may also prove effective.

Design and Analysis Issues in School-Based Intervention Research

School settings provide advantages and disadvantages for the conduct of health promotion and disease prevention research with children. These issues are discussed below with an emphasis on selected problems. Readers are encouraged to consult an evaluation text for assistance in the complete design of a school-based intervention study (Cook & Campbell, 1979; Rossi & Freeman, 1993)

Experimental Designs

One of the strongest evaluation designs available for school-based intervention research is the randomized experimental design in which the school serves as both the unit of assignment and the unit of analysis. This design requires access to a large number of schools, good cooperation with school officials who will allow random assignment to conditions, and sufficient funding to conduct a large-scale experiment. This design will rule out most threats to internal validity and will maximize conclusions that can be drawn regarding the causal effects of a program (Cook & Campbell, 1979). However, careful attention must be focused on the four threats to internal validity that are not ruled out by randomization: diffusion of treatments, differential attrition, compensatory rivalry, and compensatory equalization of treatments (Cook & Campbell, 1979). Each threat may be plausible until ruled out by design or analysis strategies. The researcher must be aware of each threat, take steps to minimize its occurrence, and include process measures to assess its occurrence. Diffusion of treatments is largely ruled out by using schools as the unit of assignment. Other factors may facilitate diffusion, such as the portability of the intervention material, the interest of students in the material, and the degree to which families from the units of assignment (e.g., schools, classrooms, individuals) interact in other settings (e.g., churches). Compensatory rivalry and compensatory equalization of treatments are most likely to occur when personnel and participants in control schools are aware of the intervention being delivered to the treatment subjects and when the program is desirable. This threat may be rendered less plausible by the use of delayed intervention controls in which schools assigned to the control condition receive the intervention after the final measures are completed, and by the use of informational controls in which the control schools receive an intervention program, but one that is unlikely to produce effects on the target behavior of interest (Cook & Campbell, 1979; Rossi & Freeman, 1993).

Quasi-Experimental Designs

A randomized experimental design may not be feasible under some conditions. For example, the school district may not allow random assignment of schools to conditions or limited resources may force the researcher to assign a small number of schools to conditions, creating nonequivalence between the treatment conditions at baseline. If conditions do not allow for the use of a randomized experimental design, various quasi-experimental designs may assist the school-based researcher in determining the effectiveness of the program. Quasi-experiments are not as strong as randomized experimental designs in ruling out threats to internal validity (Cook & Campbell, 1979). However, a well-constructed quasi-experiment may allow the researcher to draw strong conclusions about the effectiveness of a program. A comprehensive delineation of quasi-experimental designs is beyond the scope of this chapter. However, we note three types of quasi-experimental designs that may be useful, including (1) nonequivalent control group designs, (2) cohort designs, and (3) the regression discontinuity design. Nonequivalent control group designs are frequently used in school-based intervention research. They resemble experimental designs except that the units of assignment (i.e., schools, classrooms, students) cannot be randomly assigned to the study conditions. Due to the practical considerations involved in school-based research, the control of assignment of schools to conditions may not be possible, and random assignment may not be achieved. In this circumstance, a nonequivalent control group design may be created. A wide range of possible nonequivalent control group designs can be developed, with some yielding many threats to internal validity implausible. Nonequivalent control group designs can be made stronger through the use of multiple pretests, multiple dependent measures, and multiple comparison groups (West, 1985).

The cohort design is a subset of nonequivalent control group designs (Cook & Campbell, 1979; Cook et al., 1975). This design takes advantage of the fact that children move through school in age cohorts that may be largely similar on many characteristics to the cohorts that have come before and to those that will come after. This allows the researcher to use prior cohorts as a comparison group for the intervention cohort of children. This design can be readily constructed in a school-based setting and is useful when the program cannot be withheld from any of the students in the target grade level. The design can be open to threats to internal validity, particularly secular trends (history).

The regression discontinuity design allows a researcher to compare individuals who receive an intervention against those who do not receive an intervention, when the decision to give the intervention is based on some characteristics of the individual that merit their assignment to the intervention condition (Cook & Campbell, 1979; Trochim, 1984; West, 1985). For example, body mass index (BMI) might be calculated on a group of children and those with a BMI indicating obesity would be assigned to receive an obesity prevention program. All children are then measured 6 months later on BMI and those children who received the intervention are compared to those who did not use the intervention based on the cut-points on BMI. If the intervention is effective, the children at and above the cut-point will have a drop in their level of BMI at 6 months compared to those below the cut-point. This design has not been frequently utilized in school-based intervention research but might provide a good alternative design when conditions permit. The design will require the creation of special classes for intervention delivery, may be susceptible to diffusion of treatments since children within the same schools will serve as treatments and controls, may be subject to a selection by maturation threat to internal validity, and may require a large number of subjects (West, 1985).

Process Evaluation

The need to monitor the integrity of a school-based intervention is crucial. This is necessary to diagnose and fix problems in implementation, as they occur, and to understand the pattern of outcome effects that are obtained. Dose–response analyses may also be possible with a carefully completed process evaluation. The publication of process evaluation data might facilitate replication and advance the science of school-based intervention research (Flay, 1986). Several examples of process evaluation in school settings have been published with the Child and Adolescent Trial for Cardiovascular Health (CATCH) intervention trial providing examples and published evaluation forms (McGraw et al., 1994; Edmundson et al., 1994; Johnson et al., 1994; Elder et al., 1994).

Measurement Issues

A full treatment of measurement issues is beyond the scope of this chapter. As in any research study, the success of the research effort will depend on the quality of the measures employed, and the reliability and validity of measures should be carefully established (Carmines & Zeller, 1979). The school setting provides some special challenges and unique opportunities for measurement. The controlled classroom setting can facilitate the collection and editing of data. However, the completion of measures in this setting may also exacerbate social desirability response biases.

Unit of Analysis

School-based researchers typically assign entire schools to treatment conditions (1) to minimize threats to internal validity including diffusion of treatments, compensatory rivalry, and resentful demoralization (Cook & Campbell, 1979); (2) to produce environmental changes in the school; and (3) to simplify the logistics of the intervention. This type of assignment is referred to as *cluster randomization* or *group randomization* and requires a careful statistical analysis procedure that accounts for the variance that exists between clusters (e.g., schools) as well as the variance across individuals within clusters (Zucker *et al.*, 1995; Cornfield, 1978; Donner, Brown, & Brasher, 1990). Because school is the unit of assignment, it should also serve as the unit of analysis. If the researcher ignores this statistical principle, inflation in the type I error rate can occur (Zucker *et al.*, 1995; Donner *et al.*, 1990). As a result, the researcher may conclude that there were significant differences between treatment conditions when true differences did not, in fact, exist (Zucker *et al.*, 1995; Simpson, Klar, & Donner, 1995; Donner *et al.*, 1990). Various analysis strategies have been suggested and employed for studies using cluster randomization (Zucker *et al.*, 1995; Murray, Hannan, & Zucker, 1989; Donner & Klar, 1994; Donner, Birkett, & Buck, 1981). The use of the school as the unit of randomization and analysis also has implications for the calculation of required sample size and statistical power, and these calculations must account for the effects of cluster randomization (Murray & Hannan, 1990; Donner, 1992; Hsieh, 1988; Donner *et al.*, 1981). Cluster randomization may lead to larger and more costly research designs because a larger number of schools must be included in the design to ensure adequate statistical power. School-based researchers should avoid using the individual as the unit of analysis when schools are assigned to conditions (Cornfield, 1978); however, if resources do not allow for a sufficient number of schools to be analyzed at the school level, then the potential inflation of type I error that is introduced by this strategy should be carefully noted. In sum, we encourage readers to review the body of literature available on clustered randomization and to enlist the assistance of a statistician familiar with these issues.

Attrition

Attrition occurs in school-based studies for a variety of reasons. Students may leave the participating schools and enroll in nonparticipating schools or students may be absent on the day(s) that assessment is completed in the schools. Students may withdraw from the study, or their parents may withdraw consent. Finally, students may fail to complete some scales on a questionnaire. Attrition is problematic for two reasons. It can be a threat to external validity, limiting the type of student included in the evaluation and, in turn, limiting the breadth of students across which the effectiveness of the study can be generalized (Cook & Campbell, 1979). Second, if attrition occurs differentially across conditions, it can be a threat to internal validity, limiting the ability to conclude that the school-based intervention produced the changes detected in the evaluation (Cook & Campbell, 1979).

Schools provide a captive audience of children, increasing access and the ability to repeat measurements. This access should facilitate the researcher's ability to construct and complete longitudinal designs that have pre- and posttest measures on the same children and should limit attrition since the same children are present at the beginning and the end of the school year. In addition, children tend to remain enrolled in the same schools until they graduate to the next educational level. However, the stability of school enrollments varies substantially between school districts. Schools that enroll students from migrant farm families, for example, may have very high turnover, while schools in very stable middle-class neighborhoods may have low turnover. Even in the best of circumstances, you must assume that attrition will occur. Thus, procedures must be in place to track and follow-up on participants who leave the schools during your study.

A number of strategies have been developed for tracking students and limiting attrition in school-based studies (Pirie et al., 1989; Ellickson, Bianca, & Schoeff, 1988; Hansen, Collins, Malotte, Johnson, & Fielding, 1985). Lessons can also be borrowed from clinic-based studies involving children (Morrison et al., 1997). The most frequently and effectively used strategies for tracking students and completing measures have been telephone and mail procedures (Ellickson et al., 1988; Hansen et al., 1985; Pirie et al., 1989). Transfer records are a very good source of information on where students have moved and can be combined with a contact at the new school (Ellickson et al., 1988; Hansen et al., 1985; Pirie et al., 1989), and even the sending of questionnaires to the new school (Ellickson et al., 1988). Actively tracking parents as well as students can be an effective strategy using telephone and mail techniques as well as drivers license searches (Pirie et al., 1989). A commonly used strategy that has been less effective is the use of third-party information gathered on individuals who will know the whereabouts of a family or through contacting neighbors (Ellickson et al., 1988). Analyses should always be completed to determine the extent to which attrition serves as a threat to external and internal validity. Several analytic strategies have been suggested for this purpose (Hansen et al., 1985; Jurs & Glass, 1971; Siddiqui, Flay, & Hu, 1996).

Recruitment of Schools and School Districts

Effective recruitment strategies, producing an adequate and representative sample, are essential for maintaining the integrity of the sampling design as well as the external validity of the data collected (Atkins et al., 1987; Lytle et al., 1994; Petosa & Goodman, 1991). Successful recruitment is grounded on a research protocol that is "school friendly" as well as methodologically and theoretically sound. It is vital that school personnel perceive the researcher's concern and appreciation for their agenda, such as meeting state education requirements, limited resources, and time constraints. A program that has minimal impact on the day-to-day activities of the school while providing external support to the school will have a greater chance of being accepted.

No single recruitment approach will be ideal in all school districts, since decision-making processes vary across districts and schools. While some districts may only require approval at the district level, others will require approval at the principal and/or teacher level as well. Researchers must be flexible in adapting their recruitment plan to fit each situation. Petosa and Goodman (1991) present a taxonomy for school district decision making. These authors have suggested ways to address the components of the decision-making process that should enhance district or school participation. A successful recruitment plan can be theoretically guided, such as the CATCH procedure (Lytle et al., 1994) and should include several components, described below, that are tailored to each school system.

School Advocate

Identifying an advocate for the research program within the school system is a fundamental first step in the recruitment process. The advocate should have an interest in the research subject, credibility within the school system, and access to both district-level and school-level administrators. For example, the High 5 study, described earlier, used district child nutritionists as advocates for their nutrition education program, leading to enhanced cooperation by the schools (Harrington et al., 1997). The advocate can facilitate district and school recruitment by identifying decision makers at each level and coordinating presentations to them. They also may serve to identify and help overcome their system's perceived barriers to participation in the program.

Program Presentation

While some districts may request a presentation only to top administration, others request presentations for several levels of personnel. These presentations can establish rapport, answer questions, and help build grassroots support for both the recruitment and intervention activities (Petosa & Goodman, 1991). These presentations should cover the program design, emphasizing components that will directly affect the school. If completed, intervention materials and data collection instruments should be available for review. When possible, the principal investigator should participate in these presentations to lend credibility to the program (Lytle et al., 1994).

Address Perceived Barriers and Potential Benefits

It is key that the researcher address perceived barriers, such as disruption of normal school activities, burdening school staff with additional work, and time taken from core subjects. The researcher should attempt to minimize these barriers in the intervention design. The researcher should also maximize potential benefits to the school. Benefits can be tangible, such as additional teacher training or support, access to innovative curricula, additional materials, and supplemental financial support, or intangible, such as enhanced reputation for innovation or alignment with the researcher's institution (Lytle et al., 1994).

Define Roles

The recruitment plan should clearly define the obligations and responsibilities of both the researcher and the school personnel. It is worthwhile to have this definition of roles take the form of a written agreement between school administrators, such as the district superintendent as well as individual school principals, and the researcher.

Finally, a successful recruitment plan should have a timetable. Ideally, recruitment would begin early in the school year 1 year prior to program implementation (Lytle *et al.*, 1994). This allows time to complete all recruitment activities and allows schools adequate time for planning changes to class schedules necessary to accommodate the research protocol. This timetable should allow for multiple presentations, sufficient time for the decision-making process, and deadlines for contacting nonrespondents.

Comprehensive School Health Education

In 1990, the National Commission on the Role of School and the Community in Improving Adolescent Health, the National Association of State Boards of Education, and the American Medical Association made the following observation; "For the first time in the history of this country, young people are less healthy and less prepared to take their places in society than were their parents" (cited in Joint Committee on National Health Education Standards, 1995). In 1994, Seffrin noted that "children don't learn as well if they're not healthy" (p. 397). These statements are fundamental to the idea of a comprehensive or coordinated school health program (CSHP). CSHP is an idea, largely put forward by Diane Allensworth and Lloyd Kolbe, to promote student and community health through a number of avenues.

In 1984, the National Professional School Health Education Organizations came out with a definition for CSHP. They defined it as "health education in a school setting that is planned and carried out with the purpose of maintaining, reinforcing, or enhancing the health, health-related skills, and health attitudes and practices of children and youth that are conducive to their good health" (p. 312).

Kane (1993) suggests that "because health behaviors are learned, they may be shaped and changed" (p. 2). He goes on to discuss how schools are perhaps the most influential entity in society for shaping the future health of Americans (Kane, 1993). CSHPs are therefore an attempt to shape the positive health behaviors, health decision-making skills, and health promotion knowledge and skills of school-aged youth, by addressing issues from different areas within the school.

As multiple factors influence the state of health and education among today's youth, so should interventions be multiple and broad based (National Health/Education Consortium, 1990). DeGraw (1994) further suggests that broader and more comprehensive approaches to health education will increase the likelihood of positive outcomes. CSHP is designed to follow the above recommendations to address multiple problems experienced by youth (K–12) from many different avenues.

Components of CSHP

As mentioned above, CSHP attempts to address numerous health concerns of school-aged youth, by approaching these issues from multiple avenues. In 1987, Allensworth and Kolbe published a foundational article on the CSHP, in which they outlined eight specific components integral to a CSHP. These eight components broadened the traditional school health education triad of health services, health education, and a healthy environment, recognizing that student health is affected by multiple factors. The eight component model includes (Allensworth & Kolbe, 1987):

1. **School health services:** primary preventive health care and initial treatment for injuries and illnesses offered at or near school facilities.
2. **School health education:** structured learning experiences that promote students' acquisition of health knowledge, development of positive attitudes, and incorporation of health behaviors into personal lifestyles.
3. **School health environment:** school climate, condition of the physical facilities, and administrative policies that reflect health choices (i.e., abstaining from tobacco, alcohol, and drug use, violence prevention, the teaching and modeling of respect, etc.).
4. **Community health partnerships:** involvement of schools, parents, businesses, health professions, law enforcement, universities and voluntary health agencies in the integration of communitywide health programs that provide children with consistent health messages.
5. **School physical education:** structured learning experiences that promote students' cardiovascular health, muscular endurance, flexibility, strength, agility, balance, coordination, good posture, and exercise.
6. **School food service:** promotion of good health by offering low-fat, nutritious food choices in cafeterias and vending machines. Knowledge of nutritional choices.
7. **School counseling and guidance programs:** large-group guidance, small-group counseling, individual assistance, and programs about academic, social, emotional, and career development of an individual on topics such as peer pressure, decision making, personal responsibility, communication skills, self-esteem, and conflict resolution.
8. **School site health promotion program for faculty and staff:** programs that promote faculty and staff wellness so that they, as role models, set healthy examples.

Although the classroom is good for structured learning and training, these other school areas are important for reinforcing the messages learned in the classroom. They are also appropriate avenues for delivering additional health promotion messages (Allensworth, 1994).

The National Professional School Health Education Organizations (1984) made initial recommendations that the following topic areas be included in a K–12 school health curriculum: community health, consumer health, environmental health, family life, growth and development, nutritional health, personal health, prevention and control of disease and disorders, safety and accident prevention, and substance use and abuse (National Professional School Health Education Organizations, 1984). These topic areas will vary depending on state and school system mandates and recommendations by professional organizations. They can be expanded by individual school districts and states to include other topics, such as violence prevention, cancer prevention, self-esteem building, stress management, and physical activity, to name just a few (Seffrin, 1994). It is important that the selection of appropriate topic areas is needs driven, that is, driven by the current and future health needs of the students and the community (DeGraw, 1994).

National Health Education Standards

In 1995, the Joint Committee on National Health Education Standards (1996) developed standards to serve as a framework for implementing a CSHP at the state and local level. There also are performance indicators for grades 4, 8, and 11 to determine health literacy. The National Health Education Standards are as follows: (1) Students will comprehend concepts related to health promotion and disease prevention; (2) students will demonstrate the ability to access valid health information and health-promoting products and services; (3) students will demonstrate the ability to practice health-enhancing behaviors and reduce health risks; (4) students will analyze the influence of culture, media, technology, and other factors on health; (5) students will demonstrate the ability to use interpersonal communication skills to enhance health; (6) students will demonstrate the ability to use goal-setting and decision-making skills to enhance health; and (7) students will demonstrate the ability to advocate for personal, family, and community health.

Benefits and Cost-Effectiveness of CSHP

Numerous national organizations strongly advocate a CSHP to combat adolescent health problems. The American Association of School Administrators (1990) promotes CSHP and the following benefits of implementation, including (1) reduced school vandalism, (2) improved attendance by students and staff, (3) reduced health care costs, (4) reduced substitute teaching costs, (5) better family communication, even on sensitive issues such as sexuality, (6) stronger self-confidence and self-esteem, (7) noticeably fewer students using tobacco, (8) improved cholesterol levels for students and staff, (9) increased seat beat use, and (10) improved physical fitness.

A school health program can be viewed from several perspectives. It improves health behavior; it improves academic performance. But in an era of ever-tightening budgets and increased pressure for accountability, it is important to know whether or not a school health program is cost-effective. Prevention saves lives, improves the quality of life, and can save millions of dollars in immediate and long-term costs. For youth the major threats to health are death or injury due to violence, substance abuse, unplanned pregnancies, and sexually transmitted diseases. In addition, many of the leading causes of death such as heart disease, cancer, and stroke have their roots in the behaviors established during youth. School health programs have a positive impact on the immediate and future health of our children, thus saving millions of dollars. It is estimated that health education comprises less than 0.30% of classroom instruction and less than 0.20% of the total cost of public education. A conservative analysis indicates that for every $1 spent on health education, a net health benefit of $1.66 would result (Wylie, 1983). Thus, there are immediate as well as long-term cost benefits of a school health program.

Overcoming Barriers to Implementing CSHP

Although the concept of CSHP is innovative and based on sound principles, it is also potentially challenging to implement. Numerous barriers must be dealt with and overcome in order for a CSHP program to be implemented successfully. One barrier to implementing CSHP involves classroom instruction. In most school settings, classroom teachers (not specialists) are the likely teachers of health (Lohrmann, Gold, & Jubb, 1987). A major concern is that these generalist teachers are not adequately prepared to teach about complex, multifaceted health issues in a developmentally appropriate manner (Lohrmann *et al.*, 1987; Hausman & Ruzek, 1995). This will continue to be a barrier to CSHP until teachers feel more comfortable teaching about potentially sensitive topic areas and until appropriate professional preparation is in place (Hausman & Ruzek, 1995).

Unfortunately, many areas and many in health education are specifically or categorically funded. This funding barrier greatly adds to the absence of a comprehensive educational approach. Those advocating for CSHP need to put more pressure on policymakers and funding agencies that restrict opportunities to achieve "mutually desirable goals efficiently and comprehensively" (English, 1994, p. 188). Obviously it is important that the components of a CSHP curriculum be individually effective. Each component or topic area should also fit into a more comprehensive framework that is designed to address multiple areas. A health education topic area, no matter how "good" it is deemed by experts, should not operate to the exclusion of other important health topics.

A third barrier to implementing a CSHP program is proper curricula development or selection. Often curricula are selected or developed according to the agendas of a few individuals (English, 1994). Schools need a standardized procedure and a committee to select and/or develop curricula in a way which will best benefit the students. Additionally, this method will help ensure that health education curricula are as comprehensive as possible. The Joint committee on National Health Education Standards (1996) and the American Cancer Society recently developed the *National Health Education Standards,* a document designed to create standards for the development of health education curricula. These standards were many years in the making and represent the combined efforts of numerous agencies and individuals. These standards are designed as a framework for schools to use in the creation of a health education instructional program. If used appropriately, these standards will help ensure the creation of a health education curriculum that reflects all appropriate aspects of a CSHP program.

A fourth barrier is that health education is often not seen by school officials as important to the curriculum. The importance of curriculum areas is often measured against emphasis given them by standardized tests. English (1994) suggests that one way to make sure health education is viewed as important to the overall school curriculum is to develop and implement statewide assessments that measure the degree to which students are meeting preapproved standards in health education. These assessments will improve the importance of health education in the eyes of administrators and teachers alike.

A fifth and final barrier is that of the tremendous job of integrating the eight different areas of a CSHP program. Linking these areas is not an easy task and needs a dedicated person in a leadership role who can work toward achieving this task (Davis & Allensworth, 1994). Schools need to appoint a health education coordinator or a health education administrator to better handle the coordination of CSHP efforts. Both are certified in health education. The administrator, however, would have administrative powers and would manage and coordinate the integration of the eight school areas, as well as the overall health education program (Resnicow & Allensworth, 1996). In addition, schools need to form interdisciplinary teams to help facilitate a strong CSHP program (Allensworth, 1994). The teams should include representatives from each of the eight CSHP areas, top school administrators, parents, teachers, and any other interested parties including students. These teams can help maximize the CSHP efforts.

Where Things Stand on CSHP

The Centers for Disease Control and Prevention (CDC) developed and implemented in 1994 the School Health Policies and Programs Study (SHPPS) to measure policies and programs at the state, district, school, and classroom level across the multiple components of a school health program. The study found that most components were administratively separated at the state, district, and local level; thus, the data collected were component specific. The study further demonstrated that within three of the components (health education, physical education, and health services) there was a great deal of variance at the state, district, and local levels.

Every state has a person responsible for coordinating school health education, yet only half of the school districts have a person identified to direct school health education. These individuals are also responsible for drug free schools and communities program and physical education, but other components of a CSHP such as nutrition and school health services are not included in the same administrative unit as health education. The majority of states require that schools provide health education in grades K–12. Most states provide written guidance in the form of health education curricula/guidelines/frameworks and most states provide in-service training for the teachers on a variety of health topics. Few states include health education topics as a part of mandated academic testing (Collins et al., 1995).

Most states legally require physical education. The majority of the states' and half of the districts have a person responsible for directing physical education. Many of these requirements require less exposure to physical activity than recommended by the national health objectives for the year 2000, with the majority of activities being competitive team sports rather than lifetime activities. SHPPS also concluded that collaboration between physical education staff and other CSHP staff occurred most often at the state level (Pate et al., 1995).

In addition, approximately 75% of the states had a person responsible for directing school health nurse services and almost 79% of those individuals had other responsibilities. Half the states require schools to offer school health services, approximately 10% of the school districts have a school-based clinic, and 8% had a school-linked clinic (Small et al., 1995).

Examples of CSHP in Practice

The Teenage Health Teaching Modules (THTM) were developed for secondary school students by the CDC and the Educational Development Center (Nelson, Cross, & Kolbe, 1991). An evaluation of over 5000 students and 150 teachers reported that the curriculum was effective in reducing some health risk behaviors (smoking, alcohol use, and other drug use) of secondary school students. THTM consists of numerous modules on various health topics that can be covered in the classrooms. Modules can be used or deleted according to the desires of teachers, schools, school boards, and state departments of education. This curriculum is one example of a comprehensive health education curriculum that can be used within a CSHP program.

A number of states have CSHP models in place that are endorsed and partially supported at the state level, usually by the state Department of Education. These models include most if not all of the eight components of a CSHP program and sometimes contain additional components. Nebraska has a CSHP model entitled *Healthy Kids, Healthier Nebraska* (Nebraska Department of Education, 1990). Nebraska's model utilizes all eight of the traditional eight components, with the addition of one component called "program management." This program management component is a necessary aspect of any successful CSHP program whether specifically identified or not.

Iowa also has a CSHP model in place that is endorsed by the state Department of Education, entitled *Iowa . . . A Place to Grow Healthy* (Iowa Department of Education, 1992). Iowa's program also contains the eight components of CSHP; however, it is divided into four headings: school services, curriculum/instruction, environment, and community. Iowa also has an additional component entitled "administration."

It is important to reiterate that both Iowa and Nebraska use CSHP models that are endorsed by the state. Also, they add a managerial or administrative component to their state models emphasizing the importance of coordination.

Conclusions

CSHP is not only an idea who's time has come, but is also a reality in some states and districts. CSHP is a schoolwide, coordinated effort to better the health of students and, in turn, better the health of the community. It requires endorsement by the state and/or the school district, appropriate funding, sincere interest of those involved, and a coordinated effort by all parties involved. CSHP is a school-based model for improving health knowledge, skills, attitudes, and behaviors of students, and can be successful if coordinated, concerned efforts are made by all parties involved. Program success will not come overnight; however, if proper time, effort, and coordination is injected into the effort, outcomes should be positive.

School-Based Health Clinics

Health services, taken directly to children and adolescents by way of school-based or school-linked clinics, offer promise in meeting unmet health needs, particularly the unmet needs of indigent children. In this country, children increasingly face financial and nonfinancial barriers to care caused by lack of family resources, lack of a parent's employer-provided insurance, reduced time investments by adults, and lack of community resources. School-based health clinics (SBHCs) by design ease problems of access, establish routines familiar to students and sensitive to the culture of the school, employ providers focused on delivery of services to students, and facilitate compliance and follow-up. The enhanced observation of students in the school setting offers the potential for early identification of emotional, social, and mental problems and for targeted interventions (Klein & Cox, 1995; Taylor & Adelman, 1996).

When SBHCs developed at the turn of the century, public health departments and social reformers in the largest cities sought to better control communicable diseases, particularly among the children of immigrants, and to assist the immigrant children with assimilation to the new culture. In these early instances, nurses were the primary service providers, though they were often limited by state law with respect to the scope of services they could provide. Personal health services remained the domain of private medical practice and school health became most associated with limited health education or screening (Tzack, 1992).

The increasing interest in more comprehensive SBHCs in the 1970s and 1980s was based, not on a need for communicable disease control services, but on the need to address the so-called "social or lifestyle" morbidities of school-aged children and to provide adolescents with a comfortable and confidential health care "home" (Dryfoos, 1994). Particularly in adolescents, health status indicators were worsening, with increased rates of substance abuse, teen pregnancy, and sexually transmitted diseases and increased deaths due to injury, violence, suicide, and homicide. Educators recognized that the declining physical and psychological health of students was limiting their ability to learn. Nurse practitioner training programs that were starting at this time facilitated a treatment model without the costs associated with physicians. In 1991, the publication of *Healthy People 2000* (US DHHS, 1991) reinforced the need to target services to populations at highest risk, and school-linked or school-based services became recognized as a viable choice for service delivery "to detect and prevent developmental problems . . . facilitate access to basic services" (p. 54).

The growth of SBHCs was largely a grassroots effort sustained by public and private grants (Lear, Montgomery, Schlitt, & Rickett, 1996). As early models were promoted and as community leaders saw the need to responded to the problems of adolescents, replication of the successful programs increased sharply (Lear, Gleicher, St. Germain, & Porter, 1991). As summarized by Lear (1996), the numbers of schools providing clinic services grew from about 30 in the early 1980s to over 700 by the mid 1990s. Moreover, SBHCs were no longer located only in high schools but were disseminated throughout school systems. A 1994 state survey indicated that 45% of SBHCs were located in high schools, 27% in elementary schools, 16% in middle or junior high schools, and 12% in alternative or K–12 schools (Schlitt, Rickett, Montgomery, & Lear, 1994). Clinics were urban or rural, linked to or located within the schools, but most often in high-risk, low-income neighborhoods (Sells, Resnic, & Walker, 1995). States defined SBHCs as vehicles for coordinating and delivering accessible primary physical and mental health services to students.

Scope of Services

The flexibility of SBHCs in meeting the unique needs of the neighborhood developed as a hallmark of the early programs. Thus, no single design for services dominated. Programs were distinguished by the type and range of services actually provided, what entity within the community was responsible for the management of the clinic, and whether only students or students and their children benefited, or whether services were open to others at the school or community. Some programs offered day care and early intervention to assist the adolescent mother to stay in school and improve the parenting for the child. The Institute of Medicine in a report on school-based services offered a definition of comprehensive services: the "integrated set of planned, sequential, school-affiliated strategies, activities, and services designed to promote the optimal physical, emotional, social, and educational development of students" (Allensworth, Wyche, Lawson, & Nicholson, 1995, p. 18). Comprehensive services required a multidisciplinary team, integrated into the services delivery system of the community and accountable to the community for program quality and effectiveness. Since few programs met the ideal model, the report recognized the need to clarify the services provided, categorize the models, and identify which of the models had the better results (Allensworth *et al.*, 1995).

Whether SBHCs offer basic screening procedures or comprehensive medical care depends in part on the organizational structure and management of the health providers in charge of services and whether that organization is the traditional provider to the population at the school (Guernsey & Pastore, 1996). Services run by schools typically are more limited in scope and affected by school rules defining the routine procedures. In an underserved area, opposition to the clinic based on the competitive concerns of private practitioners is lessened. Traditional health providers such as community health centers, public health departments, hospitals, medical schools, and nonprofit agencies typically offer more comprehensive services and more effectively integrate school services into community networks. The ability of school-based clinics to fit into the delivery system becomes critical with the current emphasis on managed care.

According to a survey by the CDC in 1994, 59.2% of states fund school-based or -linked clinics, and at least one school-based or -linked clinic exists in 11.6% of all districts (Small *et al.*, 1995). The services that are most likely to be provided at SBHCs include administration of first aid (90.7%), administration of medication (90.7%), health screening (90%), evaluation of suspected child abuse (84%), development of the health component of individual educational plans (84%), early childhood health screening (73.7%), assessment of vital signs (69.3%), case management of chronic problems (65.3%), and clean dressing changes (58.7%) (Schlitt *et al.*, 1994). A 1995 survey of 173 urban health departments medical services were provided in 71–80% of school-based or -linked services. Mental health and social services were provided by less than half of the urban health departments. Reproductive counseling was common in over 95% of clinics; however, supplies were limited to 21% of clinics. The local debates over the appropriateness of providing reproductive health services in SBHCs have constrained their ability to meet some adolescents' health needs by limiting contraceptive services (Bullerdiek, Simpson, & Peck, 1995).

Effectiveness of School Clinics

While the successes of SBHCs are ideally determined on the basis of effectiveness in meeting the goals identified by local needs assessment, the local evaluation is rarely comprehensive and most often focuses on process rather than outcome measures. The complexities of the behaviorally determined outcomes and the inherent limitation in comparisons in school settings also hamper studies (Gomby & Carson, 1992). Three factors contributing to this difficulty include the difficulty in determination of the type of service actually provided and being studied. Clinic staff may have an impact on students through health education and health promotion in classrooms, through individual counseling, and through group counseling. The combination of the services, the differences in organization of the services, how the services were defined, and the goals of the components can affect outcomes and confuse results. Second, the schools by their nature present particular difficulties in data access and collection. In the schools with the highest risk populations, the transient nature of students introduces problems in determining the dose of services received by which students. Finally, the differences in the population groups and the methodology in finding the adequate control groups can be challenging.

Despite these concerns, SBHCs are effective in increasing utilization of services by needy youth consistent with the goals of improvement in access to health care. A study by the General Accounting Office in 1994 noted that SBHCs help to overcome financial and nonfinancial barriers that limit access to care for the groups studied, including lack of a source of routine medical care and insufficient attention of other providers to the particular needs of adolescents (US Congress Office of Technology Assessment, 1994). Students, parents, teachers, and school personnel report a high level of satisfaction with SBHCs and particularly appreciate their accessibility, convenience, and caring attitude (Marks & Marske, 1993). SBHCs are more likely to be found in communities of greatest need and to be used most by the highest-risk students who report the greatest number of health problems (Walter *et al.*, 1996). When mental health services are provided, students and families gain access to psychosocial counseling previously unavailable and have higher use of services than adolescents in the general population (Anglin, Naylor, & Kaplan, 1996).

SBHCs may have an impact on improving school performance and reducing absences (McCord, Klein, Foy, & Feathergill, 1993). Minor illnesses such as headaches, menstrual cramps, and accidents on school property can be treated in school, decreasing school absences and potentially lowering dropout rates (Klerman, 1988). For a provider familiar with dealing with adolescents, the common complaints often may be useful markers for exploring possible psychosocial problems, suggesting that school nurses need to look beyond a student's stated reasons for visits if psychosocial problems are to be addressed (Schneider, Friedman, & Fisher, 1995).

The impact of SBHCs on students' uses of other sources of health care has been variable. Students continue to see their usual providers. Inappropriate utilization of emergency rooms for primary health care services has declined in areas with school clinics (Dryfoos, Brindis, & Kaplan, 1996). Another study addressing the impact of health insurance status on adolescents' utilization of school-based clinic services found students with private insurance or health maintenance organization coverage had the highest rates of SBHC utilization and students without health insurance and with Medicaid had the lowest (Brindis, Kapphalm, McCarter, & Wolfe, 1995). School-based clinics rarely provide services on a 24-hour basis or over holidays and weekends.

In a national evaluation of the 19 clinics funded by the Robert Wood Johnson Foundation, outcome measures studied included students' knowledge of key health facts and self-reports of high-risk behavior, including sexual activity, contraceptive use, use of condoms, pregnancies, births, and health status (Kisker, Brown, & Hill, 1994). Students from the participating schools were compared to a national sample of urban youths. Although health knowledge increased among students having access to the SBHCs, the estimated impacts on health status and risky behavior were inconsistent and not statistically significant, suggesting more intensive or different services are needed if they are to significantly reduce risk taking behavior (Kisker & Brown, 1996).

SBHCs may be limited in the reproductive services that they may provide. Although many studies have focused on teen pregnancy prevention and a clinic's ability to delay the onset of intercourse, encourage consistent use of contraception in sexually active students, lower birth rates, and lower pregnancy rates, results are mixed. Some data suggest that school-based clinics have had an impact on delaying the initiation of sexual intercourse, upgrading the quality of contraceptive use, and lowering pregnancy rates. However, these health-promoting behavior changes have only been identified in programs that offer comprehensive family planning services (Kirby, Waszak, & Ziegler, 1991). Contraceptive services and condom distribution are the most likely services to be missing from an otherwise comprehensive SBHC due to the sensitivity of this issue in some communities.

Implications for Services

School-based service and prevention programs for children and adolescents are effective in reaching school-aged children and adolescents, increasing utilization of services, and increasing knowledge of behavioral risks. Programs work best that are interrelated and implemented early, before risk behavior become entrenched and more difficult to modify. Health educators working with clinic staff can schedule presentations in classes with the objectives to provide students with timely and accurate information about risk behavior and prevalent health problems, provide social skills training to avoid or reduce risky behavior, and encourage students to discuss their particular health concerns with SBHC staff. Athletic physicals, first aid, or common complaints are effective in bringing the most students to services, though special efforts may be needed to reach some youth in great need of SBHC services in order to enhance their utilization of clinic services (Santelli, Morreale, Wigten, & Grason, 1996). Such youth may be unaware of the availability and range of services that the SBHC provides or may lack the trust and rapport associated with clinic utilization.

Recent surveys show high public acceptance of SBHCs, particularly in those communities in greatest need. With the changing demographics of the American family, many of those surveyed favored use of public school facilities to provide health and social services to students, even the distribution of condoms in schools. National medical groups such as the American Medical Association and American Academy of Pediatrics strongly support SBHCs where the services are directed by a physician.

To facilitate the uniform implementation of school health services, the National Association of School Nurses (Proctor, Lord, & Sarger, 1993) developed School Nursing Practice Roles and Standards, and the American School Health Association (1995) developed guidelines for comprehensive school health programs. Service guidelines and quality standards define the recommended practice. Nurses, most often the providers, must practice under these guidelines, and the degree of nursing autonomy depends largely on state laws. Clinics continue to face the special problems of recruiting and retaining appropriately trained staff with the special interest in serving children and adolescents at SBHCs.

Future of School Clinics

The future of SBHCs, particularly in the complex and changing climate of managed care, depends on identification of stable financing mechanisms and continued community support. SBHCs historically have been supported by a mix of funding. A survey in 1990 of SBHC funding sources showed that state health departments provided 24% of support; private foundations, 18%; maternal and child health block grants, 17%; local governments, 12%; schools, 8%; community health centers, 7%; Medicaid, 2%; and private payers, less than 1% (Wazak & Neidell, 1992). Centers that lack a stable source of funding do not always have sufficient resources for meeting their patients' health needs and may have difficulty obtaining reimbursement from public and private insurers. With the increasing penetration of managed care and continuing health care reform, finding future resources may become more difficult. Some managed care groups refuse to recognize SBHCs and refuse to provide reimbursement.

A few states have passed legislation to encourage the development of school-based services and to facilitate the reimbursement for those services. In those communities where schools have become managed care providers, the schools can become the medical home if appropriate links with community providers exist and medical home standards that require 24-hour care and the ability to respond to emergencies can be met.

Greater reliance on patient care revenues is not endorsed by all SBHCs or their supporters. The blend of social supports, mental health, health education, and medical services that have distinguished many comprehensive SBHCs does not lend itself to a financing strategy that requires school-based centers to fit within a traditional medical services model. To tie the work of the SBHC to a reimbursement structure that does not recognize the nonmedical services appears to some to threaten what is most valuable about SBHCs. The large number of uninsured students using the centers increases the importance of public health dollars in funding care for the uninsured. Costs and benefits of comprehensive services delivered at the school cannot easily be compared to the costs and potential outcomes of a typical outpatient clinic visit (Lear *et al.*, 1996).

SBHCs are most likely to survive where they are recognized for the special role that they play in reaching the particularly high-risk students and where they have strong community leadership. Medicaid expansions for low-income children and the funding of services for currently uninsured populations offer opportunities for resources, but this will be beneficial to SBHCs only as they become part of comprehensive service networks. However, there may be financial incentives for managed care plans to exclude SBHCs from provider networks and administrative complexities that deter contractual relationships between insurer and SBHC. Monitoring of the system, documentation of the needs and gaps, and participation in policy discussions and political processes will determine the system of care and long-term presence of SBHC's place in future services delivery (Brellochs, Zimmerman, Zink, & English, 1996).

Conclusions

Schools are an effective setting for reaching children to promote health and reduce disease risk. Each of the three major areas of health promotion reviewed in this chapter, including school-based intervention research, comprehensive school health programs, and school-based health clinics, has a strong contribution to make to the health of children. However, several challenges must be addressed before the full potential of these school health activities can be realized. A partial list of these challenges includes (1) increasing the amount and longevity of behavior change produced by school-based intervention programs, (2) facilitating the dissemination of school-based intervention programs that are known to change behavior, (3) achieving the full implementation of comprehensive school health programs nationwide, (4) sustaining the growth of school-based health clinics nationwide, and (5) developing a better understanding of the ways in which school-based intervention research, comprehensive school health programs, and school-based health clinics can work together to increase the positive impact of these activities on the health of youth. If these and other challenges can be met, health promotion and disease prevention in school settings will become an increasingly important contributor to the good health of children and adolescents in the United States.

References

Ajzen, I. (1991). The theory of planned behavior. *Organizational Behavior and Human Decision Processes, 50,* 179–211.

Allensworth, D. A. (1994). The research base for innovative practices in school health education at the secondary level. *Journal of School Health, 64,* 180–187.

Allensworth, D. A., & Kolbe, L. J. (1987). The comprehensive school health program: Exploring an expanded concept. *Journal of School Health, 57,* 409–412.

Allensworth, D., Wyche, J. L., Lawson, E., & Nicholson, L. (1995). Committee on Comprehensive School Health Programs, Institute of Medicine. Washington, DC: National Academy Press.

American Association of School Administrators. (1990). *Healthy Kids for the year 2000: An action plan for schools.* (AASA Stock #021-00306). Arlington, VA: Author.

American School Health Association (1995). *Guidelines for comprehensive school health programs.* Kent, OH: Author.

Anglin, T. M., Naylor, K. E., & Kaplan, D. W. (1996). Comprehensive school-based health care: High school students use of medical, mental health and substance abuse services. *Pediatrics, 97,* 318–330.

Atkins, C. J., Patterson, T. L., Roppe, B. E., Kaplan, R. M., Sallis, J. F., & Nadar, P. R. (1987). Recruitment issues, health habits and the decision to participate in a health promotion program. *American Journal of Preventive Medicine, 3,* 87–94.

Baldwin, J. A., Rolf, J. E., Johnson, J., Bowers, J., Benally, C., & Trotter, R. T. (1996). Developing culturally sensitive HIV/AIDS and substance abuse prevention curricula for Native American youth. *Journal of School Health, 66,* 322–327.

Bandura, A. (1986). *Social foundations of thought and action: A social cognitive theory.* Englewood Cliffs, NJ: Prentice-Hall.

Baranowski, T., Perry, C. L., & Parcel, G. S. (1997). How individuals, environments, and health behavior interact: Social cognitive theory. In K. Glanz, F. M. Lewis, & B. K. Rimer (Eds.), *Health behavior and health education: Theory, research, and practice* (pp. 153–178). San Francisco: Jossey-Bass.

Basch, C. E., Zybert, P., & Shea, S. (1994). 5-a-Day: Dietary behavior and the fruit and vegetable intake of Latine children. *American Journal of Public Health, 84,* 814–818.

Basen-Engquist, K., O'Hara-Tompkins, N., Lavato, C. Y., Lewis, M. J., Parcel, G. S., & Gingiss P. (1994). The effect of two types of teacher training on implementation of smart choices: A tobacco prevention curriculum. *Journal of School Health, 64,* 334–339.

Berenson, G. S., Srinivasan, S. R., Webber, L. S., Nicklas, T. A., Hunter, S. M., Harsha, D. W., Johnson, C. C., Arbeit, M. L., Dalferes, E. R., Wattingney, W. A., & Lawrence, M. D. (1991). *Cardiovascular risk in early life: The Bogalusa Heart Study* (pp. 13–17). Kalamazoo, MI: Upjohn Company.

Bowen, D. J., Kinne, S., & Orlandi, M. (1995). School policy in COMMIT: A promising strategy to reduce smoking by youth. *Journal of School Health, 65,* 140–144.

Brellochs, C., Zimmerman, D., Zink, T., & English, A. (1996). School-based primary care in a managed care environment: options and issues. *Adolescent Medicine: State of the Art Reviews, 7,* 197–206.

Brindis, C., Kapphalm, C., McCarter, V., & Wolfe, A. L. (1995). The impact of health insurance status on adolescent's utilization of school based clinic services: Implications for health care reform. *Journal of Adolescent Health, 16,* 18–25.

Bullerdiek, H. W., Simpson, P. S. & Peck, M. G. (1995). *What works III: Focus on school health in urban communities.* Omaha, NE: City Match.

Bush, P. J., Zuckerman, A. E., Taggart, V. S., Theiss, P. K., Peleg, E. O., & Smith, S. A. (1989). Cardiovascular risk factor prevention in black school children: The "Know Your Body" evaluation project. *Health Education Quarterly, 16*, 229–244.

Carmines, E. G., & Zeller, R. A. (1979). *Reliability and validity assessment.* Beverly Hills, CA: Sage.

Center for Population Options. (1991). *School-based and school-linked clinics.* Update. Washington, DC: Author.

Clarke, W. R., Schrott, H. G., Leaverton, P. E., Connor, W. E., & Lauer, R. M. (1978). Tracking of blood lipids and blood pressures in school age children: The Muscatine Study. *Circulation, 58*, 626–634.

Collins, J. L., Small, M. L., Kann, L., Pateman, B. C., Gold, R. S., & Kilbe, L. J. (1995). School health education. *Journal of School Health, 65*, 302–311.

Committee on School Health, American Academy of Pediatrics. (1993). P. R. Nader (Ed.), *School health–Policy and practice.* Elk Grove Village, IL: Author.

Connel D. B., Turner, R. R., & Mason, E. F. (1985). Summary of findings of the school health education evaluation: Health promotion effectiveness, implementation, and costs. *Journal of School Health, 55*, 316–321.

Contento, I., Balch, G. I., Bronner, Y. L., Lytle, L. A., Maloney, S. K., Olson, C. M., & Swadener, S. S. (1995). Nutrition education for school-aged children. *Journal of Nutrition Education, 27*, 298–311.

Cook, T. D., & Campbell, D. T. (1979). *Quasi-experimentation: Design and analysis issues for field settings.* Boston, MA: Houghton Mifflin.

Cook, T. D., Appleton, H., Conner, R. F., Shaffer, A., Tamkin, G., & Weber, S. J. (1975). *"Sesame Street" revisited.* New York: Russell Sage Foundation.

Cornfield, J. (1978). Randomization by group: A formal analysis. *American Journal of Epidemiology, 108*, 100–102.

Davis, T. M., & Allensworth, D. D. (1994). Program management: A necessary component for the comprehensive school health program. *Journal of School Health, 64*, 400–404.

DeGraw, C. (1994). A community-based school health system: Parameters for developing a comprehensive student health promotion program. *Journal of School Health, 64*, 192–195.

Donner, A. (1992). Sample size requirements for stratified cluster randomization designs. *Statistics in Medicine, 11*, 743–750.

Donner, A., & Klar, N. (1994). Methods comparing event rates in intervention studies when the unit of allocation is a cluster. *American Journal of Epidemiology, 140*, 279–289.

Donner, A., Birkett, N., & Buck, C. (1981). Randomization by cluster. *American Journal of Epidemiology, 114*, 906–914.

Donner, A., Brown, K. S., & Brasher, P. (1990). A methodological review of non-therapeutic intervention trials employing cluster randomization 1979–1989. *International Journal of Epidemiology, 19*, 795–800.

Dryfoos, J. G. (1994). *Full-service schools: A revolution in health and social services for children, youth, and families.* San Francisco: Josey-Bass.

Dryfoos, J. G., Brindis, C., & Kaplan, D. W. (1996). Research and evaluation in school-based health care. *Adolescent Medicine: State of the Art Reviews, 7*, 207–219.

Edmundson, E. W., Luton, S. C., McGraw, S. A., Kelder, S. H., Layman, A. K., Smyth, M. H., Bachman, K. J., Pedersen, S. A., & Stone, E. J. (1994). CATCH: Classroom process evaluation in a multicenter trial. *Health Education Quarterly* (Suppl.), 2, S27–S50.

Elder, J. P., McGraw, S. A., Stone, E. J., Reed, D. B., Harsha, D. W., Greene, T., & Wambsgans, K.C. (1994). CATCH: Process evaluation of environmental factors and programs. *Health Education Quarterly*, (Suppl.) 2, S107–S128.

Ellickson, P.L., Bianca, D., & Schoeff, D.C. (1988). Containing attrition in school-based research: An innovative approach. *Evaluation Review, 12*, 331–351.

Ellison, R. C., Capper, A. L., Goldberg, R. J., Witschi, J. C., & Stare, F. J. (1989). The environmental component: Changing school food service to promote cardiovascular health. *Health Education Quarterly, 16*, 285–297.

English, J. (1994). Innovative practices in comprehensive health education programs for elementary schools. *Journal of School Health, 64*, 188–191.

Ernst, N. D., & Obarzanek, E. (1994). Child health and nutrition: Obesity and high blood cholesterol. *Preventive Medicine, 23*, 427–436.

Esobedo, L. G., Marcus, S. E., Hotzma, D., & Giovino, G. A. (1993). Sports participation, age at smoking initiation, and the risk of smoking among US high school students. *Journal of the American Medical Association, 269*, 1391–1395.

Flay, B. R. (1985). Psychosocial approaches to smoking prevention: A review of findings. *Health Psychology, 4*, 449–488.

Flay, B. R. (1986). Efficacy and effectiveness trials (and other phases of research) in the development of health promotion programs. *Preventive Medicine, 15,* 451–474.

Flay, B. R., Miller, T. Q., Hedeker, D., Siddiqui, O., Britton, C. F., Brannon, B. R., Johnson, C. A., Hansen, W. B., Sussman, S., & Dent, C. (1995). The television, school, and family smoking prevention and cessation project. *Preventive Medicine, 24,* 29–40.

Flynn, B. S., Worden, J. K., Secker-Walker, R. H., Badger, G. H., Geller, B. M., & Costanza, M. C. (1992). Prevention of cigarette smoking through mass media intervention and school programs. *American Journal of Public Health, 82,* 827–834.

Garcia, A. W., Broda, M. A. N., Frenn, M., Coviak, C., Pender, N. J., & Ronis, D. L. (1995). Gender and developmental differences in exercise beliefs among youth and prediction of their exercise behavior. *Journal of School Health, 65,* 213–219.

Gingiss, P. L. (1992). Enhancing program implementation and maintenance through a multiphase approach to peer-based staff development. *Journal of School Health, 62,* 161–166.

Gomby, D. S., & Larson, C. S. (1992). Evaluation of school linked services. In R. E. Behrman (Ed.), *The future of children, school-linked services* (pp. 68–84). Los Altos, CA: The David and Lucile Packard Foundation.

Green, L. W., & Kreuter, M. W. (1991). *Health promotion planning: An educational and environmental approach.* Mountain View, CA: Mayfield.

Guernsey, B. P., & Pastore, D. R. (1996). Comprehensive school-based health center: Implementing the model. *Adolescent Medicine: State of the Art Reviews, 2,* 181–195.

Hansen, W. B., Collins, L. M., Malotte, C. K., Johnson, C. A., & Fielding, J. E. (1985). Attrition in prevention research. *Journal of Behavioral Medicine, 8,* 261–275.

Harrington, K. F., Binkley, D., Duvall, R. C., Reynolds, K. D., Copeland, J. R., Franklin, F., & Raczynski, J. (1997). Recruitment issues in school-based research: Lessons learned from the high-5 Alabama project. *Journal of School Health, 67,* 415–421.

Hausman, A. J., & Ruzek, S. B. (1995). Implementation of comprehensive school health education in elementary schools: Focus on teacher concerns. *Journal of School Health, 65,* 81–86.

Hopper, C. A., Gruber, M. B., Munoz, K. D., & Herb, R. A. (1992). Effect of including parents in a school-based exercise and nutrition program for children. *Research Quarterly for Exercise and Sport, 63,* 1–7.

Hsieh, F. Y. (1988). Sample size formulae for intervention studies with the cluster as unit of randomization. *Statistics in Medicine, 8,* 1195–1201.

Iowa Department of Education. (1992). *Iowa . . . A Place to Grow Healthy.* Des Moines, IA: Author.

Johnson, C. C., Osganian, S. K., Budman, S. B., Lytle, L. A., Barrera, E. P., Bonura, S. R., Wu, M. C., & Nader, P. R. (1994). CATCH: Family process evaluation in a multicenter trial. *Health Education Quarterly* (Suppl.) 2, S91–S106.

Joint Committee on Health Education Terminology. (1991). Report of the 1990 joint committee on health education terminology. *Journal Health Education, 22,* 97–108.

Joint Committee on National Health Education Standards. (1995). *National health education standards.* New York: American Cancer Society.

Jurs, S. G., & Glass, G. V. (1971). The effect of experimental mortality on the internal and external validity of the randomized comparative experiment. *Journal of Experimental Education, 40,* 62–66.

Kane, W. M. (1993). *Step by step to comprehensive school health: The program planning guide.* Santa Cruz, CA: ETR Associates.

Kann, L., Collins, J. L., Collins-Pateman, B., Leavy-Small, M., Ross, J. G., & Kolbe, L. J. (1995). The school health policies and programs study (SHPPS): Rationale for a nationwide status report on school health programs. *Journal of School Health, 65,* 291–294.

Kann, L., Warren, C. W., Harris, W. A., Collins, J. L., Williams, B. I., Ross, J. G., & Kolbe, L. J. (1996). Youth risk behavior surveillance—United States, 1995. *Journal of School Health, 66,* 365–377.

Kelder, S. H., Perry, C. L., Klepp, K. I., & Lytle, L. L. (1994). Longitudinal tracking of adolescent smoking, physical activity, and food choice behaviors. *American Journal of Public Health, 84,* 1121–1126.

Kirby, D., & DiClemente, R. J. (1994). School-based behavioral interventions to prevent unprotected sex and HIV among adolescents. In R. J. DiClemente & J. L. Peterson (Eds.), *Preventing AIDS: Theories and methods of behavioral interventions* (pp. 117–139). New York: Plenum Press.

Kirby, D., Waszak, C., & Ziegler, J. (1991). Six school-based clinics: Their reproductive health services and impact on sexual behavior. *Family Planning Perspectives, 23,* 6–16.

Kisker, E. E., & Brown, R. (1996). Do school-based health centers improve adolescents access to health care, health status, and risk-taking behavior? *Journal of Adolescent Health, 18,* 335–343.

Kisker, E. E., Brown, R. S., & Hill, J. (1994). *Healthy caring: Outcomes of the Robert Wood Johnson Foundation's school-based adolescent health care program*. Princeton, NJ: Mathematica Policy Research.

Klein, J. D., & Cox, E. M. (1995). School-based health clinics in the mid-1990s. *Current Opinion in Pediatrics, 7*, 353–359.

Klerman, L. V. (1988). School absence—a health perspective. *Pediatric Clinics of North America, 35*, 1253–1256.

Krebs-Smith, S. M., Cook, A., Subar, A. F., Cleveland, L., Friday, J., & Kahle, L. L. (1996). Fruit and vegetable intakes of children and adolescents in the United States. *Archives of Pediatric and Adolescent Medicine, 150*, 81–86.

Lear, J. G. (1996). School-based services and adolescent health: Past, present, and future. *Adolescent Medicine: State of the Art Reviews, 2*, 163–179.

Lear, J. G., Gleicher, H. B., St. Germain, A., & Porter, P. J. (1991). Reorganizing health care for adolescents: The experience of the school-based adolescent health care program. *Journal of Adolescent Health, 12*, 450–458.

Lear, J. G., Montgomery, L. L., Schlitt, J. J., & Rickett, K. D. (1996). Key issues affecting school- based health centers and Medicaid. *Journal of School Health, 66*, 83–88.

Lohrmann, D. K., Gold, R. S., & Jubb, W. H. (1987). School health education: A foundation for school health programs. *Journal of School Health, 57*, 420–425.

Luepker, R. V., Perry, C. L., McKinlay, S. M., Nader, P. R., Parcel, G. S., Stone, E. J., Webber, L. S., Elder, J. P., Feldman, H. A., Johnson, C. C., Kelder, S. H., & Wu, M. (1996). Outcomes of a field trial to improve children's dietary patterns and physical activity: The Child and Adolescent Trial for Cardiovascular Health (CATCH). *Journal of the American Medical Association, 275*, 768– 776.

Lytle, L. A., & Achterberg, C. (1995). Changing the diet of America's children: What works and why? *Journal of Nutrition Education, 27*, 250–260.

Lytle, L. A., Johnson, C. C., Bachman, K., Wambsgan, K., Perry, C. L., Stone, E. J., & Budman, S. (1994). Successful recruitment strategies for school-based health promotion: Experiences from CATCH. *Journal of School Health, 64*, 405–409.

Marks, E. L, & Marzke, C. H. (1993). *Healthy caring, a process evaluation of the Robert Wood Johnson Foundation's school-based adolescent health care program*. Princeton, NJ: Mathtech.

McBride, C. M., Curry, S. J., Cheadle, A., Anderman, C. Wagner, E. H., Diehr, P., & Psaty, B. (1995). School-level application of a social bonding model to adolescent risk-taking behavior. *Journal of School Health, 65*, 63–68.

McCord, M. T., Klein, J. D. Foy, J. M., & Fothergill, K. (1993). School-based clinic use and school performance. *Journal of Adolescent Health, 14*, 91–98.

McGraw, S. A., Stone, E. J., Osganian, S. K., Elder, J. P., Perry, C. L., Johnson, C. C., Parcel, G. S., Webber, L. S., & Luepker, R. V. (1994). Design of process evaluation within the Child and Adolescent Trial for Cardiovascular Health (CATCH). *Health Education Quarterly* (Suppl.) 2, S5–S26.

Mitchell-DiCenso, A., Thomas, B. H., Devlin, M. C., Goldsmith, C. H., Willan, A., Singer, J., Marks, S., Watters, D., & Hewson, S. (1997). Evaluation of an educational program to prevent adolescent pregnancy. *Health Education and Behavior, 24*, 300–312.

Morrison, T. C., Wahlgren, D. R., Hovell, M. F., Zakarian, J., Burkham-Kreitner, S., Hofstetter, C. R., Slymen, D. J., Keating, K., Russos, S., & Jones, J. A. (1997). Tracking and follow-up of 16,915 adolescents: Minimizing attrition bias. *Controlled Clinical Trials, 18*, 383–396.

Murray, D. M., & Hannan, P. J. (1990). Planning for the appropriate analysis in school-based drug-use prevention studies. *Journal of Consulting and Clinical Psychology, 58*, 458–468.

Murray, D. M., Hannan, P. J., & Zucker, D. M. (1989). Analysis issues in school-based health promotion studies. *Health Education Quarterly, 16*, 315–320.

Nader, P. R., Sallis, J. F., Patterson, T. L., Abramson, I. S., Rupp, J. W., Senn, K. L., Atkins, C. J., Roppe, B. E., Morris, J. A., Wallace, J. P., & Vega, W. A. (1989). A family approach to cardiovascular risk reduction: Results from the San Diego Family Health Project. *Health Education Quarterly, 16*, 229–244.

National Cancer Institute. (1991). *5 a day for better health program guidebook*. Bethesda, Md: NCI.

National Center for Health Statistics. (1995). Trends in pregnancies and pregnancy rates: Estimates for the United States, 1980–1992. *Monthly Vital Statistics Report, 43*, Suppl.

National Center for Health Statistics. (1996). Advance report of final mortality statistics, 1993. *Monthly Vital Statistics Report, 44*, Suppl.

National Health/Education Consortium. (1990). *Crossing the boundaries between health and education*. Washington, DC: National Commission to Prevent Infant Mortality.

National Professional School Health Education Organizations. (1984). Comprehensive school health education. *Journal of School Health, 54,* 312–315.

Nebraska Department of Education. (1990). *Healthy kids, healthier Nebraska.* Lincoln, NE: Author.

Nelson, G. D., Cross, F. S., & Kolbe, L. J. (1991). Introduction: Teenage health teaching modules evaluation. *Journal of School Health, 61,* 20.

Nicklas, T. A., Webber, L. S., Johnson, C. C., Srinivasan, S. R., & Berenson, G. S. (1995). Foundations for health promotion with youth: A review of observations from the Bogalusa Heart Study. *Journal of Health Education, 26,* S18–S26.

Office on Smoking and Health, DASH, CDC. (1996). Tobacco use and usual source of cigarettes amonghigh school students—United States 1995. *Journal of School Health, 66,* 222–224.

Osborne, M. L., Kistner, J. A., & Helgemo, B. (1993). Developmental progression in chidren's knowledge of AIDS: Implications for education and attitudinal change. *Journal of Pediatric Psychology, 18,* 177–192.

Parcel, G. S. (1984). Theoretical models for application in school health education research. *Health Education, 15,* 39–49.

Parcel, G. S., Simons-Morton, B. G., O'Hara, N. M., Baranowski, T., Kolbe, L. J., & Bee, D. E. (1987). School promotion of healthful diet and exercise behavior: An integration of organizational change and social learning theory interventions. *Journal of School Health, 57,* 150–156.

Parcel, G. S., Simons-Morton, B., O'Hara, N. M., Baranowski, T., & Wilson, B. (1989). School promotion of healthful diet and physical activity: Impact on learning outcomes and self-reported behavior. *Health Education Quarterly, 16,* 181–199.

Pate, R. R., Small, M. L., Ross, J. G., Young, J. C., Flint, K. H., & Warren, C. W. (1995). School physical education. *Journal of School Health, 65,* 312–318.

Perry, C. L., Crockett, S. J., & Pirie, P. (1987). Influencing parental health behavior: Implications of community assessments. *Health Education, 18,* 68–77.

Perry, C. L., Luepker, R. V., Murray, D. M., Kurth, C., Mullis, R., Crockett, S., & Jacobs, D. (1988). Parent involvement with children's health promotion: The Minnesota home team. *American Journal of Public Health, 79,* 1156–1160.

Perry, C. L., Luepker, R. V., Murray, D. M., Hearn, M. D., Halper, A., Dudovitz, B., Maile, M. C., & Smyth, M. (1989). Parents' involvement with children's health promotion: A one-year follow-up of the Minnesota home team. *Health Education Quarterly, 16,* 171–180.

Perry, C. L., Stone, E. J., Parcel, G. S., Ellison, R. C., Nader, P. R., Webber, L. S., & Luepker, R. V. (1990). School-based cardiovascular health promotion: The Child and Adolescent Trial for Cardiovascular Health (CATCH). *Journal of School Health, 60,* 406–413.

Perry, C. L., Kelder, S. H., & Klepp, K. I. (1994). The rationale behind early prevention of cardiovascular disease in young people. *European Journal of Public Health, 4,* 156–162.

Petosa, R., & Goodman, R. M. (1991). Recruitment and retention of schools participating in schoolhealth research. *Journal of School Health, 61,* 426–429.

Pirie, P. L., Thomson, S. J., Mann, S. L., Peterson, A. V., Murray, D. M., Flay, B. R., & Best, J. A. (1989). Tracking and attrition in longitudinal school-based smoking prevention research. *Preventive Medicine, 18,* 249–256.

Porkka, K. V., Viikari, J. S. A., & Akerblom, H. K. (1991). Tracking of serum HDL–cholesterol and other lipids in children and adolescents: The caridiovascular risk in young Finns study. *Preventive Medicine, 20,* 713–724.

Proctor, S. T., Lordi, S. L., & Sarger, D. S. (1993). *School nursing practice roles and standards.* Scarborough, ME: National Association for School Nurses.

Resnicow, K., & Allensworth, D. (1996). Conducting a comprehensive school health program. *Journal of School Health, 66,* 59–63.

Reynolds, K. D., Raczynski, J. M., Binkley, D., Franklin, F. A., Duvall, R. C., Devane-Hart, K., Harrington, K. F., Caldwell, E., Jester, P., Bragg, C., & Fouad, M. (1998). Design of "High 5": A school-based study to promote fruit & vegetable consumption for reduction of cancer risk. *Journal of Cancer Education, 13,* 169–177.

Rickard, K. A., Gallahue, D. L., Gruen, G. E., Tridle, M., Bewley, N., & Steele, K. (1995). The play approach to learning in the context of families and schools: An alternative paradigm for nutrition and fitness education in the 21st century. *Journal of the American Dietetic Association, 95,* 1121–1126.

Rooney, B. L., & Murray, D. M. (1996). A meta-analysis of smoking prevention programs after adjustment for errors in the unit of analysis. *Health Education Quarterly, 23,* 48–64.

Rossi, P. H., & Freeman, H. E. (1993). *Evaluation: A systematic approach.* Newbury Park, CA: Sage.

Sallis, J. F. & McKenzie, T. L. (1991). Physical education's role in public health. *Research Quarterly for Exercise and Sport, 62,* 124–137.

Santelli, J., Kouzis, A., & Newcomer, S. (1996a). Student attitudes toward school-based health centers. *Journal of Adolescent Health, 18,* 349–356.

Santelli, J., Morreale, M., Wigton, A., & Grason, H. (1996b). School health centers and primary care for adolescents: A review of the literature. *Journal of Adolescent Health, 18,* 357–366.

Schaalma, H. P., Kok, G., Bosker, R. J., Parcel, G. S., Peters, L, Poelman, J., & Reinders, J. (1996). Planned development and evaluation of AIDS/STD education for secondary school students in the Netherlands: Short-term effects. *Health Education Quarterly, 23,* 469–487.

Schlitt, J. J., Ricket, K. D., Montgomery, L. L., & Lear, J. G. (1994). *State initiatives to support school-based health center: A national survey.* Washington, DC: Making the Grade National Program Office.

Schneider, M. B. Friedman, S. B., & Fisher, M. (1995). Stated and unstated reasons for visiting a high school nurse's office. *Journal Adolescent Health, 16,* 35–40.

Seffrin, J.R. (1994). America's interest in comprehensive school health education. *Journal of School Health, 64,* 397–399.

Sells,W., Resnic, M. D., & Walker, J. (1995). *School-based and school-linked clinics in rural America; a report prepared for the office of rural health policy.* Minneapolis, MN: National Adolescent Health Resource Center.

Sells, C. W., & Blum, R. W. (1996). Current trends in adolescent health. In R. J. DiClemente, W.B. Hansen, & L. E. Ponton (Eds.), *Handbook of adolescent health risk behavior* (pp. 5–34). New York: Plenum Press.

Siddiqui, O., Flay, B. R., & Hu, F. B. (1996). Factors affecting attrition in a longitudinal smoking prevention study. *Preventive Medicine, 25,* 554–560.

Simpson, J. M., Klar, N., & Donner, A. (1995). Accounting for cluster randomization: A review of primary prevention trials, 1990 through 1993. *American Journal of Public Health, 85,* 1378–1383.

Small, M. L, Majer, L. S, Allensworth, D. D., Farquhar, B. K., Kann, L., & Peteman, B. C. (1995). School health services. *Journal of School Health, 65,* 319–326.

Stein, A. D., Shea, S., Basch, C. E., Contento, I. R., & Zybert, P. (1991). Variability and tracking of nutrient intakes of preschool children based on multiple administrations of the 24–hour dietary recall. *American Journal of Epidemiology, 134,* 1427–1437.

Stiff, J. B. (1994). *Persuasive communication.* New York: Guilford Press.

Taioli, E., & Wynder, E. L. (1991). Effect of the age at which smoking begins on frequency of smoking in adulthood. *New England Journal of Medicine, 325,* 968–969.

Taylor, L., & Adelman, H. S. (1996). Mental health in schools: Promising directions for practice. *Adolescent Medicine: State of the Art Reviews, 7,* 303–317.

Trochim, W. M. K. (1984). *Research design for program evaluation: The regression-discontinuity approach.* Beverly Hills, CA: Sage.

Tzack, D. (1992). Health and social services in public schools: Historical perspectives. In R. E. Behrman (Ed.), *The future of children, school-linked services* (pp. 19–31). Los Altos, CA: The David and Lucile Packard Foundation.

US Congress, Office of Technology Assessment. (1994). *Health care reform, school-based health centers can promote access to care.* (GAO/HEHS-94-166). Washington, DC: US Government Printing Office.

US Department of Health and Human Services. (1991). *Healthy people 2000: National health promotion and disease prevention objectives.* (DHHS Publication No. PHS 91-50212). Washington, DC: US Government Printing Office.

Van Ryn, M., & Heaney, C.A. (1992). What's the use of theory? *Health Education Quarterly, 19,* 315–330.

Walter, H. J, Vaughan, R., Armstrong, B., Krakoff, R. Y., Tiezzi, L., & McCarthy, J. F. (1996). Characteristics of users and nonusers of health clinics in inner-city junior high school. *Journal of Adolescent Health, 18,* 344–348.

Wazak, C., & Neidell, S. (1992). *School-based and school-linked clinics, update 1991.* Washington, DC: Center for Population Options.

Webber, L. S., Srinivasan, S. R., Wattigney, W., & Berenson, G. S. (1991). Tracking of serum lipids and lipoproteins from childhood to adulthood—The Bogalusa Heart Study. *American Journal of Epidemiology, 133,* 884–899.

West, S. G. (1985). Beyond the laboratory experiment: Experimental and quasi-experimental designs for interventions in naturalistic settings. In P. Karoly (Ed.), *Measurement strategies in health psychology* (pp. 183–233). New York: John Wiley & Sons.

Wylie, W. E. (1983). Cost-benefit analysis of a school health education program: One method. *Journal of School Health, 53,* 371–373.

Zellerman, G. L. (1981). *The response of the schools to teenage pregnancy and parenthood.* Santa Monica, CA: The Rand Corporation.

Zucker, D. M., Lakatos, E., Webber, L. S., Murray, D. M., McKinlay, S. M., Feldman, H. A., Kelder, S. H., & Nader, P. R. (1995). Statistical design of the Child and Adolescent Trial for Cardiovascular Health (CATCH): Implications of cluster randomization. *Controlled Clinical Trials, 16,* 96–118.

CHAPTER *20*

Planning Community Health Interventions

M. Janice Gilliland and Judith E. Taylor

Introduction

Public health as a discipline came into being in the mid-19th century and soon led to improvements in the prevention of infectious, nutritional, and parasitic diseases, mainly through amelioration in living conditions for the poorer segments of society. Medical treatment also improved during the same period with the development of better training for physicians and scientific discoveries in nutrition, bacteriology, and other basic sciences (Duffy, 1979). These successes helped to bring about what Omran (1980) has termed the *epidemiological transition*. This term was coined to describe the change in patterns of human illness from a time when most morbidity and mortality was caused by infectious and communicable diseases to a period when chronic diseases became the leading causes of deaths. Unfortunately, this change has created new challenges for prevention efforts in that oftentimes chronic disease risk is highly associated with certain lifestyle behaviors that may be difficult to change.

Healthy People 2000 (USDHHS, 1990) highlights the need for more aggressive efforts in disease prevention for persons of all ages and ethnicities. The report also stresses the need for collaboration and partnering among health care affiliates to more effectively address the myriad of health needs apparent in the American population (McKenzie & Smeltzer, 1997; USDHHS, 1990). The need for collaborative health promotion and disease prevention programs is evident when noting that quality of life indicators in the United States have continued to decline over the past decade even though both longevity and health care expenditures have increased (Shultz & Young, 1997). Further evidence can be found in that of the 10 leading causes of death in the

M. Janice Gilliland • Behavioral Medicine Unit, Division of Preventive Medicine, Department of Medicine, School of Medicine, Department of Health Behavior, School of Public Health, UAB Center for Health Promotion, University of Alabama at Birmingham, Birmingham, Alabama 35294.   *Judith E. Taylor* • Mississippi University for Women, Division of Health and Kinesiology, Columbus, Mississippi 39701.

Handbook of Health Promotion and Disease Prevention, edited by Raczynski and DiClemente. Kluwer Academic/Plenum Publishers, New York, 1999.

United States (USDHHS, 1990), all arguably have a behavioral component to disease initiation and/or development.

Health-related behavior is influenced both by individual characteristics such as personality type, beliefs, knowledge, and attitudes and by the external physical and sociological environments within which the behavior occurs. These personal characteristics and external environmental systems may encourage or discourage certain types of health behaviors, and indeed, may operate in opposition to each other. For example, social norms and governmental regulations are bringing increasingly strong pressure against the use of tobacco, although governmental tobacco subsidies continue. Because behavior does not occur in isolation but is embedded within this social, political, economic, and cultural web, programs aimed at bringing about beneficial changes in health behaviors must focus not on individuals alone, but also on altering the system in ways that will support personal efforts at change. Green and Raeburn (1990) discuss the system versus the individual approach for changing behaviors and suggest that the community is the most appropriate focus for health promotion activities.

Multidimensional, community-based interventions have been documented as the most appropriate and feasible method for stimulating health enhancing behavioral modifications (Green & Raeburn, 1990). Blackburn (1997) recommends the communitywide intervention as a "potentially efficient as well as effective" prevention strategy and calls for "primordial prevention" to discourage people, particularly the young, from adopting unhealthy behaviors or lifestyles that contribute to increased risk for many chronic diseases.

Despite widespread agreement of the community as the most appropriate level at which to intervene with health prevention messages, there has been little agreement in what constitutes "community." Community has been defined in numerous ways by social science researchers, but most definitions incorporate some commonality either of geographic location, shared social institutions or interactions, and personal or health characteristics and/or interests that includes more or less homogeneous groups of people who share common goals or purposes (Haglund, Weisbrod, & Bracht, 1990; Jewkes & Murcott, 1996; Minkler, 1990). The community may also be defined by internal strata, with the levels based on biological attributes such as age, gender, or disease status, or on sociological characteristics such as education or income. Regardless of how the community is defined or subdivided, it should be remembered that communities are themselves part of the larger context of the system or society in which they exist, and are thus subject to influence from these outside forces. Nevertheless, defining a study community is a basic requirement to intervention planning in that it permits the definition of a more or less delimited setting in which to implement health-promoting activities that are geared to local needs, strengths and idiosyncrasies.

Green and Kreuter (1991, p. 263) make a distinction between "community interventions" and "interventions in a community." They define community interventions as programs designed to bring about change in most of the total community population. Interventions in the community, in comparison, attempt to bring about changes within a specific subpopulation in the community, often in a particular setting such as a work site or school. Although this distinction is useful, the ultimate purpose of public health disease intervention programs is to reduce the burden of disease and disease risks and improve the quality of life and well-being of individuals, families, and communities, whether in a targeted segment or in the entire population. Thus, as used in this chapter, community-based health interventions (CBIs) are programs designed to focus on healthful changes in either subgroups or localized populations.

Background

With the epidemiological transition (Omran, 1980) in Westernized countries from mortality and morbidity caused primarily by infectious agents spread through person-to-person contact, poor sanitary practices, or contaminated water supplies, to the condition of most illness and death occurring from chronic diseases associated more with environmental assaults, genetic factors, and lifestyle behaviors, the emphasis in public health practice has changed. Intensive public health programs aimed at improving sanitation and nutrition and promoting vaccinations against common infectious diseases, combined with the use of antibiotic therapy after World War II, led to greatly decreased threats to the general population from infectious diseases, resulting in a much improved average life span (Olshansky, Carnes, Rogers, & Smith, 1997). Although infectious diseases are still the major killers in many parts of the world and new diseases or antibiotic-resistant strains of old ones are currently emerging in many areas, the average life span is now increasing also for much of the world's non-Westernized population. Unfortunately, the price paid for increased longevity for most people is the greater importance of certain lifestyle behaviors as threats to health and well-being. To reduce the risk from diseases and conditions associated with lifestyle behaviors, multidimensional CBI are crucial.

The notion of using CBIs to improve the public health is not new. They have been used in the prevention of disease and the promotion of health by public health affiliates since the late 1800s and early 1900s (NHLBI, 1990), but the emphases and strategies have shifted as public health concerns have changed. A number of advancements in the design of community-based educational interventions have evolved over the years, especially since World War II (NHLBI, 1990). Such advancements include greater attention to multi- and interdisciplinary approaches to disease prevention, including an increased utilization of the media and related modalities to plan and broadcast more sophisticated health communication initiatives. The notion of a community intervention has evolved also from being programs imposed on the community by usually well-meaning public health officials to interventions developed with participation from the community to meet locally perceived needs.

A number of community health programs are often cited as classic references for people interested in designing community-based health interventions. Programs initiated in the United States targeting chronic disease prevention include the Stanford Three Community and Five City Project heart disease prevention studies (Schooler, Farquhar, Fortmann, & Flora, 1997); the Minnesota Heart Health Program (MHHP) (Luepker *et al.*, 1996), and the Pawtucket Heart Health Program (PHHP) (Schooler *et al.*, 1997). All of these were longitudinal, community-based clinical trials funded by the National Institutes of Health (NIH). Though many similarities exist among these three studies with regard to design, each intervention focused on a different key issue.

The Stanford Three Community and Five City studies (Schooler *et al.*, 1997) are two of the most important community intervention studies in the United States. Both studies concentrated on the use and role of mass media as a method for decreasing premature death from coronary heart disease (CHD). The Three Community study began in 1972. The communities were assigned to three different experimental conditions: mass media only, mass media plus intensive instruction in selected high-risk community residents, and a comparison community with no intervention. Results indicated significant effects on decreasing rates of smoking, high blood pressure, and cholesterol levels. Significant effects were reported also for a composite measure of

CHD risk reduction (Schooler *et al.*, 1997). The Stanford Five City study was similar. Two cities received a 5-year education program beginning in 1980. The intervention consisted of electronic and print media, small media materials, and direct education and participation in community events; however, 99% of the messages were delivered through either television or print media (Schooler *et al.*, 1997). Significant reductions were found for the total population in smoking and resting pulse rates, blood pressure and cholesterol levels, and CHD risk (Schooler *et al.*, 1997).

The MHHP was a research and demonstration project designed to decrease population rates for CHD and stroke in men and women aged 30 to 74 years by increasing levels of physical activity and reducing smoking, blood pressure, and cholesterol levels (Luepker *et al.*, 1996; Schooler *et al.*, 1997). The intervention was conducted from 1980 to 1990 and was implemented in three matched community pairs. Intervention components included community organization, and both mass media and direct education combined with specific risk factor education and screening. The MHHP focused on broad-based community involvement with message delivery primarily through in-person education and screenings (Schooler *et al.*, 1997). No significant intervention effects were found for either CHD or stroke (Luepker *et al.*, 1996). Nevertheless, population-based surveys showed an increased level of physical activity for both men and women, and a reduction in smoking rates for women (Luepker *et al.*, 1996). Other successes attributable to the intervention were evident in some components of the study, such as school programs and risk factor screenings (Schooler *et al.*, 1997).

The PHHP was implemented in one treatment city (Pawtucket) with a matched comparison city. The project began in 1984 with a 7-year campaign (Schooler *et al.*, 1997). Project components consisted of community organization, educational programs, and print media targeted to individuals, groups, and the community to decrease cardiovascular disease risks through reductions in rates of hypertension, hypercholesteremia, smoking, obesity, and physical inactivity (Schooler *et al.*, 1997). Social learning theory was the primary theoretical basis for the education program (Carleton *et al.*, 1995). The PHHP emphasized the use of volunteers to disseminate heart health promotion messages (NHLBI, 1990; Schooler *et al.*, 1997). Still, 79% of education messages were delivered through newspapers and other print media. Broadcast media were not used to deliver intervention messages in the PHHP. Treatment effects were significant for obesity and lowered CHD risk (Schooler *et al.*, 1997), but no significant differences were found between Pawtucket and the comparison city at 3 years postintervention (Carleton *et al.*, 1995).

As indicated, these large-scale community intervention programs met with varying degrees of success, but all have been landmarks in recent chronic disease CBI studies in the United States. Comparable studies have taken place in other countries with similar results (Schooler *et al.*, 1997).

Planning Community Interventions

The basic idea behind CBIs as currently envisioned is to empower the local community (however it is defined) to change lifestyle behaviors detrimental to health by altering political, social, economic, and environmental structures such that they will promote rather than hinder the changes (Guldan, 1996). CBIs are generally designed to reduce one or more given health or social morbidities and should use the concept of holistic inclusion to ensure "buy-in" by community members, increase avenues for dissemination of intervention components, promote trust between interventionists and consumers, and foster feelings of "ownership" by the community. Ownership and buy-in by the community are important considerations in that health enhancing changes are more likely to be successful and long-lasting when they are part of a community initiative rather than a program imposed from the outside (Thompson & Kinne, 1990). Community ownership also increases the likelihood that the program will be sustained in the community after the initial intervention has been completed and outside funding has ceased. Developing ownership and buy-in for the intervention usually begins with a community organization effort. Bracht and Kingsbury (1990) propose a five-stage community organization process that involves community analysis, design and initiation, implementation, maintenance and consolidation, and dissemination and reassessment of the process. A broad-based community organization is pivotal to the development of support for other components of the intervention.

As noted above, personal health behaviors are a reflection of ingrained personality and psychosocial traits and habits peculiar to the individual, but are woven into a network of social, political, economic, cultural, and other environmental and biological factors that can either promote or discourage changes in personal behaviors (Guldan, 1996). These factors make lifestyle behaviors resistant to change. Bringing about change usually requires a multifaceted assault on many fronts at once, involving multiple "hits" through many different channels before the individual, community or system can make and sustain healthful behavior changes (Flora, Saphir, Schooler, & Rimer, 1997). CBIs usually include multiple components that are designed to improve knowledge, change attitudes and behaviors, and promote health-enhancing skills within the targeted community or one or more subgroups. To be successful, the intervention may require changes in other groups or segments of the community, not just in the people exhibiting the unhealthy behaviors. For example, health care providers may need to be recruited and trained to transmit the message to their patients, or legislation may need to be enacted to promote the desired behavior change (e.g., use of bicycle helmets mandated). Irrespective of the target, program components are ordinarily most successful when delivered in a variety of ways through diverse channels to the intended audience(s).

Regardless of whether the focus is on communicable diseases, chronic diseases, or social morbidities, four factors are fundamental to the development of broad-based multidimensional community health interventions. Knowledge and understanding of these factors, as discussed below, are crucial to developing and implementing a successful CBI.

First Factor: Thorough and Comprehensive Needs Assessment

A thorough and comprehensive needs assessment should be conducted by individuals knowledgeable in community health assessment procedures. Determining the social character of the intended intervention community or target population, coupled with an analysis of educational needs, readiness, and support, serve ultimately to facilitate the design and success of the intervention. When engaging in community assessment, and when implementing and evaluating the intervention, it is important always to be sensitive to the culture, beliefs, and needs of the proposed target population. Also, it is vital to involve community members in the process as much

as possible, partly to ensure a better understanding of the community, but also to garner the local support that is essential to the success of such interventions.

Assessment procedures must include modes that ensure a multidimensional
analysis of the target community. As such, the community assessment should include, for example, data collection to provide information on social, educational, epidemiological, and organizational factors that serve to directly or indirectly influence
health status. Social issues essential to a community assessment include, but are not
limited to, socioeconomic characteristics of the proposed target population and access
to health and other support facilities. A determination of health or other needs as perceived by community members is perhaps the most important part of a needs assessment. Actual patterns of morbidity and premature mortality are identified in the
epidemiological component of the assessment. Having a theoretical framework on
which to base the needs assessment can help to insure that all relevant information is
gathered.

Second Factor: Theoretical Basis or Framework for Guiding Development, Implementation, and Evaluation

Using an appropriate theoretical framework gives structure to the intervention
and increases the likelihood of its success. Knowledge and utilization of a theoretical
framework can facilitate the assessment process as well as guide the development of
subsequent intervention components. It also increases the probability of assessing intrapersonal, interpersonal, institutional, community, and/or public policy factors that
may influence individual and community health morbidity (Glanz, Lewis, & Rimer,
1990; Haglund et al., 1990).

Planning and Analysis Models

There are a number of models that can be used to facilitate the planning, implementation, and evaluation of population-specific community health interventions.
Perhaps the most influential planning model is PRECEDE–PROCEED, developed by Green
and Kreuter (1991). PRECEDE is an acronym that stands for predisposing, reinforcing
and enabling causes in educational diagnosis and evaluation. The PROCEED component
of the model stands for policy, regulatory, organizational constructs in educational
and environmental development. This model is built on a belief in the need to engage
in a multidimensional diagnosis to more effectively determine, categorically, factors
that may influence health status in the community of focus. Use of this model can
guide the interventionist through a multidimensional diagnosis of the population, its
needs, and other factors that may influence health status in both individuals and the
community. Application of the PRECEDE–PROCEED model requires the intervention plan-
ner to evaluate social, educational, and organizational factors that can influence
health status potential. In addition, it helps with negotiating through organizational
structures to access available resources.

Community analysis using the PRECEDE–PROCEED model progresses through a series of stages or phases (Green & Kreuter, 1991). The original model (PRECEDE only)
was composed of phases 1–6. Phase 1 guides the user through social diagnosis or assessment of quality of life issues important to the community. The purpose of phase 1
is to determine a problem or problems of concern to members of the target commu-

nity. Epidemiological diagnosis of the community takes place in phase 2. This phase is concerned with identifying health issues that contribute to the problems disclosed in phase 1, not merely with collecting health statistics. The third phase examines behavioral and environmental factors and how they relate to the problems revealed in the epidemiological diagnosis phase. At this point, the community problem that is seen as most crucial and that is amenable to change is selected as the focus of the intervention. Phase 4 is concerned with the educational and organizational diagnosis, particularly with ascertaining the predisposing, reinforcing, and enabling factors that may affect behavior. Understanding these factors is crucial to developing a good, broad-based community intervention. Phase 5 deals with administration and organizational issues, and is concerned with developing the resources and support needed to implement the intervention. Phase 6 is the implementation stage, which should go smoothly if phases 1–5 have been conducted properly. Program evaluation takes place in phases 7–9, with the stages corresponding to process, impact, and outcome evaluation. Although somewhat complex, using the PRECEDE–PROCEED model ensures a thorough analysis of the community, its needs, problems, and assets, which is essential to a successful community intervention.

Another model that is often used to facilitate the development of appropriate interventions is PATCH, developed by the United States Public Health Service in 1981. PATCH is an acronym that stands for planned approach to community health, and is designed to provide a structured approach to developing interventions that are truly community programs, adapted to local characteristics and needs. The model has three major components: (1) community mobilization, (2) community diagnosis, and (3) community intervention. PATCH stresses horizontal and vertical collaborations among local, state, and federal agencies to provide the resources and support needed to implement the local community intervention (Kreuter, 1992).

MATCH (multilevel approach to community health) is a more recently originated intervention model that was developed by Simons-Morton and associates in 1988 (Simons-Morton, Greene, & Gootlieh, 1995). MATCH is similar to PATCH in that both are concerned with involving the local community in planning and implementation of community health interventions. Both PATCH and MATCH provide for a structured assessment of various factors that may influence the health status of individuals and communities alike. Each model correlates, to some degree, with PRECEDE–PROCEED. However, PRECEDE–PROCEED focuses predominantly on an extensive needs assessment, while MATCH stresses implementation of an intervention, and the PATCH model emphasizes collaboration between the community and local, state, and federal personnel (Kreuter, 1992; Simons-Morton *et al.*, 1995).

Behavioral Change Models

In addition to the planning models mentioned above, a number of theories of behavior change have been used to plan and structure CBIs. Behavioral change theories attempt to explain why and how people change from one type of behavior (usually seen as detrimental to health) to another (considered to promote health). The behavioral change models most commonly used to explain or bring about changes in individual health behaviors include the health belief model (Becker, 1974; Rosenstock, 1990), often used to predict and explain why people do or do not engage in preventive health behaviors (Janz & Becker, 1984); Bandura's (1986) social cognitive theory, which emphasizes the potential role of the environment on behavior and behavioral change; self-regulatory theory, which attempts to explain how people perceive and cope with illness episodes (Leventhal, 1970); the theory of reasoned action (Ajzen and Fishbein, 1980; Fishbein & Ajzen, 1975), which stresses the importance of attitude and the influence of a social environment on promoting behavioral change; and finally, the transtheoretical model (Prochaska, DiClemente, & Norcross 1992), which suggests that behavior change can be brought about by targeting the intervention to the individual's placement in a series of stages along which change progresses. These models are detailed in Chapter 3, and therefore, will not be discussed further here.

Implementation Models

Implementation models are used to structure and execute the intervention. Methods and techniques typically used in behavior change often focus on one-on-one counseling, or small-group intervention sessions. Although effective to a greater or lesser degree, these methods would be prohibitively expensive if applied to an entire community; hence other strategies are necessary when implementing community intervention programs. The need here is to reach a wide audience, either the general population or one or more specific target groups. Messages for a broad, diverse audience are by definition less personalized and easier for the individual to ignore. Thus, reaching a community audience requires that the message be repeated through as many channels and as often and in as many different forms as possible. Type of channel delivery and diversity of message channels is vital to reaching different audience segments. Flora and colleagues (1997) present research that suggests that print media channels produce higher-involvement cognitive processing of information than television and demonstrate larger increases in knowledge and greater behavior changes. Nevertheless, not all individuals will respond to print material either because of problems with reading and interpretation, owing to literacy or vision problems, lack of exposure, or other reasons. Therefore, it is essential to know the sociodemographic profile of the target community or group for whom the message is intended in order to design a message or messages that are pertinent and effective for a particular audience and to broadcast the message through appropriate channels in as many different forms as possible.

Two theoretical models have been used predominately to guide the implementation of CBIs: social marketing theory and diffusion of innovation. Social marketing is a strategy borrowed from business marketing theory and is a process by which specifically designed programs, messages, or ideas are promoted to a particular audience, using advertising techniques that were originally designed to sell consumer goods. Targeted messages, formulated to bring about behavioral change, are disseminated throughout a selected site and via a given mode(s) to increase their probability of acceptance by the predetermined target population (Lefebvre & Flora, 1988). Use of social marketing strategies enables greater penetration and promotion of a message to various segments of a community. The success of social marketing efforts depends on the consumer's interpretation of the message and his or her belief that the message is beneficial. Therefore, the message content, clarity, presentation, and delivery channels are vitally important and must be thoroughly researched as to appropriateness and effectiveness for the target population or group. As can be seen, knowledge of optimal communication and distribution strategies is essential for successful social marketing.

Diffusion of innovation attempts to explain how a change or innovation is disseminated throughout cultural or social systems (Oldenburg, Hardcastle & Kok, 1997; Rogers, 1983). The innovation may be an idea, a product, or a new way of doing things. It can also include ideas about appropriate health behaviors. Application of this theory centers around the distribution of a message or innovation to one or more groups or subgroups in a community over a selected and predetermined period of time. The theory suggests that change is adopted by a process of awareness of the innovation, persuasion of the benefits of the making the change, making the decision and implementing change, and finally, confirmation that the innovation is beneficial (Rogers, 1983). The diffusion process can be enhanced by identifying specific interventions, channels, methods, and modalities likely to reach the greatest proportion of the target community (Bracht, 1990). The major criticism of classical diffusion theory is that it fails to view adoption of changes as only one of many steps whereby the behavior is adopted and maintained (Orlandi, Landers, Weston, & Haley, 1990). To be successful, CBIs usually must make more than a temporary change in the targeted health behavior; the change must be permanent. Nevertheless, diffusion of innovation and social marketing techniques working together can optimize success of the intervention by ensuring that it addresses the target group's needs and barriers to change.

Third Factor: Evaluation Must Be Both a Pre- and a Corequisite Component

Evaluation must be both a pre- and a corequisite component of the community assessment process and the planning, promotion, and implementation of the intervention. Evaluation, broadly viewed, begins with the inception of an idea and continues throughout the needs assessment process as well as the development and implementation phases of the intervention. Evaluation is often subdivided into several types, each one appropriate to a certain stage of the intervention, from planning to ending activities. Freeman and Rossi (1993, p. 35) divide what they call a "comprehensive evaluation" into three major phases. The first phase is concerned with program conceptualization and design. This type of evaluation is also referred to as formative evaluation (Green & Kreuter, 1991). Possible questions addressed by formative evaluation is the appropriateness of the program materials or even whether the program should be implemented at all (Pirie, 1990). Freeman and Rossi's (1993) second phase consists of the ongoing monitoring of the program. Often referred to as process evaluation, this phase determines whether the program is being implemented as planned and if it is reaching the target audience (Pirie, 1990). The last evaluation phase is concerned with assessing program effectiveness and efficiency (Freeman & Rossi, 1993) and determines whether the program had the planned effect. Some researchers divide this part of the evaluation into impact and outcome (Green & Kreuter, 1991). Impact evaluation is concerned with measuring whether the program met intermediate objectives for behavioral and environmental changes; outcome evaluation is the assessment of the program effects on ultimate objectives; meaning, was it effective in bringing about actual changes in health or quality of life (Green & Kreuter, 1991).

Evaluations may be either quantitative or qualitative, although some combination of the two is usually desirable. Quantitative data can give a broad overview of a project, but may lack the depth required to interpret the intervention results, particularly if they are unexpected. These data are limited by the nature of the information gathering process, which means that responses are restricted to specific categories specified beforehand by the interventionist, and reduces the information collected to numerical form. Quantitative data are generally less time consuming to collect and allow information to be gathered on large numbers of variables and subjects. In addition, analysis is usually faster and the results can be more easily compared with those from other quantitative studies. Qualitative data are usually limited in scope or number of individuals responding and analysis can be time consuming. However, these data can provide a richness of detail not found in quantitative data, and may reveal unexpected findings because the responses to questions have not been preordained. Qualitative evaluations are especially useful when developing the intervention and for helping to interpret and explain unexpected findings. A number of good references are available for further study of evaluation including texts by Cook and Campbell (1979), Windsor, Baranowski, Clark, and Cutter (1984), Green and Kreuter (1991), and Freeman and Rossi (1993), all of which focus on quantitative evaluation. Qualitative evaluation texts include those by Miles and Huberman (1994), Patton (1990), and Stake (1995), among others. In addition, Shaddish, Cook, and Leviton (1991) provide an excellent background on influential practitioners and ideas in the field of program evaluation.

Evaluation efforts benefit the stakeholders, interventionists, and the intervention. A good evaluation enables consumers to see health needs that should be addressed, resources needed to support or facilitate the implementation, ways to meet program goals and objectives, and after implementation, whether those goals and objectives were actually met. It should be remembered that the most important component in a successful evaluation consists of asking the right questions. No matter how good the technical components of the evaluation (e.g., questionnaire design, data collection, and analysis), it is futile if the questions to which answers are being sought are inappropriate to collect the information necessary to make the assessment. A good, comprehensive program evaluation may be the single-most important component to ensuring a successful CBI. It can uncover problems early enough to make corrections in the intervention, and can assess the actual effect of the program on the various components and target groups. Although a good evaluation alone cannot insure a successful CBI, it can allow the interventionists and other stakeholders to determine whether the program worked as planned, and if not, why. Therefore, it is important to have a person knowledgeable in program evaluation involved in the program from inception to finish.

Fourth Factor: A Variety of Educational Methodologies Should Be Utilized

A variety of educational methodologies should be used to increase the probability that the intervention messages can reach and be understood by members of the target population. A single, well-defined goal should govern the educational component of the intervention. However, a variety of short- and long-term objectives that target cognitive, affective, and psychomotor domains related to the overall goal should be used also (Dignan & Carr, 1992). It is key to the success of the intervention that specific, measurable objectives be written that are designed to promote knowledge, create personal identification with a given health promotion/risk reduction message, and ultimately alter behaviors that may negatively affect health status.

Again, it is crucial to the potential success of a behavioral modification campaign that members from the intended target population be involved in the planning process as early and completely as possible. For example, using positive role models to convey risk reduction/health promotion messages and identifying other key community figures to collaborate with the delivery of the intervention can promote a sense of empowerment among target consumers. Messages should be relayed to the target population by diverse spokespersons, including blue- and white-collar workers and those of various ethnic backgrounds if appropriate for the targeted audience(s). The purveyors of the message should be people who are credible and respected by members of the target population, but also should be people with whom they can identify. To be most effective, messages planned for delivery during the intervention should be evaluated by public health educators, other health professionals, marketing experts, and community members, as deemed appropriate. Each message should also be pilot tested on a group as similar as possible to that of the intended target population.

An assessment of the community's media channels should have been conducted as part of the intervention planning process. A comprehensive community assessment will provide information on the number, types, and avenues for generating various media messages. Sample channels that may be used to disseminate health-enhancing messages include, but are not limited to, the following: media outlets such as radio, television, newspapers, and newsletters, and community channels such as civic organizations, work sites, health clinics and agencies, churches, schools, and social service agencies. The sequence of the messages may be important also (Flora *et al.*, 1997). Sequencing can build on previous messages to move people along to acquiring new knowledge and establishing new behavior patterns.

Knowledge of potential media channels is necessary to disseminate the message throughout all segments of the target community. No matter how narrowly defined the community may be for any one intervention, it can be further defined or divided into subgroups, based on different characteristics or refinements of the original distinguishing features. For example, if the intervention is designed to bring about behavior changes in an African-American community, further subdividing could be done on age groupings, gender, or educational levels, all of which may affect how the message is received or understood. To reach all subgroups of the target population, expert opinion should be sought to ensure that messages are delivered through the optimal mode(s) and with the best possible timing and sequencing.

Broad-based multidimensional CBIs can also be designed to involve and ultimately to be implemented in various settings, including clinics, work sites, churches, or schools. Interventionists should ideally target, as possible, occupational and/or community sites that may enhance the dissemination of intervention messages. A prerequisite to the implementation of a clinical health education/health promotion intervention effort involves gaining the support of and preparing via training a variety of allied health professionals. For example, a clinical intervention designed to decrease time to pharmacological treatment of acute myocardial infarction should involve collaboration among emergency department personnel, primary care physicians, cardiologists, cardiac rehabilitation personnel, and emergency medical service providers. Regardless of the topic addressed, education departments in local hospitals should be recruited and involved in the community intervention efforts if at all possible. Other hospital personnel should be involved also, when appropriate, to assist with disseminating a broad-based community intervention. Collateral, nonclinical employees can be important members of the intervention team. These people may ultimately serve as major advocates for the intervention in both the hospital and the subcommunities in which they reside.

Limitations to Community-Based Interventions

Although CBIs have shown some success in bringing about behavioral changes, there are a number of limitations involved. Some of these limitations are a result of the process itself and some from the way in which such programs have been implemented. Guldan (1996), in a recent article, discusses nine obstacles to community health promotion programs. These obstacles can be grouped into three general categories. The first category of obstacles is related to impediments in the health care system. These are obstacles caused by the lack of training that physicians and most other health care professionals receive in health promotion, primarily because the medical model for health care still focuses on curing the individual, not promoting community health. A second category of limitations is composed of deficiencies in leadership, including the absence of a clear statement regarding the importance of social and community health issues and solutions, and low political salience that results in poor funding for health promotion activities. Most obstacles, however, are a function of problems inherent in the way in which interventions have been implemented. These include failure to engage the community or target groups in the intevention, inability to maintain interest in the program and health promotion activities over time, and poor evaluations that fail to show the relevance of the interventions. According to Guldan (1996), these obstacles must be overcome to make progress toward improved health for the entire community.

Another limitation is that CBIs can be expensive and may be cost-effective only if the behavioral risk factor(s) and the disease(s) that are the focus of the intervention are serious and relatively prevalent in the community. For example, approximately 25% of the US population are current cigarette smokers (American Cancer Society, 1998), and smoking is a strong risk factor for cardiovascular diseases and several types of cancer. Reducing smoking rates, even by a small percentage, could have substantial repercussions on rates of cardiovascular disease and cancer with subsequent reductions in associated morbidity and mortality.

Summary and Conclusions

Public health prevention concerns in the 20th century have shifted from a focus on infectious diseases to an emphasis on chronic diseases such as coronary or vascular diseases and cancer. These diseases are the major causes of morbidity and mortality in the late 20th century, and all are strongly influenced by lifestyle behaviors. This change in public health concerns has required alterations in intervention methods. The public health can no longer be protected by increasing vaccination rates or ensuring sanitary water supplies. Although CBIs have been utilized in a variety of settings throughout much of our nation's history, only recently have they been used to address concerns at a community level health that result from individual lifestyle behaviors.

CBIs have emerged in the United States and other countries as a useful strategy to reduce overall disease morbidity and mortality and to improve the quality of health in a community by changing individual risk factors through behavioral modification. The fundamental premise or rationale for using multidimensional CBIs is that disease etiology stems from multiple sources, and thus requires many different approaches to prevention. For example, a given morbidity may be traced to family social or genetic history, personal behaviors, external environmental factors, or more often a combination of all three. In other words, a variety of personal and /or social norms may affect one's health status or quality of life.

Large-sample US community intervention programs include the Stanford Three Communities Study and Five City Projects, the Minnesota Heart Health Project, and the Pawtucket Healthy Heart Program (Schooler *et al.*, 1997). Community intervention studies have produced mixed results, possibly because of methodological and other limitations in most of the ones conducted to date. Nevertheless, CBIs have shown successes in changing some detrimental lifestyle behaviors. The success of CBIs is dependent on reaching individuals and helping them to make permanent changes in behaviors. This can be best accomplished by broad-based interventions that are supported and embraced by the target community.

The four essential elements for conducting good CBIs are: (1) a comprehensive needs assessment; (2) use of a theoretical framework to design the intervention; (3) extensive and ongoing program evaluation; and (4) multiple educational strategies to disseminate the message. Attention to these four basic elements will improve the odds on implementing a successful intervention. Success is also likely to be dependent on how much community involvement the intervention generates. No intervention can be successful without being accepted by the audience for which it was designed. People often want to make health enhancing changes in lifestyle behaviors, but find it difficult to change on their own. Community-based interventions are one way of providing people with the knowledge, tools, and justification for making the change.

References

Ajzen, I., & Fishbein, M. (1980). *Understanding attitudes and predicting social behavior*. Englewood Cliffs, NJ: Prentice-Hall.

American Cancer Society. (1998). *Cancer facts and figures—1998*. Atlanta, GA: Author.

Bandura, A. (1986). *Social foundations of thought and action: A social cognitive theory*. Englewood Cliffs, NJ: Prentice-Hall.

Becker, M. H. (1974). The health belief model and personal health behavior. *Health Education Monographs, 2*, 324–473.

Blackburn, H. (1997). Epidemiological basis of a community strategy for the prevention of cardiopulmonary diseases. *Annals of Epidemiology, 7* (Suppl. 7), S8–S13.

Bracht, N. (1990). *Health promotion at the community level*. Newbury Park, CA: Sage.

Bracht, N., & Kingsbury, L. (1990). Community organization principles in health promotion: A five-stage model. In N. Bracht (Ed.), *Health promotion at the community level* (pp. 66–88). Newbury Park, CA: Sage.

Carleton, R. A., Lasater, T. M., Assaf, A. R., Feldman, H. A., McKinlay, S., & The Pawtucket Heart Health Program Writing Group. (1995). The Pawtucket Heart Health Program: Community changes in cardiovascular risk factors and projected disease risk. *American Journal of Public Health, 85*(6), 777–785.

Cook, T. D., & Campbell, D. T. (1979). *Quasi-experimentation design and analysis issues for field settings*. Boston: Houghton Mifflin.

Dignan, M. B., & Carr, P. A. (1992). *Program planning for health education and promotion* (2nd ed.). Philadelphia: Lea and Febiger.

Duffy, J. (1979). *The healers: A history of American medicine.* Urbana: University of Illinois Press.

Fishbein, M., & Ajzen, I. (1975). *Belief, attitude, and behavior: An introduction to theory and research.* Reading, MA: Addison-Wesley.

Flora, J. A., Saphir, M. N., Schooler, C., & Rimal, R. N. (1997). Toward a framework for intervention channels: Reach, involvement, and impact. *Annals of Epidemiology, 7* (Suppl. 7), S104–S112.

Freeman, P. H., & Rossi, H. E. (1993). *Evaluation: A systematic approach* (5th ed.). Newbury Park, CA: Sage.

Glanz, R., Lewis, B., Rimer, B. (1990). *Health behavior and health education—Theory, research, and practice.* San Francisco: Jossey-Bass.

Green, L. W., & Kreuter, M. W. (1991). *Health promotion planning: An educational and environmental approach* (2nd ed.). Palo Alto, CA: Mayfield.

Green, L. W., & Raeburn, J. (1990). Contemporary development in health promotion: Definitions and challenges. In N. Bracht. (Ed.), *Health promotion at the community level* (pp. 29–34). Newbury Park, CA: Sage.

Guldan, G. S. (1996). Obstacles to community health promotion. *Social Science and Medicine, 43* (5), 689–695.

Haglund, B., Weisbrod, R. R., & Bracht, N. (1990). Assessing the community: Its services, needs, leadership, and readiness. In N. Bracht. (Ed.), *Health promotion at the community level* (pp. 91–108). Newbury Park, CA: Sage.

Janz, N. K., & Becker, M. H. (1984). The health belief model: A decade later. *Health Education Quarterly, 11,* 1–47.

Jewkes, R., & Murcott, A. (1996). Meanings of community. *Social Science and Medicine, 43* (4), 555–563.

Kreuter, M. W. (1992). PATCH: Its origin, basic concepts, and links to contemporary public health policy. *Journal of Health Education, 23* (3), 135–139.

Lefebvre, R. C., & Flora, J. A. (1988). Social marketing and public health intervention. *Health Education Quarterly, 15,* 299–315.

Leventhal, H. (1970). Findings and theory in the study of fear communications. *Advances in Experimental Social Psychology, 5,* 119–186.

Luepker, R. V., Råstam, L., Hannan, P. J., Murray, D. M., Gray, C., Baker, W. L., Crow, R., Jacobs, Jr. D. R., Pirie, P. L., Mascioli, S. R., Mittelmark, M. B., & Blackburn, H. (1996). Community education for cardiovascular disease prevention. *American Journal of Epidemiology, 144* (4), 351–362.

McKenzie, J. F., & Smeltzer, J. L. (1997). *Planning, implementing, and evaluating health promotion programs: A primer* (2nd ed.). Boston: Allyn and Bacon.

Miles, M. B., & Huberman, A. M. (1994). *Qualitative data analysis.* Thousand Oaks, CA: Sage.

Minkler, M. (1990). Improving health through community organization. In K. Glanz, F. M. Lewis, & B. K. Rimer. (Eds.), *Health Behavior and Health Education* (pp. 257–287). San Francisco: Jossey-Bass.

National Heart, Lung, & Blood Institute (NHLBI). (1990). Three community programs change heart health across the nation. *INFOMEMO.* Bethesda, MD: DHAS/NIH.

Oldenburg, B., Hardcastle, D. M., & Kok, G. (1997). Diffusion of Innovations. In K. Glanz, F. M. Lewis, & B. K. Rimer (Eds.), *Health behavior and health education theory, research, and practice* (2nd ed., pp 270–276). San Francisco: Jossey-Bass.

Olshansky, S. J., Carnes, B., Rogers, R. G., & Smith, L. (1997). Infectious diseases—New and ancient threats to world health. *Population Bulletin, 52*(2), 2–52.

Omran, A. R. (1980). Epidemiologic transition in the United States: The health factor in population change. *Population Bulletin, 32*(2), 1–45 (updated report).

Orlandi, M. A., Landers, C., Weston, R., & Haley, N. (1990). Diffusion of health promotion innovations. In K. Glanz, F. M. Lewis, & B. K. Rimer (Eds.), *Health behavior and health education* (pp. 288–313). San Francisco: Jossey-Bass.

Patton, M. Q. (1990). *Qualitative evaluation and research methods* (2nd ed.). Newbury Park, CA: Sage.

Pirie, P. L. (1990). Evaluating health promotion programs: Basic questions and approaches. In N. Bracht (Ed.), *Health promotion at the community level* (pp. 201–208). Newbury Park, CA: Sage.

Prochaska, J. O., DiClemente, C. C., & Norcross, K. C. (1992). In search of how people change. Applications to addictive behaviors. *American Psychologist, 47* (9), 1102–1114.

Rogers, E. M. (1983). *Diffusion of innovations* (3rd ed.). New York: Free Press.

Rosenstock, I. M. (1990). The health belief model: Explaining health behavior through expectancies. In K. Glanz, F. M. Lewis, & B. K. Rimer (Eds.), *Health behavior and health education* (pp. 39–62). San Francisco: Jossey-Bass.

Schooler, C., Farquhar, J. W., Fortmann, S. P., & Flora, J. A. (1997). Synthesis of findings and issues from community prevention trials. *Annals of Epidemiology* (Suppl. 7), S54–S68.

Shaddish, W. R., Jr., Cook, T. R., & Leviton, L. C. (1991). *Foundations of program evaluation*. Newbury Park, CA: Sage.

Shultz, H. A., & Young, K. M. (1997). *Health care USA: Understanding its organization and delivery*. Gaithersburg, MD: Aspen Publishers.

Simons-Morton, B. G., Greene, W. H., & Gootlieh, N. H. (1995). *Introduction to health education and health promotion* (2nd ed.). Prospect Heights, IL: Waveland Press.

Stake, R. E. (1995). *The art of case study research*. Thousand Oaks, CA: Sage .

Thompson, B., & Kinne, S. (1990). Social change theory: Applications to community health. In N. Bracht (Ed.), *Health promotion at the community level* (pp. 45–65). Newbury Park: Sage.

US Department of Health and Human Services (USDHHS). (1990). *Healthy people 2000*. (DHHS Publication No. PHS 91-50212). Washington, DC: US Government Printing Office.

Windsor, R., Baranowski, T., Clark, N., & Cutter, G. (1984). *Evaluation of health promotion and evaluation programs*. Palo Alto, CA: Mayfield Publishing.

CHAPTER 21

Health Promotion in Health Care Settings

Molly Engle and Polly P. Kratt

Introduction

Health care settings appear to be attractive sites for health promotion activities with patients. Providers and staff in these settings see a high volume of individuals, many of whom are at higher risk for disease or disability. Patients are also frequently seen on a recurrent basis, which provides opportunities for monitoring and reinforcing behavior modification. Patients also traditionally have given their provider essentially absolute authority over their health care so that recommendations from providers are a strong motivation for attempting behavior change. However, it is often necessary to intervene in health care settings in order to persuade and educate providers and staff to deliver prevention messages. Such interventions must disseminate health promotion information as well as proactively assist providers in changing professional practice patterns to include health promotion activities.

In this chapter we will describe the variety of health care settings, the challenges of implementing interventions in such settings, strategies for successful dissemination and implementation, and examples of interventions implemented in such settings.

Health Care Settings

Health care settings include clinics, physician offices, hospitals, and any other location where health care providers interact with patients. Clinic sites are either inpatient or outpatient, private, or community-based. Physician offices may remain private practice or, increasingly, be involved with managed care or health maintenance

Molly Engle • Department of Public Health, College of Health and Human Performance, Oregon State University, and Oregon State Extension Service, Corvallis, Oregon 97331.   *Polly P. Kratt* • Behavioral Medicine Unit, Division of Preventive Medicine, School of Medicine, UAB Center for Health Promotion, University of Alabama at Birmingham, Birmingham, Alabama 35294.

Handbook of Health Promotion and Disease Prevention, edited by Raczynski and DiClemente. Kluwer Academic/Plenum Publishers, New York, 1999.

organizations. One recent trend for physician offices is the merging of individual practices into a large group practice and the resulting group developing a clinic of specialized care. Hospitals capitalize on the critical mass of consumers and have developed extensive patient and in-service education departments and programs. In urban areas these sites are usually staffed by physicians and support staff. However, in rural and underserved areas, nurse practitioners and physician assistants are often the only staff and provide the primary care to the consumer. Nurse practitioners are also the primary care provider in schools. Home health care is provided by nurse specialists or home health care specialists working out of public health departments, hospitals, or large clinics. Providers and staff at each of these sites have opportunities to address prevention activities with patients. Each type of site also presents specific challenges to interventionists attempting to establish, enhance, and/or promote health promotion activities at that site.

Challenges of Implementing Interventions

While few, if any, would question providers' intentions to provide the best care and best advice for their patients, the difficulties faced by providers to remain current with the literature and incorporate changes in information, guidelines, and techniques into practice patterns have been amply acknowledged in the literature (Bass & Elford, 1988; Lewis, 1988; Oxman, Thomson, Davis, & Haynes, 1995; Williams, Eckert, Epstein, Mourad, & Helmick, 1994). Barriers to incorporating prevention activities into practice patterns comprise challenges to the interventionist. The challenges are classified into two broad areas: challenges related to existing professional preparation and practice activities and challenges of dissemination methodology.

Challenges in Professional Preparation and Practice Activities

Although providers may be a logical choice for a health promotion channel, providers have been somewhat less than enthusiastic about dispensing health promotion messages to their patients. Prevention activities do not follow the medical model and were not included in medical school curricula until the early 1990s (Glanz & Gilboy, 1992; Phillips, Rubeck, Hathaway, Becker, & Boehlecke, 1993; Scott & Neighbor, 1985). The science of prevention and considerations of the impact of lifestyle on health are relatively new in the literature. Prevention guidelines have only recently become available and are still not available for all problems or diagnosis groups. They are also not without controversy. For example, the age at which women should begin having an annual mammogram as well as the age at which women should stop having mammograms are not universally agreed upon (Leitch, 1995; Zyzanski et al., 1994).

The type of practice influences the amount of health promotion activity with primary care providers, such as family practice physicians, obstetricians, and internists, being more likely to offer prevention guidance than the more specialized providers (Davis, 1994). More prevention activities tend to occur in primary care settings (such as clinics and offices) rather than tertiary care settings (such as hospitals). In general, physicians engage in health promotion messages in varying degrees depending on the risk factor behavior addressed and the provider's personal health promotion habits.

For example, internists who are physically active are more likely to counsel on the benefits of physical activity; however, certain behaviors, such as wearing seat belts in automobiles, are rarely addressed by any providers (Schwartz *et al.*, 1991).

Prescribing tests or treatments not covered by insurance deters providers from using the natural authority inherent in the profession from recommending them. Although some preventive measures, such as cancer screening by Pap tests and mammograms, are now covered by many insurance plans, physician visits for preventive purposes are typically not reimbursable by either public or private insurance. Physicians' and other care providers' inconsistent prescribing patterns for preventive measures are likely to continue until preventive measures are routinely reimbursed by third-party payers.

For many health promotion topics, no natural triggers exist in office practice to cue the provider to practice prevention activities. Occasional smoking or alcohol binges by a patient may not be known or obvious to the provider. Physicians appear to be uncomfortable with dispensing advice on lifestyle behavior change. Physicians express the attitude that it is important to intervene with smokers, yet most believe they are not effective with the attempts they make (Glynn, 1988; Wechsler, Levine, Idelson, Rohman, & Taylor, 1983; Wells, Lewis, Leake, & Ware, 1984). Limited provider compliance with mammography screening guidelines has been reported to exist because of the physician's lack of confidence in their ability to persuade patients to be screened and in their perceptions of patients' fear of the tests, fear of cancer, concerns over cost, or simply lack of interest (Rimer *et al.*, 1990; Weinberger *et al.*, 1991). Regardless of the intent to furnish prevention guidelines to the consumer, having adequate time and energy to address lifestyle behaviors will be difficult for most providers.

Challenges of Dissemination Methodology

Dissemination of research findings and medical information has been traditionally viewed as continuing medical education (CME), and often is limited to pharmaceutical marketing, literary/research journals, and/or conferences. These CME offerings are rarely based on the results of educational needs assessments that reflect the physician's perspective and the context of physician-expressed needs. Rather, they are often based on perceived needs, and the evidence from the literature suggests that the impact on practice patterns is low. For example, these traditional didactic approaches focus on knowledge, with little or no skill or performance base attached. This was supported by Ashbaugh and McKean (1976), who found that 94% of deficiencies in patient care were performance based, while the remaining 6% resulted from lack of knowledge. Davis, Thomson, Oxman, and Haynes (1992) stated that didactic CME delivery methods have little impact on improving professional practice, and that objective determination of practice and/or learning needs is a necessary prerequisite for effective education.

Strategies for Successful Dissemination

The difficulties of changing practice patterns in health care settings have spawned research efforts into how providers change (Fox, Mazmanian, & Putnam, 1989; Greco & Eisenberg, 1993) and to determine methods that successfully and efficiently assist the provider in modifying behavior to be proactive in promoting health with patients (Davis *et al.*, 1992, 1995; Oxman *et al.*, 1995). A summary of findings that appear to be effective for health promotion applications are described in the following classifications of design considerations and implementation considerations.

Design Considerations

Enhance CME Offerings

Although the traditional CME has limited dissemination outcomes, Davis *et al.* (1992) expanded the definition of CME to include all ways by which physician learning and clinical practice may be altered by educational or persuasive means, including academic detailing, opinion leaders, audit with feedback, chart review or chart-stimulated recall, and reminders. Their review of literature investigating the effectiveness of educational strategies designed to change physician performance and health care outcomes indicated that physician performance, and to a lesser extent health care outcomes, may be altered by many of the CME interventions. The most promising such CME interventions included those that used practice-enabling strategies [such as an individual in the practice who facilitates behavior change (an office facilitator) or patient educational materials/methods], or reinforcing methods (such as reminders) with disseminating strategies. If an intervention included an opinion leader (a recognized professional peer whose opinion is valued), peers were able to observe application of an intervention in an environment conducive to adoption. Techniques often mentioned as effective in changing provider practice include opinion leaders (Lomas *et al.*, 1991; Stross & Bole, 1980; Stross, Hiss, Watts, Davis, & Mac-Donald, 1983), academic detailing (Daly *et al.*, 1993), and chart reviews (Everett, DeBlois, Chang, & Holets, 1983; Martin, Wolf, Thibodeau, Dzau, & Braunwald, 1980; Meyer, Van Kooten, Marsh, & Prochazka, 1991). One example of excellent patient educational materials for dissemination is the catalogue, *Healthy Moms, Healthy Babies, Healthy Families: Helping your Patients Quit Smoking* (Winders, Raczynski, Gallagher, Westfall, & Gerald, 1997), which, following evaluation of the materials available, selected and published an annotated sample from which the provider may choose.

Davis *et al.* (1995) attempted to discover components consistent with successful and not successful interventions. Expanding on Davis and colleagues (1992), Davis and colleagues (1995) concluded that a combination of predisposing, enabling, and reinforcing strategies leads to greater success in promoting behavior change among physicians. Key to success with these three strategies is the focus on both knowledge and skill. Predisposing strategies (such as physician performance, health care, or patient outcomes) were less apt to result in performance change and even less likely to influence health care outcomes when used alone. Enabling strategies (like patient education and computerized practice-based information) work better in tandem with one of the other two strategies. Reinforcing strategies (such as feedback and reminders) appear to overcome many of the logistical and sociological barriers to change, yet are not sufficient to ensure change. However, when all strategies are used in combination, the probability of behavior change enduring increases.

An apparent relationship between the intensity of the intervention and the degree of outcome change was reported by Davis (1994). In studies using only predisposing activities, the researchers reported negative or inconclusive results. In studies using a combination of enabling and/or reinforcing activities, researchers reported positive results. Combinations of successful strategies included patient education materials used with academic detail visits, other printed material, and/or health status questionnaires or interviews. Lomas *et al.* (1991) reported that the use of specific practice protocols used with printed materials and workshops changed physician performance in family practice, as did computer-generated information in two studies by Tierney, McDonald, Hui, and Martin (1988) and Tierney, Miller, and McDonald (1990). Another example includes feedback and/or reminders coupled with didactic presentations, workshops, academic detail visits, and/or printed materials. Combining workshops, patient education materials, other printed materials, and reminders has also been effective (Davis *et al.*, 1992).

Kottke, Battista, DeFriese, and Brekke (1988) conducted a meta-analysis investigating 108 interventions in 39 controlled smoking cessation trials to discover attributes that predicted success. They concluded that the most effective interventions employed more than one modality for initiating abstinence, and involved both physicians and other health professionals in individualized face-to-face effort providing multiple messages over the longest period of time. This combination of factors proved successful 12 months after the intervention, although not to the degree reported after 6 months.

Incorporate Providers In Dissemination Research

Research that seeks to change physician behavior tends to be a better product and more applicable to incorporation into physician practices if the research occurs in a practice setting and utilizes provider recommendations. However, recruiting providers to participate in a behavior changing activity may be difficult (Borgiel *et al.*, 1989; Dietrich *et al.*, 1990; Green, Niebauer, Miller, & Lutz, 1991; Kottke *et al.*, 1990; Selby, Riportella-Muller, Sorenson, Quade, & Luchok, 1992; Taylor, 1992; Tierney, Hui, & McDonald, 1986; Trynor *et al.*, 1993; Ward, 1994). Rokstad's and Fugelli's (1993) model for successful recruitment and participation in multipractice studies employed the following activities to assure success: (1) multiple personal visits by a project leader that fostered an equal relationship between the university-based researchers and the practitioners; (2) tailoring study procedures to practice characteristics and routines; and (3) accurately estimating practice work load to prevent attrition.

Other factors to which they attributed success included using a reminder system, encouraging continuous contact with the study participants, a personal reward system providing feedback and serving as an effective incentive, and engaging the entire practice staff in study decisions. Rokstad and Fugelli concluded that this combination could be used successfully and would consistently result in multisite, practice-based research with few problems in recruiting, participation, compliance, or attrition. The reasons reported by Nazarian, Maiman, and Becker (1989) for success in recruiting 90 physicians from a physician population of 97 supported the Rokstad and Fugelli findings. Nazarian and colleagues (1989) also reported that the value in minimizing the participation requirements for the physician and the patient, identifying a liaison physician who facilitated communication between the investigators and the practitioners, and establishing a formal, ongoing relationship between the sponsoring academic institution and the community physicians appeared to contribute to success of their study.

The requirement for study guidelines, methodological rigor, and evaluation of results is a special need in dissemination research (Windsor *et al.*, 1990, 1993).

Link Challenges to Theory

The effectiveness of these strategies can be strengthened by linking the challenges with one of the several existing theories of behavior modification and have been addressed in this volume (see Chapter 3, this volume). For example, the recent theory of behavior change, the transtheoretical model (Prochaska &DiClemente, 1986), has recently been used to try and explain why dissemination efforts have not been consistent across practitioners, settings, or behaviors. Cohen, Halvorson, and Gosselink (1994) applied the Prochaska and DiClemente (1986) stages of change, or transtheoretical, model to physician behavior. Cohen and colleagues (1994) suggest that a physician's behavior change to include a health promotion messages to patients may be expedited by first identifying the stage of readiness to change behavior (precontemplation, contemplation, preparation, action, and maintenance). Methods appropriate to the specific stage and to moving the provider toward action and maintenance would then apply. These conclusions support the conditions necessary for change described by Prochaska and DiClemente, specifically, restructuring the environment and providing social support and record systems fostering the behavior change.

Capitalize on Patient-Initiated Approaches

A frequently overlooked mechanism for changing physician behavior is change initiated by patients. Patients appear to expect their physicians to counsel about all aspects of health, including preventive behavior (Brody *et al.*, 1989; Price, Desmond, & Losh, 1991). Patients are frequently willing to act on their provider's advice. Studies that document the provider's recommendation as the most important trigger for women getting a mammogram is one example (Fox, Murata, & Stein, 1991; Lackland, Dunbar, Keil, Knapp, & O'Brien, 1991). Although generating public demand for a procedure would be difficult to organize in a limited time period, secular trends toward healthy (or unhealthy) behaviors occur as social marketing or news dissemination through the media generates questions from patients. Such questions from patients can change provider behavior. Taylor *et al.* (1996) found this to be the case in a community-based intervention to increase mammography screening that increased provider recommendations for screening. Secular trends for mammography screening in the late 1980s and early 1990s were also fueled by major changes that removed a number of barriers to both patient and physician. Reimbursement for screening became more common and substantial funding from the federal government programs increased screening. The increased media attention to breast cancer and mammography contributed heavily to the secular trend.

Implementation Considerations

In addition to appropriate design strategies, it is imperative that the office support staff be included in the intervention activities as well as the physician. Engle and co-workers (1996) reported that excluding the staff when attempting to change practice patterns resulted in decreased physician participation. Further, despite the physicians overall tacit authority, the duration and intensity of the staff's contact with the patients is often greater than that of the physician, and it is the staff who will frequently be implementing the changed practice behavior.

Other factors that need to be considered and incorporated into the intervention include the organizational structure of the setting. The administrative hierarchy of a hospital is generally more dense than that of a clinic or private practice. Identifying the key individual to facilitate and identifying that individual as a liaison between the practice staff and physicians and the intervention staff helps assure ease of implementation.

A health care setting has its own culture, and sensitivity to that culture is vital both in the content of the intervention and the implementation. If the presentation is presented in a manner that is foreign to the practice, the practice will not be able to implement the intervention successfully and practice patterns will not change. This is especially true in clinics dealing with a multicultural population, as is increasingly common today.

Pride of ownership results in empowerment of the individual. By tailoring the presentation of the intervention to the needs, schedule, and protocols of the practice, the likelihood for success is increased (Greco & Eisenberg, 1993; Karuza et al., 1995). Much is written today about the empowerment movement; suffice it to say, that practice behavior changes will occur more readily if the providers can view the intervention as being consistent with their own circumstances. Other characteristics of empowerment include adapting each intervention to the type of physician and practice as well as to the stage of the physician and practice and the behavior being addressed.

Last, there is some evidence that incentives and/or sanctions are of little value in changing behavior (Hickson, Altemeier, & Perrin, 1987; Hillman, Pauly, & Kerstein, 1989; Kahn et al., 1990). Incentives devalue the need for introducing the intervention and sanctions increase resistance to adopting the intervention.

Examples of Successful Interventions

Although there are numerous examples of prevention interventions occurring in practice settings, we will only provide one for each setting. For clinics, an example of an intervention in dental clinics to incorporate smokeless tobacco cessation into routine dental hygiene is presented (Stevens, Severson, Lichenstein, Little, & Leben, 1995). For community-based practices, the Engle et al. (1997c) study of substance abuse awareness intervention for community obstetric practices will be summarized. For hospitals, the antenatal corticosteroid dissemination study (Leviton et al., 1999) study will be summarized.

Clinic Example: Implementing Smokeless Tobacco Cessation Intervention in the Dentist's Office

Introductory Comment

This study was conducted in the Kaiser Permanente Dental Care Program, a prepaid group practice health maintenance organization. Although the primary intent of the study was to determine the effectiveness of a health promotion message by dentists and dental hygienists on the quit rate of smokeless tobacco users (STU), the study also provides an excellent example of a successful dissemination methodology. The intervention with the dental staff was brief (about 2 hours) and the time requirements were minimal for incorporation of the health prevention message into ongoing practice patterns. As a result, providers and staff successfully added the health promotion message into their clinic protocol. The study also is able to demonstrate the linkage between the patients' outcomes of quitting the use of smokeless tobacco to the health promotion intervention with the providers.

Study Example

Because over half of the adult population was reported to receive dental care annually [US Department of Health and Human Services (USDHHS), 1988] and the immediate effects of the use of smokeless tobacco can frequently be seen, dental offices were advocated for delivery of messages to reduce the use of smokeless tobacco (Little & Stevens, 1991). The Kaiser Permanente study was designed to test this theory.

Eight Kaiser Permanente dental care program clinics were selected for this study. All males over 15 years of age who came in for a routine dental hygiene visit completed a questionnaire on tobacco use. Those patients that reported using smokeless tobacco became participants in the study and were randomly assigned to the treatment group or to the usual care group. Three additional clinics were later added to provide a preintervention control group.

Dissemination of the study methodology required a one-time 2-hour training for receptionists, hygienists, and dentists at the eight clinics. A project team member also visited each clinic weekly to assess progress and provide ongoing training and quality control. The intervention was designed to fit easily into routine dental practice. Receptionists used a questionnaire to determine the use of tobacco. The hygienists performed routine examination, cleaning, and education activities on STUs assigned to usual care. Use of smokeless tobacco may or may not have been addressed by the hygienist, depending on that provider's usual care protocol. Hygienists recorded study data and directly advised the patient to quit using smokeless tobacco and other tobacco products. In addition, they provided the usual care examination and other prophylactic and education tasks to STUs assigned to the treatment group. The treatment intervention added 2–4 minutes to the hygienists' usual care activities.

Dentists, who see patients following the hygienist, pointed out lesions and any other harmful effects of smokeless tobacco and advised the patient to stop tobacco use. The treatment intervention added about 30 seconds to the dentists' usual care activities.

Messages to the patient were direct and unambiguous. If lesions were present, they were linked to use of tobacco. A 9-minute video was also shown to patients who were agreeable to watch it. Patients were persuaded to set a quit date and given a self-help quit kit containing oral substitutes. Telephone calls to support quitting efforts were made after about a week. Other mailings were made on a monthly basis and resources such as tobacco telephone hotline numbers and support group numbers were made available. A formal 3- and 12-month follow-up were made, with a free oral examination offered at the 12-month call.

At the 3-month follow-up, patients in the treatment group reported significantly higher abstinence (32.2%) than patients in the usual care group (21.3%). Similarly, patients in the treatment group reported significantly higher abstinence (33.5%) than usual care patients (24.5%) at the 12-month follow-up. The lower abstinence rates reported in the three clinics of the preintervention group suggested that the training provided by the project may have sensitized dental care providers to STU, resulting in changes to the usual care practices. Also, patients at the highest risk for disease and those with lesions and greatest substance use were the least likely to abstain following the intervention.

Patient response to the dental care health promotion message was positive. Response rates by participants to mailings and telephone interviews were good. The response rate at 12 months was lower than at 3 months but was still a healthy 83%.

Provider compliance with the intervention was high, with 95% of dentists and 97% of hygienists reporting advising patients to quit.

Office Example: Substance Abuse Awareness Intervention for Community Obstetric Practices

Introductory Comment

This study with community-based obstetric practices demonstrates the use of multiple strategies in successfully changing provider practice behaviors. Providers have traditionally not adequately addressed substance use and abuse (tobacco, alcohol, or other substances) in pregnant women, perhaps because of the intractability of the patient problem. However, this intervention increased the confidence of providers to assess, manage, and refer women who use and/or abuse substances by providing the practice staff with strategies that support (predispose), enable, and reinforce desired assessment, management, and referral behaviors.

Study Description

In 1993, the National Institute of Drug Abuse funded the "Substance Abuse Intervention for Community Obstetric Practices." The purpose of this study was to develop, implement, and evaluate a practice (office)-based intervention for obstetricians and their staffs to increase the frequency of assessment, management, and referral behaviors with pregnant women who use or abuse substances. Ten community-based practices ranging in size from a 2-physician practice to a 12-physician practice were recruited and randomly assigned to an immediate or delayed intervention group. Prior to the intervention implementation, all individuals employed in the practice were requested to complete a knowledge and self-efficacy survey dealing with substance use (tobacco, alcohol, and other substances) and to identify a liaison who would work closely with the intervention team. In addition, two, blind-to-intervention-group record reviewers were employed to document the providers' baseline assessment, management, and referral behaviors in charts of women who had delivered in the previous 12 months. The intervention was then implemented in the immediate group (six practices) and 18 months later in the delayed group (two practices). One practice withdrew from participation after the baseline data collection and another practice agreed to records review but declined participation in the intervention (Engle et al., 1996).

The intervention consisted of a 1-hour orientation (a predisposing strategy) delivered at a time convenient to the practice (either first thing in the morning or over the lunch break). Then the practice was provided with feedback from the knowledge and self-efficacy scales (a reinforcing strategy) and provided with a list of available topics related to assessment, management, and referral of women who use or abuse substances. From this list, based on the feedback, the group chose six (or occasionally seven) 1-hour special topic presentations. These varied in format and included didactic presentations, case studies, practice sessions, and discussion (predisposing and enabling strategies). The intervention included the use of patient education materials, other print materials, enabling activities such as use of stickers and reminders, and regular contact with the intervention team.

At the end of the 6 months, surveys were completed again and records were reviewed. A delay of 6 months was instituted to allow for a sufficient time for establishing durability of the intervention and to increase the number of available records of women who could have been affected by the change in practice behavior. The delayed group was then presented with the intervention following the same protocol as with the immediate group. At the conclusion of the delayed group intervention, surveys were again completed and records reviewed.

Preliminary data analysis indicates that the combination of predisposing, enabling, and reinforcing strategies and the liaison between the intervention team and the practice resulted in an increase in assessing, managing, and referring behaviors on the part of practice providers (Engle *et al.*, 1997a), and self-efficacy (Schumacher *et al.*, 1997), and knowledge also increased (Engle *et al.*, 1997b).

The one finding of this study that has implications for future interventions with providers in practice settings is that with the advent of managed care, the availability of time to implement such an extensive intervention on the part of the intervention team was severely limited. It is the intention of the team to package the intervention in such a manner that it can be presented to practices in a 1-hour detailing package coupled with telephone resource support. We found that, in the future, interventions in the office need to be presented in such a way that the practice can incorporate them with little effort, little time, and with maximum effect.

Hospital Example: Antenatal Corticosteroid Dissemination Study—Low Birthweight Port

Introductory Comment

The Low Birthweight Patient Outcomes Research Team PORT study offers an excellent design and implementation strategy for a dissemination study. The study used an experimental design in order to appropriately test the study hypotheses. Behavioral theory and the research experience recorded in the literature was used to formulate the initial dissemination strategy. Obstetricians' opinions on how best to disseminate the information and incorporate it into obstetric practice were also integrated into the strategy. Additional qualitative and quantitative data on the obstetrician attitudes, beliefs, and behaviors were also collected in the planning phase to inform the prevention message to be disseminated.

Study Description

The PORT on Low Birthweight in Minority and High Risk Women has focused on the multiple etiologies of term and preterm low birthweight. One study that addressed dissemination methods to physicians dealt with the appropriate use of corticosteroid agents in threatened preterm labor. Specifically, the dissemination focused on the importance of antenatal corticosteroid agents for improving outcomes in very preterm deliveries where a woman was threatening delivery at 24–34 weeks gestation. The study arose from the available evidence on the effectiveness of appropriate treatment and the reported variation in the use of the therapy among obstetricians (Bronstein & Goldenberg, 1995; Vermont–Oxford Trials Database Project Investigators, 1993).

In order to better understand the variations in physician practice patterns, the team undertook a series of key informant interviews and focus groups with obstetricians around the country. Data gathered suggested that certain beliefs, such as a misperception of treatment benefits or risks and certain practices delay or interfere with the appropriate use of corticosteroid agents (Leviton, Baker, Hassol, & Goldenberg, 1995). Additional information on relevant clinical practices and outcomes was gathered from analysis of secondary databases.

The key informant interviews and focus groups also suggested strategies that could increase timely steroid use. These included several modes of influence such as consultation with a respected colleague, consensus among colleagues, policies in group practices and hospitals, and continuing medical education. Because dissemination research literature recommends that combining dissemination strategies and using multiple modes of influence is most effective, the dissemination design strategy included continuing medical education that incorporated local opinion leader education, academic detailing, a reminder system aimed at reducing delays in steroid administration, and reinforcement of the recommended practice guidelines through peer group discussion and collective feedback.

For the medical education component, an obstetrician knowledgeable about antenatal corticosteroid use and willing to act in the role of local opinion leader was selected at each hospital site. This obstetrician also agreed to host and promote a grand rounds on the evidence of corticosteroid use and to develop supplemental videotape and written material for distribution and use.

The reminder system was implemented by a nurse selected at each hospital who placed a reminder sticker on the charts of all women admitted to labor and delivery at risk of preterm delivery. The reminder prompted the physician to consider steroids and to refer to recommendations for use on the provided chart insert.

The third component of the dissemination strategy involved collective feedback to participating obstetricians at all hospitals that received the special dissemination. Case studies were developed for use by the local opinion leader in a group discussion format. These case studies illustrated the use of corticosteroid agents with special populations and were devised to ferret out any areas of disagreement or uncertainty among the group regarding recommended use. Although no individualized practice feedback was given, logs maintained by nurses provided hospital-level feedback for information to the opinion leaders and also to the project team to monitor implementation.

Twenty-eight hospitals that delivered large numbers of preterm babies were selected and randomized to treatment or control groups (one treatment hospital was later lost to follow-up). Obstetricians in the treatment hospitals that delivered preterm babies received the dissemination intervention. The control hospitals were exposed only to the materials on steroid use that are disseminated to the general medical audience. Maternal records were reviewed at each study hospital for the 12 months prior to the general release of corticosteroid information by National Institutes of Health and for the 12 months following intervention. A hierarchical linear model approach to analysis was used with patients nested within hospitals. The change in use of corticosteriod agents was the primary outcome measure, although variations such as appropriate steroid use versus nonuse versus inappropriate use were also investigated. Independent variables included hospital and physician characteristics as well as preintervention levels of steroid use. A number of environmental and process variables were also gathered to inform the dissemination process and results. These include site visits and opinion leader interviews, narrative reports from nurse coordinators, and grand rounds evaluation sheets.

Note: These results indicate a significant improvement in steroid use in the hospitals that received the dissemination intervention. Use in these treatment hospitals increased 2.1-fold compared to a 1.8-fold increase in the control hospitals.

Summary and Conclusions

Although the physician may have received the disseminated information, incorporating that information into practice is less than perfect. Interventions designed to change physician's behavior have varying degrees of success, for although the knowledge is incorporated and knowledge change could be measured, being able to put that knowledge into practice may not be possible.

Many gains have been made in disseminating information so that the likelihood that change in practice patterns will occur is increased. Identifying current and pressing needs and incorporating a combination of practice-based predisposing, enabling, and reinforcing strategies in disseminating information will increase that likelihood. Including these strategies means that the information must be disseminated in an interactive, proactive manner, something that is often difficult to accomplish. Imposing the information by fiat, or attaching sanctions to the lack of desired behavior has been demonstrated to be less than effective in affecting desired behavior change. Unfortunately, with the advent and growth of managed care, even the best intentions are often unsuccessful.

However, there are several dissemination methods that have not been adequately studied, including journal reading, use of opinion leaders, chart reviews, academic detail visits, and staged intervention activities. These methods need to be studied using well-controlled studies with a variety of practice settings. Studies that focus on the clinical imperative of clinical outcomes also need to be conducted.

References

Ashbaugh, D. G., & McKean, R. S. (1976). Continuing medical education. The philosophy and use of audit. *Journal of the American Medical Association, 236*, 1485–1488.

Bass, M. J., & Elford, R. W. (1988). Preventive practice patterns of Canadian primary care physicians. *American Journal of Preventive Medicine, 4(Suppl. 4)*, 17–23.

Borgiel, A. E., Dunn, E. V., Lamont, C. T., MacDonald, P. J., Evensen, M. K., Bass, M. J., Spasoff, R. A., & Williams, J. I. (1989). Recruiting family physicians as participants in research. *Family Practice, 6*, 168–172.

Brody, D. S., Miller, S. M., Lerman, C. E., Smith, D. G., Lazaro C. G., & Blum, M. J. (1989). The relationship between patients' satisfaction with their physicians and perceptions about interventions they desired and received. *Medical Care, 27,* 1027–1035.

Bronstein, J. M., & Goldenberg, R. L. (1995). Practice variations in the use of corticosteroids: A comparison of eight data sets. *American Journal of Obstetrics and Gynecology,* (Special Suppl.), *173,* 296–298.

Cohen, S. J., Halvorson, H. W., & Gosselink, C. A. (1994). Changing physician behavior to improve disease prevention. *Preventive Medicine, 23,* 284–291.

Daly, M. B., Balshem, M., Sands C., James J., Workman S., & Engstrom, P. F. (1993). Academic detailing: A model for in-office CME. *Journal of Cancer Education, 8,* 273–280.

Davis, D. A. (1994). The dissemination of information: Optimizing the effectiveness of continuing medical education. In E. V. Dunn, P. G. Norton, M. Stewart, F. Tudiver, & M. J. Bass (Eds.), *Disseminating research/Changing practice* (pp. 139–150). Thousand Oaks, CA: Sage.

Davis, D. A., Thomson, M. A., Oxman, A. D., & Haynes, R. B. (1992). Evidence for the effectiveness of CME: A review of 50 randomized controlled trials. *Journal of the American Medical Association, 268,* 1111–1117.

Davis, D. A., Thomson, M. A., Oxman, A. D., & Haynes, R. B. (1995). A systematic review of the effect of continuing medical education strategies. *Journal of the American Medical Association, 274,* 700–705.

Dietrich, J. A., O'Conner, G., Keller, A., Carney-Gersten, P., Levy, D., Nelson, E., Simmins J., Barrett, J., & Landgraf, J. M. (1990). Will community physicians participate in rigorous studies of cancer control? The methodology and recruitment of a randomized trial of physician practices. In P. F. Engstrom, B. Rimer, & L. E. Mortenson (Eds.), *Advances in cancer control: Screening and prevention research* (pp. 373–381). New York: Wiley-Liss.

Engle, M., Phelan, S., Kohler, C., Schumacher, J. E., Raczynski, J. M., & Reynolds, K. (1996, December). *Recruiting provider practices for participation in office-based health promotion research.* Paper presented at the annual meeting of National Institute for the Clinical Applications of Behavioral Medicine, Hilton Head, SC.

Engle, M., Schumacher, J. E., Kohler, C., Mukherjee, S., Houser, S. H., Phelan, S., Raczynski, J. M., Reynolds, K., & Caldwell, E. (1997a). Changing assessment, management and referral practice behaviors of community-based obstetric practices: results of a randomized clinical trial. Unpublished manuscript. Oregon State University, Corvallis, OR.

Engle, M. Schumacher, J. E., Kohler, C., Mukherjee, S., Houser, S. H., Phelan, S., Raczynski, J. M., Reynolds, K., & Caldwell, E. (1997b). Changing obstetric providers knowledge about substance use and abuse: The results of an practice-based intervention. Unpublished manuscript. Oregon State University, Corvallis, OR.

Engle, M., Schumacher, J. E., Kohler, C., Phelan, S., Raczynski, J. M. & Reynolds, K., & Hogerman, G. S. (1997c). A practice-based substance use/abuse awareness intervention for community obstetric practices. Unpublished manuscript. Oregon State University, Corvallis, OR.

Everett, G. D., DeBlois, C. S., Chang, P. F., & Holets, T. (1983). The effect of cost education, cost audits, and faculty chart review on the use of laboratory services. *Archives of Internal Medicine, 143,* 942–944.

Fox, R. D., Mazmanian, P. E., & Putnam, R. W. (1989). A theory of learning and change. In R. D. Fox, P. E. Mazmanian, & R. W. Putnam (Eds.), *Change and learning in the lives of physicians* (pp. 161–176). New York: Praeger Publishers.

Fox, S. A., Murata, P. J., & Stein, J. A. (1991). The impact of physician compliance on screening mammography for older women. *Archives of Internal Medicine, 151,* 50–56.

Glanz, K., & Gilboy, M. B. (1992). Physicians, preventive care, and applied nutrition: Selected literature. *Academic Medicine, 67,* 776–781.

Glynn, T. J. (1988). Relative effectiveness of physician-initiated smoking cessation programs. *Cancer Bulletin, 40,* 359–364.

Greco, P. J., & Eisenberg, J. M. (1993). Changing physicians' practices. *New England Journal of Medicine, 329,* 1271–1274.

Green, L. A., Niebauer, L. J., Miller, R. S., & Lutz, L. J. (1991). An analysis of reasons for discontinuing participation in a practice-based research network. *Family Medicine, 23,* 447–449.

Hickson, G. B., Altemeier, W. A., & Perrin, J. M. (1987). Physician reimbursement by salary or fee-for-service: Effect on physician practice behavior in a randomized prospective study. *Pediatrics, 80,* 344–350.

Hillman, A. L., Pauly, M. V., & Kerstein, J. J. (1989). How do financial incentives affect physicians' clinical decisions and the financial performance of health maintenance organizations? *New England Journal of Medicine, 321,* 86–92.

Kahn, K. L., Keeler, E. B., Sherwood, M. J., Rogers, W. H., Draper, D., Bentow, S. S., Reinisch, E. J., Rubenstein L. V., Kosecoff, J., & Brook, R. H. (1990). Comparing outcomes of care before and after implementation of the DRG-based prospective payment system. *Journal of the American Medical Association, 264*, 1984–1988.

Karuza, J., Calkins, E., Feather, J., Hershey, C. O., Katz, L. P., & Majeroni, B. (1995). Enhancing physician adoption of practice guidelines: Dissemination of influenza vaccination guideline using a small-group consensus process. *Archives of Internal Medicine, 155*, 625–632.

Kottke, T. E., Battista, R. N., DeFriese, G. H., & Brekke, M. L. (1988). Attributes of successful smoking cessation interventions in medical practice. *Journal of the American Medical Association, 259*, 2883–2889.

Kottke, T. E., Solberg, L. I., Conn, S., Maxwell, P., Thomasberg, M., Brekke, M. L., & Brekke, M. J. (1990). A comparison of two methods to recruit physicians to deliver smoking cessation interventions. *Archives of Internal Medicine, 150*, 1477–1481.

Lackland, D. T., Dunbar, J. B., Keil, J. E., Knapp, R. G., & O'Brien, P. H. (1991). Breast cancer screen in a biracial community: The Charleston tricounty experience. *Southern Medical Journal, 84*, 862–866.

Leitch, A. M. (1995). Controversies in breast cancer screening. *Cancer, 76*(Suppl. 10), 2064–2069.

Leviton, L., Baker, S., Hassol, A., & Goldenberg, R. L. (1995). An exploration of opinion and practice patterns affecting the use of antenatal corticosteroids. *American Journal of Obstetrics and Gynecology* (Special Suppl.), *173*, 312–316.

Leviton, L. C., Goldenberg, R. L., Baker, C. S., Freda, M., *et al.* (1999). Methods to encourage the use of antenatal corticosteroid therapy for fetal maturation: Randomized controlled trial. *Journal of the American Medical Association, 281*, 46–52.

Lewis, C. E. (1988). Disease prevention and health promotion practices of primary care physicians in the United States. *American Journal of Preventive Medicine, 4*(Suppl. 4), 9–16.

Little, S. J., & Stevens, V. J. (1991). Dental hygiene's role in reducing tobacco use: A literature review and recommendation for action. *Journal of Dental Hygiene, 65*, 346–350.

Lomas, J., Enkin, M., Anderson, G. M., Hannah, W. J., Vayda, E., & Singer, J. (1991). Opinion leaders versus audit and feedback to implement practice guidelines. *Journal of the American Medical Association, 265*, 2202–2207.

Martin, A. R., Wolf, M. A., Thibodeau, L. A., Dzau, V., & Braunweld, E. (1980). A trial of two strategies to modify the test-ordering behavior of medical residents. *New England Journal of Medicine, 303*, 1330–1336.

Meyer, T. J., Van Kooten, D., Marsh, S., & Prochazka, A. V. (1991). Reduction of polypharmacy by feedback to clinicians. *Journal of General Internal Medicine, 6*, 133–135.

Nazarian, L. F., Maiman, L. A., & Becker, M. H. (1989). Recruitment of a large community of pediatricians in a collaborative research project. *Clinical Pediatrics, 28*, 210–213.

Oxman, A. D., Thomson, M. A., Davis, D. A., & Haynes, R. B. (1995). No magic bullets: A systematic review of 102 trials of interventions to improve professional practice. *Canadian Medical Association Journal, 153*, 1423–1431.

Phillips, B., Rubeck, R., Hathaway, M., Becker, M., & Boehlecke, B. (1993). Preventive medicine: What do future practitioners really need? Are they getting it in medical school? *Journal of the Kentucky Medical Association, 91*, 104–111.

Price, J. H., Desmond, S. M., & Losh, D. P. (1991). Patients' expectations of the family physician in health promotion. *American Journal of Preventive Medicine, 7*, 33–39.

Prochaska, J. O., & DiClemente, C. C. (1986). Toward a comprehensive model of change. In W. R. Miller & N. Heather (Eds.), *Treating addictive behaviors* (pp. 3–27). New York: Plenum Press.

Rimer, B. K., Trock, B., Balshem, A., Engstrom, P. F., Rosan, J., & Lerman, C. (1990). Breast screening practices among primary physicians—reality and potential. *Journal of the American Board of Family Practice, 3*, 26–34.

Rokstad, K., & Fugelli, P. (1993). How to succeed in a multipractice study. *Family Medicine, 25*, 461–464.

Schumacher, J. E., Engle, M., Reynolds, K., Houser, S. H., Mukherjee, S., Phelan, S., Raczynski, J. M., Kohler, C., & Caldwell, E. (1997). Substance use assessment and management self-efficacy among obstetric practices. Unpublished manuscript. University of Alabama School of Medicine, Behavioral Medicine Unit, Birmingham, AL.

Schwartz, J. S., Lewis, C. E., Clancy, C., Kinosian, M. S., Radany, M. H., & Koplan, J. P. (1991). Internists' practices in health promotion and disease prevention. *Annals of Internal Medicine, 114*, 46–53.

Scott, C. S., & Neighbor, W. E. (1985). Preventive care attitudes of medical students. *Social Science and Medicine, 21*, 299–305.

Selby, M. L., Riportella-Muller, R., Sorenson, J. R., Quade, D., & Luchok, K. J. (1992). Increasing participation by private physicians in the EPSDT program in rural North Carolina. *Public Health Reports, 107*, 561–568.

Stevens, V. J., Severson, H., Lichenstein, E., Little, S. J., & Leben J. (1995). Making the most of a teachable moment: A smokeless-tobacco cessation intervention in the dental office. *American Journal of Public Health, 85,* 231–235.

Stross, J. K., & Bole, G. G. (1980). Evaluation of continuing education program in rheumatoid arthritis. *Arthritis Rheumatism, 23,* 846–849.

Stross, J. K., Hiss, R. G., Watts, C. M., Davis, W. K., & MacDonald, R. (1983). Continuing education in pulmonary disease for primary-care physicians. *American Review of Respiratory Diseases, 127,* 739–746.

Taylor, K. M. (1992). Physician participation in a randomized clinical trial for ocular melanoma. *Annals of Ophthalmology, 24,* 337–344.

Taylor, V. M., Taplin, S. H., Urban, N., White, E., Mahloch, J., Majer, K., McLerran, D., & Peacock, S. (1996). Community organization to promote breast cancer screening ordering by primary care physicians. *Journal of Community Health, 21,* 277–291.

Tierney, W. M., Hui, S. L., & McDonald, C. J. (1986). Delayed feedback of physician performance vs. immediate reminders to perform preventive care. *Medical Care, 24,* 659–666.

Tierney, W. M., McDonald, C. J., Hui, S. L., & Martin, D. K. (1988). Computer predictions of abnormal test results. Effects on outpatient testing. *Journal of the American Medical Association, 259,* 1194–1198.

Tierney, W. M., Miller, M. E., & McDonald, C. J. (1990). The effect on test ordering of informing physicians of the charges for outpatient diagnostic tests. *New England Journal of Medicine, 322,* 1499–1504.

Trynor, V., Neary, S., Bridges-Webb, C., Miles, D. A., Britt, H., & Charles, J. (1993). Recruiting general practitioners for survey research. *Australian Family Practice, 22,* 790–795.

US Department of Health and Human Services (USDHHS). (1988). *Use of dental services and dental health: United States, 1986.* (PHS publication 88-1593, National Health Survey Series 10, No. 165). Washington, DC: Author.

Vermont–Oxford Trials Database Project Investigators. (1993). The Vermont–Oxford Trials Network: Very low birthweight outcomes for 1990. *Pediatrics, 91,* 540–545.

Ward, J. (1994). General practitioners' experience of research. *Family Practice, 11,* 418–423.

Wechsler, H., Levine, S., Idelson, R. K., Rohman, M., & Taylor, J. O. (1983). The physician's role in health promotion—A survey of primary-care practitioners. *New England Journal of Medicine, 308,* 97–100.

Weinberger, M., Saunders, A. F., Samsa, G. P., Bearon, L. B, Gold, D. T., Brown, J. T., Booher, P., & Loehrer, P. J. (1991). Breast cancer screening in older women: Practices and barriers reported by primary care physicians. *Journal of the American Geriatrics Society, 39,* 22–29.

Wells, K. B., Lewis, C. E., Leake, B., & Ware, J. E., Jr. (1984). Do physicians preach what they practice? A study of physicians' health habits and counseling practices. *Journal of the American Medical Association, 252,* 2846–2848.

Williams, P. T., Eckert, G., Epstein, A., Mourad, L., & Helmick, F. (1994). In-office cancer-screening education of primary care physicians. *Journal of Cancer Education, 9,* 90–95.

Winders, S., Raczynski, J. M., Gallagher, E. A., Westfall, E., & Gerald, J. K. (1997). *Healthy moms, healthy babies, healthy families—Helping your patients quit smoking.* Madison, WI: Wisconsin Clearinghouse for Prevention Resources.

Windsor, R. A., Dalmat, M. E., Orleans, C. T., & Gritz, E. R., (1990). *A handbook to plan, implement, and evaluate smoking cessation programs for pregnant women.* New York: March of Dimes Foundation.

Windsor, R. A., Li, C. Q., Lowe, J. B., Perkins, L. L., Ershoff, D., & Glynn, T. (1993). The dissemination of smoking cessation methods for pregnant women: Achieving the year 2000 objectives. *American Journal of Public Health, 83,* 173–178.

Zyzanski, S. J., Stange, K. C., Kelly, R., Flocke, S., Shank, J. C., Chao, J., Jaen, C. R., & Smith, C. K. (1994). Family physicians' disagreements with the US Preventive Services Task Force recommendations. *Journal of Family Practice, 39,* 140–147.

CHAPTER 22

Health Promotion and Disease Prevention at the Work Site

Kathleen C. Brown, Michael T. Weaver, Lynn M. Artz, and James C. Hilyer

Introduction

National medical care expenditures reached $949 billion in 1994, resulting in unprecedented employee medical benefits costs [Health Care Financing Administration (HCFA), 1996]. With annual expenses increasing 12–20% per year, employer costs for medical benefits are limiting company profits and necessitating major cost control initiatives. Total national medical expenditures have risen at more than twice the rate of inflation to $111 billion in just the 3 years from 1991 to 1994 (HCFA, 1996; National Center for Health Statistics, 1996). With employers paying 55–80% of national medical expenditures, controlling the rising costs of medical benefits represents a key challenge for employers in both the public and private sectors (Kizer, Pelletier, & Fielding, 1995).

In an effort to control costs, companies have turned to several cost-containment strategies. Among these strategies are health promotion and disease prevention programs, managed care, and health insurance plan redesign. Companies have adopted employee health promotion programs as a means to minimize costs through improving health and reducing health risks [US Department of Health and Human Services (USDHHS), 1993]. The role of these health promotion programs in capitated managed care has resulted in heightened interest among employers to develop health promotion programs (Pelletier, 1996).

Kathleen C. Brown • Nursing Graduate Programs, School of Nursing, University of Alabama at Birmingham, Birmingham, Alabama 35294.   *Michael T. Weaver* • Nursing Graduate Programs, School of Nursing, UAB Center for Health Promotion, University of Alabama at Birmingham, Birmingham, Alabama 35294.   *Lynn M. Artz* • Department of Epidemiology, School of Public Health, University of Alabama at Birmingham, Birmingham, Alabama 35294.   James C. Hilyer • Division of Preventive Medicine, School of Medicine, University of Alabama at Birmingham, Birmingham, Alabama 35294.

Handbook of Health Promotion and Disease Prevention, edited by Raczynski and DiClemente. Kluwer Academic/Plenum Publishers, New York, 1999.

Broadened View of Health Promotion

In a July 29, 1993, manuscript in the *New England Journal of Medicine,* James Fries, C. Everett Koop, Mary Jane England (Institute of Medicine), and members of the Health Project Consortium proposed a concept of health promotion that encompassed all strategies to improve physical health of individuals and reduce health care costs. When these strategies are implemented within the workplace, the resulting initiatives include efforts to further awareness, change lifestyles, and develop company policies, incentives, and environments that promote health (O'Donnell, 1994).

This broad view of health promotion includes not just strategies to change individual lifestyles but also interventions to improve appropriate use of medical visits, programs on self-care for chronic illness, and interventions to reduce high cost medical conditions (e.g., low-birth weight babies). *Healthy People 2000* (USDHHS, 1991) also defines health promotion and disease prevention in its broadest sense and identifies clinical preventive services, such as counseling, screening, immunizations, and other interventions delivered to individuals in a health care setting as a priority.

An expanded perspective of health promotion is also necessary to correct one of the limitations in health promotion efforts to date. Work site health promotion or wellness programs, usually emphasizing primary prevention, have often been isolated from the medical care system (Stokols, Pelletier, & Fielding, 1995). A closer collaboration between work site health programming and medical providers in the primary care system should be actualized. For example, providers could refer cardiac and injured employees to their work site health and fitness facilities for rehabilitation. In addition, insurers and employers could develop coordinated health promotion initiatives to target employee risk factors. A comprehensive work site health promotion program that involves collaboration with insurers, providers, workers, and managers should be our future model of health promotion.

Work Site Health Promotion and Potential for Cost Savings

One of the major incentives for instituting health promotion at the work site arises from the recognition that 50–70% of illnesses and the concomitant costs are preventable (Fries, Bloch, Harrington, Richardson, & Beck, 1993; McGinnis & Foege, 1993). Preventable causes underlie eight of the nine leading morbidity categories and are responsible for almost 1 million deaths annually (USDHHS, 1991; Fries *et al.,* 1993). In spite of these statistics, only 3% of total health care expenditures are marked for prevention.

Empirical evidence is mounting that risky health habits are expensive. Although the longevity of smokers is decreased, their lifetime medical costs exceed nonsmokers by one third (Hodgson, 1992; Leigh & Fries, 1992). Claims costs for employees with three or more risk factors in one large corporation were twice as high as costs for those employees without risk factors (Sokolov, 1992a,b). Likewise, other researchers have reported that individuals at high risk had average annual claims of $1,550 as compared to low-risk individuals' claims which averaged $190 (Yen, Edington, & Witting, 1991). In a university employee group, employees at high risk accounted for 43% of the medical claims costs (Kingery, Ellsworth, Corbett, Bowden, & Brizzolara, 1994). Human resource managers, therefore, are convinced that risky health behaviors cost money.

Additionally, an ever-expanding body of literature provides evidence that work site health promotion programs reduce costs yielding returns between $2 and $3 for every $1 invested. Absenteeism, hospitalization costs, and ambulatory care costs have been found to be lower in groups participating in work site health intervention as compared to nonparticipants (Golaszewsik, Snow, Lynch, Yen, & Solomita, 1992; Harvey, Whitmer, Hilyer, & Brown, 1993; Jones, Bly, & Richardson, 1990; Kingery *et al.*, 1994; Oldenburg, Owen, Parle, & Gomel, 1995). Pelletier (1993) conducted a review of 31 investigations of health promotion programs and found that the savings in these programs were three times more than costs.

The city of Birmingham, Alabama, initiated its Good Health program, along with other cost-containment measures, in 1984, as a result of medical benefits costs that increased 19% per year from $1.5 million in 1974 to $7.6 million in 1983 (Harvey *et al.*, 1993). Objectives were set to lower medical benefits costs below the per employee state average and to reduce the number of hospital admissions and hospital days. Today the program consists of an all-employee health screen, contests, campaigns and events, interventions, posters, tip sheets and payroll messages, and a fitness center (Brown, Hilyer, Artz, Glasscock, & Weaver, 1995). After the Good Health program was initiated, costs in the years 1985 to 1990 remained stable. Many employers in the area who were similarly introducing managed care were experiencing annual increases of 11 to 14%, while the city of Birmingham experienced virtually no increases. Per employee annual medical benefits costs were $397 above the state average in 1985, and by 1990, city costs per employee were $922 below state average costs. As an annual expense, the 1985 cumulative costs were $1.5 million above state averages. In 1990, savings were $3,688,000. Accumulated total medical expenses between 1987 and 1990 amounted to $7,146,878 below state averages. Annual fitness testing and prescribed fitness programs for police officers and firefighters reduced job-related injuries and injury medical costs over 10% per year (Hilyer & Artz, 1992; Hilyer, Brown, Sirles, & Peoples, 1990). Between 1985 and 1990, a 55% reduction in hospital days and a 38% decline in admissions were accomplished. In the first year of the Good Health program, expenses were 22% below forecasted costs and in the fifth year, expenses were 57% below forecast. When actual costs were compared to forecasted costs, the city of Birmingham had saved millions of dollars over a 5-year period, saving about $10 for every $1 invested. Success in containing costs has continued to the present. In 1985, medical insurance costs were 11.6% of the payroll compared to 10.9% of the payroll in 1996. Similarly, medical insurance costs relative to percent of the benefits budget has remained stable. In 1985, medical insurance costs were 40.2% of the benefits budget and in 1996 these costs were 39.3% of the benefits budget.

Effectiveness of Work Site Interventions

A number of randomized intervention trials have provided scientific evidence on the efficacy of work site interventions specifically for reducing health risks. Because cardiovascular disease continues to be the leading cause of morbidity and mortality, the literature reviewed below is restricted to recent work site intervention studies designed to reduce cardiovascular risks (National Center for Health Statistics, 1996; Thomas & DeKeyser, 1996).

In a randomized controlled trial ($n = 159$) to lower blood pressure, an intervention that included work site counseling, personalized mailings, and a referral to a physician was found to be more effective than physician referral alone in decreasing blood pressure (Fielding, Knight, Mason, Klesges, & Pelletier, 1994). In a less well-designed study, claims costs for hypertensive employees at three experimental sites receiving work site monitoring and counseling were found to be lower than claims for employees at the control site (Foote & Erfurt, 1991). Another study of employees with hypertension, obesity, and cigarette smoking risks demonstrated that work sites that received either an intervention of health education plus follow-up, or a combined of health education, follow-up, and work site health promotion intervention, were nine to ten times more cost-effective in engaging employees in treatment and five to six times more cost-effective at reducing risks or preventing relapse than was the site that received only health education (Erfurt & Foote, 1991).

A 1-year work site health promotion trial of 2198 university employees reported that interventions composed of health risk appraisal only, health promotion only, or combined health promotion and health risk appraisal were equally effective in significantly lowering systolic blood pressure (Connell, Sharpe, & Gallant, 1995). In a prevalence study of 1390 textile workers, a subset of 544 workers with elevated blood pressure were administered a nurse-delivered counseling intervention (Harrell, Cornetto, & Stutts, 1992). Blood pressures dropped significantly and those with cholesterol levels beyong 240 mg/dl had a mean drop of 10.5 mg/dl ($P = 0.003$). Findings from this study must be viewed cautiously in that no control group or random assignment was utilized and the interventionist was different at each of the 11 industry sites.

Using a work site counseling and mailing intervention program for cholesterol control among high-risk employees, 365 subjects with cholesterol levels greater than 240 mg/dl were assigned to either the experimental group or a control group that received referral to a physician only (Fielding, Mason, Knight, Klesges, & Pelletier, 1995). At 1-year posttesting, a significantly greater percentage of subjects in the experimental group (36%) had achieved a reduction in cholesterol below 240 mg/dl than those in the control group (21%). Other work site intervention trials to reduce cholesterol have resulted in 3.8–5% reductions in total cholesterol; however, most of these studies did not use control groups and varied widely in content, length, and provider (Angotti & Levine, 1994; Baer, 1993; Gomel, Oldenburg, Simpson, & Owen, 1993; Hartman, McCarthy, & Hime, 1993; Hartman, Himes, McCarthy, & Kushi, 1995; Masur-Levy, Tavris, Elsey, & Pica, 1990).

An integrative review of the literature on 10 work site exercise intervention studies revealed that, in all but one of the studies, work site strategies increased adherence to exercise behaviors (Blue & Conrad, 1995). Only one study included blue-collar workers and only two studies used a true experimental design. In a study conducted in the United Kingdom, male police officers were assigned to either an aerobic training group, an anaerobic training group, or a control group to determine the physiological and psychological effects of work site exercise programs (Norris, Carroll, & Cochrane, 1990). At posttest, subjects in the aerobic group had significantly improved fitness level, heart rate, blood pressure, and self-reports of stress and well-being.

A review of scientific evidence on health promotion programs was recently conducted with funding from the Centers for Disease Control and Prevention (CDC) (Wilson, Holman, & Hammock, 1996). Using over 300 studies published between 1968 and 1994, the reviewers concluded that, in the majority of health promotion areas, evidence for effectiveness of these programs was suggestive, indicative, acceptable, or conclusive (Eddy, Fitzhugh, Wojtowicz, & Wang, 1997; Glanz, Sorenson, & Farmer, 1996; Heaney & Goetzel, 1997; Hennrikus & Jeffery, 1996; Murphy, 1996; Roman & Blum, 1996; Shephard, 1996). Hypertension control and multicomponent programs were found to have the most conclusive support (Wilson *et al.*, 1996). Reviews of stress management, weight control, nutrition, and cholesterol interventions were judged to be indicative of effectiveness, and exercise, seat belt, and alcohol work site interventions were suggestive of effectiveness. A review of the smoking cessation intervention literature has not yet been reported.

Findings from these work site intervention studies are often difficult to apply, because different types of interventions were tested, different providers delivered the interventions, some studies were lacking in control groups and random assignment, and some used self-report rather than physiological measures. Generalizations of health promotion study findings are further limited because of potential selection bias, in that healthier or more health-conscious employees may participate in the exercise, smoking cessation, and other health promotion activities at the work site. Equivalence between groups should be determined at baseline and statistical controls employed to correct for differences.

Difficulties also exist in the selection and measurement of outcomes for evaluation of effectiveness. Rather than use of self-report, direct measures of fitness, smoking status, body composition, and absenteeism should be employed. These measures should provide levels of validity and reliability that can better withstand scientific scrutiny and provide improved generalizability. Small sample sizes limit these studies, often because employers are concerned that a study may disrupt work production. Health promotion investigations with women and different subpopulations of workers are needed to identify appropriate, effective work site interventions and incentives (Blue & Conrad, 1995). Additional studies are required to identify correct doses of the intervention and long-term effects of work site health promotion. Further studies using randomized controlled trials and interventions designed for specific worker populations are needed to examine the influence of work site interventions for improving employee health promotion, disease prevention, and health care cost outcomes.

Work Site as an Optimal Setting for Health Promotion

The work site is considered the optimal setting for health promotion and disease prevention efforts because of the large audience, frequent and long-term contact with the target population, peer support, and reduced cost and travel barriers. The majority of Americans, an estimated 136 million workers, can be reached at the work site, and therefore the work site represents the key channel for systematically providing health promotion interventions for the adult population (US Department of Labor, 1997). Since health behavior changes may be incremental, the work site is ideal because employees can receive interventions over a long period of time and are a relatively captive audience. In addition, peer support and peer pressure at the work site can foster changes in health behavior and a culture of wellness. Work site programs, at little or no cost to the employee, can be offered during work hours, at lunch breaks, or before or after work, thus minimizing cost, time, and travel barriers.

Other factors in favor of work site health promotion programs involve almost two decades of these programs at the work site and enthusiastic support by the majority of employers and employees. In a recent USDHHS (1993) survey of 1507 work sites with 50 or more employees, 81% of these employers now offer wellness programs as compared to 66% in 1985. Nutrition, fitness, weight control, high blood pressure, and stress management programs have increased in that same time frame in order to support the burgeoning interest in wellness. One of the major factors contributing to the recent growth in work site health promotion programs is the advent of managed care and the key role of health promotion in managed care initiatives (Pelletier, 1996)

Both employers and employees benefit from health promotion offerings in the occupational setting. Direct economic benefits include reduced health, life, disability, and workers' compensation insurance costs. In addition, improved productivity from reduced absenteeism, less turnover, and enhanced job performance are directly beneficial to workers and employers. The work site is also considered a desired site for health promotion programs because of indirect benefits such as improved employee job satisfaction, more motivated employees, and a positive, employee-oriented company image.

Scope of Work Site Health Promotion

Traditionally, work site health programs were limited to established services such as providing physical examinations, first aid and injury care, blood pressure screenings, some safety training, and obtaining health and hospitalization benefits for employees. As the fields of occupational health and personnel benefits advanced, comprehensive programs of work site health promotion, injury prevention, hazard surveillance, and employee assistance programs were initiated. Early innovators in work site health promotion included Ford Motor Company, which developed hypertension treatment programs, Standard Oil Company, which provided mental health programs, and Johnson and Johnson, Dupont, Boeing, Pepsico, and Kimberly Clark, which expanded their services into fitness, nutrition, stress management, and other comprehensive wellness topics. A comprehensive approach now includes health screening and health risk appraisal, programs on exercise, nutrition, and weight control, smoking cessation, hypertension screening and follow-up, back care, cancer awareness, employee assistance and stress management, injury prevention, and requires management and coordination of efforts with the occupational safety and health professionals, insurers, and primary care providers. Thus, work site health promotion has evolved through the following four generations: Early programs that were developed for nonhealth reasons, subsequent programs aimed at a single health risk or population, intervention programs for multiple risks and the entire employee group, and finally, the comprehensive approaches of today that encompass all programs and policies that influence the health of employees and families (Goldbeck, 1984).

Although OSHA (Occupational Safety and Health Act of 1970) dictates safety and hazard communications in the workplace, no federal, state, or local legislation requires health promotion in the workplace. Health policy, health promotion interventions, and reimbursement guidelines have not been developed for worker aggregates as for other populations, that is, schools, health departments, and the Medicare population. Most effort in work site health promotion is voluntary and aimed at primary prevention to eliminate or reduce health risks and costs. Other more stringent approaches use company policy to change behavior at the individual or group level, for example, mandatory work site exercise programs for public safety workers (firefighters and police officers), smokefree and drugfree workplaces to restrict substance use on the job, and employer-paid health benefits contingent on participation in health risk appraisal and screening.

Employers have also used redesign of health insurance benefits to promote healthy lifestyles and prevent disease. Employer coalitions have developed to establish contracts with insurers that emphasize health and medical cost control. Such pressure is needed to shift health insurers from an emphasis on reimbursement for illness care to a focus on health. To decrease their reliance on insurers that provide limited coverage for routine physical examinations or access to preventive services, employers have contracted with health maintenance organizations (HMOs), only to learn that focusing on health promotion and disease prevention is also a continuing challenge for HMOs (Widra & Fottler, 1992). The delivery of health promotion and clinical preventive services remains a weakness in our current health care system, and employers are intent on forming alliances with insurers and providers who are in the business of making employee participation in recommended health promotion and clinical preventive services an incentive. Such approaches combine work site health promotion efforts with strategic planning to develop reduced copayments, rebates, and special packages to encourage positive health behaviors.

The limited ability of insurers to satisfy employers' health promotion needs and to report specific health risks and outcomes of interest to employers, for example, the proportion of the employer's population that participated in age- and gender-specific preventive services (Dolinsky & Caputo, 1991; Gold, 1991; McNeil, Pederson, & Gatsonis, 1992), also has implications for redesign of health insurance systems. Employers are concerned with outcome measures because perception of quality influences employee participation in needed health promotion and disease prevention services. Patient satisfaction has been empirically linked to other patient outcomes such as intention to return for care, participation in referrals, and having received or been offered preventive care (Schweikhart & Strasser, 1994; Ware, Snyder, & Wright, 1983; Weingarten *et al.*, 1995). Personnel benefits managers, insurers, and occupational health professionals are partnering to develop ideal systems of health care that do not just focus on cost outcomes but also focus on innovation, quality, and health-promotion-related outcomes (Wennberg, 1992; Wolford, Brown, & McCool, 1993).

Even though health insurance benefits are available to employees, research has demonstrated that employee participation in preventive services is not guaranteed because of obstacles such as cost-sharing and physician lack of interest in or knowledge about recommended preventive services (Fielding, Knight, Goetzel, & Laouri, 1991; Kottke, Brekke, & Solberg, 1993). As a part of work site health promotion efforts, insurers, and occupational health professionals are identifying panels of providers who are more health oriented, collaborating with them to develop joint health promotion efforts at the work site, and creating systems to reduce barriers so that employees obtain preventive services on schedule.

Common Elements of Successful Work Site Programs

Coordination and a company commitment to health promotion and disease prevention are characteristics of successful work site programs (Table 1). In collaborative strategic planning meetings, management, workers, insurers, and occupational health and safety personnel create visions and objectives for the program. *Healthy People 2000* and similar documents developed at the state level can be used to guide program components and set achievable objectives. Management has the responsibility to establish company policy in regard to health promotion and commit resources for staffing, program implementation, and evaluation. Conceptually, the successful program is an all-employee benefit that becomes visible through name identification and various in-house media.

Table 1. Health Promotion Strategies and Topic Areas

Strategy	Topic area
Contest and competitions	Exercise
Events	National Employee Fitness Day
Posting outcomes on bulletin boards	Smoking rates by departments
Paycheck tip sheets	Heart disease prevention tips
Posters in all work locations	Healthy lifestyles
Incentives for behavior change—days off, trips, sports tickets	Smoking cessation
Peer leaders	Weight loss, exercise
Wellness articles in company newsletter	Immunizations
Videos at various work site locations	Back injury prevention
Speakers for small groups, e-mail	Stress management
Ongoing exercise/aerobic classes, Fitness Center, fitness trails	Fitness
Health screenings/risk counseling	Hypertension
Health fairs	Vision protection
Self-help materials, cookbooks, self-care books	Cholesterol management
Company policy	Smoking policy, healthy cafeteria, and vending machine choices

Innovative programming to promote health includes multicomponent programs, companywide awareness and policy efforts, peer group leaders or cheerleaders, teams and campaigns, flexible continually changing programs at the work location, visual aids, and incentives (Erfurt, Foote, & Heirich, 1991). Health risk appraisals and screens, a health and fitness center, occupational health and safety professionals, creative interventionists, an employee assistance program, and a data management component are essential elements of successful work site programs.

Successful programs include analysis of available data to identify high-risk groups in the work site population, periodically report trends to the employer and employees, and project future health trends. Program directors cannot underestimate the data management component and need for a professional statistician from the beginning of the project. Small- and medium-sized companies should contract with a statistician to ensure that data-based evaluations of the project are available to the employer. Because of the capabilities of desktop computers, all companies can create databases with relevant measures of outcomes of the wellness program. Integration of health risk, medical claims, injury, physical performance, and personnel databases and the time invested in data management ensures a quality program. Strategic planning, implementation, evaluation, and communication among employer, worker, insurer, and occupational health and safety personnel are all dependent upon the data management effort.

Developing Work Site Health Promotion Programs

A number of strategies have been identified that can be recommended for successful work site health promotion programs. Each program would optimally include careful risk assessment, employee and supervisor participation in setting goals and identifying operational procedures, marketing, and implementing an ongoing variety of all-employee programs and programs targeted for high-risk groups. Other strategies include establishing passive interventions or company policy and evaluation with individual feedback as well as company and department trend information (Stokols *et al.*, 1995). Specifics on how to develop a successful work site health promotion program are included below.

Assess the Risk Factors in the Employee Population

Assessing the risk factors in a company involves gathering statistics regarding the demographics, medical claims costs, injury costs, health risks, and health promotion interests of the employee population. One should be attuned to the age, gender, socioeconomic status, and ethnic/racial distributions of the company work force. For example, an insurance company staffed with many computer operators, claims analysts, and clerical personnel may include a large proportion of females in childbearing years. Special initiatives directed at women's and children's health would need to dominate the health promotion programming. *Healthy People 2000* alerts us to disparities in health status among African Americans, Hispanics, and other minority groups; companies with large minority populations would direct their health promotion and disease prevention programs to reducing cardiovascular risks. A workplace with low turnover and mature workers may need to focus on issues regarding cancer awareness, prevention, and early detection.

Administrative data including medical claims costs for hospitalizations and ambulatory services are available through the company's insurer. The managers of the personnel benefits department and occupational health services should request insurer information about the company's top five to ten medical costs to identify target areas for the health promotion and disease prevention effort. Other data including absenteeism, injury costs, workers' compensation claims analysis, and evaluative data from observations and consultant walk-throughs of the work site can be helpful in setting priority areas for prevention.

Results from health risk appraisal questionnaires and physiological measurement of individual employees also can be aggregated to create information about health risks of the employee population. Individual reports, reports by department, and overall population statistics can help target departments, identify prevalent risks, and offer feedback to individuals regarding the areas they need to change. Health risk appraisal and company trend reports also can be used to motivate behavior change. Work site screenings are necessary because these data usually cannot be obtained from employees' primary care providers. To optimally care for employees with significant findings at the screen, the work site health screening staff should refer and follow-up to ascertain whether these employees subsequently participated in recommended primary care services. One advantageous combined approach would involve the employee seeking primary care services to obtain physiological data, submitting that data to the work site wellness program, and subsequently participating in the work site screen for a thorough health risk appraisal.

Confidentiality of data is an employee concern that is often addressed by the use of vendors. For example, the city of Birmingham contracts health promotion and data management services with the School of Nursing at the University of Alabama at Birmingham. In this way, health risk appraisal data are located offsite, and supervisors do not have access to individual data. Aggregate data only should be provided to supervisors, department heads, and managers in the form of trends and analysis reports. Individual personalized health risk appraisal results with comparisons over a 5-year period can be used to promote behavior change and should be returned to employees in confidential sealed envelopes.

Employee surveys, in which employees indicate their health promotion interests or intent to participate in programs, are the least reliable mechanism for gaining participation in health promotion programs. Thorough marketing efforts and special challenging programs, conveniently located at the individual's work site, may be more effective than surveys.

Set Goals, Mission, Resources

Strategic planning includes setting companywide goals to direct health promotion programming. Managers, worker representatives, and occupational health professionals can use *Healthy People 2000* (USDHHS, 1991) and data previously described to determine plans for the next year and beyond. A mission statement, objectives, and assigned responsibilities are developed. For example, one objective may be to offer a 6-week cholesterol reduction campaign each year over the next 3 years in four different departments.

To fully develop a program, management commitment must be strong and work site health policies should be developed. Establishing an annual budget to support the program is essential. In addition, a committee of employee volunteers from the work force in all departments and managers, who may be cheerleaders for the wellness effort, should meet monthly. Some time also must be devoted to identifying effective interventions, community resources, speakers, and resource materials that represent the best materials for each area. Planning, with employee assistance program staff, medical providers, and insurers, will result in new insights and coordinated, innovative programming.

The feasibility of offering programs and events on work time, at lunch time, and before or after work should be explored. Consider short programs offered at the time clock, at new employee screening, annual evaluations, when new personnel or product procedures are being introduced, or at the health screening. Programs offered on company time or involving strong incentives are more likely to be well attended than those offered on employee time.

Implementation

Implementation of work site health promotion may include many of the activities listed in Table 2. An emphasis should be placed on creative programming and large group efforts. Plan to go to the employees at their work sites and training or staff meetings rather than expect them to come to a central location for health promotion. The goal is to establish a work site wellness culture with multiple initiatives that are visible, fun, encouraging, and rewarding. A steady stream of events, messages, partial copayment for self-help programs, health insurer newsletters, and reminders for preventive services create a positive approach to change. Workplace changes in cafeteria foods, vending machines, no-smoking policy, and fitness trails promote health without placing the entire burden for health promotion on the indi-

Table 2. Smoking Cessation Strategies at the Work Site

Smoke-free workplace policy
No cigarettes in vending machines
Health risk appraisals with smoking status questions
Advise all smokers to quit
Determine smoker's willingness to quit
Motivate to promote quit attempts
Encourage nicotine replacement therapy
Provide self-help materials, nicotine replacement starter kits
Work site system to identify smokers, document attempts to quit
Individual and group counseling advice on successful quitting
Follow-up contact in person or telephone
Pamphlets, booklets, audiotapes, videotape library
Smoking cessation campaigns with incentives
Posters, tip sheets on hazards of smoking
Social support from ex-smoker or telephone support hotline
Referral to smoking cessation community groups
Reimbursement for smoking cessation treatments

---

vidual. Support and encouragement from a company culture makes it more likely that the individual will succeed.

Evaluation

The most successful work site health promotion programs are those that plan from the beginning to evaluate their outcomes. The strongest plan is one in which you create an integrated database of individual health risk data, injury data, absenteeism data, and medical claims data. Impact evaluation measures of health care utilization, health costs, and absenteeism are also important elements. Because health outcome data would not be available in the administrative data from insurers, the health promotion program instead must plan to directly obtain measurable data immediately following an intervention or at regularly scheduled screenings to determine smoking rates, exercise participation, weight, and so forth. Try to get physiological measures (e.g., fitness levels of police officers) rather than self-report.

Specific Work Site Health Promotion Initiatives

Smoking cessation and stress management are two initiatives that are especially important for work site health promotion. Specific strategies for individual and group interventions for smoking cessation are included in Table 2.

Smoking Cessation

Tobacco use is the major cause of mortality in the United States, accounting for 400,000 deaths per year and contributing to unnecessary cancer, heart disease, stroke, and chronic obstructive lung disease morbidity. Smoking cessation should be the priority initiative for most work site health promotion programs. Approximately 25% of Americans still smoke despite scientific evidence and widespread publicity regarding its health effects. The increasing prevalence of smoking among adolescents is adding every day to the numbers addicted to tobacco.

In the past two decades, health behavior experts have developed improved interventions and further understanding of smoking cessation. Nicotine replacement therapy, self-help kits, work site interventions, and no-smoking policies have become highly regarded interventions. In addition, clinicians acknowledge that smokers usually engage in a lengthy cessation process that may involve multiple quit attempts and relapses.

With mounting scientific evidence regarding the dangers of secondhand smoke, work site policies against smoking have proliferated. Employers, nonsmokers, and health care providers have supported organizational efforts to control smoking. Smokers have responded by attending employer-sponsored smoking cessation programs before and subsequent to the initiation of no-smoking policies.

Recently, an expert panel convened by the Agency for Health Care Policy and Research disseminated clinical practice guidelines on smoking cessation (Fiore *et al.*, 1996). The following work site health promotion recommendations were adapted from the clinical practice guidelines:

1. Effective smoking cessation treatments are available, and work site programs should alert employees about nicotine replacement therapy, social support programs, and self-help aids and techniques on achieving and maintaining abstinence and provide access to one or more of these treatments for every employee who smokes.
2. Work site programs should document the tobacco-use status of every employee and provide targeted intervention programs for tobacco users.
3. During visits to the occupational health clinic, health providers should urge every smoker to quit and should develop a quit plan in collaboration with the smoker. A personalized, clear, and strong manner is most effective for conveying this message. After counseling and determination of a quit plan, the health care provider should schedule follow-up and telephone support. The guideline recommends that the smoking cessation intervention last as long as possible because the longer the person-to-person counseling or intervention, the more effective the treatment. Individual treatment of four to seven sessions has been found to be especially effective. Even brief counseling interventions (sessions lasting 3-10 minutes) have been found to be superior to no-contact interventions.
4. Finally, employers should encourage health insurance/managed care providers to offer smoking cessation treatments (both pharmacotherapy and counseling) as paid benefits to subscribers. With little or no cost barriers, smokers are more likely to attempt cessation interventions.

Stress Management

Another important initiative for work site health promotion is stress reduction. Recent downsizings, mergers, transfers, automation, and job redesigns are contributing to excessive stress in American workplaces (Stokols *et al.*, 1995). Although the influence of moderate stress is often negligible, high stress levels have been found to be correlated with absenteeism, heart disease, alcoholism, workplace violence, suicide, burnout, and job dissatisfaction. Stress refers to internal as well as external stimuli that demand biophysiological adaptation. Multiple stress-producing situations occur on the job, including multiple demands, quotas and rush deadlines, difficult co-workers, job redesign and layoffs, isolated work conditions, limited resources, uncomfortable temperatures, noise, and hazardous work conditions requiring constant vigilance. Other occupational stresses include having more work than can be managed, monotonous jobs, feeling devalued, job ambiguity, lack of performance feedback, poor supervision, and shiftwork. On a more personal note, external stresses such as holidays, aged parents, child and teen issues, taxes, finances, and transportation problems also contribute to the stress quotient.

Signs and symptoms of high levels of stress include increased use of sick time, increased injuries, decreased productivity and quality of work, decreased use of vacation time, negativism, dissatisfaction, emotionality, increased turnovers, substance abuse, and hypertension. Employees in high work demand and low control jobs such as air traffic controllers, clerical workers, and production workers are among those groups of workers who experience high levels of occupational stress.

Work site health promotion interventions at both the individual level and organizational level are appropriate to address occupational stress (Murphy, 1996). Work site sports/fitness programs and stress management programs that emphasize progressive muscle relaxation, imagery, time management, and assertiveness have been found to be helpful work site interventions. Individual counseling regarding the need to play, laugh, exercise, participate in hobbies, listen to music, and not take work home may assist some employees to control stress in their lives.

At the organizational level, employee involvement and management support are essential to control stress. Employee groups who best know the jobs should negotiate and determine reasonable workloads. Job rotation, frequent breaks, and cross-training are interventions that have the potential to minimize monotony, isolation, and uncomfortable conditions. Ergonomic redesign is useful to improve lighting, ventilation, and noise control and reduce hazards. Company newsletters, supervisors trained in stress management techniques, and social activities such as picnics, bowling teams, and recognition luncheons also promote positive well-being at the work site. Relocation services to assist employees whose jobs are transferred or eliminated should be available. Finally, employers and occupational health professionals can rely on contracted employee assistance programs that provide onsite stress management programs and offsite confidential treatment for troubled employees and their families. Ongoing evaluations and investigations are needed to determine the effectiveness of stress management strategies for the occupational setting.

Conclusions

In the future, work site health promotion programs will expand to reach more American workers, and successful programs will serve as models for companies in the United States and internationally. The next avenue for promoting health will involve innovations that reach spouses or dependents of workers through home mailings, invitations to participate in programs, and incentives for family health. Incentives programs will be developed that provide monetary rewards for employees and their families who actively work to control personal risk levels. Administrative efforts, such as nonsmoking policies and required demonstrations of physical abilities to perform essential job functions, will become more common. Management will assume a more aggressive position in employee health matters and a more active role in health promotion activities. More demands will be placed on the work force to adopt health behaviors that will reduce health care costs. We will have a greater understanding of cultural influences on health promotion and disease prevention and more health promotion materials that incorporate cultural influences and strategies. Coordination of work site health promotion programs with health insurers and occupational safety programs will continue to evolve into collaborative targeted plans. Finally, goal setting in all health promotion programs will improve, with increased emphasis on data collection and better integration of databases to measure outcomes from our work site health promotion effort.

References

Angotti, C., & Levine, M. (1994). Review of five years of a combined dietary and physical fitness intervention for control of serum cholesterol. *Journal of the American Dietetic Association, 94*, 634–638.

Baer, J. (1993). Improved plasma cholesterol levels in men after a nutrition education program at the worksite. *Journal of the American Dietetic Association, 93*, 658–663.

Blue, C., & Conrad, K. (1995). Adherence to worksite exercise programs: An integrative review of recent research. *American Association of Occupational Health Nurses Journal, 43*(2), 76–86.

Brown, K., Hilyer, J., Artz, L., Glasscock, L., & Weaver, M. (1995). The Birmingham Good Health Program: Meeting Healthy People 2000 objectives. *Health Values: Journal of Health Behavior, Education, and Promotion, 19*, 45–53.

Connell, C., Sharpe, R., & Gallant, M. (1995). Effect of a health risk appraisal on health outcomes in a university worksite health promotion trial. *Health Education Research, 10*(2), 199–209.

Dolinsky, A., & Caputo, R. (1991). An assessment of employers' experiences with HMOs: Factors that make a difference. *Health Care Management Review, 16*, 25–31.

Eddy, J., Fitzhugh, E., Wojtowicz, G., & Wang, M. (1997). The impact of worksite-based safety belt programs: A review of the literature. *American Journal of Health Promotion, 11*(4), 281–289.

Erfurt, J., & Foote, A. (1991). The cost-effectiveness of worksite wellness programs for hypertension control, weight loss, and smoking cessation. *Journal of Occupational Medicine, 33*(9), 962–970.

Erfurt, J., Foote, A., & Heirich, M. (1991). Worksite wellness programs: Incremental comparisons of screening and referral alone, health education, follow-up counseling, and plant organization. *American Journal of Health Promotion, 5*(6), 438–448.

Fielding, J., Knight, K., Goetzel, R., & Laouri, M. (1991). Utilization of preventive health services by an employed population. *Journal of Occupational Medicine, 33*, 985–990.

Fielding, J., Knight, K., Mason, T., Klesges, R., & Pelletier, K. (1994). Evaluation of the IMPACT blood pressure program. *Journal of Occupational Medicine, 36*(7), 743–746.

Fielding, J., Mason, T., Knight, K., Klesges, R., & Pelletier, K. (1995). A randomized trial of the IMPACT worksite cholesterol reduction program. *American Journal of Preventive Medicine, 11*, 120–123.

Fiore, M., Bailey, W., Cohen, S., Dorfman, S. F., Goldstein, M., Gritz, E., Heyman, R., Holbrook, J., Jaen, C., Kottke, T., Lando, H., Mecklenberg, R., Mullen, P., Nett, L., Robinson, L., Stitzer, M., Tommasello, A., Villejo, L., & Wewers, M. (1996). *Smoking cessation clinical practice guideline no. 18.* AHCPR Publication No. 96-0692. Rockville, MD: US DHHS, Public Health Service, Agency for Health Care Policy and Research.

Foote, A., & Erfurt, J. (1991). Benefit to cost ratio of work-site blood pressure control programs. *Journal of the American Medical Association, 265*(10), 1283–1286.

Fries, J., Bloch, D., Harrington, H., Richardson, B., & Beck, R. (1993). Two-year results of a randomized controlled trial of a health promotion program in a retiree population: The Bank of America study. *American Journal of Medicine, 94*, 455–462.

Glanz, K., Sorenson, G., & Farmer, A. (1996). The health impact of worksite nutrition and cholesterol intervention programs. *American Journal of Health Promotion, 11*(2), 109–111.

Golaszewsik, T., Snow, D., Lynch, W., Yen, L., & Solomita, B. (1992). A benefit-to-cost analysis of a work-site health promotion program. *Journal of Occupational Medicine, 34*, 1164–1172.

Gold, M. (1991). HMOs and managed care. *Health Affairs, 4*, 189–206.

Goldbeck, W. (1984). Foreword. In M. O'Donnell & T. Ainsworth (Eds.), *Health promotion in the workplace* (p. v). New York: John Wiley and Sons.

Gomel, M., Oldenburg, B., Simpon, J., & Owen, N. (1993). Worksite cardiovascular risk reduction: A randomized trial of health risk assessment, education, counseling and incentives. *American Journal of Public Health, 83*, 1231–1238.

Harrell, J., Cornetto, A., & Stutts, N. (1992). Cardiovascular risk factors in textile workers. *American Occupational Health Nurses Journal, 40*, 581–589.

Hartman, T., McCarthy, P., & Hime, J. (1993). Use of eating pattern messages to evaluate changes in eating behavior in a worksite cholesterol education program. *Journal of the American Dietetic Association, 93*, 1119–1123.

Hartman, T., Himes, J., McCarthy, P., & Kushi, L. (1995). Effects of a low fat, worksite intervention on blood lipids and lipoproteins. *Journal of Occupational and Environmental Medicine, 37*(6), 690–696.

Harvey, M., Whitmer, R., Hilyer, J., & Brown, K. (1993). The impact of a comprehensive medical benefit cost management program for the city of Birmingham: Results at five years. *American Journal of Health Promotion, 7*, 296–303.

Health Care Financing Administration. (1996). *1996 HCFA statistics*. US Bureau of Data Management. HCFA Publication No. 03394. Baltimore, MD: Health Care Financing Administration, US DHHS.

Heaney, C., & Goetzel, R. (1997). A review of health-related outcomes of multi-component worksite health promotion programs. *American Journal of Health Promotion, 11*(4), 291–307.

Hennrikus, D., & Jeffery, R. (1996). Worksite intervention for weight control: A review of the literature. *American Journal of Health Promotion, 10*(6), 471–498.

Hilyer, J., & Artz, L. (1992). Physical fitness for emergency responders. In L. Andrews (Ed.), *Emergency responders training manual* (pp. 443–472). Center for Labor Education and Research. New York: Van Nostrand Reinhold.

Hilyer, J., Brown, K., Sirles, A., & Peoples, L. (1990). A flexibility intervention to reduce the incidence and severity of joint injuries among municipal firefighters. *Journal of Occupational Medicine, 32*, 631–637.

Hodgson, T. (1992). Cigarette smoking and lifetime medical expenditures. *Milbank Quarterly, 70*, 81–125.

Jones, R., Bly, J., & Richardson, J. (1990). A study of a worksite health promotion program and absenteeism. *Journal of Occupational Medicine, 32*, 95–99.

Kingery, P., Ellsworth, C., Corbett, B., Bowden, R., & Brizzolara, J. (1994). High-cost analysis. A closer look at the case for work-site health promotion. *Journal of Occupational Medicine, 36*, 1341–1347.

Kizer, K., Pelletier, K., & Fielding, J. (1995). Work-site health promotion programs and health care reform. *Western Journal of Medicine, 162*, 467–468.

Kottke, T., Brekke, M., & Solberg, L. (1993). Making time for preventive services. *Mayo Clinic Proceedings, 68*, 785–791.

Leigh, J., & Fries, J. (1992). Health habits, health care use and costs in a sample of retirees. *Inquiry, 29*, 44–54.

Masur-Levy, P., Tavris, D., & Elsey, P. (1990). Cardiovascular risk changes in a worksite health promotion program. *Journal of the American Dietetic Association, 90*, 1427–1428.

McNeil, B., Pederson, S., & Gatsonis, C. (1992). Current issues in profiling quality of care. *Inquiry, 29*, 298–307.

Murphy, L. (1996). Stress management in work settings: A critical review of the health effects. *American Journal of Health Promotion, 11*(2), 112–135.

National Center for Health Statistics. (1996, October 4). Births and deaths: U.S. 1995. *Monthly Vital Statistics Report, 45*(3), Suppl. 2.

Norris, R., Carroll, D., & Cochrane, R. (1990). The effects of aerobic and anaerobic training on fitness, blood pressure, and psychological stress and well-being. *Journal of Psychosomatic Research, 34*(4), 367–375.

O'Donnell, M. (1994). Preface. In M. O'Donnell & J. Harris (Eds.), *Health promotion in the workplace* (p. ix). Albany, NY: Delmar.

Oldenburg, B., Owen, N., Parle, M., & Gomel, M. (1995). An economic evaluation of four work site based cardiovascular risk factor interventions. *Health Education Quarterly, 22*(1), 9–19.

Pelletier, K. (1993). A review and analysis of the health and cost-effective outcome studies of comprehensive health promotion and disease prevention programs at the worksite 1991–1993. *American Journal of Health Promotion, 8*, 50–62.

Pelletier, K. (1996). A review and analysis of the health and cost-effective outcome studies of comprehensive disease prevention and health promotion programs at the worksite: 1993–1995 update. *American Journal of Health Promotion, 10*(5), 380–388.

Roman, P., & Blum, T. (1996). Alcohol: A review of the impact of worksite health interventions on health and behavioral outcomes. *American Journal of Health Promotion, 11*(2), 136–149.

Schweikhart, S., & Strasser, S. (1994). The effective use of patient satisfaction data. *Topics in Health Information Management, 15*(2), 49–60.

Shephard, R. (1996). Worksite fitness and exercise programs: A review of methodology and health impact. *American Journal of Health Promotion, 10*(6), 436–452.

Stokols, D., Pelletier, K., & Fielding, J. (1995). Integration of medical care and worksite health promotion. *Journal of the American Medical Association, 273*(14), 1136–1141.

Thomas, S., & DeKeyser, F. (1996). Blood pressure. *Annual Review of Nursing Research, 15*, 3–22.

US Department of Health and Human Services. (USDHHS). (1991). *Healthy people 2000: National health promotion and disease prevention objectives.* Washington, DC: US Government Printing Office.

US Department of Health and Human Services. (USDHHS). (1993). *National survey of worksite health promotion activities.* Washington, DC: US Government Printing Office.

Ware, J., Snyder, M., & Wright, R. (1983). Defining and measuring patient satisfaction with medical care. *Evaluation and Program Planning, 6*, 247–263.

Weingarten, S., Stone, E., Green, A., Pelter, M., Nessim, S., Huang, H., & Kristopaitis, R. (1995). A study of patient satisfaction and adherence to preventive care practice guidelines. *American Journal of Medicine, 99*(6), 590–596.

Wennberg, J. (1992, Winter). Perspective: AHCPR and the strategy for health benefit packages for health promotion and health care reform. *Health Affairs, 4*, 67–71.

Widra, L, & Fottler, M. (1992). Determinants of HMO success: The case of complete health. *Health Care Management Review, 17*, 33–44.

Wolford, G., Brown, M., & McCool, B. (1993). Getting to go in managed care. *Health Care Management Review, 18*, 7–19.

Yen, L., Edington, D., & Witting, P. (1991). Associations between health risk appraisal scores and employee medical claims costs in a manufacturing company. *American Journal of Health Promotion, 6*, 46–54.

PART VII

Special Populations and Issues

CHAPTER 23

Promoting the Health of Women and Children

Lorraine V. Klerman

Introduction

The health of women and children is the result of interaction among many factors including genetic endowment, economic status, education, nutrition, physical and emotional environment, medical care, and personal behaviors. Too many Americans believe that their health is the responsibility of their physician or of the public health system. The truth is that much of the illness and injury experienced by Americans is the result of actions they have taken or not taken.

This is particularly true for women during their reproductive years (generally 15–44 years of age) and for infants, children, and adolescents, because these populations suffer less from the chronic diseases that require ongoing medical care. The personal health behaviors that affect the health of women and children include not only lifestyle behaviors, such as eating, exercise, smoking, and drinking, but also effective and timely seeking of medical care, compliance with the recommendations of health care providers, avoidance of safety hazards, and political action to improve the environment.

Sweat and Denison (1995), in a review of human immunodeficiency virus (HIV) interventions, noted that modification of individual-level factors dominates most prevention efforts and urged the incorporation of superstructural, structural, and environmental factors into prevention programs. The same can be said of many other health promotion interventions. These health-influencing factors are often not considered in the development of health promotion and disease prevention programs. However, without system changes, health promotion strategies are less likely to be successful or optimally effective.

Because health promotion and disease prevention activities for women and children cover a wide array of behaviors, the author has chosen to use examples from each of four periods in the lives of women and children. This chapter will examine each of

Lorraine V. Klerman • Department of Maternal and Child Health, School of Public Health, UAB Center for Health Promotion, University of Alabama at Birmingham, Birmingham, Alabama 35294.

Handbook of Health Promotion and Disease Prevention, edited by Raczynski and DiClemente. Kluwer Academic/Plenum Publishers, New York, 1999.

these examples in terms of the factors that influence whether the individual chooses to perform the health-enhancing activity or to avoid the health-reducing one. While the conventional individual-level problems, such as fear, insufficient or inaccurate information, and inadequate motivation, will be described, considerable attention will be given to system-level problems, such as health system barriers and legislation and regulation.

The Preconception Period: Prevention of Unintended Pregnancies and Births

The prevention of an unintended pregnancy or birth is an important activity in women's lives. The average age of menarche is now between 12 and 13, and most women remain fertile though the middle or late 40s. Sexual activity for many women starts relatively early: 10% have had their first sexual experience by age 15. By age 18, 52% of women are sexually experienced, and by age 20, 76%. Because the average age at marriage for women is now between 24 and 25, the average woman has a period of almost 12 years (between menarche and marriage) in which she should try to avoid out-of-wedlock pregnancies, which are the most likely to be unintended (Alan Guttmacher Institute, 1994).

Healthy People 2000 (Public Health Service, 1990), the federal Department of Health and Human Services' health promotion and disease prevention objections for the nation by the year 2000, has an objective in the area of unintended pregnancy: Reduce to no more than 30% the proportion of all pregnancies that are unintended.

Epidemiology of Unintended Pregnancy

Most studies use the definition of unintended pregnancy developed by the federal government for its periodic National Survey of Family Growth (NSFG). This definition includes both unwanted pregnancies, where the woman did not want this pregnancy at this time or at any time in the future, and mistimed pregnancies, where the woman wanted to become pregnant later. Pregnancies that were wanted earlier are grouped with intended pregnancies. While the NSFG only reports the pregnancy intendedness of women who have borne a live child and therefore its statistics reveal the number of unintended births, most studies include abortions among the unintended pregnancies. Including abortions, the Institute of Medicine study of unintended pregnancies concluded that in 1987, only 43% of pregnancies were intended at the time of conception. Of the 57% that were unintended, 20% were mistimed and resulted in live births, 8% were unwanted and also resulted in live births, and 29% were either mistimed or unwanted and were terminated by abortions (Brown & Eisenberg, 1995). Henshaw's (1998) analysis of the 1995 NSFG revealed that, excluding miscarriages, 49% of the pregnancies concluding in 1994 were unintended and that 54% of these unintended pregnancies ended in abortion.

Unintended pregnancies occur more often among women at both ends of the reproductive age range, among unmarried, poor, and minority women, and among those with less education. But unintended pregnancies are not unknown among women of all ages, marital statuses, and social classes. Women with unintended pregnancies are more likely than those with intended pregnancies to seek care late in pregnancy, to smoke, and possibly to drink during pregnancy. Children resulting from unwanted births are more likely to be neglected or abused (Brown & Eisenberg, 1995).

Health Promotion and Disease Prevention Strategies

Health System Barriers

Many studies have shown that adult women, as well as teenagers, have difficulty adhering to a contraceptive regimen. Some of this is due to health system issues, such as the cost of contraceptives and difficulty in accessing a family planning facility because of transportation or time problems. A related factor is the absence of a suitable contraceptive for most teenagers who have sex infrequently. In addition, access to abortions is severely limited in many states.

Legislation and Regulation

Legislation and regulation in the area of family planning reflect this nation's ambivalence about reproductive health care, particularly in relation to minors, unmarried women, and abortions. Several federal laws provide funds that enable low-income women to obtain family planning services free or at reduced cost; however, such services are not an entitlement except for women who are Medicaid eligible. This means that family planing services sometimes may be restricted.

Interestingly, the federal family planning act specifies that teenagers must be allowed to obtain contraceptive services at facilities that receive funds under this act. The Reagan administration tried to reduce teenage access through regulation, the so-called "squeal rule," which would have required clinics receiving federal family planning funds to advise parents if their children sought contraceptives. This proposed regulation never took effect, but many experts believe that during the period when it was being considered and even after it was withdrawn, adolescents were reluctant to attend family planning clinics because they did not want their parents to know that they were sexually active.

Although abortion is legal in all states because of the Supreme Court's decision in *Roe v. Wade*, many states have erected substantial legal barriers to its availability. These include, for adolescents, parental consent and, for women of any age, waiting periods and paternal notification. As a result of these actions and terrorist activities at abortion clinics, abortion facilities are not available in many areas. Many women must travel long distances if they want an abortion. Only 69% of women live in counties with an abortion provider (Matthews, Ribar, & Wilhelm, 1997).

Also, the Hyde amendment to the Medicaid law prohibits the use of federal Medicaid funds for an abortion. A few states use state funds, but many women find abortions unavailable because of their expense, including not only the medical cost but also time lost from work to travel to the clinic and have the procedure. More time is lost if the state requires a waiting period between a first, informational visit and the actual procedure. According to the *New York Times*, however, abortion rights advocates have been successful in many cases involving increased access to abortions that have been heard in state courts (Holmes, 1998).

Individual-Level Barriers

Fear. Fear of the possible side effects of several of the contraceptives is another barrier to family planning. Some women believe that the pill causes cancer. And many women, particularly adolescents, fear or find distasteful the pelvic examination required before contraceptives are prescribed. Another very realistic fear is of confrontation with members of "Right to Life" groups at abortion facilities. While the Supreme Court has ruled that such activities can be limited, they have not been eliminated and such harassment can be a deterrent to seeking abortions. The violence experienced by several abortion clinics also may add to discomfort.

Information and Education. The level of incorrect information among many adolescents is very high and many adult women are also relatively uninformed about pregnancy and birth prevention. Adolescents often believe that they are too young to become pregnant or that if they have escaped pregnancy after the first few acts of intercourse that they are infertile. Despite the high rates of teenage pregnancies and births, many school systems refuse to allow family life education programs in schools. Even in those school systems that allow such health education programs, they often start too late, for example, in senior high school after a large percentage of the youth have initiated sexual activity; or a school board may restrict what can be taught, particularly methods of contraception, which is what most youth want to learn. Discussion of abortion as an option is unthinkable in many school systems. Increasing attention is also being paid to the issue of intelligence and literacy. It is very possible that some women do not understand the instructions that they are given in regard to the use of contraceptives (Parker, Williams, Baker, & Nurss, 1996).

Motivation. Many of the reasons given in response to survey questions suggest a lack of motivation for family planning among both younger and older women. Although they may not want to raise a child, they may be unwilling to expend the considerable time, effort, and expense essential to avoid pregnancy or birth; or other activities may seem more important than avoiding pregnancy or birth. Teenagers are likely to say that they had intercourse because they did not want to hurt their boyfriend's feelings by saying "no." Teenagers and adult women also report becoming pregnant in order to maintain a relationship.

Most experts believe that family life education and easier availability of contraceptives and abortion are necessary but not sufficient conditions to the reduction of unintended births. What is also needed, particularly but not exclusively for teenagers, both men and women, is a vision of the future that would be more difficult or even impossible to attain if the woman became a mother.

Pregnancy Prevention Programs

Unintended births can be prevented by total or periodic abstinence, the proper and consistent use of contraceptives, and abortions. Abstinence should be encouraged among young teenagers. The federal government and many state governments are urging abstinence as the only way of preventing unintended pregnancies, as well as sexually transmitted diseases. A few school- and community-based programs have been successful in delaying sexual initiation among young teenagers, but they have had little success in achieving abstinence among teenagers who are already sexually active. Moreover, the programs that are the most effective in preventing pregnancies use a dual approach. They stress abstinence but also provide information about the effectiveness of various contraceptives, how to use them, and where to obtain them. The effective programs also use many behavioral techniques including role playing, peer modeling, personalizing risk information, and providing practice in communication skills, especially those related to refusal and negotiation (Kirby, 1997).

School-based or school-linked health centers are often considered an approach to the prevention of unintended pregnancies among adolescents. Although such centers have many other positive features, only a few demonstration projects have supported this assumption. One reason why many centers are unable to prevent pregnancies is their inability to prescribe and provide contraceptives on-site, usually because of the opposition of local school boards (Peak & McKinney, 1996).

In order to attract more teenagers to family planning clinics before they become pregnant, many such facilities now provide birth control pills or an initial Depo-Provera injection without a pelvic examination. The examination is conducted when they return after 3 months for additional pills or the next injection (Armstrong & Stover, 1994).

The difficulties encountered in trying to prevent pregnancies, presumably unintended, among teenagers was shown in a demonstration project that offered a monetary incentive to women under 18 years of age who already had one child if they would participate in a peer-support group. While the incentive of a dollar for each day they were not pregnant increased participation in the groups, it did not effect subsequent pregnancies (Stevens-Simon, Dolgan, Kelly, & Singer, 1997).

The Prenatal Period: Seeking Prenatal Care

Pregnant women are universally urged to seek prenatal care early, usually defined as within the first trimester, and to make and keep appointments according to the schedule developed by the American College of Obstetricians and Gynecologists, if they are at low risk. High-risk women are usually seen more often (American College of Obstetricians and Gynecologists, 1996). There seems little doubt that prenatal care received on this schedule and of high quality has reduced the rate of maternal morbidity and mortality. It may also have reduced the incidence of infants born with congenital anomalies or genetic conditions and of intrauterine growth-retarded infants, because interventions during pregnancy can prevent these conditions in women and their infants. There is little evidence, however, that even the best prenatal care can prevent spontaneous or induced preterm delivery; and the conditions associated with preterm delivery, including low birth weight, are the major causes of infant mortality and morbidity (Alexander & Korenbrodt, 1997). Infant mortality in this country has been significantly reduced over the past 30 years because interventions before and immediately following birth have made it possible to save infants born too soon and too little, who formerly would have died. *Healthy People 2000* (Public Health Service, 1990) also has an objective in the area of prenatal care: Increase to at least 90% the proportion of all pregnant women who receive prenatal care in the first trimester of pregnancy.

Epidemiology of Prenatal Care

Despite public education about the importance of prenatal care, in 1996, 4.0% of women who had live births started their care in the third trimester or received no care at all; 81.9% started care in the first trimester, and the remainder in the second.

But these figures hide some real problems in specific areas. For example, over 11% of mothers in the District of Columbia and in the Virgin Islands and over 6% in Arizona, Nevada, and New Mexico started care in the third trimester or received no care. Teenagers are less likely to start care early, as are black, Hispanic, and Native American women. The median number of visits was 12.3 (Ventura, Martin, Curtin, & Mathews, 1998).

Health Promotion and Disease Prevention Strategies

Health System Barriers

The 1988 Institute of Medicine report on prenatal care (Brown, 1988) listed financing as the major barrier to quantitatively adequate prenatal care. Women who believed that they would be unable to pay for prenatal care and/or intrapartum care (labor and delivery) did not seek care at all, sought it late, or did not make and keep the recommended number of appointments. Other health systems barriers suggested in the report were inadequate transportation, long waiting periods in offices and clinics, limited provider availability, and dislike of physicians. Financial barriers have been reduced since the federal govenrment required states to provide Medicaid coverage for prenatal care and labor and delivery for all women with family incomes up to 133% of the federal poverty level and up to 185% at state option. Some states have chosen to cover women at over the 200% level.

Legislation and Regulation

Women are not required by law to obtain prenatal care nor is prenatal care a right except for those eligible for Medicaid. But, as noted below, laws and regulations regarding drug abuse and child abuse may cause women to hesitate before seeking care.

Individual-Level Barriers

Fear. Fear of prenatal care per se is not usually a major barrier, although dislike of some obstetrical procedures, including those involving the taking of blood samples, may delay care. Fear of having others learn that they are pregnant, however, does appear to delay seeking care. This is a particular problem for teenagers, whose concern is usually about their parents' reaction, but may also be about their partner's; but unmarried women may also experience this fear.

Another type of fear is related to cultural beliefs. Women in some cultures may not feel that it is appropriate to be cared for by a male (Byrd, Mullen, Selwyn, & Lorimor, 1996). Still another type of fear is related to substance abuse. Smokers usually are aware that they will be strongly urged to stop smoking during pregnancy and after. Women who are heavy drinkers have the same concern. And, perhaps most important, women who use illegal drugs are not only concerned that they will be told to stop, but also that the health care providers may inform the police about their habits, and, what is usually the worst fear, that when their infants are born they will not be allowed to take them home. They will be considered unfit mothers, ones who may neglect or even abuse or allow others to abuse their children. In many states, children of drug abusers are placed in foster care by child protection agencies (Besharov, 1994). In some areas, pregnant drug abusers have been jailed in order to prevent them from "delivering an illegal drug" to their fetuses.

Information and Education. The absence of information or education about the importance of prenatal care is not a major barrier. Most women seem to know that they should seek care early and periodically, even those who do not. Women with low levels of education and those in some cultural subgroups, however, may be uninformed or unconvinced about the value of prenatal care, particularly early care. Some women believe that they need not seek care until "quickening," when the fetus starts to move. For most women, pregnancy is a healthy state and infants can be born healthy with little professional assistance. Thus, some women believe that they need not seek care unless something seems to be wrong, for example, they are not gaining weight, their ankles are swelling, or they have headaches. This attitude also probably accounts for the fact that with each succeeding pregnancy, unless there has been a pregnancy loss or a poor pregnancy outcome, women tend to seek care later. Having experienced one uneventful pregnancy, they believe that they know what they need to know and can care for themselves for much of the prenatal period.

Motivation. The major barrier to adequate prenatal care appears to be motivation. Women with unintended pregnancies, whether they be mistimed or unwanted, seek care later. It is reasonable that a women who actively is seeking to have a child will recognize her pregnancy quickly and seek care early and regularly to ensure the infant's health, while one who does not want to have a child at all or at that time may ignore the signs of pregnancy and procrastinate about seeking care. Lack of motivation may also take the form of denial. In a Missouri study, 15.1% of women who had given birth reported that early in pregnancy they had not wanted to think about being pregnant, had not wanted others to know about the pregnancy, or had not known that they were pregnant (Sable *et al.*, 1997.) Teenagers and very obese women, both of whom may have irregular menstrual cycles, may genuinely not realize that they are pregnant until several months have passed.

Infancy and Early Childhood: Immunization

Many of those reading this chapter have never experienced a group of diseases that were relatively commonplace at the turn of the century and for many years after. Measles, mumps, rubella (German measles), and pertussis (whooping cough) occur infrequently. Polio is close to being eradicated in this country. The decline in these diseases and others is due to the development and use of vaccines, starting with the smallpox vaccine. Smallpox is now eradicated from the entire world and vaccination to prevent it is no longer needed. Despite the availability of vaccines to prevent the common childhood illnesses, many children are not appropriately immunized.

Healthy People 2000 (Public Health Service, 1990) also has several objectives in the area of childhood immunization. One set of objectives calls for reducing to zero indigenous cases of the following vaccine-preventable diseases: diphtheria and tetanus (among people aged 25 and younger), polio (wild-type virus), measles, and rubella; and reducing mumps cases to 500 and pertussis cases to 1000. The objectives also call for increasing to at least 90% the percentage of children under age 2, and to at least 95% the percentage of children in licensed day care facilities and kindergarten through postsecondary education institutions, who have completed the basic immunization series.

Epidemiology of Immunizations

As a result of laws requiring immunization before entering school or day care, outbreaks of vaccine-preventable diseases are relatively infrequent in school age populations, with the exception of those populations that are exempt from these regulations because of religious beliefs, such as the Amish (Centers for Disease Control, 1991). In the late 1980s and early 1990s, however, there were several serious outbreaks of vaccine-preventable diseases, largely among preschool children. Most dramatically, in 1989 and 1990, there were 55,000 cases of measles and 132 measles-related deaths (Orenstein, Atkinson, Mason, & Bernier, 1990). Investigations by the Centers for Disease Control and Prevention and state and local health departments revealed that preschool children were often not up-to-date on their immunizations. Federal and state programs now stress that all children should be appropriately immunized by age 2.

Health Promotion and Disease Prevention Strategies

Health System Barriers

Once again, financing is an important barrier. Although in most areas, immunizations can be obtained free or on a sliding fee scale from health department clinics, some parents are dismayed by the high cost of immunizations in a private physician's office and in some areas there are no clinics.

Another health system barrier is inadequate record keeping. Children who are seen for well-child supervision almost always receive the immunization appropriate for their age. But children are often seen for illnesses or injuries and if their record does not clearly indicate that they are due for an immunization, the provider may care for the presenting complaint and not use the opportunity to immunize. Many clinics and health maintenance organizations (HMOs) now put the child's immunization record at the very top of the child's file or even on the file cover itself, in order not to miss an opportunity for immunization regardless of the reason for the visit.

Some clinics and private physicians have a policy not to provide immunizations except when the child is being seen for that purpose or for a well-child visit. In these cases, the parents of the children seen for other reasons are told to return later with the children for their immunization. This may or may not happen. If it does not, an opportunity has been wasted. Whether due to office convenience, that is, the office is not set up for an immunization at that time or there are time pressures, or even the desire to charge for an additional office visit, these policies should be changed (Taylor *et al.*, 1997)

Legislation and Regulation

For many years, all states have required that children be immunized before they enter school and usually before they enter a licensed child care facility. Up-to-date immunizations are required of all children in the federal Head Start program.

Individual-Level Barriers

Fear. Infrequently children have life-threatening or even fatal reactions to an immunization. The pertussis vaccine has been the one most likely to cause such reactions. The public health and medical professions believe that far more lives are saved as a result of vaccines than are lost and they continue to advocate immunization even while the pharmaceutical companies are developing vaccines with fewer side effects. Nevertheless, after the media described the problems with the pertussis vaccine, the number of children immunized dropped sharply. Concern about one vaccine often spreads to concerns about vaccines in general and leads to a failure to seek immunization.

Physicians' concern about parental reactions to multiple vaccinations may also lead to underimmunized children. When health professionals find that a child is behind on several immunizations, present guidelines call for giving multiple "shots," even though the child may protest. Public health professionals believe that if only one immunization is given and the parent is told to return later with the child for additional ones, that the parent may not keep the subsequent appointment. Rather than again risk underimmunization, multiple shots are recommended. Nevertheless, some physicians report that parents do not want to see their children endure the discomfort that such procedures involve and, rather than lose their patients, the physicians delay the additional immunizations needed.

Information and Education. Misinformation is a major barrier to up-to-date immunizations. If you ask the average parent whether immunizations are important for children, the overwhelming majority say "yes." Queried further, however, most would probably note that children should be immunized before attending school and that their physicians or clinics will notify them when their children need their "shots." Both of these statements are likely to be untrue. Immunizations are essential before age 2 and many physicians and clinics do not routinely remind parents of their children's need for immunization.

Inadequate provider information has also led to underimmunization. Many physicians and nurses have been reluctant to immunize a child who had an illness, a rash, or other conditions. Current guidelines indicate that the only major impediment to immunization is a child who is immunocomprised, that is, has an inadequate immune system.

Motivation. Lack of motivation is not a major reason for inadequate immunization. As noted earlier, most parents realize the important of this measure for their children and will seek it even when other barriers exist.

Immunization Promotion Programs

The concern aroused by the epidemics of 1989–1990 has created several new programs to increase immunization levels. Many state and local health departments now have reminder systems using postcards, letters, phone calls, and even home visits. Georgia has had success in increasing preschool immunizations using computer-generated telephone reminder and recall messages (Linkins, Dini, Watson, & Patriarca, 1994). Because many managed care monitoring systems use percentage of children appropriately immunized as a measure of the quality of care, many HMOs now use similar methods to ensure that their enrollees are immunized. Also, the federal government has increased its efforts to increase immunization rates through educational campaigns and financing and monitoring efforts, as well as additional assistance to states.

The British have achieved childhood immunization levels that are much higher than this country's partially by using a provider incentive system. Providers receive a minimum payment if at least 70% of all children in their practices due for immunizations during the quarter are immunized and a larger payment if their immunization rates are 90% or higher (Durch, 1994).

Late Childhood and Early Adolescence: Unintentional Injuries

The number one cause of death and hospitalization among children 5 to 14 years of age is injury. *Healthy People 2000* (Public Health Service, 1990) has many objectives related to unintentional injuries and to violence. Examples include: (1) increase use of occupant protection systems, such as safety belts, inflatable safety restraints, and child safety seats, to at least 85% of motor vehicle occupants; and (2) extend to 50 states laws requiring safety belt and motorcycle helmet use for all ages.

Epidemiology of Unintentional Injuries among Children and Adolescents

Motor vehicle crashes kill the most children, 5.4 deaths per 100,000 children aged 5 to 14 in 1996; but firearms, drowning, fire and burns, and suffocation together killed 3.6 per 100,000. Even more alarming is the fact that over half of the firearms deaths were homicides (Maternal and Child Health Bureau, 1998). Parents must assume most of the responsibility for the safety of young children; but by age 14, this responsibility is shared with the young adolescent.

Health Promotion and Disease Prevention Strategies

Health System Barriers

There are no health system barriers per se to the behaviors essential to prevent childhood injuries. However, parents who do not have easy access to physicians or clinics because of financial constraints or physical or cultural distance and children who are not served by adequate school health services may not receive the education essential to the development of preventive behaviors.

Legislation and Regulation

Legislation and regulation have been and continue to be very important in reducing injuries. Requirements for auto restraints have reduced crash injuries, fire-retardant clothing has reduced burns, window guards have reduced falls, and pool fencing has reduced drowning, to name just a few examples. More regulations and stricter enforcement of existing ones, including those related to gun control, would further reduce injuries.

Individual-Level Barriers

Fear. Fear is not a major reason for failure to adopt preventive behaviors by parents or children; in fact, a greater level of concern might increase preventive behaviors. In young adolescents, it may be the need to show oneself as fearless that leads to risky behaviors such as unsupervised swimming, riding a bicycle without a helmet, or playing with a firearm.

Information and Education. Periodically, the federal government adds a health promotion segment to its National Health Information Survey. The questions generally ask about behavior rather than information; nevertheless, the responses suggest that parents are either ill-informed or, if informed, are taking unnecessary risks. The 1990 survey revealed that approximately two-thirds of children under 17 years of age lived in households that claimed to have a functional smoke detector, but fewer than 10% lived in households where the water temperature was known to be below the level that would cause scalding. Less than half of children under 10 years of age lived in households that knew the number of the poison control center and only about a quarter in households that claimed to have ipecac syrup (poison control measures). Finally, less than three fifths of the children under 5 years of age were reported to always use a car safety seat (Mayer & LeClere, 1994).

Motivation. Lack of motivation to adopt injury-preventing behaviors appears to be the major impediment to reducing injuries among children and particularly among adolescents. While some children may still listen or be cajoled, bribed, or threatened into wearing bicycle helmets or using seat belts, adolescents frequently suffer from a feeling of invulnerability: "It can't (or won't) happen to me." Helping adolescents realistically assess danger is a challenge to parents, teachers, and group workers.

Injury Prevention Programs

Studies have shown that counseling about health-promoting activities by health care providers can increase injury prevention activities, yet teachable moments in a physician's office or clinic are often missed. For example, the American Academy of Pediatrics' Back to Sleep campaign appears to have reduced significantly the number of deaths due to sudden infant death syndrome (SIDS). Yet physicians report a reluctance to ask certain questions in their offices, such as about gun possession in the household or physical abuse of the mother (often associated with abuse of a child as well), that would enable them to detect and possibly prevent injury; or to offer anticipatory guidance about hazards such as drowning (O'Flaherty & Pirie, 1997).

Rivara and Grossman (1996) reviewed traumatic deaths in children between 1978 and 1991. Death rates for unintentional injuries decreased by 39% during that period. They believe that the application of currently available strategies could further reduce deaths significantly. Among the strategies that they suggest to reduce automotive-related injuries and deaths are child restraints, protection from side impacts, and measures to reduce car speed, decrease traffic volume, and move traffic away from residential areas. Bicycle helmet use would reduce trauma and death; fencing and latching of pools and adult supervision of children in or near water, including natural sites, pools, and bathtubs, would reduce drowning; self-extinguishing cigarettes, smoke detectors, and residential sprinkler systems would reduce fire-related injuries; and deaths due to carbon monoxide poisoning could be reduced by smoke and carbon monoxide detectors, adequate ventilation of heating equipment, inspection of motor vehicle exhaust systems, and not allowing children to ride in the back of enclosed pickup trucks.

Summary and Conclusions

This review of four areas in which personal behaviors could improve the health of women and children suggests several ways to encourage health-promoting action. The facts should make very clear that changing individual behavior is not totally dependent on education and information, regardless of how persuasive the message, how credible the individual or medium that delivers it, or how appropriate its theoretical basis. Many years ago health educators learned a lesson from industry, that it is more effective to modify the injury-producing machine than to educate the worker about how to avoid being injured by the machine. A barrier that prevents the worker from inserting his hand into a machine press to realign the piece being formed is more effective than instruction about why the hand should not be inserted.

Public health professionals who want to change the behaviors of reproductive age women, parents of both genders, and children should use a multifaceted approach. They should focus both on individual-level factors and system-level factors, or structural factors in Sweat and Denison's (1995) terms. If there are formidable financial or health system barriers to behaving in a health-promoting manner, these must be removed or at least reduced if education is to be effective. While no one wants to live in an overregulated society, reasonable legislation and regulation that require parents and adolescents to "do the right thing," while not convincing everyone, at least make the educational task easier. A law without education is often broken and education in the absence of a law is often ineffective.

It is essential to remember that it is not only parents and children who need education, it is providers as well. Pediatricians and other primary care practitioners for women and children need to be taught how to provide counseling that will improve health-related behaviors. Many find it difficult to ask questions or advise about gun possession, abuse, and similar matters. Attention to these issues in medical school, residencies, and continuing medical education programs would increase these important counseling activities. Additional consideration of cultural factors would also improve providers' ability to modify behavior.

Professionals in the maternal and child health field spend large amounts of time and effort trying to convince women, parents, children, and adolescents to avoid health-compromising behaviors and to adopt health-promoting ones. In the last few decades they have received much assistance from specialists in health behavior who have helped make their messages more effective. A notable example is the use of the stages of change approach in smoking cessation programs for pregnant women. Nevertheless, the field cannot place total responsibility on the adults and children whose behavior is to be molded. Doing so would be to "blame the victim." Maternal and child health practitioners must be alert to factors other than lack of information and education that influence behavior. Reducing structural barriers is as integral a part of health promotion as are educational efforts.

ACKNOWLEDGMENT. The preparation of this chapter was made possible, in part, by grant MCJ 9040 from the federal Maternal and Child Health Bureau.

References

Alan Guttmacher Institute. (1994). *Sex and America's teenagers.* New York: Author.

Alexander, G. R., & Korenbrodt, C. C. (1997). The role of prenatal care in preventing low birth weight. *Future of Children, 5,* 103–120.

American College of Obstetricians and Gynecologists. (1996). *Guidelines for women's health care.* Washington, DC: Author.

Armstrong, K. A., & Stover, M. A. (1994). Smart Start: An option for adolescents to delay the pelvic examination and blood work in family planning clinics. *Journal of Adolescent Health, 15,* 389–395.

Besharov, D. J. (Ed.). (1994). *When drug addicts have children.* Washington, DC: Child Welfare League of America.

Brown, S. S. (Ed.). (1988). *Prenatal care. Reaching mothers, reaching infants.* Washington, DC: National Academy Press.

Brown S. S., & Eisenberg, L. (Eds). (1995) *The best intentions. Unintended pregnancy and the well-being of children and families.* Washington, DC: National Academy Press.

Byrd, T. L., Mullen, P. D., Selwyn, B. J., & Lorimor, R. (1996). Initiation of prenatal care by low-income Hispanic women in Houston. *Public Health Reports, 111,* 536–540.

Centers for Disease Control. (1991). Outbreaks of rubella among the Amish. *Morbidity and Mortality Weekly Report, 40,* 264–265

Durch, J. S. (Ed.). (1994). *Overcoming barriers to immunization. A workshop summary.* Washington, DC: National Academy Press.

Henshaw, S. K. (1998). Unintended pregnancy in the United States. *Family Planning Perspectives, 30,* 24–29, 46.

Holmes, S. A. (1998). Right to abortion quietly advances in state courts. *The New York Times,* (12/6/98).

Kirby, D. (1997). *No easy answers: Research findings on programs to reduce teen pregnancy.* Washington, DC: National Campaign to Prevent Teen Pregnancy.

Linkins, R. W., Dini, E. F., Watson, G., & Patriarca, P. A. (1994). A randomized trial of the effectiveness of computer-generated telephone messages in increasing immunization visits among preschool children. *Archives of Pediatric and Adolescent Medicine, 148,* 908–914.

Maternal and Child Health Bureau. (1998). *Child Health USA 1998.* Washington, DC: US Government Printing Office.

Matthews, S., Ribar D., & Wilhelm, M. (1997). The effects of economic conditions and access to reproductive health services on state abortion rates and birthrates. *Family Planning Perspectives, 29,* 52–60.

Mayer, M. S., & LeClere, F. B. (1994). Injury prevention measures in households with children in the United States, 1990. *Advance Data from Vital and Health Statistics of the National Center for Health Statistics No. 250.* Hyattsville, MD: National Center for Health Statistics.

O'Flaherty, J. E., & Pirie, P. L. (1997). Prevention of pediatric drowning and near-drowning: A survey of members of the American Academy of Pediatrics. *Pediatrics, 99,* 169–174.

Orenstein, W. A., Atkinson, W., Mason, D., & Bernier, R. H. (1990). Barriers to vacinating preschool children. *Journal of Health Care for the Poor and Underserved, 1,* 315–330.

Parker, R. M., Williams, M.V., Baker, D. W., & Nurss, J. R. (1996). Literacy and contraception: Exploring the link. *Obstetrics and Gynecology, 88* (Suppl. 3), 72S–77S.

Peak, G. L., & McKinney, D. L. H. (1996). Reproductive and sexual health at the school-based/school-linked health center: An analysis of services provided by 180 clinics. *Journal of Adolescent Health, 19,* 276–281.

Public Health Service. (1990). *Healthy people 2000* (DHHS Publication No. (PHS) 91-5021). Washington, DC: US Government Printing Office.

Rivara, F. P., & Grossman, D.C. (1996). Prevention of traumatic deaths to children in the United States: How far we have come and where do we need to go? *Pediatrics, 97,* 791–797.

Sable, M. R., Spencer, J. C., Stockbauer, J. W., Schramm, W. F., Howell, V., & Herman, A. A. (1997). Pregnancy wantedness and adverse pregnancy outcomes: Differences by race and Medicaid status. *Family Planning Perspectives, 29,* 76–81.

Stevens-Simon, C., Dolgan, J. I., Kelly, L., & Singer, D. (1997). The effect of monetary incentives and peer support groups on repeat adolescent pregnancies. *Journal of the American Medical Association, 277*, 977–982.

Sweat M. D., & Denison J. A. (1995). Reducing HIV incidence in developing countries with structural and environmental interventions. *AIDS, 9* (Suppl. A), S251–S257.

Taylor, J. A., Darden, P. M., Slora, E., Hasemeier, C. M., Asmussen, L., & Wasserman, R. (1997). The influence of provider behavior, parental characteristics, and a public policy initiative on the immunization status of children followed by private pediatricians: A study from pediatric research in office settings. *Pediatrics, 99*, 209–215.

Ventura, S. J., Martin, J. A., Curtin, S. C., & Mathews, T. J. (1998). Report of final natality statistics, 1996. *Monthly Vital Statistics Report, 46* (No. 11, Suppl.). Hyattsville, MD: National Center for Health Statistics.

CHAPTER *24*

Adolescent Health Promotion and Disease Prevention

Ralph J. DiClemente and Brenda Cobb

Introduction

Adolescence has traditionally been conceptualized as a period of transition between childhood and adulthood. While adolescence is less studied and less understood than other developmental periods, activities that youth begin to experience during this transition have been described as risky behavior predisposing adolescents to injury and illness. Thus, the development of interventions to promote the adoption and maintenance of healthy behaviors requires a careful consideration of the developmental characteristics of adolescence.

In accomplishing the maturational transition from childhood to adolescence, increasing autonomy and identity formation are key developmental goals. For some youth, the need for social acceptance may outweigh the perceived dangers of participating in activities that place them in situations that could prove life-threatening. While risk taking among adolescents has been noted as a necessary process in the healthy development of youth (Jessor, 1991), many of these activities can also result in devastating consequences for the individual, their family and society in general.

This chapter describes the factors that contribute to the vulnerability of adolescents, reviews the characteristics of risky behaviors in which adolescents engage, and presents models that attempt to explain the initiation and maintenance of risky behaviors. Health promotion interventions designed to either prevent adolescents' involvement in risky behaviors or reduce negative consequences of these behaviors are also presented. And, finally, we describe directions for future research in the area of adolescent health promotion and disease prevention.

Ralph J. DiClemente • Department of Behavioral Sciences and Health Education, Rollins School of Public Health, Emory University, and Emory/Atlanta Center for AIDS Research, Atlanta, Georgia 30322. *Brenda Cobb* • School of Nursing, UAB Center for Health Promotion, University of Alabama at Birmingham, Birmingham, Alabama 35294.

Handbook of Health Promotion and Disease Prevention, edited by Raczynski and DiClemente. Kluwer Academic/Plenum Publishers, New York, 1999.

Sociodemographics of American Adolescents

The United States Bureau of the Census estimates that, as of December 1996, the number of youth between ages 10 and 19 years was almost 38 million, representing approximately 14% of the total US population; more than half (51%) were male. This number has grown by 1.2 million since 1990. Most of this growth is among teenagers 10 to 14 years. Further, the proportion of minorities has increased over the past six years (US Bureau of the Census, 1997a).

Family constellations have changed markedly over the past several decades. Children living in single-parent families have increased from 11.3% in 1970 to 24.5% in 1994; this change is most prominent among African Americans, changing from 33.6% in 1970 to 59.5% in 1994 (US Bureau of the Census, 1996a,b). These changes have been predominately toward a growing number of mother-only families and have implications for the availability of financial resources for youth. In 1995, the proportion of married persons with children under 18 years of age living in poverty was 8.7% compared with 44.8% of female-headed families with children (Baughner & Lamison-White, 1996). In 1995, 13.8% of the total population were living below poverty (Baughner & Lamison-White, 1996). Table 1 displays the ethnic/racial distribution by family type. Overall, poverty disproportionately plagues minority populations and female-headed households.

Children in married families among all ethnic/racial groups have a greater economic advantage relative to those from single-parent families. In addition to single-parent families, there also is an increasing number of mothers who work outside the home (Bianchi, 1995), creating opportunities for youth to participate in risky activities as a result of a lack of parental supervision during large portions of the day.

The poverty rate for children under the age of 18 was 20.8%, higher than any other age group (Baughner & Lamison-White, 1996) and has increased from 17.1% in 1975 (US Bureau of the Census, 1997b). While the majority of poor children are white, the rates for whites are markedly lower (11.7%) relative to African American (42%) and Hispanic (40%) children (Baughner & Lamison-White, 1996). Youth under 18 years of age were particularly vulnerable in the South, as this region had the highest poverty rates for this age group (23.5%).

Poverty may not, in and of itself, create a risk factor for adolescents' participation in risky activities. However, poverty can force families to live in neighborhoods in which there is a high prevalence of crime, violence, and substance use, which may negatively impact the development of youth (Brooks-Gunn, Duncan, Klebanov, & Sealand, 1993; Crane, 1991). Approximately 5% of all children in the United States live in poor neighborhoods [US Department of Health and Human Services (USDHHS),

Table 1. Ethnic/Racial Distribution by Family Type

	Caucasian	African American	Hispanic
Population below poverty level	11.2%	29.3%	30.3%
Two-parent families below poverty level	9.6%	28.5%	29.2%
Single-parent families below poverty level	29.7%	48.2%	52.8%
Youth < 18 years old below poverty level	16.2%	41.9%	40.0%
Married couple with child < 18 years old	7.0%	9.9%	22.6%
Female head of household with child < 18	35.6%	53.2%	7.3%

1996a]. Those most vulnerable are African-American children and youth who live in single-parent households.

Adolescent Mortality and Morbidity

Mortality rates for the US population have generally declined. However, this decline has not been as marked for youth 5–24 years of age (Rosenberg, Ventura, Maurer, Heuser, & Freedman, 1996). In fact, the overall mortality rate for youth has changed little over the past 15 years (Singh & Yu, 1996). However, mortality rates vary markedly by gender and ethnicity/race. While the mortality rate for females declined approximately 45% between 1950 and 1993, this was not the case for males. Analysis of the effects of ethnicity/race indicated that, in 1950, there was a significant racial difference among males, with mortality rates for African-American males twice as high as that of white males. Although this disparity narrowed through the 1960s and 1970s, in 1984, the difference again began to increase. Mortality for females followed a similar ethnicity/racial pattern, but was not as marked as that of males.

The leading cause of adolescent death is accidental injury; 75% of the deaths due to injury are the result of a motor vehicle accident (Rosenberg *et al.*, 1996). However, while injury mortality due to accidents (motor vehicle and non–motor vehicle) have declined since 1968, death rates due to firearm injuries, homicide, and suicide have increased annually at 1.91%, 2.18%, and 1.85%, respectively (Singh & Yu, 1996). Mortality rates for US youth are higher than those in other industrialized countries, primarily due to factors related to violence (Singh & Yu, 1996), with African Americans and Hispanics between 15 and 24 years of age at greatest risk for homicide (Singh, Kochanek, & MacDorman, 1996). Moreover, it is estimated that for every fatal injury due to violence, there are about 100 nonfatal injuries (US Department of Justice, 1988). Motor vehicle accidents, other unintentional injury, homicide, and suicide contribute to 72% of the mortality of youth 5 to 24 years of age (Centers for Disease Control, 1996).

Mortality rates for male adolescents are significantly higher than that of females, with greater than a 2:1 male–female ratio for youth 10 to 19 years of age and greater than a 3:1 ratio for those 20 to 24 years of age (US Department of Health and Human Services, 1996b). African-American males are disproportionately affected. While mortality rates for other groups have remained fairly stable, rates for African Americans ages 15 to 24 years continue to rise (Singh *et al.*, 1996). This is particularly true for homicide mortality rates, which has reached epidemic proportions for Afrcian-American adolescents.

Morbidity data on nonfatal injuries have been more difficult to quantify. Most of this information is gathered through data collected from hospital emergency departments (Gallagher, Finison, Guyer, & Goodenough, 1984) or self-report (Cobb, Cairns, Miles, & Cairns, 1995). Studies have suggested that nonfatal injuries for youth occur more often in males versus females (Cobb *et al.*, 1995; Scheidt *et al.*, 1995) and severity generally increases with age (Scheidt *et al.*, 1995). Among the major contributing factors to nonfatal injuries for 10- to 17-year-old males and females is their participation in sports activities, being struck, cut, or falling (Scheidt *et al.*, 1995). Motor vehicle accidents are also cited as a contributing factor to nonfatal injuries among youth, particularly males (Cobb *et al.*, 1995).

Many of the negative health consequences reflected in both mortality and morbidity statistics have been the result of youth participating in risk taking. These activities have been characterized as posing some form of potential danger to their health and well-being. Youth often engage in these activities while in a state of intoxication or other mind-altered state, thus escalating the possibility for negative outcomes.

To understand the complex interpaly between a host of environmental, intrapersonal, and interpersonal factors, a number of theroetical models of adolescents' risk behavior have been developed and tested. Below we briefly review some of these models and key constructs.

Models of Adolescent Risk Behavior

Risky behavior has been described as activities that have the potential for some type of loss (Furby & Beyth-Maron, 1990). Many conceptual models have been used to frame studies of adolescent risk behavior and the issues surrounding this period of development. Empirical work on adolescent risk behavior involves the search for linkages between characteristics of the individual and the contextual factors that create their living environment, such as biopsychosocial factors, ecological factors, and cultural norms.

Legal statutes in the United States help to create an age-appropriate behavior trajectory that defines when specific activities can be safely negotiated by youth. However, in their attempt to push the boundaries established for them, young people have been known to frequently break the legal lines that were drawn for their protection. In addition, laws also have been established to define the excesses of a particular activity for all groups in society, such as blood alcohol level and speed limit, which could result in dangerous consequences.

Some researchers suggest that we should not assume adolescents have less ability to distinguish between potential negative and positive outcomes than adults (Shaklee & Fishoff, 1990). Misunderstandings such as those pertaining to human immunodeficiency virus (HIV) risk have been known to fluctuate across socioeconomic and ethnic groups (Anderson et al., 1990; DiClemente, Boyer, & Morales, 1988), but differences pertaining to perception of risk of negative experiences did not vary between 18- and 65-year-old study participants (Weinstein, 1987). Therefore, it is more likely that poor judgment is based on misperceptions of the potential consequences rather than magical thinking (Quadral, Fishoff, & Davis, 1993).

It is difficult for youth to imagine images far into their future that are less than ideal. Studies have shown that adolescents are more concerned with consequences that affect their immediate lives as opposed to the remote possibility of long-term outcomes (Kegeles, Adler & Irwin, 1988; Greening & Dollinger, 1991). In their efforts to establish themselves as a person separate from their family and have an identity with which they feel comfortable, youth will sometimes appear "on the fringe." The troubling part of this is that this need for adolescents to appear unconventional has been linked to participation in problem behaviors (Jessor & Jessor, 1977).

Piaget described the cognitive development of adolescents as a transition from "formal operations" to abstract and socially focused thinking (Flavell, 1963). A lack of practical experience in applying this method of decision making results in immaturity, a key antecedent in adolescents' perceived invulnerability: a denial that the risks apply to them (Millstein & Irwin, 1988). On the other hand, youth can be expected to participate in some aspect of risky behavior (Elliott, 1993). Jessor (1991) has explained that participating in risk-taking behavior has a developmental and maturational advantage. Many of the risky activities will provide a mechanism for youth to explore their abilities to function within the adult world. In addition, participating in activities such as smoking, drinking alcohol, and risky driving may be viewed as a developmental task in which youth explore the world (Jessor, 1982). Through participating in such activities, they gain respect from their peers and autonomy from parental control and other types of authority; risk taking also helps them establish their identity and marks their passage from childhood toward becoming an adult (Jessor, 1991). In their psychosocial development, adolescents look toward their peers for guidance in their attempts to gain independence from their family (Millstein & Irwin, 1988).

Irwin and Millstein (1986) synthesized risk activities into a biopsychosocial model to explain the interrelationships among risk-taking behaviors. They posit that biological maturation affects adolescent's psychosocial functioning in terms of their (1) cognitive ability, (2) perception of themselves, (3) perception of their social environment, and (4) personal values. These factors, in turn, affect who they choose as their peer group and their perceptions of risk and serve as mediating factors for risk-taking behavior.

Biological Domain

The biological domain is a key factor in adolescent development, particularly in light of the hormonal surges that begin to occur (Udry, 1990). Development of individuals that is not in synch with their peers can create a myriad of difficulties. The adoption of adultlike behaviors by early-maturing young women has been associated with their involvement in cigarette smoking, alcohol drinking (Brooks-Gunn, 1988), and sexual intercourse (Brooks-Gunn, 1988; Phinney, Jensen, Olsen & Cundick, 1990). These behaviors prove a greater risk for young adolescents who likely do not have the psychosocial skills to negotiate protective behaviors and who are known to take chances that may pose a threat to their well-being (Millstein *et al.*, 1992). Using testosterone as a primary force in the biological domain that affects behavior, Udry (1990), in his biosocial model of problem behaviors in male adolescents, found that, when analyzed separately, social and biological variables contributed the same amount of variance to male problem behavior (24%) (Udry, 1994). However, analysis of the combination of social and biological variables yielded a much different picture: 30% of the variance in male problem behavior was explained with the social variables contributing only 6% of that variance. Although social situations and opportunities create a pathway for biological expression, the adolescent's biological mechanisms help to create those situations and opportunities.

Other biological substances, such as adrenaline, have been implicated as predictive in long-term criminal behavior (Magnusson, Klinteberg, & Stattin, 1994). The hypothesis of a genetic link to alcoholism has been supported by study findings that suggest the propensity for children of alcoholics to abuse alcohol more often than children of nonalcoholics (Adger, 1991; Marlatt, Baer, Donovan, & Kivlahan, 1988; Cloniger, 1987).

Biology also plays an important part in individuals being susceptible to acquiring disease. For example, the development of cervical cellular structures in postpubescence early adolescent females renders them vulnerable to acquiring particular sexually transmitted diseases (STDs) such as gonorrhea and chlamydia (Harrison, Phil, & Costin, 1985).

Psychological Factors

Psychological factors are also key in the biopsychosocial model. One rationale for adolescent risk taking was adolescent egocentrism proposed by Elkind (1967). He suggested two avenues of cognitive processing of risks: (1) the imaginary audience and (2) the personal fable. Adolescents perceive themselves as central to other people's worlds as they are to their own. On the other hand, adolescents perceive themselves as superior to and unique from others. Both these perspectives provide a rationale for perception of invulnerability among youth. However, this perspective remains largely untested.

Sensation seeking has been defined as a personality "trait defined by the need for varied, novel, and complex sensations and experiences and the willingness to take physical and social risks for the sake of such experiences" (Zuckerman, 1979, p. 10). For both males and females, sensation seeking tends to increase during early childhood and decline after an individual reaches 20 years of age. Sensation seeking has been linked to risky sexual activity (Fisher & Misovich, 1990; Kalichman, Heckman, & Kelly, 1996; Newcomb & McGee, 1991; Seal & Agostinelli, 1994; Sheer & Cline, 1995). Zuckerman (1979) linked sensation-seeking trait of adolescents to risk-taking behavior and suggests that individuals perceive risk-taking activities differently, depending on their level of sensation seeking.

Other psychological variables associated with adolescent problem behavior include self-esteem (Orr, Wilbrandt, Brack, Rauch, & Ingersoll, 1989), alienation, and rebelliousness (Jessor & Jessor, 1977). Low self-esteem among young adolescent girls has been associated with participation in sexual intercourse (Orr *et al.*, 1989).

Social Factors

Social influences are also pertinent to the risk behaviors of adolescents. Family relationships influence the behavior of adolescent offspring. For example, young people who live in single-parent family situations are more likely to become involved in sexual intercourse and substance use (Turner, Irwin, Tschsann, & Millstein, 1993). Interpersonal skills, such as communication, is also key to adolescent's participation in risky behaviors. For example, the ability of an individual to discuss condom use (Wilson, Kastrinakis, D'Angelo, & Getson, 1994) and other aspects of sexuality (Cobb, 1997) play a key role in the adoption of sexually protective practices.

Neighborhoods in which youth are raised have been found to be influential in the way children and adolescents engage in risky behaviors (Brooks-Gunn *et al.*, 1993). Exposure to violence adversely affects the way youth choose to deal with problems (Kolbo, 1996). Adolescents who participate in violent behavior are more likely to have been exposed to violence in their neighborhood or family (DuRant, 1994; Farrell, 1997). Communities where primarily low-paid workers reside tend to have more adolescents drop out of school (Crane, 1991).

Peer Relationships

Jessor and Jessor (1977) emphasize the idea that participation in problem behavior by adolescents is associated with the failure of conventional bonding to the family, the school, and community systems. In the absence of this conventional bonding, peer bonding to deviant peer subgroups may occur. Other theorists emphasize violence and criminality as survival strategies for the urban underclass who are economically deprived (Leibow, 1967). Still other theorists look at the combination of a tolerant social environment and the availability of behavior models (Dembo, Blount, Schmeidler & Burgos, 1986). In a similar vein, disorganization theory (Gartner, 1990; Merton, 1957) emphasizes the disorganization that accompanies crime-ridden neighborhoods.

Scope of Adolescent Risk Behaviors

Adolescents participate in activities that result in health-compromising events or conditions that can have both short- and long-term adverse health consequences. However, they are more likely to view this participation from a positive perspective, focusing more on the benefits as opposed to the risks (Lavery, Siegle, Cousins, & Rubovits, 1993). Some risks have devastating consequences due to lack of skills/ability of adolescents to successfully negotiate activities that place them in danger and/or judgment necessary to accurately evaluate the real danger. Thus, in general, threats to the well-being of adolescents in the United States are, for the most part, a result of participating in risky behaviors. These risk behaviors, in turn, are preventable (Ginzberg, 1991). Modifying adolescents' willingness to engage in risk behaviors is a critical challenge that has long-term rewards, both for adolescents and society in general. Below, we address more specifically some of the prominent health threats for adolescents. And, while an exhaustive review is beyond the scope of this chapter, we refer readers to DiClemente, Hansen, and Ponton (1996), the *Handbook of Adolescent Health Risk Behaviors*, for a more thorough analysis and exposition.

Injury

Annually, almost one third of youth in the United States between 5 and 17 years of age are injured (Scheidt *et al.*, 1995). In 1995, for example, the mortality rate for adolescents 15 to 24 years of age was 37.6 per 100,000; 75% of those fatalities were due to injuries associated with motor vehicle accidents (Rosenberg *et al.*, 1996). Unintentional injury is the leading cause of death among adolescents (Schwartz, 1993); circumstances leading to those deaths include motor vehicle accidents, drowning, firearm use, sports, and work-related accidents. Many factors have been cited as contributing to the mortality and morbidity statistics for youth. Among the most common contributing factors for injury due to vehicular accidents include lack of seat belt use and lack of helmet use when riding a bicycle or motorcycle (US Department of Health and Human Services, 1995). Alcohol is also a major contributing factor to deaths due to motor vehicle accidents in the United States (US Department of Health and Human Services, 1990; Mahew, Donelson, Beirness, & Simpson, 1986). Alcohol has contributed to approximately one half of deaths on the nation's highways (National Highway Traffic Safety Administration, 1991), particularly among youth, and continues to be a significant threat to adolescents' health (US Department of Health and Human Services, 1995).

Homicide and suicide, defined as intentional injuries, are the second and third leading causes of death for adolescents 15 to 24 years of age (Rosenberg *et al.*, 1996). However, for African-American males, homicide, one aspect of violence, is the leading cause of death. Intentional injuries are associated with carrying a weapon, history of fighting, participating in other types of violent activities, and suicide attempts or ideation. Violence among youth has markedly increased over the past decade between 1988 and 1994, arrest rates for violent offenders (murder, rape, robbery, and aggravated assault) for youth 10–17 years of age almost doubled for females and increased 60% for males (Snyder, 1998).

Suicide has risen to the third leading cause of death among adolescents 15–24 years of age (Singh et al., 1996). Although suicide is more likely to be attempted by females, males are more likely to succeed (Rosenberg, Smith, Davidson & Conn, 1987). Suicide is more often the cause of death for older (15–24 years old) than for younger adolescents (5–14 years old) (Singh et al., 1996). White adolescents are more likely than blacks to attempt suicide.

Unintentional Injury Prevention

One encouraging trend has been the observed decline of deaths due to motor vehicle accidents over the past several decades. The number of youth who died due to injuries sustained in a traffic accident decreased 38% between 1979 and 1992 (National Center for Health Statistics, 1993; National Safety Council 1993). Graham (1993) suggests that the primary factors contributing to a decline in traffic accident deaths were improvements in roads, automobiles, and emergency medical rescue services. Restrictions in alcohol use, changes in the legal limit of a persons's blood alcohol level, enforcement of seat belt use (Lescohier & Gallagher, 1996), raising the legal drinking age to 21 years (DuMouchel, Williams, & Zador, 1987; Hingson, Merrigan, & Heeren, 1985; Womble, 1989), and imposing curfews on adolescents (Williams, 1985) have been cited as contributing to the decline of traffic-related mortality. Unfortunately, seat belt use, although receiving increasing recognition for its role in injury prevention and often mandated in many locales, remains inconsistent. For example, only 34.2% of high school students reported that they always use a seat belt as a passenger in a car (USDHHS, 1995). Improvements in traffic-related death rates can also be attributed to community involvement from groups such as Mothers Against Drunk Drivers (MADD) and Students Against Drunk Drivers (SADD), a community-oriented approach that encourages both the adoption of nondrinking norms among the public and enforcement of legal liability for those intoxicated (Graham, 1993; Lescohier & Gallagher, 1996). According to Haddon and Baker (1981), injury prevention involves education of individuals, employers, and public officials, careful design of equipment used in the workplace, sports, and other equipment used by consumers, and public laws designed to regulate and enforce safety standards.

Intentional Injury Prevention/Violence

The prevention of intentional injury (homicide and suicide) is embedded in the issues related to violence in this country. Since most of the victims of homicide among 5- to 24-year-old adolescents have been killed by guns (Singh et al., 1996), legislation that provides for gun control has been favored as one strategy of decreasing the incidence of violence (Wintemute, 1987). The escalating level of homicide and other violent activities among youth suggests that the current level of gun control legislation may not be effective at prohibiting adolescents' access to weapons.

Although violence in the United States is escalating, particularly among youth, there have been few prevention interventions attempting to curb this growing problem (Wilson-Brewer, Cohen, O'Donnell, & Goodman, 1991). In general, the focus of violence prevention has rested with the judicial and, by extension, the penal system, specifically placement of juvenile offenders in institutions after a crime has been committed. However, this method of deterrence has not proven successful.

Few, if any, violence prevention programs that have been developed have been evaluated in terms of their effectiveness in preventing violence in either specific populations or communities. One program, the Kansas City Project, was a 3-year violence control strategy that involved community agencies and targeted youth who had a history of violence (Mitchell, 1991). Using conflict resolution training and anger control skills, efforts were made to prevent adolescents from engaging in violent activities such as homicide. However, evaluation data are not yet available to assess the program's effectiveness. A second program, the Boston Violence Prevention Project, involved a community-based approach using a 10-session educational approach to present information on violence, teach conflict resolution techniques, and create a nonviolent environment to serve as a role model (Prothrow-Sith, 1991). While attitudes toward violence changed, behavioral outcomes did not. Other strategies have been attempted in the form of early intervention with families of aggressive children in an attempt to enhance nonviolent attitudes and master positive interpersonal skills, both for children and their families. However, these programs have not undergone long-term follow-up to evaluate effectiveness.

Suggestions for curbing homicide and other types of violence include: working with teenagers to help them deal with their anger in less destructive ways, identifying youth who may be at-risk for perpetrating violent activities (those with low self-esteem, carrying weapons, etc.), and making referrals for youth who may be in a high-risk category for violence (Runyan & Gerken, 1989). Dr. James Mason (1991), former Director of the Centers for Disease Control, in his closing remarks at the Forum on Youth, Violence and Minority Communities: Setting the Agenda for Prevention, suggested the need for (1) grassroots efforts with individuals working with troubled adolescents in their communities; (2) improvement in family commitment to each other; and (3) providing opportunities for youth to participate in constructive activities within their communities. At the same conference, Dr. Louis Sullivan (1991) recommended that the issue of violence be taken out of the total jurisdiction of the criminal justice system and shared with the public health sector.

Suicide Prevention

Suicide prevention programs began on a large scale in the 1960s with the establishment and rapid growth of prevention centers (Miller, Coombs, Leeper, & Barton, 1984). However, there is little evidence that confirm the efficacy of these programs. A meta-analysis of suicide prevention centers revealed that, while these centers attract high-risk individuals, there was no evidence that they were successful in reducing suicide rates (Dew, Bromet, Brent & Greenhouse, 1987). Miller and colleagues (1984) found that the group who gained the most from this type of preventive intervention was Caucasian adolescent females. However, knowledge of these services may not have reached other adolescents (Shaffer, Garland, Gould, Fisher, & Trautman, 1988).

School-based strategies to prevent suicide have included education programs of some type. Shaffer and colleagues (1988) reviewed suicide prevention programs and found that most attempted to increase awareness of the problem of suicide, open up avenues of communication between peers regarding potential suicide, enhance coping among youth regarding stress, and inform students of support services in mental health. Shaffer, Garland, Underwood, and Whittle (1987) did find that students in their school-based program identified themselves as needing help, but there were no major changes in attitudes toward suicide. Some programs designed to prevent adolescents from reaching the point of suicide have also included skills training aimed at helping youth to be self-reflective regarding their feelings and encouraging them to discover ways to cope with difficulties and seek help (Joan, 1986).

Prevention programs in schools have shown mixed results in enhancing adolescents' knowledge regarding suicide. Shaffer *et al.* (1987) found no increase in knowledge about suicide risk factors, although students at risk were identified. Further work by Shaffer and colleagues (1988) revealed that few school-based suicide prevention programs included a coping skills component. In general, the effectiveness of such programs have yet to be established.

One suicide prevention strategy is to restrict access to firearms among youth (Eddy, Wolpert, & Rosenberg, 1987; Runyan & Gerken, 1989). Other strategies include identifying youth that may be at high risk for suicide, enhanced treatment for those that attempt suicide and school screening (Eddy *et al.*, 1987). Reducing the availability of firearms has been suggested as effective in some studies (Brent, Perper, Moritz, Baugher & Allman, 1993; Brent, Perper, & Allman, 1987; Brent *et al.*, 1991; Oliver & Hertzel, 1972).

Cohen, Spirito, and Brown (1996) recommend that suicide prevention programs be located in close proximity to communities in which one would expect higher rates or risk of suicide: poverty, violence, substance use, and areas with a high prevalence of school dropouts, and so forth. Moroever, health professionals need to be better prepared to both screen for risk factors and either intervene or refer for intervention to prevent suicide among adolescents (Blumenthal & Kupfer, 1986; Holinger, 1989). This includes mental health professionals, many who have not had adequate training to effectively intervene with youth (Bongar & Harmatz, 1989).

Risky Sexual Activities

Teen pregnancy has gained some measure of social acceptance, with increasing numbers of programs developed to meet the needs of this high-risk situation. About 60.9% of never-married youth between 14 and 21 years of age reported ever experiencing sexual intercourse (58.2% white; 79.2% African American; and 56.5% Hispanic) (USDHHS, 1995). High-risk sexual behaviors can result in pregnancy or sexually transmitted diseases, including HIV infection. The number of young women between 15- and 19-years-old becoming pregnant has increased 23% from 1972 to 1990 (Henshaw, 1994), while live births to young women in this same age group increased from 53.0/1000 in 1980 to 58.9/1000 in 1994 (Ventura, Martin, Mathews, & Clark, 1996).

Additionally, approximately 25% of sexually active youth acquire an STD each year (Alan Guttmacher Institute, 1994). STDs, including HIV, occur more frequently among African Americans than other racial groups (DiClemente, 1996; Webster,

Berman, & Greenspan, 1993). HIV disease was the sixth leading cause of death for minority group members aged 15 to 24 years of age and seventh for Caucasians in that same age group (Peters, Kochanek, & Murphy, 1998).

Sexual debut is occurring at increasingly younger ages. Between 1971 and 1988, the number of sexually active women 15-19 years old who reported six or more sexual partners doubled, from 7% to 14% (Kost & Forrest, 1992). While the use of barrier protection methods has increased among adolescents (Forrest & Singh, 1990), the consistency of use remains low and a major challenge (Cobb, 1995; USDHHS, 1995). One study reports that 29% of high school virgins reportedly engaged in genital sexual activities that could place them at risk for disease transmission (Schuster, Bell, & Kanouse, 1996).

Predictors of inconsistent condom use include having an older sex partner (greater than 5 years older), smoking, and more lifetime sex partners (D'Angelo & DiClemente, 1996). On the other hand, consistent condom use was strongly associated with communication between partners about acquired immunodeficiency syndrome (AIDS), sexual negotiation skills, condom self-efficacy, and the perception of peer norms supporting condom use (DiClemente, 1991, 1992, 1996; Joffe, 1993).

Prevention of Sexual Risks

While abstinence is the only certain way to prevent pregnancy and STDs, including HIV infection, many adolescents become sexually active while in high school (Kann *et al.*, 1991); therefore, the use of protective mechanisms is essential to prevent unwanted and adverse outcomes of sexual activity. While correct and consistent use of latex condoms is the most effective strategy for preventing the transmission of STDs (Cates & Stone, 1992; Van de Perre, Jacobs, & Sprecher-Goldberger, 1987), prevention of pregnancy offers more options [e.g., birth control pills, Depo Provera, intrauterine devices (IUDs), etc.]. However, even though the use of chemical contraceptives are extremely effective at preventing pregnancy, they offer no protection from STD/HIV infection.

Many of the sexual risk prevention programs are based on the assumption that increased knowledge will lead to improved preventive practices among adolescents. It has become increasingly clear, however, that while knowledge of pregnancy and STD/HIV risk factors is necessary, it may not be sufficient to motivate the adoption and maintenance of protective behaviors (DiClemente, 1993, 1997). Based on these findings, a variety of prevention programs have been developed, implemented, and evaluated. Most frequently, these programs are tailored to school-based youth (Kirby & DiClemente, 1994).

One school-based sexual risk reduction program included not only risk information and perceived vulnerability, barriers/benefits of practicing prevention, and perceived acceptability for practicing prevention activities, but also focused on enhancing self-efficacy and sexual negotiation skills (Walter & Vaughan, 1993). Evaluation based on a 3-month follow-up indicated that, compared to a control group, program participants reported fewer sexual contacts with high-risk partners, fewer partners, and increase in consistent condom use. Another school-based approach included sexuality and contraception education, counseling techniques, and professional services for junior and senior high students (Zabin, Hirsch, Smith Streett, & Hardy, 1986). While knowledge was enhanced, changes in risky sexual attitudes were less apparent, as many adolesents may have already held the opinion that it was beneficial to delay childbearing and use contraception. The behavioral outcome for this 3-year project did demonstrate delay in sexual debut. Likewise, a skills-based intervention was found to increase knowledge about HIV and enhanced adolescents' intentions to use safer sex practices (Main *et al.*, 1994). These skills were included in a 15-session program based on social cognitive theory and the theory of reasoned action. At a 6-month follow-up, sexually active students reported having fewer partners, using condoms more frequently, and intended to engage in sex less frequently. No changes were noted, however, in students' frequency of sex or frequency of substance use prior to sexual activity. Another recent program, Safer Choices, is a school-based program designed to reduce risky sexual behavior (unprotected sexual activity, multiple sex partners) and substance use and encourage students who have participated in risky behavior to seek counseling (Coyle *et al.*, 1996). In addition to the students, this program targeted multiple facets of the student environment: school teachers and staff, parents, peers and community. Evaluation is currently underway to determine the effectiveness of the intervention as well as the success of the implementation process.

School-based programs have traditionally included sex education or family life information (Moore *et al.*, 1995). While knowledge is increased in the area of sexuality, it is not entirely clear what impact this information has on the sexual activities of youth. In Kirby's (1992) analysis of school-based sex risk reduction efforts, knowledge-only and values-based programs were largely ineffective. However, theoretical-based skill-building programs such as Reducing the Risk (Barth, 1989), show delays in sexual debut for some adolescents.

Community-based programs also have been used to complement school-based programs by accessing a hard-to-reach adolescent population. In a community-based program targeted toward runaways, youth in an intervention group participated in workshops, coping skills training, and counseling sessions (Rotheram-Borus, Koopman, Haignere & Davies, 1991; Rotherman-Borus, Feldman, Rosario, & Dunne, 1994). Results indicate that these youth used condoms more consistently and engaged in high-risk sexual behaviors less frequently both at a 6-month and 2-year follow-up. Similarly, a community-based intervention tailored to African-American aodolescent males using visual and interactive educational strategies (games, exercises, and videotapes) and found that the intervention group engaged in less risky sexual activities (less frequent sexual intercourse, fewer partners, and more consistent condom use) than did young men in the control group (Jemmott, Jemmott, & Fong, 1992). Similarly, a community-based program, a Focus on Kids, was designed to decrease HIV risk among low-income, urban, African-American youth (Galbraith *et al.*, 1996). This program integrated skill-building strategies to enable young people to resist drugs and manage sexual activities and included community involvement in the form of consultants from the study community organizations, an advisory board with parents, educators, government officials, and other key community officials associated with either housing and health services. Community members also assisted in the delivery of the intervention. Most of the organization meetings and interventions were located in the community. At 6-months postintervention, there was a significant increase in condom use and intention to use condoms, in comparison to the control group; however, this change was not sustained at the 12-month follow-up (Stanton *et al.*, 1996).

In addition to school- and community-based interventions, clinics are an important venue for accessing high-risk youth. Prevention efforts using counseling strategies by physicians and other health care providers have resulted in decreased sexual activity and greater condom use among adolescents attending an adolescent medicine clinic (Mansfield, Conroy, Emans, & Woods, 1993). Similarly, the use of peer educators has achieved significant reductions in risk behavior (Slap, Plotkin, Khalid, Michelman, & Forke, 1991). Unfortunately, however, while clinics are an important access point for reaching adolescents, they remain underused. Clinics could be more effective and offer an opportunity to provide individually tailored interventions for some of the highest risk adolescents (DiClemente & Brown, 1994).

Overall, the accumulation of findings indicate that theory-based approaches that include skills training, are based on social learning theory, and address salient and pervasive peer, social, and media pressures to engage in risky sexual behavior can be effective (Kirby & DiClemente, 1994). Moroever, programs that are culturally sensitive, developmentally appropriate, and gender specific (Wingood & DiClemente, 1992; Airhihenbuwa, DiClemente, Wingood, & Lowe, 1992; Fullilove, Fullilove, Bowser, & Gross, 1990) are more likely to be effective in reaching their intended target audience and creating an environment conducive to behavior change. While modifying adolesents' sexual behavior has posed a formidable challenge, evidence developed incremenatlly over the past decade, spurred by the emergence of HIV disease, suggests that reducing sexual risk behaviors and their adverse sequelae is achievable.

Smoking

Approximately 89% of smokers began smoking by age 18 (Institute of Medicine, 1994), and it is estimated that 50% of youth between 16 and 17 years old who have started smoking cigarettes recently will continue to smoke well into adulthood (Pierce & Gilpin, 1996). Although the sale of cigarettes to youth younger than 18 years of age has been illegal, many adolescents continue to have unimpeded access to cigarettes and many (72.3%) have tried smoking cigarettes (CDC, 1996). About 14% of both male and female high school students reported in the 1993 Monitoring the Future survey that they smoked frequently (Johnston, O'Malley, & Bachman, 1995). A survey of high school seniors revealed that 30% reported that they had smoked within the past 30 days, and 19% said that they were regular smokers (Institute of Medicine, 1994).

Smoking Prevention

Smoking prevention has been elevated to a new level of priority within the United States, particularly among youth. Laws have recently been passed that require cigarette vendors to ensure that anyone who looks to be 27 years old or younger must provide proof of their age to purchase cigarettes. This legislation was in response to cigarette companies' direct targeting of adolescents as a marketing strategy to increase sales. Previous attempts at limiting access to cigarettes for adolescents included efforts to ban cigarette vending machines, a primary source for cigarette purchases among adolescents (DiFranza, Savageau & Aisquith, 1996; Forster, Hourigan, & McGovern; 1992; Hoppock & Houston, 1990).

Perry and Staufacker (1996) have idenified two successful approaches to smoking prevention: affective education and social influence. Early smoking prevention programs used education as its primary influential tactic and were based on the assumption that if youth knew the dangers of smoking, they would not smoke (Thompson, 1978). Fear appeals were also added to these educational programs and included pictures of lungs damaged from smoking. Affective education strategies were based on the belief that young people smoked because they identified with smoking (Durell & Bukoski, 1984). These programs focused on increasing self-worth in an effort to empower adolescents to abstain from smoking cigarettes (Hansen & Malotte, 1986).

Social influence strategies for preventing smoking need to include skills-building methods. Adolescents are influenced by cigarette advertising and their friends (peers) who smoke (Botvin, Goldberg, Botvin, & Dusenbury 1993). Therefore, programs were needed to empower youth to resist social pressures including advertising and peers. An example of one of these programs was a 15-session curriculum that included well-prepared teachers to deliver a cognitive component (consequences of smoking, ways to improve self-image, and advertising awareness), decision-making exercises, relaxation training, and assertiveness training (Botvin, Renick, & Baker, 1983). Findings indicate a 50% reduction in smoking. The addition of a "booster" session 1 year after the initial program was completed was found to further enhance smoking reduction. Unfortunately, even the best smoking prevention programs that do not include follow-up programs either in schools, communities, or media have shown erosion of treatment effects over time (Botvin et al., 1983; Perry , Klepp, & Shultz, 1988; Botvin & Botvin, 1992; Pentz et al., 1989; Ellickson, Bell, & McGuigan, 1993).

School-based smoking prevention programs have been somewhat successful in delaying the initiation of smoking among youth (Glynn, 1989). The key components to school-based programs to prevent smoking include early intervention, peer–parent and teacher education and involvement, and social influence processes. Hansen, Collins, Johnson, and Graham (1985) found that high school students who had started smoking but quit on their own were more likely to be influenced by their moral beliefs about smoking, their nonsmoking friends, and not thinking that smoking would lead to positive outcomes. However, continuing to be a nonsmoker was enhanced by the belief in the negative long-term effects of smoking, a conformist self-image, and a nonsmoking family environment.

Other smoking prevention programs have used social influence models to build their interventions. Long-term follow-up (5–6 years) by Murray, Pirie, Luepker, and Pallonen (1989) on their smoking prevention program, which used a combination of teaching and practicing skills that could assist youth to resist the social pressures of smoking, compared adult-led versus peer-led programs. Similar to other smoking prevention programs based in schools, there were short-term gains. However, the long-term effects have not been as positive.

An emerging health threat has been adolescents' use of smokeless tobacco. Most of the programs that target smokeless tobacco have been a part of smoking prevention programs (Perry & Staukacker, 1996). Knowledge about the physical outcomes of using smokeless tobacco appear to have a restraining ability (Sussman et al., 1993). A telephone follow-up strategy and newsletters for ninth graders designed to enhance and reinforce prevention messages have been successful in preventing smokeless tobacco use in a 3-year follow-up evaluation (Elder et al., 1993).

Overall, findings from a recent meta-analysis of smoking prevention programs suggest that intervention outcomes could be improved if they included early initiation of the educational strategies. Further, program effectiveness could be enhanced by using trained peer leaders. And, finally, smoking prevention programs need to be part of a multidimensional health promotion program that includes follow-up sessions (boosters) to reinforce and amplify initial intervention effects (Rooney & Murray, 1996).

Alcohol Use

Denise Kandel (1985) has identified alcohol as a "gateway" substance, antecedent to marijuana use and other illegal substances. Across 140 college campuses, drinking was related to smoking cigarettes, using marijuana, and having several sex partners within the last month (Wechsler, Dowdall, Davenport & Castillo, 1995). Alcohol use is more common among males and Caucasians than among females and African Americans (Cobb *et al.*, 1994).

Although alcohol use by high school seniors has declined slightly (Johnston, O'Malley, & Bachman, 1994), it continues to be frequently used by adolescents: 80.4% of students have tried drinking some type of alcoholic beverage (CDC, 1996). Although binge drinking decreased for high school students over the 1980s, an upward trend was noted in the 1994 Monitoring the Future data: from 27.5% in 1993 to 29.8% in 1995, high school seniors reported having five or more drinks in a row during the previous 2 weeks (Johnston *et al.*, 1995). Binge drinking among college students (defined as five drinks for males, but only four drinks for females per drinking episode) was much more prevalent, occurring in 50% of the males and 39% of females (Wechsler *et al.*, 1995).

Alcohol Prevention

Programs designed to prevent the use and abuse of alcohol have been categorized into several levels of support systems (Windle, Shope, & Bukstein, 1996). Family-focused programs, such as the Parent Communication Project (Shain, Suurvali, & Kilty, 1980), have focused on parental skills development in an effort to better listen to their adolescents, to open communication, and enable youth to make better informed decisions about alcohol use. Although this project showed immediate positive changes, these improvements declined over the 2-year follow-up.

Other family-focused programs have emphasized family strengthening to encourage parents to be both involved and supportive of their adolescents (Hawkins, Catalano, & Miller, 1992). Poor parenting, high family conflict, and low parent–child bonding have been found to contribute to problem behavior, including alcohol use among adolescents (Brook, Brook, Gordon, Whiteman, & Cohen, 1990). Although parent modeling should be considered in prevention programs for adolescent alcohol use, this focus has not been widely implemented. Other alcohol prevention programs have emphasized the development of individual skills. These have included anger management strategies and improvement of self-esteem appear to show some effectiveness (Windle *et al.*, 1996).

At schools, teachers have been educated to identify potential drinking problems of their students, including the parents who drink (McLaughlin, Holcomb, Jibaja-Rusth, & Webb, 1993). Programs that target early risk factors among adolescents (e.g., anger, poor school achievement) have been effective. Successful approaches identitfied in Hawkins and co-workers' (1992) review article included engaging students in an interactive and proactive manner. While community-based programs have targeted psychological factors such as self-esteem and supervised activities (homework, play, acting), these programs have proven unsuccessful except in identifying an interaction between student's self-esteem and scores on standardized tests (Ross, Saavedra, Shur & Winters, 1992).

Other indirect measures of preventing alcohol use and abuse among adolescents have been focused toward legal restrictions. Suggestions have been made to increase the age at which young people can drive, restrict licenses, and limit the hours that youth can drive (Williams, Karps, & Zador, 1983), thus supposedly eliminating drinking and driving among youth. Raising the age at which youth can purchase alcohol has been found to reduce alcohol-related traffic deaths (Decker & Graitcer, 1988; Saffer & Grossman, 1987). Lowering the legal blood alcohol level and strengthening legal consequences for driving with blood alcohol level above the legal limit have resulted in lower traffic fatalities among youth (Hingson, 1993). Areas that have increased taxes on beer also have observed lower traffic mortality rates for young people (Saffer & Grossman, 1987).

For late adolescents, harm reduction strategies have been developed to target those youth who are expected to consume alcohol. For example, a brief intervention (15 minutes) was conducted with college students prior to spring break (Cronin, 1996) in an attempt to reduce the adverse consequences of drinking activities that generally occur during this annual event. Rather than present the information to students as a deviant behavior, they were approached with the potential problems often associated with alcohol use (i.e., hangover, sexual risks, interpersonal conflict, etc.). Findings suggested that those who participated in this brief intervention were less likely to have experienced alcohol-related problems. However, additional studies in this area are limited and the need for further research in the area of alcohol use prevention and harm reduction is critical, given the prevalence and health-damaging consequences of this behavior.

Substance Use

Fewer students have reported using other substances at some point in their lifetime: marijuana (42.4%), cocaine (7%), steroids (3.7%), injected drugs (2%), other illegal drugs (16%), and inhalants (20.3%) (CDC, 1996). However, drug use, particularly marijuana, in this country is increasing among youth (Johnston et al., 1994). In 1991, among high school students 3.2% of eighth graders, 8.7% of tenth graders, and 13.8% of twelfth graders reported using marijuana during the previous 30 days; these percentages increased in 1995 to 9.1%, 17.2%, and 21.2%, respectively (Monitoring the Future Study press release of 12/4/95 at University of Michigan). This fact is particularly unsettling because marijuana has been shown to lead to other drugs that have a far greater potential for health-damaging consequences.

Substance Use Prevention

In an early review of the substance use prevention strategies, Durell and Bukoski (1984) identified primary prevention strategies as media campaigns, school programs, and generic programs that target adolecents' affective domain. Initial media strategies that attempted to inform the public about the harmful effects of drugs were deemed ineffective, and in fact drug use continued to rise. School-based drug prevention programs represent perhaps the largest segment of interventions targeted towards youth.

Most of the school programs of the 1960s and 1970s, also using information-providing strategies, were found to be ineffective in reducing drug use among youth. An affective–educational approach attempted to use findings from correlation studies of factors that were identified as contributing to drug use. Therefore, programs were established that targeted adolescents' general self-esteem, interpersonal interactions, and coping with authority figures (Durell & Bukoski, 1984).

In a meta-analysis of drug use prevention programs, Tobler (1992) found that both the knowledge-only and affective-only drug prevention strategies are ineffective in reducing drug use among adolescents. However, peer group methods that combine a knowledge component with skill-building strategies that are developmentally appropriate (more structured at younger ages) were most effective. The Safe Haven Program is a primary prevention strategy that was developed for substance use prevention among African-American families in which there is a substance using parent (Aktan, Kumpfer & Turner, 1996). The program is composed of three components: parent training to increase their coping ability and positive interactions with their children; skills training for children to assist them to make decisions, control anger, and cope with feelings, loneliness, and peer pressure; and family skills training to enable the parents to more effectively set limits and acknowledge good behaviors in their children. The primary success of this program was in the enhanced parenting skills, improved behavior among their children, and less substance use among the parents and their families.

The All Stars program (Hansen, 1996) was designed to provide an interactive environment in which students during eight class sessions would examine mediators that have been found to be significant in the study of problem behavior: (1) ideals that are incompatible with participating in risky behavior, (2) normative beliefs about risky behavior, and (3) commitment to avoid participating in risky behavior. This pilot study found that these mediators were modified by the program. However, the long-term outcome of problem behavior will require continued follow-up and evaluation to adequately assess program impact.

Access to Health Care Services for Youth

In a study investigating health concerns of adolescents, high school students perceived other teenagers to be more concerned about health risk behaviors (sexual and substance use) than they were concerned about their own health risk behaviors (Weiler, 1992). While a large proportion of young people emerge from their youth having experienced only minor health problems, this is not the case for many others who have not be so fortunate.

Health services for youth include school-based health clinics, community adolescent services, community clinics, and private pediatricians who may or may not specialize in adolescent care. Approximately 75% of adolescents reported that they had received care within a 2-year period (U.S. Congress, Office of Technology Assessment, 1991); however, 15% lacked any type of medical insurance (Newacheck,

McManus, & Gephart, 1992), and youth from Southern communities are the least likely to have insurance coverage.

Although there are major health problems among our youth, many health professionals are ill-prepared to address those problems in their practice. While the American Medical Association publication, *Guidelines for Adolescent Prevention Services* (GAPS) (Elster & Kuzsets, 1994), outlined specific recommendations for the delivery of preventive health care by health professionals, adolescents receive little preventive teaching in medical offices (Igra & Millstein, 1993). This may be a consequence of the lack of specialized training for health professionals in the care of adolescents (Bearinger & Gephart, 1987; Bearinger, Widley, Gephart, & Blum, 1992; Cohen, 1994).

The Interrelatedness of Adolescent Health-Threatening Behaviors

The initiation of health-threatening risk behaviors usually begins with experimentation in youth. These risk behaviors appear to cluster together (Donovan, Jessor & Costa, 1988, 1991; Irwin & Millstein, 1986; Jessor & Jessor, 1977). Young people who participate in one type of risk activity are likely to participate in other risk behaviors. Over the duration of adolescence, participation in this experimentation tends to increase. For example, the 1992 National Health Interview Survey—Youth Risk Behavior Supplement presented a cumulative risk index showing that participation in problem behavior (dropped out of school, experienced sexual intercourse, used illegal drugs, had five or more alcoholic beverages in a row in the past month, and stayed out all night without permission during previous year) increased with age. While 55% participated in at least one risk behavior at age 15 years, 84% reported engaging in problem behaviors at age 18 (62% reported two or more risks).

Alcohol has been normalized as an activity that almost all youth will at least try once. However, excessive drinking has been shown to be a culprit for many devastating outcomes when paired with driving, sexual activity, and other recreational activities. For example, alcohol use during adolescence has been shown to be closely related to fatal injuries from motor vehicle accidents for persons 12 to 24 years of age (Friedman, 1985) and boating accidents and adolescent drownings (Wintemute, 1990).

In addition, substance use among adolescents is correlated with delinquency and sexual risk taking (Gruber, DiClemente, Anderson, & Lodico, 1996; Neumark-Sztainer *et al.*, 1996), teen pregacy, school misbehavior, and school dropout (Elliott, Huizinga, & Menard, 1989; Jessor & Jessor, 1977; Zabin, Hardy, Smith & Hirsch, 1986). Substance use has also been connected with eating disorders and relationship difficulties. Young women who diet frequently are more likely to drink alcohol and smoke cigarettes; these factors are also associated with decreased connectedness to others and binge eating (French, Story, Downes, Resnick & Blum, 1995).

Nonsexual risky activities have been linked to sexual activities of adolescents. Youth, 15–17 years of age, who had experienced sexual intercourse were more likely (1.5–4 times) than virgins to also be involved in nonsexual problem behaviors (theft, school suspension/expulsion, personal violence, drug use) (Ketterlinus, Lamb, Nitz, & Elster, 1992). Drug use does appear to be related to the risk of having had a sexually transmitted disease. This may be the result of drug use altering the decision-making skills of an acutely intoxicated individual, may alter their sex drive, or may be the result of adolescents trading sex for drugs, which in turn may expose the adolescent to multiple sex partners (Jemmott & Jemmott, 1993; Shafer, et al., 1993; Fullilove et al., 1990).

There have been attempts to determine the antecedents and consequences of problem behavior among adolescents. However, most studies have looked at cooccurrence through either retrospective studies or cross-sectional designs, therefore limiting the ability to identify causal relationships. Through this work we do know that youth who participate in problem behaviors are known to fail to achieve academically and are not likely to participate in religious activities (Bachman, Johnston, & O'Malley, 1981; Donovan, Jessor & Costa, 1988; Jessor & Jessor, 1977). They also place more value on personal independence, have greater tolerance for deviance, and are bonded more strongly to peers than parents (Jessor & Jessor, 1977). Adolescents who participate in school-based extracurricular activities were less likely to become involved in risky behaviors (drop out of school, drug use, pregnancy, smoke cigarettes, get arrested) except for drinking alcohol (Zill, Nord, & Loomis, 1995).

Peer influence is strongly associated with adolescent cigarette smoking (Conrad, Flay, & Hill, 1992); however, parental influence is particularly strong for young Caucasians and adolescent females (Bauman, Foshee, Linzer, & Koch, 1990; Chassin, Presson, Montello, Sherman, & McGrew, 1986; Sussman, Dent, Stacy, & Flay, 1987). Adolescents who are less likely to smoke cigarettes achieve academically (Gerber & Newman, 1989; Chassin, Presson, Sherman, 1990), develop health-promoting activities such as nutritional eating exercise habits (Kelder, 1992), and can resist invitations to smoke cigarettes (Conrad et al., 1992). Using smokeless tobacco is also associated with engaging in other risky behaviors and poor academic status (Dent, Sussman, Johnson, Hansen, & Flay, 1987; Jones & Moberg, 1988)

Methodological Gaps in the Study of Adolescent Health Promotion/Disease Prevention

According to Runyan and Gerken (1989), we have little information on morbidity data and the information that is available is not always defined consistently. Further, there is a lack of information on the relationship of exposure to risk versus negative outcome of that exposure. And, finally, there is a paucity of empirical data describing the perspectives of adolescents. There also are few longitudinal studies. This limits the ability to reliably identify antecedents and consequences of behavior. The use of self-report data with surveys and questionnaires can call into question the validity of the data (Pattishall, 1994), particularly in evaluating sexual risk reduction intervention (O'Leary, DiClemente, & Aral, 1997).

Future Directions for Adolescent Health Promotion

Research

Overall, more funding needs to be allocated toward prevention research. Adolescent health researchers have suggested the need for a behavioral Framingham approach to the study of adolescence using multidisciplinary and longitudinal designs accomplished through collaborative efforts of public and private agencies (Pattishall,

1994). This would enable the inclusion of intraindividual variability for behavioral concepts. This approach also would enable a propsective examination of a broad array of ecological factors that contribute to the behavior of adolescents (Bronfenbrenner, 1979). In addition, developmental transitions could be more effectively linked to behavior (Zaslow & Takanishi, 1993). These studies need to be conducted with participants who are nationally representative (Dryfoos, 1990) and need to emerge from an interdisciplinary research perspective (Zaslow & Takanishi, 1993). Moroever, as Dr. Robert DuRant (1995), the former president of the Society for Adolescent Medicine, noted, not only are we concerned with identifying determiants of adolescent risk behavior, but we need to know more about the characteristics that enhance resiliency for adolescents faced with health threats and how to share appropriate and effective prevention programs to communities where there is an identified need.

With respect to methodological issues, Kirby (1992) recommends that research designs to study adolescent risky behavior include rigorous methods such as random assigment to treatment and control groups, statistical analysis to determine sample size needed to gain power, follow-up procedures to determine long-term effectiveness, and appropriate assessment of behavior. Theory-driven research would also strengthen the body of knowledge in adolescent risk behavior by providing an overarching framework from which to orient research and program development.

Prevention Programs

Programs that are focused on the prevention of risky behaviors among adolescents need to adopt a comprehensive approach that links behaviors and that is developmentally and culturally appropriate. This approach must include not only individual characteristics of the adolescent, but also the immediate context within which the young person exists: family, peers and community. Stiffman and colleagues (1996) have suggested that the most important and realistic intervention for violence prevention would involve enlisting the cooperation of the media in reducing the social acceptability of violence, and supporting opportunites for youth to develop a productive and positive lifestyle. Violence among adolescents has reached an alarming level and requires intervention that cannot reach only the adolescent from the inner-city ghettos, but also the rural areas and so-called "safe" suburban neighborhoods.

Haffner (1996) reported that the National Commission on Adolescent Sexual Health recommended interactive approaches in sexuality programs and that these programs be offered across the youth age span (kindergarten through college). No issues should be banned from these programs and leaders must be well-prepared to facilitate these programs.

Most of the information that discusses approaches or presents research findings on adolescent risky behavior prevention programs suggest the need for evaluation. A recent study of HIV risk behaviors among African-American adolescents concluded that interventions must target culturally specific motivation factors and barriers that affect the adoption of prevention activities (Grinstead, Peterson, Faigeles & Catania, 1997). Therefore, there is an urgent need to develop tools that effectively determine the quality of the process and outcome of these programs. These instruments must address the requirements of being developmentally appropriate and culturally sensitive to adequately assess the program under study. In addition, prevention interventions need to be offered where adolescents live—in their environment, their language, and at their comfort level.

Conclusions

The future health status for today's children and adolescents is worrisome due to several realities. Families that are stuck in poverty and thus in neighborhoods in which many types of deviant behaviors are the norm provide a poor environment from which youth glean their role models. Family structure has changed, leaving one parent, usually the mother, with all of the responsibility of raising the children and providing financial support to keep the basic needs of the family met. The parent's availability to provide emotional support and guidance may be lacking. Therefore, older children are left to raise their younger siblings, creating a scenario for early participation in risk behaviors.

On an individual level, adolescents, in striving to meet their proximal goals of social acceptance, are generally not looking down the road toward their future, much less the potential long-term negative consequences of today's actions. However, there are notable problems, both at the individual and societal level. The financial costs of (1) rehabilitation and other types of health needs necessary to care for problems that result from injuries; (2) treating fertility problems and cervical cancer associated with STDs; and (3) chronic conditions due to smoking, alcohol and drug use. Societal consequences include: (1) lack of adequately educated work force due to dropping out of school or poor school performance/achievement; (2) family stress and strain when there are special needs resulting from premature death of a family member or for chronic care; and (3) inadequate parenting due to children having children with less than adequate maturity and financial and social resources.

A "Call to Arms"—Developing a Comprehensive and Coordinated Research Agenda

To avert further increases in adolescent risk behaviors and the adverse health and social consequences that accompany these behaviors, development of effective prevention and treatment interventions are urgently needed. To facilitate this research effort, a comprehensive and coordinated infrastructure is critical to conceptualize, stimulate and support the continuum of adolescent health promotion research (Di-Clemente, Ponton, & Hansen, 1996). One clear advantage of this systematic approach is that it avoids development of isolated prevention and treatment programs that have impeded cross-fertilization of information and the sharing of new and effective prevention and treatment strategies between investigators and practitioners working with different risk behaviors. Furthermore, this approach would also permit more rapid integration of findings derived from longitudinal cohort studies focused on identifying the determinants of specific risk behaviors to be consolidated into existing and planned prevention and treatment programs. Finally, a systematic approach encourages continued rigorous evaluation of prevention and treatment programs as one mechanism of identifying efficacious programs and eliminating ineffective approaches. Without a defined, structured response to the problem of adolescent risk behaviors, many adolescents will experience the pain and suffering that is often the consequence of these behaviors.

References

Adger, H. (1991). Problems of alcohol and other drug abuse in adolescents. *Journal of Adolescent Health, 12*, 606–613.

Airhihenbuwa, C. O., DiClemente, R. J., Wingood, G. M., & Lowe, A. (1992). HIV/AIDS education and prevention among African-Americans: A focus on culture. *AIDS Education and Prevention, 4*, 251–260.

Alan Guttmacher Institute. (1994). *Sex and America's teenagers*. New York: Author.

Aktan, G. B., Kumpfer, K. L., & Turner, C. W. (1996). Effectiveness of a family skills training program for substance use prevention with inner city African-American families. *Substance Use and Misuse, 31*(2), 157–175.

Anderson, J., Kann, L., Holtzman, D., Arday, S., Truman, B., & Kolbe, L. (1990). HIV/AIDS knowledge and sexual behavior among high school students. *Family Planning Perspectives, 22*, 252–255.

Bachman, J. G., Johnston, L. D., & O'Malley, P. M. (1981). *Monitoring the future: Questionnaire responses from the nation's high school seniors—1980*. Ann Arbor, MI: Institute for Social Research, University of Michigan.

Barth, R. (1989). *Reducing the risk: Building skills to prevent pregnancy*. Santa Cruz, CA: Newark Publications.

Baughner, E., & Lamison-White, L. (1996). US Bureau of the Census, Current Population Reports, Series P60-194, *Poverty in the United States: 1995*. Washington, DC: US Government Printing Office.

Bauman, K. E., Foshee, V. A., Linzer, M. A., & Koch, G. G. (1990). Effect of parental smoking classification on the association between parental and adolescent smoking. *Addictive Behaviors, 15*, 413–422.

Bearinger, L., & Gephart, J. (1987). Priorities for adolescent health: Recommendations of a national conference. *American Journal of Maternal Child Nursing, 12*, 161–164.

Bearinger, L. H., Widley, L., Gephart, J., & Blum, R. W. (1992). Nursing competence in adolescent health: Anticipating future needs of youth. *Journal of Professional Nursing, 8*, 80–86.

Bianchi, S. M. (1995). Changing economic roles of women and men. In I. R. Farley (Ed.), *State of the union: Americans in the 1990s* (Vol. I, pp.; 107–154). New York: Russell Sage Foundation.

Blumenthal, S. J., & Kupfer, D. J. (1986). Generalizable treatment strategies for suicidal behavior. *Annals of the New York Academy of Science, 487*, 327–340.

Bongar, B., & Harmatz, M. (1989). Graduate training in clinical psychology and the study of suicide. *Professional Psychology: Research and Practice, 20*, 209–213.

Botvin, G. J., & Botvin, E. M. (1992). Adolescent tobacco, alcohol, and drug abuse: Prevention strategies, empirical findings, and assessment issues. *Journal of Development and Behavioral Pediatrics, 13*, 290–301.

Botvin, G. J., Renick, N. L., & Baker, E. (1983). The effects of scheduling format and booster sessions on a broad-spectrum psychosocial approach to smoking prevention. *Journal of Behavioral Medicine, 6*, 359–379.

Botvin, G. J., Goldberg, C. J., Botvin, E. M., & Dusenbury, L. (1993). Smoking behavior of adolescent exposed to cigarette advertising. *Public Health Reports, 108*, 217–224.

Brent, D. A., Perper, J. A., & Allman, C. J. (1987). Alcohol, firearms, and suicide among youth: Temporary trends in Allegheny County, Pennsylvania, 1960–1983. *Journal of the American Medical Association, 257*, 3369–3372.

Brent, D., Perper, J., Allman, C., Moritz, G., Wartella, M., & Zelenak, J. (1991). The presence and availability of firearms in the homes of adolescent suicides: A case–control study. *Journal of the American Medical Association, 266*, 2989–2995.

Brent, P. A., Perper, J., Moritz, G., Baugher, M., & Allman, C. (1993). Suicide in adolescents with no apparent psychopathology. *Journal of the American Academy of Child and Adolescent Psychiatry, 32*, 494–500.

Bronfenbrenner, U. E. (1979). *The ecology of human development: Experiments by nature and by design*. Cambridge, MA: Harvard University Press.

Brook, J. S., Brook, D. W., Gordon, A. S., Whiteman, M., & Cohen, P. (1990). The psychosocial etiology of adolescent drug use: A family interactional approach. *Genetic Social and General Psychology Monography, 116*, 111–267.

Brooks-Gunn, J. (1988). Antecedents and consequences of variations in girls maturational timing. *Journal of Adolescent Health Care, 9*, 1–9.

Brooks-Gunn, J., Duncan, G. J., Klebanov, P. K., & Sealand, N. (1993). Do neighborhoods influence child and adolescent development? *American Journal of Sociology, 99*, 353–395.

Cates, W., & Stone, K. M. (1992). Family planning, sexually transmitted diseases and contraceptive choice: A literature update—part I. *Family Planning Perspectives, 24*, 75–84.

Centers for Disease Control (CDC) (1996). Youth risk behavior surveillance—United States, 1995. *Morbidity and Mortality Weekly Report, 45*(SS-4), 1–84.

Chassin, L., Presson, C. C., Montello, D., Sherman, S. J., & Mcgrew, J. (1986). Changes in peer and parent influence during adolescence: longitudinal versus cross-sectional perspectives on smoking initiation. *Developmental Psychology, 22,* 327–334.

Chassin, L., Presson, C. C., & Sherman, S. J. (1990). Social psychological contributions to the understanding and prevention of adolescent cigarette smoking. *Personality and Social Psychology Bulletin, 16,* 133–151.

Cloniger, C. R. (1987). Neurogenetic adaptive mechanisms in alcoholism. *Science, 236,* 410–416.

Cobb, B.K. (1995). HIV-related protection used by college women during sexual transition in a heterosexual relationship. Presented at the *Ninth Annual Conference of the Southern Nursing Research Society,* February 16–18, 1995, Lexington, KY.

Cobb, B. K. (1997). Communication types and sexual protective practices of college women. *Public Health Nursing, 14,* 291–299.

Cobb, B. K., Cairns, R.B., Cairns, B.D., & Greene, S. (1994). Factors related to adolescent substance use. Presented at the *American Public Health Association 122nd Annual meeting,* October 30–November 3, 1994, Washington, DC.

Cobb, B. K., Cairns, B. D., Miles, M. S., & Cairns, R. B. (1995). A longitudinal study of the role of sociodemographic factors and childhood aggression on adolescent injury and "close calls". *Journal of Adolescent Health, 17,* 381–388.

Cohen, M. (1994). A youth portriat gallery: Its problems, its prospects and some new paradigms. In K. Holt, K. Langlykke, & S. Panzarine (Eds.), *Reaching youth: A public health responsibility* (pp. 1–12). Arlington, VA: National Center for Education in Maternal and Child Health.

Cohen, Y., Spirito, A., & Brown, L. K. (1996). Suicide and suicide behavior. In R. J. DiClemente, W. B. Hanson, & L. E. Ponton (Eds.), *Handbook of adolescent health risk behaviors* (pp. 193–224). New York: Plenum Press.

Conrad, K. M., Flay, B. R., & Hill, D. (1992). Why children start smoking cigarettes: Predictors of onset. *British Journal of Addiction, 87,* 1711–1724.

Coyle, K., Kirby, D., Parcel, G., Basen-Engquist, K., Banspach, S., Rugg, D., & Weil, M. (1996). Safer choices: A multicomponent school-based HIV/STD and pregnancy prevention program for adolescents. *Journal of School Health, 66,* 89–94.

Crane, J. (1991). The epidemic theory of ghettos and neighborhood effects on dropping out and teenage childbearing. *American Journal of Sociology, 96,* 1226–1259.

Cronin, C. (1996). Harm reduction for alcohol-use-related problems among college students. *Substance Use and Misuse, 31,* 2029–2037.

D'Angelo, L. J., & DiClemente, R. J. (1996). Sexually transmitted diseases including human immunodeficiency virus infection. In R. J. DiClemente, W. B. Hanson, & L. E. Ponton (Eds.), *Handbook of adolescent health risk behaviors* (pp. 333–368). New York: Plenum Press.

Decker, M. D., & Graitcer, P. L. S. (1988). Reduction in motor vehicle fatalities associated with an increase in the minimum drinking age. *Journal of the American Medical Association, 260,* 3604–3610.

Dembo, R., Blount, W. R., Schmeidler J., & Burgos, W. (1986). Perceived environmental drug use risk and the correlates of drug use and non-use among inner-city youths: The motivated actor. *International Journal of the Addictions, 21,* 977–1000.

Dent, C. W., Sussman, S., Johnson, C. A., Hansen, W. B., & Flay, B. R. (1987). Adolescent smokeless tobacco incidence: Relations with other drugs and psychosocial variables. *Preventive Medicine, 16,* 422–431.

Dew, M. A., Bromet, E. J., Brent, D., & Greenhouse, J. B. (1987). A quantitative literature review of the effectiveness of suicide prevention centers. *Journal of Consulting and Clinical Psychology, 55,* 239–244.

DiClemente, R. J. (1991). Predictors of HIV-preventive sexual behavior in a high-risk adolescent population: The influence of perceived peer norms and sexual communication on incarcerated adolescents' consistent use of condoms. *Journal of Adolescent Health, 12,* 385–390.

DiClemente, R. J. (1992). Psychosocial determinants of condom use among adolescents. In R. J. DiClemente (Ed.), *Adolescents and AIDS: A generation in jeopardy* (pp. 34–51). Newbury Park, CA: Sage.

DiClemente, R. J. (1993). Preventing HIV/AIDS among adolescents: Schools as agents of change. *Journal of the American Medical Association, 270,* 760–762.

DiClemente, R. J. (1996). Adolescents at-risk for acquired immune deficiency syndrome: Epidemiology of AIDS, HIV prevalence and HIV incidence. In S. Oskamp & S. Thompson (Eds.), *Understanding and preventing HIV risk behavior* (pp. 13–30). Newbury Park, Ca: Sage.

DiClemente, R. J. (1997). Looking forward: Future directions for prevention of HIV among adolescents. In L. Sherr (Ed.), *AIDS and adolescents* (pp. 189–199). Reading, Berkshire, United Kingdom: Harwood Academic Publishers.

DiClemente, R. J., & Brown, L. K. (1994). Expanding the pediatrician's role in HIV prevention for adolescents. *Clinical Pediatrics, 32,* 1–6.

DiClemente, R. J., Boyer, C., & Morales, E. (1988). Minorities and AIDS: Knowledge, attitudes and misconceptions among black and Latino adolescents. *American Journal of Public Health, 78,* 55–57.

DiClemente, R. J., Ponton, L.E., & Hansen, W. (1996). New directions for adolescent risk prevention and health promotion research and interventions. In R.J. DiClemente, W. Hansen, & L.E. Ponton (Eds.), *Handbook of adolescent health risk behavior* (pp. 413–420). New York: Plenum Press.

DiFranza, J. R., Savageau, J. A., & Aisquith, B. F. (1996). Youth access to tobacco: The effects of age, gender, vending machine locks, and "It's the Law" programs. *American Journal of Public Health, 86,* 221–224.

Donovan, J., Jessor, R., & Costa, F. M. (1988). Syndrome of problem behavior in adolescence: A replication. *Journal of Consulting and Clinical Psychology, 56,* 762–765.

Donovan, J. E., Jessor, R., & Costa, F. M. (1991). Adolescent health behavior and conventionality–unconventionality: An extension of problem–behavior theory. *Health Psychology, 10,* 52–61.

Dryfoos, J. G. (1990). *Adolescents at risk.* New York: Oxford University.

DuMouchel, W., Williams, A. F., & Zador, P. (1987). Raising the alcohol purchase age: Its effects on fatal motor vehicle creashes in 26 states. *Legal Studies, 16,* 249–266.

DuRant, R. H. (1994). Exposure to violence and victimization and fighting behavior by urban black adolescents. *Journal of Adolescent Health, 15,* 311–318.

DuRant, R. H. (1995). Adolescent health research as we proceed into the twenty-first century. *Journal of Adolescent Health, 17,* 199–203.

Durell, J., & Bukoski, W. (1984). Preventing substance abuse: The state of the art. *Public Health Reports, 99,* 23–31.

Eddy, D. M., Wolpert, R. L., & Rosenberg, M. L. (1987). Estimating the effectiveness of interventions to prevent youth suicides. *Medical Care, 25,* S57–S65.

Elder, J. P., Wildey, M., Demoor, C., Sallis, J. F., Eckhardt, L., & Edwards, C. (1993). Long-term prevention of tobacco use among junior high school students through classroom and telephone interventions. *American Journal of Public Health, 83,* 1239–1244.

Elkind, D. (1967). Egocentricism and adolescence. *Child Development, 38,* 1025–1034.

Ellickson, P. L., Bell, R. M., & McGuigan, K. (1993). Preventing adolescent drug use: Long-term results of a junior high program. *American Journal of Public Health, 83,* 856–862.

Elliott, D. B., Huizinga, D., & Menard, S. (1989). Multiple problem youth: Delinquency, substance use, and mental health problems. New York: Springer-Verlag.

Elliott, D. S. (1993). Health-enhancing and health compromising lifestyles. In S. G. Millstein, A. C. Peterson, & E. O. Nightingale (Eds.), *Promoting the health of adolescents: New directions for the twenty-first century* (pp. 119–145). New York: Oxford University Press.

Elster, A., & Kuzsets, N. (1994). *AMA guidelines for adolescent preventive services (GAPS).* Baltimore: Williams & Wilkins.

Farrell, A. D. (1997). Impact of exposure to community violence on violent behavior and emotional distress among urban adolescents. *Journal of Clinical Child Psychology, 26,* 2–14.

Fisher, J. D., & Misovich, S. J. (1990). Evolution of college students' AIDS-related behavioral responses, attitudes, knowledge, and fear. *AIDS Education and Prevention, 2,* 322–337.

Flavell, J. H. (1963). *The developmental psychology of Jean Piaget.* Princeton, NJ: Van Nostrand.

Forrest, J. D., & Singh, S. (1990). The sexual and reproductive behavior of American women. *Family Planning Perspectives, 22,* 206–214.

Forster, J. L., Hourigan, M., & McGovern, P. (1992). Availability of cigarettes to underage youth in three communities. *Preventive Medicine, 21,* 320–328.

French, S. A., Story, M., Downes, B., Resnick, M. D., & Blum, R. W. (1995). Frequent dieting among adolescents: Psychosocial and health behavior correlates. *American Journal of Public Health, 85,* 695–701.

Friedman, I. M. (1985). Alcohol and unnatural deaths in San Francisco youths. *Pediatrics, 76,* 191–193.

Fullilove, R. E., Fullilove, M. T., Bowser, B. P., & Gross, S. A. (1990). Risk of sexually transmitted disease among black adolescent crack users in Oakland and San Francisco, Calif. *Journal of the American Medical Association, 263,* 851–855.

Furby, L., & Beyth-Maron, R. (1990). *Risk taking in adolescence: A decision making perspective.* Washington, DC: Carnegie Council on Adolescent Development.

Galbraith, J., Ricardo, I., Stanton, B., Black, M., Feigelman, S., & Kaljee, L. (1996). Challenges and rewards of involving community in research: An overview of the "Focus on Kids" HIV risk reduction program. *Health Education Quarterly, 23,* 383–394.

Gallagher, S. S., Finison, K., Guyer, B., & Goodenough, S. (1984). The incidence of injuries among 87,000 Massachusetts children and adolescents: Results of the 1980–81 statewide childhood injury prevention program surveillance system. *American Journal of Public Health, 74,* 1340–1347.

Gartner, R. (1990). The victims of homicide: A temporal and cross-national comparison. *American Sociological Review, 55,* 92–106.

Gerber, R. W., & Newman, I. M. (1989). Predicting future smoking of adolescent experimental smokers. *Journal of Youth and Adolescence, 18,* 191–201.

Ginzberg, E. (1991). Adolescents at risk conference: Overview. *Journal of Adolescent Health, 12,* 588–590.

Glynn, T. J. (1989). Essential elements of school-based smoking prevention program. *Journal of School Health, 59,* 181–188.

Graham, J. D. (1993). Injuries from traffic crashes: Meeting the challenge. *Annual Review of Public Health, 14,* 515–543.

Greening, L., & Dollinger, S. (1991). Adolescent smoking and perceived vulnerability to smoking related causes of death. *Journal of Pediatric Psychology, 16,* 687–699.

Grinstead, O. A., Peterson, J. L., Faigeles, B., & Catania, J. A. (1997). Antibody testing and condom use among heterosexual African Americans at risk for HIV infection: The National AIDS Behavioral Surveys. *American Journal of Public Health, 87,* 857–859.

Gruber, E., DiClemente, R.J., Anderson, M.N., & Lodico, M. (1996). Early drinking onset and its association with alcohol use and problem behavior in late adolescence. *Preventive Medicine, 25,* 293–300.

Haddon, W., & Baker, S. P. (1981). Injury control. In D. Clark & B. MacMahon (Eds.), *Preventive and community medicine* (pp. 000–000). Boston: Little Brown.

Haffner, D. W. (1996). Sexual health for America's adolescents. *Journal of School Health, 66,* 151–152.

Hansen, W. B. (1996). Pilot test results comparing the All Stars Program with seventh grade D.A.R.E.: Program integrity and mediating variable analysis. *Substance Use and Misuse, 31,* 1359–1377.

Hansen, W. B., & Malotte, K. (1986). Perceived personal immunity: The development of beliefs about susceptibility to the consequences of smoking. *Preventive Medicine, 15,* 363–372.

Hansen, W. B., Collins, L. M., Johnson, C. A., & Graham, J. W. (1985). Self-initiated smoking cessation among high school students. *Addictive Behaviors, 10,* 265–271.

Harrison, H. R., Phil, D., & Costin, M. (1985). Cervical *Chlamydia trachomatis* infection in university women: Relationship of history of contraception, ectopy, and cervicitis. *American Journal of Obstetrics and Gynecology, 153,* 344–251.

Hawkins, J. D., Catalano, R. F., & Miller, J. Y. (1992). Risk and protective factors for alcohol and other drug problems in adolescence and early adulthood: implications for substance abuse prevention. *Psychological Bulletin, 112,* 64–105.

Henshaw, S. K. (1994). *U.S. teenage pregnancy statistics.* New York: The Alan Guttmacher Institute.

Hingson, R. (1993). Prevention of alcohol-impaired driving. *Alcohol Health and Research World, 17,* 28–34.

Hingson, R., Merrigan, E., & Heeren, T. (1985). Effects of Massachusetts raising the legal drinking age from 18 to 20 on deaths from teenage homicide, suicide and nontraffic accidents. *Pediatric Clinics of North America, 32,* 221–232.

Holinger, P. C. (1989). Epidemiologic issues in youth suicide. In C. Pfeffer (Ed.), *Suicide among youth: Perspectives on risk and prevention* (pp. 41–62). Washington, DC: American Psychiatric Press.

Hoppock, K. C., & Houston, T. P. (1990). Availability of tobacco products to minors. *Journal of Family Practice, 30,* 174–176.

Igra, V., & Millstein, S. G. (1993). Current status and approaches to improving preventive services for adolescents. *Journal of the American Medical Association, 269,* 1408–1412.

Institute of Medicine. (1994). *Growing up tobacco free: Preventing nicotine addiction in children and youths.* Washington, DC: National Academy Press.

Irwin, C. E., & Millstein, S. G. (1986). Biopsychosocial correlates of risk-taking behaviors during adolescence. *Journal of Adolescent Health Care, 7,* 82S–96S.

Jemmott, J. B., & Jemmott, L. S. (1993). Alcohol and drug use during sexual activity: Predicting the HIV-risk related behaviors of inner-city black male adolescents. *Journal of Adolescent Research, 8,* 41–57.

Jemmott, J. B., Jemmott, L. S., & Fong, G. T. (1992). Reductions in HIV risk-associated sexual behaviors among black male adolescents: Effects of an AIDS prevention intervention. *American Journal of Public Health, 82,* 372–377.

Jessor, R. (1982, May). Problem behavior and developmental transition in adolescence. *Journal of School Health, 52*, 295–300.

Jessor, R. (1991). Risk behavior in adolescence: A psychosocial framework for understanding and action. *Journal of Adolescent Health, 12*, 597–605.

Jessor, R., & Jessor, S. L. (1977). *Problem behavior and psychosocial development: A longitudinal study of youth.* New York: Academic Press.

Joan, P. (1986). *Preventing teenage suicide: The living alternative handbook.* New York: Human Sciences Press.

Joffe, A. (1993). Adolescents and condom use. *American Journal Diseases of Children, 147*, 746–754.

Johnston, L. D., O'Malley, P. M., & Bachman, J. G. (1994). *National survey results from the Monitoring the Future Study, 1975–1993. Vol. I—Secondary school students.* Rockville, MD: National Institute on Drug Abuse.

Johnston, L. D., O'Malley, P. M., & Bachman, J. G. (1995). *National survey results on drug use from Monitoring the Future Study, 1975–1994.* Rockville, MD: National Institute on Drug Abuse.

Jones, R. B., & Moberg, D. P. (1988). Correlates of smokeless tobacco use in a male adolescent population. *American Journal of Public Health, 78*, 660–666.

Kalichman, S. C., Heckman, T., & Kelly, J. A. (1996). Sensation seeking as an explanation for the association between substance use and HIV-related risky sexual behavior. *Archives of Sexual Behavior, 25*, 141–154.

Kandel, D. B. (1985). On processes of peer influences in adolescent drug use: A developmental perspective. *Advances in Alcohol and Substance Abuse, 4*, 139–163.

Kann, L., Anderson, J. E., Holtzman, D., Ross, J., Truman, B. I., Collins, J., & Kolbe, L. J. (1991). HIV-related knowledge, beliefs, and behaviors among high school students in the United States: Results from a national survey. *Journal of School Health, 61*, 397–401.

Kegeles, S.M., Adler, N.E., & Irwin, C.E. (1988). Sexually active adolescents and condoms: Changes over one year in knowledge, attitudes and use. *American Journal of Public Health, 78*, 460–461.

Kelder, S. H. (1992). *Youth cardiovascular disease risk and prevention: The Minnesota Heart Health Program and the Class of 1989 Study.* Unpublished dissertation, University of Minnesota, Minneapolis, MN.

Ketterlinus, R. D., Lamb, M. E., Nitz, K., & Elster, A. B. (1992). Adolescent non-sexual and sex-related problem behaviors. *Journal of Adolescent Research, 7*, 431–456.

Kirby, D. (1992). School-based programs to reduce sexual risk-taking behaviors. *Journal of School Health, 62*, 280–287.

Kirby, D., & DiClemente, R.J. (1994). School-based interventions to prevent unprotected sex and HIV among adolescents. In R. J. DiClemente & J. Peterson (Eds.), *Preventing AIDS: Theories and methods of behavioral interventions* (pp. 117–139). New York: Plenum Press.

Kolbo, J. R. (1996). Risk and resilience among children exposed to family violence. *Violence and Victims, 11*, 113–128.

Kost, K., & Forrest, J. D. (1992). American women's sexual behavior and exposure to risk of sexually transmitted diseases. *Family Planning Perspectives, 24*, 244–254.

Lavery, B., Siegel, A. W., Cousins, J. H., & Rubovits, D. S. (1993). Adolescent risk-taking: An analysis of problem behaviors in problem children. *Journal of Experimental Child Psychology, 55*, 277–294.

Leibow, E. (1967). *Tally's corner: A study of Negro street corner men.* Boston: Little, Brown.

Lescohier, I., & Gallagher, S. S. (1996). Unintentional injury. In R. J. DiClemente, W. Hansen, & L. E. Ponton (Eds.), *Handbook of adolescent health risk behavior* (pp. 225–258). New York: Plenum Press.

Magnusson, D., Klinteberg, B., & Stattin, H. (1994). Juvenile and persistent offenders: Behavioral and physiological characteristics. In R. D. Ketterlinus & M. E. Lamb (Eds.), *Adolescent problem behaviors: Issues and research* (pp. 81–91). Hillsdale, NJ: Erlbaum.

Mahew, D. R., Donelson, A. C., Beirness, D. J., & Simpson, H. M. (1986). Youth, alcohol and relative risk of crash involvement. *Accident Analysis and Prevention, 18*, 273–287.

Main, D. S., Iverson, D. C., McGloin, J., Banspach, S. W., Collins, J. L., Rugg, D. L., & Kolbe, L. J. (1994). Preventing HIV infection among adolescents: Evaluation of a school-based education program. *Preventive Medicine, 23*, 409–417.

Mansfield, C. J., Conroy, M. E., Emans, S. J., & Woods, E. R. (1993). A pilot study of AIDS education and counseling of high-risk adolescents in an office setting. *Journal of Adolescent Health, 14*, 115–119.

Marlatt, G. A., Baer, J. S., Donovan, D. M., & Kivlahan, D. R. (1988). Addictive behaviors: Etiology and treatment. *Annual Review of Psychology, 39*, 223–252.

Mason, J. (1991). Prevention of violence: A public health commitment. *Public Health Reports, 106*, 265–268.

McLaughlin, R. J., Holcomb, J. D., Jibaja-Rusth, M. L., & Webb, J. (1993). Teacher ratings of student risk for substance use as a function of specialized training. *Journal of Drug Education, 23*, 83–95.

Merton, R. K. (1957). *Social theory and social structure.* New York: Free Press.

Miller, H. L., Coombs, D. W., Leeper, J. D., & Barton, S. N. (1984). An analysis of the effects of suicide prevention facilities on suicide rates in the United States. *American Journal of Public Health, 74,* 340–343.

Millstein, S. G., & Irwin, C. E. (1988). Accident-related behaviors in adolescence: A biopsychosocial view. *Alcohol, Drugs and Driving, 4,* 21–29.

Millstein, S. G., Irwin, C. E., Adler, N. E., Cohn, L. D., Kegeles, S. M., & Dolcini, M. M. (1992). Health-risk behaviors and health concerns among young adolescents. *Pediatrics, 89,* 422–428.

Mitchell, M. (1991). The Kansas City project. *Public Health Reports, 106,* 237.

Moore, K. A., Miller, B. C., Sugland, B. W., Morrison, D. R., Glei, D. A., & Blumenthal, C. (1995). *Beginning too soon: Adolescent sexual behavior, pregnancy and parenthood: A review of research and interventions.* Washington, DC: US Department of Health and Human Services.

Murray, D. M., Pirie, P., Luepker, R. V., & Pallonen, U. (1989). Five- and six-year follow-up results from four seventh-grade smoking prevention strategies. *Journal of Behavioral Medicine, 12,* 207–218.

National Center for Health Statistics. (1993). Monthly vital statistics report. *Advance report of final mortality statistics, 1991, 42*(2, Suppl.) Hyattsville, MD: Public Health Service.

National Highway Traffic Safety Administration. (1991). *Drunk driving facts.* Washington, DC: US Department of Transportation, National Highway Traffic Safety Administration.

National Safety Council. (1993). Accident facts. Itasca, IL: Naitonal Safety Council.

Neumark-Sztainer, D., Story, M., French, S., Cassuto, N., Jacobs, D. R., & Resnick, M. D. (1996). Patterns of health-compromising behaviors among Minnesota adolescents: Sociodemographic variations. *American Journal of Public Health, 86,* 1599–1606.

Newacheck, P. W., McManus, M. A., & Gephart, J. (1992). Health insurance coverage of adolescents: A current profile and assessment of trends. *Pediatrics, 90,* 589–596.

Newcomb, M. D., & McGee, L. (1991). Influence of sensation seeking on general deviance and specific problem behaviors from adolescence to adulthood. *Journal of Personality and Social Psychology, 61,* 614–628.

Office of the Inspector General. (December, 1992). Youth access to tobacco. Washington, DC: US Department of Health and Human Services. Report No. OEI-02-92-00880.

O'Leary, A., DiClemente, R. J., & Aral, S. (1997). Reflections on the design and reporting of STD/HIV behavioral intervention research. *AIDS Education & Prevention, 9* (Suppl. A), 1–14.

Oliver, R. G., & Hertzel, B. S. (1972). Rise and fall of suicide rates in Australia: Relation to sedative availability. *Medical Journal of Australia, 2,* 919–923.

Orr, D. P., Wilbrandt, M. L., Brack, C. J., Rauch, S. P., & Ingersoll, G. M. (1989). Reported sexual behaviors and self-esteem among young adolescents. *American Journal of Diseases of Children, 143,* 86–90.

Pattishall, E. G. (1994). A research agenda for adolescent problems and risk-taking behaviors. In R. D. Ketterlinus & M. E. Lamb (Eds.), *Adolescent problem behaviors: Issues and research* (pp. 209–215). Hillsdale, NJ: Erlbaum.

Pentz, M. A., MacKinnon, D. P., Dwyer, J. H., Wang, E. Y. I., Hansen, W. B., Flay, B. R., & Johnson, C. A. (1989). Longitudinal effects of the Midwestern Prevention Project on regular and experimental smoking in adolescents. *Preventive Medicine, 18,* 304–321.

Perry, C. L., & Staufacker, M. J. (1996). Tobacco use. In R. J. DiClemente, W. Hansen, & L. E. Ponton (Eds.), *Handbook of adolescent health risk behavior* (pp. 53–82). New York: Plenum Press.

Perry, C. L., Klepp, K. I., & Shultz, J. M. (1988). Primary prevention of cardiovascular disease: Communitywide strategies for youth. *Journal of Consulting and Clinical Psychology, 56,* 358–364.

Peters, K. D., Kochanek, K. D., & Murphy, S. L. (1998). Deaths: Final data for 1996. *National vital statistics reports, 47*(9). Hyattsville, MD: Public Health Service.

Phinney, V. G., Jensen, L. C., Olsen, J. A., & Cundick, B. (1990). The relationship between early development and psychosexual behaviors in adolescent females. *Adolescence, 98,* 321–332.

Pierce, J. P., & Gilpin, E. (1996). How long will today's new adolescent smoker be addicted to cigarettes? *American Journal of Public Health, 86,* 253–256.

Prothrow-Sith, D. (1991). Boston's violence prevention project. *Public Health Reports, 106,* 237–239.

Quadral, M. J., Fishoff, B., & Davis, W. (1993). Adolescent (in)vulnerability. *American Psychologist, 48,* 102–116.

Rooney, B. L., & Murray, D. M. (1996). A meta-analysis of smoking prevention programs after adjustment for errors in the unit of analysis. *Health Education Quarterly, 12,* 48–64.

Rosenberg, H. M., Ventura, S. J., Maurer, J. D., Heuser, R. L., & Freedman, M. A. (1996). Births and deaths: United States, 1995. *Monthly Vital Statistics Report, 45*(3, Suppl. 2). Hyattsville, MD: National Center for Health Statistics.

Rosenberg, M. L., Smith, J. C., Davidson, L. E., & Conn, J. M. (1987). The emergence of youth suicide: An epidemiologic analysis and public health perspective. *Annual Review of Public Health, 8,* 417–440.

Ross, J. G., Saavedra, P. J., Shur, G. H., & Winters, F. (1992). The effectiveness of an afterschool program for primary grade latchkey students on precursors of substance abuse. *Journal of Community Psychology, Special Issue: Programs for Change,* 22–38.

Rotheram-Borus, M. J., Koopman, C., Haignere, C., & Davies, M. (1991). Reducing HIV sexual risk behaviors among runaway adolescents. *Journal of the American Medical Association, 266,* 1237–1241.

Rotheram-Borus, M. J., Feldman, J., Rosario, M., & Dunne, E. (1994). Preventing HIV among runaways: Victims and victimization. In R. J. DiClemente & J. Peterson (Eds.), *Preventing AIDS: Theories and methods of behavioral interventions* (pp. 175–188). New York: Plenum Press.

Runyan, C. W., & Gerken, E. A. (1989). Epidemiology and prevention of adolescent injury: A review and research agenda. *Journal of the American Medical Association, 262,* 2273–2279.

Saffer, H., & Grossman, M. (1987). Beer taxes, the legal drinking age, and youth motor vehicle fatalities. *Journal of Legal Studies, 16,* 351–374.

Scheidt, P. C., Harel, Y., Trumble, A. C., Jones, D. H., Overpeck, M. D., & Bijur, P. E. (1995). The epidemiology of nonfatal injuries among US children and youth. *American Journal of Public Health, 85,* 932–938.

Schuster, M. A., Bell, R. M., & Kanouse, D. E. (1996). The sexual practices of adolescent virgins: Genital sexual activities of high school students who have never had vaginal intercourse. *American Journal of Public Health, 86,* 1570–1576.

Schwarz, D. (1993). Adolescent trauma: Epidemiologic approach. *Adolescent Medicine: State of the Art Reviews, 4,* 11–22.

Seal, D. W., & Agostinelli, G. (1994). Individual differences associated with high-risk sexual behaviour: Implications for intervention programmes. *AIDS Care, 6,* 393–397.

Shafer, M. A., Hilton, J. F., Ekstrand, M., Keogh, J., Gee, L., DiGiorgio-Haag, L., Shalwitx, J., & Schachter, J. (1993). Relationship between drug use and sexual behaviors and occurrence of sexually transmitted diseases among high-risk male youth. *Sexually Transmitted Diseases, 20,* 307–313.

Shaffer, D., Garland, A., Underwood, M., & Whittle, B. (1987). *An evaluation of three youth suicide prevention programs in New Jersey.* Trenton: New Jersey State Department of Health and Human Services.

Shaffer, D., Garland, A., Gould, M., Fisher, P., & Trautman, P. (1988). Preventing teenage suicide: A critical review. *Journal of the American Academy of Child and Adolescent Psychiatry, 27,* 675–687.

Shain, M., Suurvali, H., & Kilty, H. (1980). *The Parent Communication Project: A longitudinal study of the effects of parenting skills on children's use of alcohol.* Toronto: Addiction Research Foundation of Ontario.

Shaklee, H., & Fishoff, B. (1990). The psychology of contraceptive surprises: Judging the cumulative risk of contraceptive failure. *Journal of Applied Psychology, 20,* 385–403.

Sheer, V. C., & Cline, R. J. W. (1995). Individual differences in sensation seeking and sexual behavior: Implications for communication intervention for HIV/AIDS prevention among college students. *Health Communication, 7,* 205–223.

Singh, G. K., & Yu, S. M. (1996). Trends and differentials in adolescent and young adult mortality in the United States, 1950 through 1993. *American Journal of Public Health, 86,* 560–564.

Singh, G. K., Kochanek, K. D., & MacDorman, M. F. (1996). Advance report of final mortality statistics, 1994. *Monthly Vital Statistics Report, 45*(3, Suppl.). Hyattsville, MD: National Center for Health Statistics.

Slap, G. B., Plotkin, S. L., Khalid, N., Michelman, D. F., & Forke, C. M. (1991). A human immunodeficiency virus peer education program for adolescent females. *Journal of Adolescent Health, 12,* 434–442.

Snyder, H. (December 10, 1998). Male and female juvenile arrest rates for violent crime index offenses, 1981–1997. *OJJDP Statistical Briefing Book.* Online: http://ojjdp.ncjrs.org/ojstatbb/qa004.html.

Stanton, B. F., Li, X., Ricardo, I., Galbraith, J., Feigelman, S., & Kaljee, L. (1996). A randomized, controlled effectiveness trial of an AIDS prevention program for low-income African-American youths. *Archives of Pediatrics and Adolescent Medicine, 150,* 363–372.

Stiffman, A. R., Earls, F., Dore, P., Cunningham, R., & Farber, S. (1996). Adolescent violence. In R. J. DiClemente, W. B. Hansen, & L. E. Ponton (Eds.), *Handbook of adolescent health risk behaviors* (pp. 289–312). NY: Plenum Press.

Sullivan, L. (1991). Forum on youth violence in minority communities. The prevention of violence—a top HHS priority. *Public Health Reports, 106,* 268–269.

Sussman, S., Dent, C. W., Stacy, A. W., Sun, P., Craig, S., & Simon, T. R. (1993). Project towards tobacco use: 1-year behavior outcomes. *American Journal of Public Health, 83,* 1245–1250.

Thompson, E. L. (1978). Smoking education programs, 1960–1976. *American Journal of Public Health, 68,* 250–257.

Tobler, N. S. (1992). Drug prevention programs can work: Research findings. *Journal of Addictive Diseases,* 11, 1–28.

Turner, R. A., Irwin, C. E., Tschsann, J. M., & Millstein, S. G. (1993). Autonomy, relatedness, and the initiation of health risk behaviors in early adolescence. *Health Psychology,* 12, 200–208.

Udry, J. R. (1990). Biosocial models of adolescent problem behaviors. *Social Biology,* 37, 1–10.

Udry, J. R. (1994). Integrating biological and sociological models of adolescent problem behaviors. In R. D. Ketterlinus & M. E. Lamb (Eds.), *Adolescent problem behaviors: Issues and research* (pp. 93–107). Hillsdale, NJ: Erlbaum.

US Bureau of the Census. (1996a). *Current population reports: Household and family characteristics, various years* (P-20). Washington, DC: US Department of Commerce.

US Bureau of the Census. (1996b). *Current population reports: Marital status and living arrangements* (Nos. 433, 445, 450). Washington, DC: US Department of Commerce.

US Bureau of the Census. (1997a). *Resident population of the United States: Estimates by age and sex.* (PPL-57). Washington, DC: US Department of Commerce.

US Bureau of the Census, Poverty and Health Statistics Branch. (1997b). *March current population survey.* Washington, DC: US Department of Commerce.

US Congress, Office of Technology Assessment. (1991). *Adolescent health—Volume III: Cross-cutting issues in the delivery of health and related services.* Washington, DC: US Government Printing Office. No. OTA-H-467.

US Department of Health and Human Services (USDHHS). (1990). *Healthy people 2000: National health promotion and disease prevention objectives.* Washington, DC: Public Health Service.

US Department of Health and Human Services (USDHHS). (1995). *Vital and health statistics, Health-risk behaviors among our nation's youth: United States, 1992.* Hyattsville, MD: National Center for Health Statistics.

US Department of Health and Human Services (USDHHS). (1996a). Trends in the well-being of America's children and youth: 1996. In P. A. Jargowski (Ed.), *1990 census summary tape,* File 3A (pp. 30). Washington, DC: General Printing Office, PSO24853.

US Department of Health and Human Services (USDHHS). (1996b). *Vital and health statistics, leading causes of death by age, sex, race and Hispanic origin: United States, 1992.* Hyattsville, MD: National Center for Health Statistics.

US Department of Justice. (1988). *Criminal victimization in the United States, 1986: A national crime survey report* (NJC-111456). Washington, DC: Bureau of Justice Statistics.

Van de Perre, P., Jacobs, D., & Sprecher-Goldberger, S. (1987). The latex condom, an efficient barrier against sexual transmission of AIDS-related viruses. *AIDS,* 1, 49–52.

Ventura, S. J., Martin, J. A., Mathews, T. J., & Clark, S. C. (1996). Advance report of final natality statistics, 1994. *Monthly Vital Statistics Report,* 44(11S), p. 31 . Hyattsville, MD: National Center for Health Statistics.

Walter, H. J., & Vaughan, R. D. (1993). AIDS risk reduction among a multiethnic sample of urban high school students. *Journal of the American Medical Association,* 270, 725–730.

Webster, L. A., Berman, S. M., & Greenspan, J. R. (1993). Surveillance for gonorrhea and primary and secondary syphilis among adolescents, United States. 1981–1991. *Morbidity and Mortality Weekly Report,* 42, 1–11.

Wechsler, H., Dowdall, G. W., Davenport, A., & Castillo, S. (1995). Correlates of college student binge drinking. *American Journal of Public Health,* 85, 921–926.

Weiler, R. M. (1992). Health concerns of rural high school students and their beliefs about the health concerns of their best friends and other teenagers. Paper presented at the *120th Annual meeting of the American Public Health Association,* Washington, DC.

Weinstein, N. D. (1987). Unrealistic optimism about susceptibility to health problems: Conclusions from a community-wide sample. *Journal of Behavioral Medicine,* 10, 481–500.

Williams, A., Karps, R., & Zador, P. (1983). Variations in minimum licensing age and fatal motor vehicle crashes. *American Journal of Public Health,* 73, 1401–1403.

Williams, A. F. (1985). Nighttime driving and fatal crash involvement of teenagers. *Accident Analysis and Prevention,* 17, 1–5.

Wilson, M. D., Kastrinakis, M., D'Angelo, L. J., & Getson, P. (1994). Attitudes, knowledge, and behavior regarding condom use in urban black adolescent males. *Adolescence,* 113, 13–26.

Wilson-Brewer, R., Cohen, S., O'Donnell, L., & Goodman, I. (1991). *Violence prevention for young adolescents: A survey of the state of the art.* Washington, DC: Carnegie Council.

Windle, M., Shope, J. T., & Bukstein, O. (1996). Alcohol use. In R.J. DiClemente, W. Hansen, & L.E. Ponton (Eds.), *Handbook of adolescent health risk behavior* (pp. 115–160). New York: Plenum Press.

Wingood, G. M., & DiClemente, R. J. (1992). Cultural, gender and psychosocial influences on HIV-related behavior of African-American female adolescents: Implications for the development of tailored prevention programs. *Ethnicity and Disease, 2*, 381–388.

Wintemute, G. H. (1987). Firearms as a cause of death in the United States, 1920–1982. *Journal of Trauma, 27*, 532–536.

Wintemute, G. J. (1990). Childhood drowning and near-drowning in the United States. *American Journal of Diseases of Children, 144*, 663–669.

Womble, K. (1989). *The impact of minimum drinking laws on fatal crash involvement: An update of the NHTSA analyses.* Washington, DC: National Highway Traffic Safety Administration.

Zabin, L. S., Hirsch, M. B., Smith, E. A., Streett, R., & Hardy, J. B. (1986a). Evaluation of a pregnancy prevention program for urban teenagers. *Family Planning Perspectives, 18*, 119–126.

Zabin, L. S., Hardy, J. B., Smith, E. A., & Hirsch, M. B. (1986b). Substance use and its relation to sexual activity among inner-city adolescents. *Journal of Adolescent Health Care, 7*, 320–331.

Zaslow, M. J., & Takanishi, R. (1993). Priorities for research on adolescent development. *American Psychologist, 48*, 185–192.

Zill, N., Nord, C. W., & Loomis, L. S. (1995). *Adolescent time use, risky behavior and outcomes: An analysis of national data.* Report prepared for the Office of the Assistant Secretary for Planning and Evaluation, US Department of Health and Human Services.

Zuckerman, M. (1979). *Sensation seeking: Beyond the optimal level of arousal.* Hillsdale, NJ: Lawrence Erlbaum.

CHAPTER *25*

Older Populations

Melissa M. Galvin, Marilyn M. Gardner, and Molly Engle

Introduction

At the turn of the 20th century, life expectancy for humans was 47 years. Few individuals lived into their 70s, and only 1 in 10 individuals lived past the age of 65. Today, at the turn of the 21st century, life expectancy has reached the mid-70s. Many individuals, however, are living well past that point; over 8 in 10 can now expect to live into their late 70s. Today, approximately 1 in 8 Americans is over the age of 65 (13%). By the year 2030, it is estimated that 1 in 5, or 20% of the population, will be age 65 or older.

To keep pace with the specific needs of the aging population, it is important to understand the challenges and implications of these changing demographics. The implications to the nation's health care system, for example, are staggering. Chronic diseases such as heart disease, cancer, and stroke now account for 7 of every 10 deaths in the older US population. These chronic conditions contribute to the elderly's increased use of health services: People over the age of 65 visit a doctor eight times a year as compared to five times for the general public. Further, those age 65 and older are hospitalized three times more often than those under the age of 65 and stay 50% longer and use twice as many prescriptions.

The provision of health care for the elderly must extend beyond palliative care and concerns with life expectancy, to include issues related to quality of life. Health promotion strategies hold great potential in enhancing quality of life among the elderly. Because risk factors for common diseases become more complex during the aging process, it is imperative that health promotion and disease prevention activities be tailored to meet the specific needs of this population.

In this chapter, we discuss the changing demographic picture and the complexity of risk factors among older populations. We look at how these risk factors relate to health promotion strategies and how these strategies differ for older adults.

Melissa M. Galvin and Marilyn M. Gardner • Department of Health Behavior, School of Public Health, University of Alabama at Birmingham, Birmingham, Alabama 35294.   *Molly Engle* • Department of Public Health, College of Health and Human Performance, Oregon State University, and Oregon State Extension Service, Corvallis, Oregon 97331.

Handbook of Health Promotion and Disease Prevention, edited by Raczynski and DiClemente. Kluwer Academic/Plenum Publishers, New York, 1999.

Epidemiology: Demographic Upheaval

In the 1880s, Germany's Chancellor von Bismarck established the universal military retirement age at 65 years. Since that time, age 65 has become a commonly accepted benchmark that indicates the beginning of an individual's "third age." Yet, as is often the case with policy decisions, there were political and economic ramifications surrounding the choice of 65 years. Life expectancy at that time was around 45 years. Almost 90% of the population could expect to die before age 65. As such, von Bismarck shrewdly chose 65 as the retirement age, thus assuring that the state did not have to pay lengthy and expensive retirement income to the army (Dychtwald, 1986).

As mentioned earlier, approximately one in eight Americans today is over the age of 65 (13%). The fastest-growing segment of this older population is among the oldest-old, those aged 85 and older (Fig. 1). This burgeoning segment of the older population is having a major impact on the nation's health care and its social service delivery, as well as on family systems.

To illustrate the impact of this changing age distribution, one need only look at the shift in the percentages of older persons compared to those under the age of 18 (Fig. 2). At the turn of the century, only 4% of the population was over the age of 65, while 40% was under age 18. Anticipated projections for 2030 suggest that 22% of the population will be over the age of 65 and 21% will be under age 18. This "population squaring" is the result of the baby boom generation (those individuals born between 1946 and 1964) moving into the third age as society moves into the third millennium.

In addition to people living longer, family size has declined as people are electing to have fewer children. At the turn of the century, the average family had four children. Today the average is less than two. This shrinking size of the American family is changing the shape of the elderly–support ratio, the number of people aged 65 and older compared to the number of people of working age, 18 to 64 years. In the

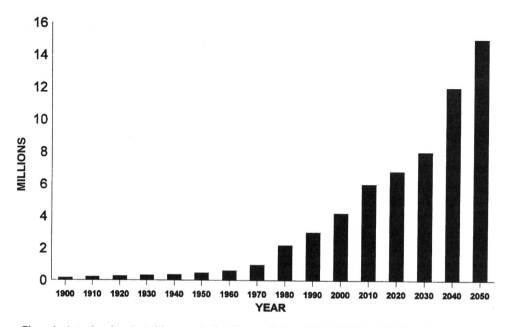

Figure 1. Actual and projected increase in the 85+ population: 1900–2050. From USDHHS (1991, p. 12).

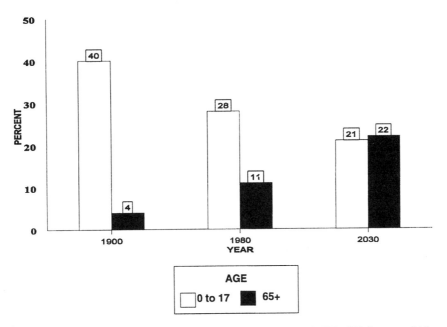

Figure 2. Percent of children and elderly in the population: 1900, 1980, and 2030. 1900 figures, which exclude Alaska, Hawaii, and Armed Forces overseas, from US Bureau of the Census (1965). 1980 and 2030 figures, from USDHHS (1991, p. 9).

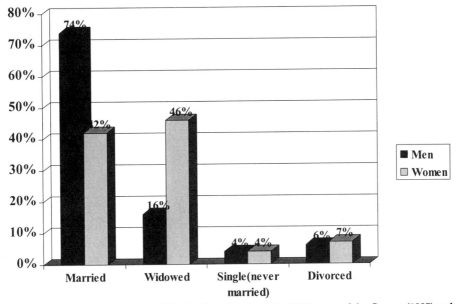

Figure 3. Marital status of persons 65+: 1995. Based on data from the US Bureau of the Census (1995) and Profile of Older Americans (1997).

early 1900s, the elderly–support ratio was 7 per 100. Elderly–support ratio projections for year 2030 are 38 per 100. Because services for and to the elderly are supported primarily through publicly funded entitlement programs, the policy implication of this shift are far reaching (US Senate Special Committee on Aging, 1991). Programs such

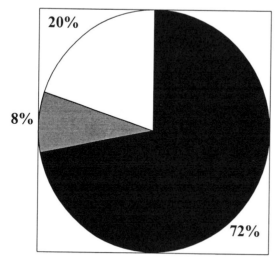

20%

8%

72%

Men

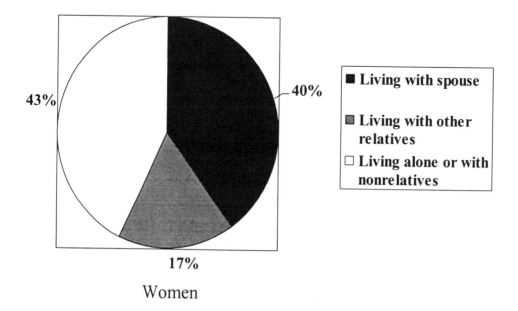

43%

40%

■ Living with spouse

▨ Living with other relatives

☐ Living alone or with nonrelatives

17%

Women

Figure 4. Living arrangements of persons 65+: 1995. Based on data from US Bureau of the Census (1995).

as Social Security and Medicare will need major restructuring to accommodate this burgeoning cohort.

The increasing overall percentage of elderly affects other demographic considerations as well. The most notable perhaps is gender distribution. Men generally have higher death rates than women at every age. Consequently, most elderly, especially the oldest-old, are women. By age 65, women outnumber men 3 to 2. By age 85, more than 7 out of 10 (72%) of the US population in this age group are women (US Senate Special Committee on Aging, 1991).

This gender disparity is also noted in marital status and living arrangements. Older men, for example, spend the latter years of their life married (76%) and in family settings (81%). More women, however, spend their latter years as widows (47%) and live alone or with nonrelatives (44%) (Figs. 3, 4). Less than a third (30%) of the noninstitutionalized elderly live alone. Yet, only an average of 4% of those 65 and older live in nursing homes. This percentage increases with age: 1% for ages 65–74, 5% for ages 75–84, and 15% for ages 85+ (US Senate Special Committee on Aging, 1991).

The elderly are also concentrated in geographic locations. Over half (52%) of the elderly live in nine states: California, Florida, New York, Texas, Pennsylvania, Ohio, Illinois, Michigan, and New Jersey. They are divided fairly evenly among urban (30%), suburban (46%), and rural (24%) areas (US Senate Special Committee on Aging, 1991).

Today, the elderly population is predominately white. However, beginning in the next century, older adults of color are expected to increase more rapidly than the older white population, resulting in a much more ethnically and racially diverse elderly group. Between the late 1990s and the year 2050, the number of elderly black are expected to more than triple, and the number of Hispanic elderly are expected to increase 11 times (Siegel, 1996).

Behavioral Risk Factors and the Older Adult

Understanding the overall health status of the elderly is an essential component of designing, implementing, and evaluating health promotion programs for older adults. Overall health declines with advancing age as chronic conditions, such as arthritis, hypertension, hearing impairment, and heart disease increase (Table 1) (USDHHS, 1991). Memory and other cognitive functioning are affected, with Alzheimer's disease being the leading cause of cognitive impairment. Social functioning changes over time as well, as society changes around the older adult. Yet despite these changes, most older adults (71.4%) describe themselves in good health (USDHHS, 1991). As illustrated in Table 2, an individual's health is directly related to his or her income, with 26% of those elderly with incomes over $35,000 describing their health as excellent compared to 10% of those with incomes less than $10,000.

Promoting Health among Older Populations

Behavioral risk factors commonly associated with diseases in adults under 65, such as diet, activity, smoking, drinking, are still contributory to diseases in adults 65 and over (Fig. 5). Yet because these risk factors are often overshadowed and com-

Table 1. Number of Elderly People and Percent Distribution by Respondent-Assessed Health Status, by Sex and Family Income, 1989[a]

Characteristic	All persons[c] (000s)	Respondent-assessed health status[b]					
		All health status[d]	Excel- lent	Very good	Good	Fair	Poor
All persons 65+[e]	29,219	100.0	6.4	23.1	31.9	19.3	9.2
Sex:							
Men	12,143	100.0	16.9	23.2	30.8	18.4	10.7
Women	17,076	100.0	16.1	23.0	32.8	20.0	8.1
Family income:							
Under $10,000	5,612	100.0	10.3	19.4	29.7	25.0	15.6
$10,000 to $19,999	8,002	100.0	14.8	21.7	33.9	21.1	8.5
$20,000 to $34,999	5,242	100.0	20.2	25.7	32.5	15.7	5.9
$35,000 and over	3,484	100.0	26.0	26.8	30.3	11.7	5.1

[a] USDHHS (1991, p. 109). Data are based on household interviews of the civilian, noninstitutionalized population.
[b] Excludes unknown health status.
[c] Includes unknown health status.
[d] The categories related to this concept result from asking the respondent, "Would you say health is excellent, very good, good, fair, or poor?" As such, it is based on the respondent's opinion and not directly on any clinical evidence.
[e] Includes unknown family income.
NOTE: Percentages may not add to 100 percent due to rounding.

Table 2. Personal Health Characteristics for People 18+: 1985[a]

Characteristic (%)	Sleeps 6 hours or less	Never eats breakfast	Smokes every day[b]	Less physically active than contem- poraries	Had 5 or more drinks on any one day[c]	Current smoker	30% or more above desirable weight[d]
All people 18+[e]	22.0	24.3	39.0	16.4	37.5	30.1	13.0
AGE							
18 to 29 years old	19.8	30.4	42.2	17.1	54.4	31.9	7.5
30 to 44 years old	24.3	30.1	41.4	18.3	39.0	34.5	13.6
45 to 64 years old	22.7	21.4	37.9	15.3	24.6	31.6	18.1
65+ years	20.4	7.5	30.7	13.5	12.2	16.0	13.2
65 to 74 years old	19.7	9.0	32.4	15.8	NA	19.7	14.9
75+ years	21.5	5.1	27.8	9.8	NA	10.0	10.3

[a] US National Center for Health Statistics, unpublished data. Based on National Health Interview Survey.
[b] Percent of current smokers.
[c] Percent of drinkers who had five or more drinks on any one day in the past year.
[d] Based on 1960 Metropolitan Life Insurance Company standards. Data are self-reported.
[e] Excludes people whose health practices are unknown.

pounded by the presence of one or more chronic conditions, health care tends to be palliative. In spite of their overall positive, self-reported health status, there are no data that suggest that older populations are immune from the benefits associated with health promotion and prevention activities. Understanding the complex and myriad risk factors influencing health promotion for older populations is not simple but is important if risk factors are to be modified.

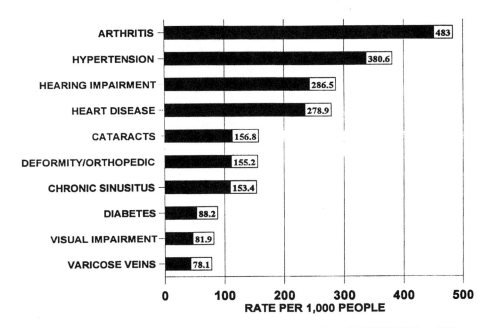

Figure 5. The top ten chronic conditions for people 65+: 1989. From USDHHS (1991, p. 113).

Adapting Theory: A Case for Self-Efficacy

Although behavior change theories abound, as noted in other chapters of this volume, the challenge when working with the older adult lies in adapting theory to meet the special needs of an aging population. Though there is no singular theory that is without limitations, Bandura's self-efficacy theory (1977) is now widely acknowledged as a key construct when working with the elderly (Strecher, DeVellis, Becker, & Rosenstock, 1986; Schunk & Carbonari, 1984). Self-efficacy, defined as "beliefs in one's capabilities to organize and execute the courses of action required to produce given attainments" (Bandura, 1997, p. 3), is closely associated with changes in and maintenance of behaviors that promote the physical, cognitive, and social functional areas related to health (Waller & Bates, 1992; Strecher *et al.*, 1986). Waller and Bates (1992) speculate that higher generalized self-efficacy increases the probability of that older adults will benefit from health promotion programs.

Efficacy beliefs influence behaviors through cognitive, affective, and motivational processes. As we note throughout this chapter, the strength of efficacy influences both perceptions and performance. For example, people with a high health efficacy, that is, who believe health is within their personal control and therefore modifiable, rather than biologically predetermined, are more active participants in health-promoting and -protecting behaviors (Waller & Bates, 1992).

Although self-efficacy is a key variable in behavioral change, elderly individuals vary in how they respond to opportunities to exercise personal control. Generally, the elderly express less desire for control than their younger counterparts (Woodward & Wallston, 1987), even though such personal efficacy promotes health and aids in the physical and social recovery from injuries common to older people [e.g., hip fractures, coronary artery surgery (Carrol, 1995; Ruiz, 1992)].

Self-Efficacy and Functional Areas

Evidence exists supporting the influence of the individuals generalized self-efficacy on physical, cognitive, memory, and social functional areas. Each functional area is discussed below.

Physical Functioning

Advancing age is generally associated with changes in physiological functioning and biological decay. Losses with advancing age are noted in immune, cardiovascular, endocrine, renal, and pulmonary systems. Moreover, evidence exists that suggests that there is a biologically fixed, upper limit of the life span (Hayflick, 1968; Fries & Crapo, 1981). Biological reserves in organ systems far exceed what is needed given the upper limit of the life span. As such, biological degeneration does not necessarily impair one's functional capability (Fries & Crapo, 1981). The disparity between the biological degeneration and ones functional capability explains at least some of the great variability in the aging process and geriatric disease patterns among older individuals.

Little research has been published on the healthy elderly. In fact, standard definitions of health are not always applicable to the elderly, due to the presence of at least one chronic disease in a majority of this population (Lichtenstein & Thomas, 1987). Thus, researchers have often measured the health status of the elderly using individual's perceived and functional health (Lichtenstein & Thomas, 1987), as well as through proximal measures such as medical service delivery and days of hospitalization (or length of stay) (German, 1981; Kane & Kane, 1981). The inferences drawn from these proximal measures can negatively influence perceptions of individual physical health, and thus, hasten his or her biological decline.

Research on aging has largely focused on pathological states. Thus, we are provided primarily with a descriptive analysis of the aging process rather than an understanding of the biological mechanisms of aging. As research on aging discovers more about the mechanisms and processes of aging, a knowledge base serving as a foundation for health initiatives aimed at disease prevention and health enhancement for the older adult is being created.

Complementing this expanding knowledge base is a shift away from the traditional biomedical model emphasizing palliative care toward a broader psychosocial approach. This psychosocial approach, which moves beyond measuring health as the absence of disease and physical impairment, views both health and morbidity as being psychosociobiological in nature. Health and morbidity are considered the product of interactions between biological and psychosocial factors, with prevention and health enhancement as vital tenets. A key product of this interaction is self-efficacy specifically as it relates to personal control (Bandura, 1997).

Relinquishing personal control has an impact on physical functioning. At the individual level, physical states take on increasing importance as indicators of physical capability as one ages. As an individual ages, more attention is paid to normal aches and pains, interpreting them as signs of decline or functional loss. While this supposition is not supported by research, it can and often does initiate a spiral of decline by lessening physical efficacy, the amount of confidence an individual has in her or his physical abilities. Lowered physical efficacy, in turn, influences the amount of effort exerted or whether an effort is exerted at all (Bandura, 1997).

Individual beliefs and cognitive function are often cited as the cause of declines in physical functioning. Too often, however, these declines are misattributed to biology by both the aging individuals and those around them. For example, although declines in physical stamina are frequently blamed on aging, researchers have reported that physical stamina can be reduced by lowering perceived physical efficacy (Weinberg, Gould, & Jackson, 1979; Weinberg, Yukelson, & Jackson, 1980). This lowered physical efficacy likely reduces the amount and type of physical activity in which older people engage. Lowered physical efficacy may contribute to the fact that only about 8% of those aged 65 or over engage in regular physical activity, and an alarming 43% are sedentary, in spite of the fact that regular physical activity is known to be a means of improving health and extending life (Caspersen, Christenson, & Pollard, 1986).

Consequently, physical inactivity has a detrimental impact on health, resulting in impaired physiological functioning and biological decay. Notably, physical inactivity produces many similar declines in biological functions as those commonly experienced by the older adult and attributed to the aging process (Bortz, 1982). Conversely, those with a high physical efficacy are more consistently physically active (McAuley, 1993), and thus, experience less physical decline.

Cognitive Functioning

Cognitive functioning encompasses a host of capabilities and processes. There is great variability in how these change during aging. The speed and flexibility during information processing and psychomotor facility, for example, tend to decline over time. Processes that require accumulated expert knowledge, such as reasoning, problem solving, and wisdom, however, tend to remain stable or increase into old age (Baltes & Smith, 1990).

Cross-sectional comparisons of different age groups reveal a significant decline in intellectual functioning between the young and old. Longitudinal cohort studies, however, reveal no pervasive or general decline in intellectual functioning until the very advanced years (Baltes & Labouvie, 1973; Schaie, 1995). This suggests that differences are attributable more to generational differences than to biological aging (Schaie, 1995). Further, cross-sectional studies of same-aged adults show an increase in cognitive functioning over generations, thus supporting the view that many "declines" in cognitive functioning are actually misattributed to aging.

Cognitive functioning varies greatly across individuals. Examination of elders who maintained high levels of cognitive functioning revealed a positive association with certain psychosocial determinants, including education and the pursuit of intellectually stimulating activities as well as adaptability and satisfaction with life accomplishments in mid-life. Elders whose lifestyle promoted and maintained physical health also maintained a high level of cognitive functioning (Schaie, 1995).

An exhaustive longitudinal analysis of successful cognitive aging identified four independent contributors to the preservation of cognitive functioning in the elderly from a vast array of sociodemographic, psychosocial, lifestyle, and physiological factors. They were educational level, pulmonary capacity, a physically active lifestyle, and a sense of efficacy to influence daily life (Albert et al., 1995). Since these contributors can all be modified, it follows that cognitive functioning can be modified even into advanced old age. Teaching the elderly strategies to make better use of their cognitive capabilities result in substantially improved levels of cognitive functioning

(Baltes & Lindenberger, 1988). Even brief training in cognitive strategies can create gains in cognitive functioning (Willis & Schaie, 1986).

Memory Functioning

Memory is a cognitive function that warrants special consideration. Memory decline is of major concern to the elderly, who frequently view memory performance as an indicator of intellectual capability (Berry, 1989). As such, normal lapses in memory are often distorted and assume great significance as a sign of cognitive decline. In reality, there are different types of memory that are affected differently by biological aging. Some do, indeed, decline with aging, such as those requiring active processing or restructuring of materials. Others, however, remain stable, such as long-term memory.

Memory function is often regarded as being a finite entity that diminishes with biological aging. This belief fosters the notion that people have little or no control over memory functioning. The perceived lack of control over memory functioning serves as a disincentive for even trying, thus setting into motion a rather vicious cycle. The more the elderly disbelieve in their ability to influence memory, the less use they make of their cognitive capabilities. This reduced effort then contributes to forgetfulness, regardless of cognitive capabilities (Lachman, Bandura, Weaver & Elliott, 1995). This cycle results in lowered efficacy in the elderly, which can contribute to feelings of doubt about abilities to solve problems and live independently and to depression. For some, it also raises concern over the possibility that the perceived memory loss experienced signals the onset of Alzheimer's disease.

In marked contrast, those who believe memory is a controllable skill devote more time to cognitively processing memory (Berry, 1996). This increased processing effort results in better memory performance. It is this segment of the population that displays more confidence in ability to improve memory, solve problems, and live independently. Memory self-efficacy is also associated with low depression (Bandura, 1997).

Social Functioning

Aging occurs within the broader context of society, which shapes expectations and constructs social realities. An often overlooked factor in this equation of social realities is the fact that societies age as people do. Therefore, what was true of older people in the past may not hold true for older people today or for those in the future. That societal change influences social functioning is of great importance, yet research in this area is sorely lacking. When research on aging separates individuals' social functioning from the larger social context, there is an inherent danger of misattributing declines in social functioning, in whole or in part, to biological aging (Bandura, 1997).

Today's generation of elderly is aging more successfully than past generations. Unfortunately, the existing social systems have not kept pace (Riley, Kahn, & Foner, 1994). Failing to accommodate the expanded potential of the elderly introduces constraints that affect the potential of the older adult living a healthy, productive life and fosters functional declines. Consequently, it is reasonable to suggest that problems faced by the elderly are at least partially attributable to the failure of social systems.

At an individual level, people tend to age more successfully when discontinuity or disruption in their major life pursuits are minimal (Bandura, 1997). As people age, however, life is typically fraught with changes and interruptions. Retirement, the "empty nest," and death each bring about changes in or loss of productive roles, self-identification, and personal relationships and limit access to stimulating or challenging activities. The more limited the elderly are by these environmental constraints, the greater their decline in functioning (Schooler, 1987).

Aging also brings about periods of self-examination, reflection, and evaluation as people transition to their third age. Aging occurs against the backdrop of perceptions and stereotypes of aging held by the individual, based on past generations of elderly, and of other sources of social comparison. In the media, for example, advertisements targeting the elderly abound, most highlighting the problems of "biological" decline. Further, the elderly are typically portrayed as comical or eccentric characters, rather than as vital people living productive, stimulating lives. Such social comparisons contribute to the minimalization by others of the significant contributions the elderly can make and alters the aging individual's social functioning (Bandura, 1997).

Once age assumes great personal significance, changes in social functioning are often misattributed to biological aging. Contributing sociocultural factors, such as shifting cultural mores, role attributions, and expectations, are downplayed or disregarded. As with physical and cognitive functioning, there is great variability in social functioning with aging and in individuals' responses to the stress and challenges of later life. The way in which these challenges are handled is influenced by the individual's social efficacy, the confidence one has in her or his ability to function socially (Bandura, 1997).

Persons with low social efficacy perceive that they are unable to control or influence important life events. This low social efficacy fosters feelings of despondency (Marshall & Lang, 1990) and predicts depression even when multiple controls are applied for differences in social support, faulty automatic thinking, and preexisting depression (Olioff, Bryson, & Wadden, 1989). These feelings of despondency further lower social efficacy (Kavanaugh & Bower, 1985), thus creating a spiral of social decline.

Lowered social efficacy further increases susceptibility to stress and depression indirectly by hampering the development of supportive social relationships. Conversely, a strong sense of social efficacy facilitates the development of relationships that are socially supportive (Holahan & Holahan, 1987a,b). Engaging in such socially supportive relationships is a vital part of successful aging. Supportive relationships serve an enabling function that enhances individuals' perceived coping efficacy (Major *et al.*, 1990) and helps mitigate the depression associated with many of the changes associated with aging.

Socially supportive relationships reduce depressive reaction to chronic life stressors and increase personal and social efficacy (Holahan & Holahan, 1987a), through many interrelated and interdependent processes. Socially supportive relationships, for example, model successful coping attitudes and skills and provide incentives and resources for engaging in health enhancing activities. These relationships can also inspire others by illustrating that difficulties can be overcome through perseverance (Major *et al.*, 1990).

Socially supportive relationships can positively affect an aging individual's functioning, be it social, cognitive, or physical, by assisting with change efforts. Attitudes and behaviors subject to strong normative influences are especially susceptible to change. This normative influence, however, can have a negative influence, as well, when social relationships inadvertently or overtly slow or thwart change efforts. Therefore, the sociocultural realities that help or hinder personal control must be taken into consideration and addressed if success of health promotion efforts is to be achieved (Bandura, 1997).

Examples of Health Promotion Programs for an Older Population

The adoption and maintenance of health-promoting behaviors and the reduction or cessation of health-detracting behaviors have the potential to influence both the prevention of disease and the day-to-day management of chronic health conditions. There is a paucity of information, however, regarding these behaviors across the course of a lifetime, most notably among the elderly.

Value and Efficacy of Behaviorally Focused Programs

The value and efficacy of behaviorally focused preventive interventions targeted to the elderly is a topic of debate for two broad reasons. First, problems are incurred when trying to generalize the influence of various risk factors across ages. Although treating hypertension, for example, reduces risk for cardio- and cerebrovascular disorders among middle-aged and young-old populations, findings reveal little benefit of treatment for people over age 80 (Amery, 1986).

Second, older adults receive very few preventive services and in fact are frequently excluded from other health promotion programs. In empirical studies, this exclusion is often attributed to the potential confound of comorbidities. In practice, however, it perhaps reflects the pervasiveness of that old adage, "you can't teach an old dog a new trick," in medical and health education circles.

There are some studies that report that when preventive services are made available to older adults, however, many do engage in the programs, lower their health risks, and achieve better overall health (Grembowski et al., 1993). The extent to which these preventive services and behavioral interventions can reverse or delay morbidities among and within various segments of the elderly certainly warrants careful examination. Opponents and skeptics of behavioral interventions in this population would do well to remember, however, that despite astronomical increases in health care expenditures, only a slight positive impact on life expectancy is associated with medical advances (Fuchs, 1974). And, while these advances may ameliorate some of the negative effects of morbidity, they cannot restore the loss of functioning that results from morbidities associated with behaviors that are modifiable. To illustrate, though surgical procedures may expand physical capabilities, most often there are no resultant functional improvements in the physical and social aspects of everyday life (Allen, Becker, & Swank, 1990).

Aside from genetic predisposition, lifestyle behaviors and environmental conditions are the most salient determinants of physical health and longevity. Those with healthier lifestyles are likely to raise the level of psychosociobiological function and slow the rate of biological aging. This health enhancement not only influences longevity, but augments vitality as well. The quality of the later years is improved by delaying the onset of health dysfunction, thus shortening the length of time between morbidity and mortality (Butler & Brody, 1995; Fries, 1980).

This "compression of morbidity," whereby the physical problems are condensed into a short period at the very end of the life span, does not hold true among the old-old. Despite increases in longevity among this segment of the elderly, there does not appear to be the same compression of morbidity as among the young-old. In fact, more dramatic increases in the need for medical care services are evidenced (Schneider & Brody, 1983), which calls attention to the need to enhance health rather than merely extend life. Health promotion activities targeting older populations should be viewed as a means of enhancing health.

Self-Efficacy, Smoking Cessation, and the Elderly

The health risks of smoking are well documented. These risks are especially pronounced among the elderly, who tend to have high levels of smoking-related health problems. An American Association of Retired Persons (AARP) survey of smokers over the age of 50 revealed higher nicotine addition and cigarette consumption than is found in younger cohorts (Orleans, Rimer, & Cristinzio, 1991; Rimer, Orleans, & Keintz, 1990). Further, older smokers reported more social contacts who are smokers: 57% reported their spouses were smokers and 19% stated that most of their social contacts were smokers. Of those sampled, 11% smoked an average of 46 years.

There are benefits to quitting smoking at any age. The risk of smoking-related illness is reduced 50% within 15 years, if smoking is ceased before age 50 (USDHHS, 1990). Male smokers, aged 60–64, who quit smoking reduce risk by 10%, thus potentially expanding life expectancy 2 or 3 years (USDHHS, 1990). Many older smokers, however, do not believe that quitting will improve their health. Many perceive decreased health as a normal consequence of aging and not a result of their smoking (Orleans *et al.*, 1991; Rimer *et al.*, 1990).

Unfortunately, physicians may inadvertently or overtly support these fallacies. Physicians appear less likely to assess and counsel older adults on their smoking, perhaps because they doubt the benefits of cessation in later life or have little confidence in their patients' ability to quit (Cox, 1993). An optimal time for physicians and other health professionals to encourage smoking cessation is after the diagnosis of a smoking-related disorder. A study of myocardial infarct patients demonstrated that 63% of smokers receiving specific advice to quit smoking remained abstinent at 1 year, as compared to 25% in the control group (Burt, Thornley, & Illingsworth, 1974).

Almost 65% of the older smokers in the AARP study stated they were seriously contemplating quitting within the next year, yet only a third of those were confident in their ability to quit (Orleans *et al.*, 1991; Rimer *et al.*, 1990). Increasing efficacy to quit smoking among the older smokers may prove to be especially challenging, given the constraints of their belief systems, the degree of nicotine addiction, and lack of social and medical support for change.

There are many challenges in designing and implementing smoking cessation programs for the elderly. Behavioral interventions must address the perceived and actual barriers to smoking cessation, which can differ quite significantly from those found in younger cohorts. Behavioral training, for example, has been shown to be more effective in older, chronic smokers when nicotine gum is used. The gum, however, may present problems by interfering with dental appliances (Cox, 1993).

Despite the challenges and barriers, it is well within the older smoker's ability to quit smoking successfully and within the interventionist's ability to design effective strategies to help them. The key is in empowering older smokers with skills and belief in their capabilities, so that they will be better able to achieve a healthier, smoke-free life.

Self-Efficacy, Falls, and the Elderly

Applying the concept of physical efficacy, Tinetti, Mendes de Leon, Doucette, and Baker (1994) developed the Falls Efficacy Scale. According to Tinetti *et al.* (1994), "falls efficacy represents the degree of confidence a person has in performing common daily activities without falling" (p. M141). Determining falls efficacy avoids the psychological implications of "fear" as applied to activities of daily living. Efficacy also appears to predict behavior and functioning (Bandura, 1987; Mischel, 1968) and indicates a complex and multidirectional relationship among efficacy, ability, and behavior (Bandura, 1987). With this in mind, Tinetti *et al.* (1994) collected data from a community-living cohort of elderly adults and described the "distribution of the fear of falling and fall-related efficacy," and examined "the relationship of fear of falling and fall-related efficacy with measures of basic and instrumental activities of daily living as well as higher levels of functioning represented by physical and social activities" (p. 140).

Using a stratified sampling technique, a cohort of 1103 eligible subjects agreed to participate and were enrolled. Each subject was interviewed and underwent a physical assessment of physical performance. The interview covered frequency of falls and injuries in the past year, fear of falling and the Falls Efficacy Scale. This study sets the stage for the application of efficacy in intervention studies of physical and specifically falls efficacy, as the authors found an independent association between falls efficacy and function. Such studies could involve prevention activities related to the changing physical functioning of the older adult as well as older adults in rehabilitation. The concept of falls efficacy could be developed into an efficacy building program.

Self-Efficacy and Caregivers

Not only is self-efficacy an important determinant for the older adult, it has also been demonstrated to be a factor in the caregiver's ability to cope with the burden of caring for an older adult. Many caregivers experience physical health problems, emotional problems (primarily depression and social isolation), and overwhelming feelings of burden related to their role, while other caregivers experience a great deal of satisfaction. A study of caregivers of the cognitively impaired elderly indicated that it is high self-efficacy of the caregiver rather than the condition of the patient that determine the well-being of the caregiver (Mowat & Spence Laschinger, 1994).

Characteristics of Successful Programs

Although there are many theories of health behavior, as noted in other chapters, that can be used to provide a foundation for designing health promotion activities, we have focused on the theoretical framework of self-efficacy (Bandura, 1977, 1986, 1997). Planners must recognize and effectively overcome the physical, cognitive, and social constraints posed by the aging process. Planners should also recognize the interrelatedness of these constraints. Changes in one inevitably influence the others. Therefore, the most effective strategies will be those that tackle all areas. The challenge to planners lies in adapting a chosen model or theory to meet the special health promotion needs of the older adult.

That said, however, we identify seven specific considerations that, if included in a health promotion program, can enhance the acceptability of the program (Galvin, 1986). These considerations are: (1) making materials appealing, readable, and understandable; (2) using appropriate media; (3) fostering a sense of personal value of the program, that is, relate the benefits in personal terms; (4) offering class at times and places that are accessible, convenient, and safe; (5) providing activities at low or no cost; (6) taking the weather into consideration; and (7) avoiding stereotypical views of the older adult. The older adult population is not homogeneous and activities need to address that fact (Galvin, 1986; Engle, 1990).

Conclusion

In conclusion, more is not known about health promotion for the older adult than is known. Continued research is essential if health promotion activities for the older adult are to be successfully implemented into the third millennium.

References

Albert, M. S., Savage, C. R., Blazer, D., Jones, K., Berkman, L., Seeman, T., & Rowe, J. W. (1995). Predictors of cognitive change in older persons: MacArthur studies of successful aging. *Psychology and Aging, 10,* 578–589.

Allen, J. K., Becker, D. M., & Swank, R. T. (1990). Factors related to functional status after coronary artery bypass surgery. *Heart Lung, 19,* 337–343.

Amery, A. (1986). Efficacy of antihypertensive drug treatment according to age, sex, blood pressure, and previous cardiovascular disease in patients over the age of 60. *Lancet, 2,* 589–592.

Baltes, P. B., & Labouvie, G. V. (1973). Adult development of intellectual performance: Description, explanation, and modification. In C. Eisdorfer & M. Lawton (Eds.), *The psychology of adult development and aging* (pp. 157–219), Washington DC: American Psychological Association.

Baltes, P. B., & Lindenberger, U. (1988). On the range of cognitive plasticity in old age as a function of experience: 15 years in intervention research. *Behavior Therapy, 19,* 282–300.

Baltes, P. B., & Smith, J. (1990). Toward a psychology of wisdom and its ontogenesis. In R. J. Sternberg (Ed.), *Wisdom: Its nature, origins, and development* (pp. 87–120). New York: Cambridge University Press.

Bandura, A. (1977). *Social learning theory.* Englewood Cliffs, NJ: Prentice-Hall.

Bandura, A. (1986). *Social foundations of thought and action: A social cognitive theory.* Englewood Cliffs, NJ: Prentice-Hall.

Bandura A. (1987). Reflections on self-efficacy. In S. Rachman (Ed.), *Advances in behavior research and therapy* (pp. 237–269). Oxford: Pergamon.

Bandura, A. (1997). *Self-efficacy: The exercise of control.* New York: W. H. Freeman.

Berry, J. M. (1989). A life span development perspective. *Developmental Psychology, 35,* 683–735.

Bortz, W. M. (1982). Disuse and aging. *Journal of the American Medical Association, 248,* 1203–1208.

Burt, A., Thornley P., & Illingsworth, D., (1974). Stopping smoking after myocardial infarction. *Lancet, 1,* 304–306.

Butler, R. N., & Brody, J. A. (1995). *Delaying the onset of late-life dysfunction.* New York: Springer.

Caspersen, C. J., Christenson, G. M., & Pollard, R. A. (1986). Status of the 1990 physical fitness and exercise objectives: Evidence from NHIS 1985. *Public Health Report, 101,* 587–592.

Carrol, D. L. (1995). The importance of self-efficacy expectations in elderly patients recovering from coronary artery bypass surgery. *Heart and Lung, 24,* 50–59.

Cox, J. L. (1993). Smoking cessation in the elderly patient. *Clinics in Chest Medicine, 14,* 423–428.

Dychtwald, K. (1986). *Wellness and health promotion for the elderly.* Rockville, MD: Aspen Publication.

Engle, M. (1990). Little old ladies are much maligned: Diversity reconsidered. *Educational Gerontology, 16,* 339–346.

Fries, J. F. (1980). Aging, natural death, and the compression of morbidity. *New England Journal of Medicine, 303,* 130–135.

Fries, J. F., & Crapo, L. M. (1981). *Vitality and aging: Implications of the rectangular curve.* San Francisco: W. H. Freeman.

Fuchs, V. (1974). *Who shall live? Health, economics and social choice.* New York: Basic Books.

Galvin, M. (1986). *Adapting community health promotion programs for older people.* Birmingham, AL: UAB.

German, P. (1981). Measuring functional disability in the older population. *American Journal of Public Health, 71,* 1197–1199.

Grembowski, D., Patrick, D., Diehr, P., Durham, M., Beresford, S., Kay, E., & Hecht, J. (1993). Self-efficacy and health behavior among older adults. *Journal of Health and Social Behavior, 34,* 89–104.

Hayflick, L. (1968) Human cells and aging. *Scientific American, 218*(3), 32–37.

Hobbs, F. B., & Damon, B. L. (1996). 65+ in the United States. US Department of Commerce Bureau of the Census. Washington, DC: US Government Printing Office.

Holahan, C. K., & Holahan, C. J. (1987a). Self-efficacy, social support, and depression in aging: A longitudinal analysis. *Journal of Gerontology, 42,* 65–68.

Holahan, C. K., & Holahan, C. J. (1987b). Life stress, hassles, and self-efficacy in aging: A replication and extension. *Journal of Applied Psychology, 17,* 574–592.

Kane, R. A., & Kane, R. L. (1981). *Assessing the elderly.* Lexington, MA: Lexington Books.

Kavanaugh, D. J., & Bower, G. H. (1985). Mood and self-efficacy: Impact of joy and sadness of perceived capabilities. *Cognitive Therapy and Research, 9,* 507–525.

Lachman, M., Bandura, A., Weaver S. L., & Elliott, E. (1995). Assessing memory control beliefs: The memory controllability inventory. *Aging and Cognition, 2,* 67–84.

Lichtenstein, R., & Thomas, J. (1987). A comparison of self-reported measures of perceived health and functional health in an elderly population. *Journal of Community Health, 12,* 213–230.

Major, B., Cozzarelli, C., Sciacchitano, A. M., Cooper, M. L., Testa, M., & Mueller, P. M. (1990). Perceived social support, self-efficacy, and adjustment to abortion. *Journal of Personality and Social Psychology, 59,* 452–463.

Marshall, G. N., & Lang, E. L. (1990). Optimism, self-mastery, and symptoms of depression in women professionals. *Journal of Personality and Social Psychology, 59,* 132–139.

McAuley, E. (1993). Self-efficacy, physical activity and aging. In J. R. Kelly (Ed.), *Activity and aging: Staying involved in later life* (pp. 187–206). Newbury Park, CA: Sage.

Mischel, W. (1968). *Personality and assessment.* New York: Wiley.

Mowat, J., & Spence Laschinger, H. K. (1994). Self-efficacy in caregivers of cognitively impaired elderly people: A concept analysis. *Journal of Advanced Nursing 19,* 1105–1113.

Olioff, M., Bryson, S. E., & Wadden, N. P. (1989). Predictive relation of automatic thoughts and student efficacy to depressive symptoms in undergraduates. *Canadian Journal of Behavioural Science, 21,* 353–363.

Orleans, C. T., Rimer, B. K., & Cristinzio, S. (1991). Smoking cessation and severity of disease: The coronary artery smoking intervention study. *Health Psychology 2,* 119–126.

Riley, M. W., Kahn, R. L., & Foner, A. (Eds.). (1994). *Age and structural lag.* New York: Wiley.

Rimer, B. K., Orleans, C. T., & Keintz, M. K., (1990). The older smoker: Status, challenges and opportunities for intervention. *Chest, 97,* 547–553.

Ruiz, B. A. A. (1992). Hip fracture recovery in older women: The influence of self-efficacy, depressive symptoms and state anxiety. Ph. D. dissertation, University of California, San Francisco. Dissertation Abstracts International. 54-03B, 1337.

Schaie, K. W. (1995). *Intellectual development in adulthood: The Seattle longitudinal study.* New York: Cambridge University Press.

Schooler, C. (1987). Psychological effects of complex environments during the life span: A review and theory. In C. Schooler & K. W. Schaie (Eds.), *Cognitive functioning and social structure over the life course* (pp. 24–29). Norwood, NJ: Ablex.

Schneider, E., & Brody, J. (1983). Aging, natural death and the compression of morbidity: Another view. *New England Journal of Medicine, 309,* 854–856.

Schunk, D., & Carbonari, J. (1984). Self-efficacy models. In J. Matarazzo, S. Weiss, J. Herd, N. Miller, & S. Weiss (Eds.), *Behavioral health* (pp. 230–247). New York: John Wiley and Sons.

Siegel, J. (1996). Aging into the 21st century. Washington, DC: Administration on Aging, US Department of Health and Human Services.

Strecher, V., DeVellis, B., Becker, M., & Rosenstock, I. (1986). The role of self-efficacy in achieving health behavior change. *Health Education Quarterly, 13*, 73–91.

Tinetti, M. E., Mendes de Leon, C. F., Doucette, J. T., & Baker, D. I. (1994). Fear of falling and fall-related efficacy in relationship to functioning among community-living elders. *Journal of Gerontology: Medical Sciences, 49*, M140–M147.

US Department of Health and Human Services (USDHHS). (1990). The health benefits of smoking cessation: A report of the Surgeon General. (DHHA publication No (CDC) 90-8416. Bethesda, MD: US Department of Health and Human Services. Public Health Service. Centers for Disease Control. Centers for Chronic Disease Prevention and Health Promotion, Office on Smoking and Health.

US Department of Health and Human Services (USDHHS). (1991). Aging in America: Trends and Projections. USHHS Publication No. (FcoA) 91-28001. Washington, DC: US Government Printing Office.

US Department of Health and Human Services (USDHHS). (1998). Profile of older Americans: 1998. Washington, DC: Administration on Aging.

Waller, K. V., & Bates, R. C. (1992). Health locus of control and self-efficacy beliefs in a healthy elderly sample. *American Journal of Health Promotion, 6*, 302–309.

Weinberg, R. S., Gould, D., & Jackson, A. (1979). Expectations and performance: An empirical test of Bandura's self-efficacy theory. *Journal of Sport Psychology, 1*, 320–333.

Weinberg, R. S., Yukelson, D., & Jackson, A. (1980). Effect of public and private efficacy expectations o competitive performance. *Journal of Sport Psychology, 2*, 340–349.

Willis, S. L., & Schaie, K. W. (1986). Training the elderly on the ability factors of spatial orientation and inductive reasoning. *Psychology and Aging, 1*, 239–247.

Woodward, N. J., & Wallston, B. S. (1987). Age and health care beliefs: Self-efficacy as a mediator of low desire for control. *Psychology and Aging, 2*, 3–8.

CHAPTER 26

Women's Health and Health Behaviors

Carol E. Cornell, M. Janice Gilliland, and Cora E. Lewis

Women and Health Care Research

Prior to the 1980s, the scientific community paid little serious attention to gender-specific health issues. Most clinical trials conducted before 1980 failed to include women. When women were included, gender differences were typically not reported and presumably not assessed. Findings from studies of men were generalized to women with little regard for the possibility that the results might lack validity across genders. This situation has finally begun to change, as reflected in events such as the 1986 National Institutes of Health (NIH) mandate that government-funded research include women and the 1990 formation within the NIH of the Office of Research on Women's Health (Stanton, 1995).

In addition to requiring inclusion of women in government-supported research, the NIH, along with other public and private institutions, has begun to sponsor studies that exclusively target women's health. The scientific literature on women's health has expanded rapidly to accommodate the results of these studies, and regional and national conferences on women's health are becoming more common. Despite these promising developments, numerous and voluminous gaps still exist in our knowledge about women's health. This chapter will overview gender-related issues for the major disease killers and cripplers of women, and will discuss ongoing research designed to close the knowledge gaps in women's health.

Carol E. Cornell • Behavioral Medicine Unit, Division of Preventive Medicine, Department of Medicine, School of Medicine, Department of Health Behavior, School of Public Health, UAB Center for Health Promotion, University of Alabama at Birmingham, Birmingham, Alabama 35294.   *M. Janice Gilliland* • Behavioral Medicine Unit, Division of Preventive Medicine, Department of Medicine, School of Medicine, UAB Center for Health Promotion, University of Alabama at Birmingham, Birmingham, Alabama 35294. *Cora E. Lewis* • Division of Preventive Medicine, School of Medicine, UAB Center for Health Promotion, University of Alabama at Birmingham, Birmingham, Alabama 35294.

Handbook of Health Promotion and Disease Prevention, edited by Raczynski and DiClemente. Kluwer Academic/Plenum Publishers, New York, 1999.

The Major Disease Killers and Cripplers of Women

Cardiovascular disease (CVD), cancer, and osteoporosis are the greatest overall causes of morbidity and mortality in women. The latest statistics show that CVD killed 505,440 women in 1995 (American Heart Association, 1998) and that cancer killed 250,529 women in 1993 (Parker, Tong, Bolden, & Wingo, 1997). Osteoporosis is a major cause of disability in older women and the lifetime risk of dying from hip fracture has been estimated to be equal to that of dying from breast cancer for white, postmenopausal women (Cummings, Black, & Rubin, 1989). The incidence of these chronic diseases increases with age for both men and women. However, women's overall risk for morbidity and mortality rises sharply after menopause. Studies of women using hormone replacement therapy (HRT) suggest that while some of the increased incidence in chronic disease is due to the aging process itself, the hormonal changes that accompany menopause play an important role in the increased risk of CVD and osteoporosis faced by older women.

Estrogen exposure appears to play a role in women's risk for CVD, cancer, and osteoporosis. A number of studies have shown that current HRT use is associated with reduced risk for CVD and osteoporosis (e.g., Cauley, 1995; Lindsay, 1991; Writing Group for the PEPI Trial, 1995), but with increased risk for breast cancer (e.g., Colditz et al., 1995). A recent prospective study indicated an inverse relationship between bone mineral density (an indicator of osteoporosis) and breast cancer and implicated endogenous estrogen levels as responsible for this association (Cauley et al., 1996). The available data suggest that endogenous and exogenous estrogens affect risk for osteoporosis, CVD, and breast cancer and provide an important link between these significant causes of morbidity and mortality in women.

Some behavioral prevention strategies are also common to CVD, cancer, and osteoporosis. Interventions designed to help women quit smoking, modify dietary habits, and become more physically active may decrease risk for all three of these diseases. Changes in these three health behaviors have been most extensively documented as decreasing risk for the major killer of women: CVD.

Women and Cardiovascular Disease

Coronary heart disease (heart attack) and cerebrovascular disease (stroke) are the most common forms of CVD. Coronary heart disease (CHD) is responsible for more than 50% of CVD deaths and is the leading cause of death for women. Cerebrovascular disease accounts for almost 16% of CVD deaths, and stroke is the third-leading cause of death in women, ranking behind all cancers combined (American Heart Association, 1997).

CVD Risk Factors

Most known risk factors for CVD are similar for women and men as discussed in Chapter 12. However, gender differences exist in the distribution of factors and the level at which a factor confers risk (NHLBI, 1994). For example, low-density lipoprotein (LDL) is a stronger predictor of risk for men than it is for women (e.g., Eaker & Castelli, 1987), and high triglyceride levels increase CVD risk in postmenopausal women but are not associated with risk for men at any age (e.g., Austin, 1988; Castelli,

1986). The effects of psychosocial risk factors may similarly differ for women and men. For example, social support is generally associated with decreased CVD morbidity and mortality for women as well as men (e.g., Berkman & Syme, 1979; Chandra, Szklo, Goldberg, & Tonascia, 1983; Seeman & Syme, 1987). However, in only one study have the data for women been unequivocal (Berkman & Syme, 1979), and social support has actually been associated with increased mortality for some age groups of women (e.g., Shumaker & Hill, 1991). Moreover, negative social interactions may have a greater impact on risk for women than for men. For example, Cornell and colleagues (Cornell, Norvell, Slater, Lindholm, & Limacher, 1994) found that high levels of social conflict were associated with increased risk for CHD in women, but not for men.

Other risk factors are more common in women than men. For example, more women than men are obese, which increases risk for CVD and other associated conditions, including hypertension, diabetes, and hyperlipidemia (e.g., Folsom, et al., 1993; Levy & Kannel, 1988; Manson et al., 1990; Spelsberg, Ridker, & Manson, 1993; Van Itallie, 1985; Wood, Stefanick, & Williams, 1991). Women suffer from depression at higher rates than men (e.g., Cleary, 1987; Weissman & Klerman, 1977), which may place them at increased risk due to the direct effects of depression on CVD etiology, progression, and outcome and to indirect effects on CVD risk behaviors, such as increased cigarette smoking and physical inactivity. Levels of physical activity are also lower for women than men, and women become even less active as they age (Casperson, Christenson & Pollard, 1986; Pate et al., 1995). Thus, women may be at increased risk due to independent effects of physical inactivity on CVD risk and to indirect effects on other risk factors including obesity, hypertension, dyslipidemia, diabetes, stress, and depression.

Menopause and CVD Risk

Premenopausal women have significantly lower risk of CVD compared with same-aged men. However, the incidence of CVD in women quickly increases following menopause, and after age 75, the gender differences are small (e.g., American Heart Association, 1998; Lerner & Kannel, 1986). Much of the postmenopausal increase in CVD mortality results from dramatic changes in CVD risk factors. These include increases in total cholesterol and triglyceride levels (Hjortland, McNamara, & Kannel, 1976; Lindquist, 1982; Lindquist, & Bengtsson, 1980), including higher low density lipoprotein-cholesterol (LDL-C), and lower high density lipoprotein-C (HDL-C) (Matthews et al., 1989). Psychosocial variables also may interact with menopause-induced physiological changes to increase risk for CVD. Specifically, psychological stress is associated with cardiovascular and neuroendocrine changes that are thought to alter lipids. Studies comparing responses to stress suggest that postmenopausal women exhibit greater increases in systolic blood pressure, heart rate, and/or norepinephrine in response to behavioral stress tests than premenopausal women (Lindheim et al., 1992; Matthews, 1992), and that these responses are blunted by estrogen therapy (Lindheim et al., 1992). These data suggest that stress may accelerate the effects of menopause on lipid levels and may thus increase CVD risk (Matthews, 1992).

The effects of menopause on CVD risk factors may differ between African-American and white women. Cross-sectional analyses from several large studies have found significantly higher levels of serum cholesterol in white postmenopausal relative to premenopausal women, while showing no significant differences for naturally menopausal African-American women (Baird, Tyroler, Heiss, Chambless, & Hames, 1985; Demirovic, Sprafka, Folsom, Laitinen, & Blackburn, 1992). The Minnesota Heart Study reported, however, that African-American women who had undergone surgical menopause had higher postmenopausal than premenopausal cholesterol levels (Demirovic et al., 1992). Data from the Atherosclerosis Risk in Communities (ARIC) study suggest a similar pattern for LDL-C, with white premenopausal women having lower LDL-C levels than postmenopausal women, but no clear differences for African-American women (Brown et al., 1993). These studies have found no significant differences in HDL-C levels between menopausal groups in white or African-American women.

Prevention of CVD in Women

Chapter 12 overviews behavioral strategies for decreasing CVD risk in both women and men. The general areas for intervention (e.g., smoking cessation, increased physical activity, dietary changes, and alteration of psychosocial risk factors) are similar for both genders. However, specific prevention strategies are likely to differ. For example, smoking cessation programs are likely to be most successful with women if they include personal contact approaches such as formal smoking cessation groups and telephone counseling; emphasize gradual reductions in smoking, delayed quitting, relapse prevention strategies, and skill acquisition; and avoid aversive conditioning methods (Mermelstein & Borelli, 1995). These findings are in contrast to strategies that may be most effective with men. Fewer data are available regarding successful intervention approaches for women for nutrition, physical activity, and psychosocial factors. More research is needed to identify promising behavioral intervention methods for reducing these CVD risk factors in women.

HRT holds promise for prevention of CVD in postmenopausal women (e.g., Barrett-Connor & Bush, 1989; Writing Group for the PEPI Trial, 1995), but the data suggesting that HRT may reduce cardiovascular risk are plagued by methodological problems including small sample sizes, selection bias, and lack of long-term follow-up data (Matthews et al., 1997). Prescription of HRT for individual women is also complicated by findings from observational studies of an association between long-term and/or current use of HRT and an increased risk for breast cancer (e.g., Colditz et al., 1995; Matthews et al., 1997, for review). Several large clinical trials, including the Women's Health Initiative described later in this chapter, will provide more definitive data than are currently available regarding the effects of HRT on CVD, breast cancer, and other diseases. Until the results of these trials are available, physicians are cautioned to "be conservative about prescribing estrogens" (Rossouw, 1996, p. 2894) as a means of reducing coronary heart disease (CHD) risk in individual women and to focus instead on encouraging lifestyle changes and prescribing medications (such as lipid-lowering drugs) with known risk-reducing efficacy (Rossouw, 1996).

Changes in lifestyle behaviors also play a role in tertiary prevention efforts (e.g., Ades, Waldermann, Polk, & Coflesky, 1992; Allan & Scheidt, 1996; Balady, Fletcher, & Froelicher, 1994; Cannistra, Balady, O'Malley, Weiner, & Ryan, 1992; Lavie & Milani, 1995; Smith et al., 1995) and cardiac rehabilitation programs are a primary resource for assistance in making behavioral changes for many cardiac patients. Unfortunately, women are less likely than men to enroll in cardiac rehabilitation programs (Thomas et al., 1996) and more likely to drop out (Cannistra et al., 1992). Studies suggest variations in physician encouragement and preferences of women for specific program features as possible reasons for this gender difference (Ades et al., 1992; Moore & Kramer, 1996). Mosca et al. (1997) call for additional studies addressing barriers to participation in cardiac rehabilitation programs by women. Research should also investigate other possible avenues for assisting women with CVD in making needed behavioral changes.

Diagnosis and Treatment of CVD in Women

Diagnosis of CHD in women is complicated by a variety of factors, including gender differences in symptom presentation and inadequacy of diagnostic instruments for women. Chest pain is less predictive of CHD for women than for men (e.g., Kennedy et al., 1982; Lerner & Kannel, 1986) and women who have CHD may present with non-chest pain symptoms more often than men. For example, data from the Myocardial Infarction Triage and Intervention Registry (MITI) trial showed that women experiencing myocardial infarction (MI) were more likely than men to report nausea, fatigue, abdominal pain, and dyspnea. These symptoms were accompanied by complaints of chest pain for most (90%) but not all of these women (Kudenchuk, Maynard, Martin, Wirkus, & Weaver, 1996).

Diagnostic tests for CHD, such as exercise treadmill testing, are also less accurate for women (e.g., Cerqueira, 1995; Marmor & Zeira, 1993; Mosca et al., 1997). For example, standard exercise treadmill testing has limited diagnostic value in women (e.g., Glazer & Hurst, 1987), and although accuracy of exercise testing in women is improved using radioisotopes such as thallium, these procedures are complicated for many women by attenuation artifacts due to overlying breast tissue (Gibbson, 1993).

There also are gender differences in receipt of treatment for CVD. Several recent clinical trials have documented that women with CHD are less likely than men to receive coronary revascularization interventions even after the data are adjusted for clinical and demographic characteristics (Kudenchuk et al., 1996; Mosca et al., 1997; Stone et al., 1996; Weitzman et al., 1997). Some studies suggest that women experience more complications and greater procedure-related morbidity than men for some revascularization procedures, while other studies have failed to find gender differences (e.g., Eysmann & Douglas, 1993; Mosca et al., 1997 for overviews). Overall, more large clinical trials are needed to evaluate the efficacy of these procedures for women.

To receive maximum benefit from medical therapies for CVD, individuals must seek early treatment for symptoms. Although findings are mixed (e.g., Matthews, Siegel, Kuller, Thompson, & Varat, 1983; Maynard et al., 1989), studies have reported that women wait longer than men to seek treatment for acute cardiac symptoms (e.g., Schmidt & Borsch, 1990; Turi et al., 1986) for at least some phases of the treatment-seeking process (Alonzo, 1986). For example, Alonzo (1986) reported that women spent more time than men attempting to evaluate and treat their symptoms alone, which resulted in increased delays in obtaining medical evaluation and care. Individuals who delay in obtaining medical care for acute cardiac symptoms are less likely to benefit from thrombolytic and other artery-opening therapies that are most effective when given within the first hours following MI. Gender bias in referral patterns also has been reported, so women may have more advanced disease when they are finally referred for interventional procedures (e.g., Khan et al., 1990; Steingart et al., 1991). Chapter 6 in this volume discusses additional issues related to gender differences in health-care-seeking behaviors. Future studies should address the various reasons for women's increased treatment-seeking delay times and intervene appropriately to induce women to seek medical attention more rapidly for possible cardiac symptoms.

Women and Cancer

Cancer is the second-leading overall killer of women in the United States and is the leading cause of death among women aged 35–74 (Parker, Tong, Bolden, & Wingo, 1996). Breast cancer has the highest incidence in women, followed by lung and colorectal cancers; however, lung cancer kills the most women (American Cancer Society, 1998). This chapter will overview gender issues related to these cancers in women, with a focus on breast cancer. Issues surrounding gender differences in lung, colorectal, and other cancers are discussed in more detail in Chapter 13 in this volume.

Colorectal Cancer

Colorectal cancer is typically diagnosed in women and men who are over age 50, and screening is recommended beginning at that age (US Preventive Services Task Force, 1996). Screening procedures for both genders include testing for blood in stools, digital rectal exams, and proctoscopy (US Preventive Services Task Force, 1996). For women, colorectal screening procedures are used less often than breast and cervical cancer procedures, perhaps due in part to less consensus regarding screening policies (Rozenberg, Liebens, Kroll, & Vandromme, 1996). While colorectal cancer is an important health problem for women and should not be overlooked, this is not an area where significant gender differences are apparent.

Lung Cancer

Lung cancer accounts for only 13% of cancer incidence among women, but kills more women than any other cancer (Parker *et al.*, 1997). Lung cancer among women has increased more than 550% in the past 40 years (Ernster, 1996), and it is estimated that by the year 2000, more women than men in the United States will die from this disease (Itri, 1987). Relatively little has been written on women and lung cancer, reflecting the bias in women's health research toward gynecological health problems. Since 1987, however, more research attention is being paid to lung cancer in women and prevention efforts are beginning to focus more on women.

The prognosis for diagnosed lung cancer is not encouraging, with an overall survival rate of less than 15% (Parker *et al.*, 1997). The high mortality rates associated with lung cancer can largely be attributed to late diagnosis. Nevertheless, widespread screening for lung cancer is not a cost-effective strategy (US Preventive Task Force, 1996). Intervention programs therefore must focus on primary prevention.

Tobacco intervention must be the primary focus of lung cancer prevention efforts because cigarette smoking is responsible for more than 80% of all lung cancers in women (Ernster, 1996). Although smoking prevention and cessation interventions are needed for both men and women, gender differences in smoking are apparent and intervention efforts for women require consideration of these differences. Smoking rates have dropped for women and men (Weiss, 1997), but the decrease for women has been substantially less than that for men (Centers for Disease Control, 1987; Weiss, 1997). Moreover, the total number of women smokers has actually *increased* from 22 million in 1965 to 25.3 million in 1985 (USDHHS, 1980). Women are also smoking more heavily and beginning to smoke at younger ages than ever before (Centers for Disease Control, 1991; USDHHS, 1989). Women with lower income and educational levels have higher rates of smoking than more educated and affluent women (Baldini & Strauss, 1997). Ethnicity also plays a role with higher prevalences in Native American, white, and African-American rather than Hispanic and Asian-American women (Mermelstein & Borrelli, 1995). Importantly, adolescent women with lower educational levels are beginning to smoke at higher and higher rates (Pierce, Fiore, Novotny, Hatziandreu, & Davis, 1989), while smoking initiation rates for other segments of the population are dropping (USDHHS 1989).

Special intervention efforts are needed to encourage more women to quit smoking and to counteract the trend toward increasing smoking rates among specific groups. As noted earlier in this chapter, studies have suggested specific characteristics of tobacco intervention programs that are likely to appeal to women (Mermelstein & Borelli, 1995). Other findings also should be considered in designing interventions for women. These include indications that increased smoking initiation among adolescent girls parallels increased tobacco advertising targeted to women, so prevention programs should include policies to influence these types of advertising campaigns (Geronimus, Neidert, & Bound, 1993). Although the data are mixed (French, Jeffery, Pirie, & McBride, 1992; Gritz, Wellisch, Siau, & Wang, 1990), some studies have also suggested that worry about weight gain is a factor in women's concerns about quitting, especially for white adolescent girls (Camp, Klesges & Reylea, 1993). However, actual weight gained following smoking cessation is very small (only 1 kg for women as well as men) (Williamson *et al.*, 1991). Thus, prevention programs also might include education about the actual relationship between smoking cessation and weight gain. Additional outcomes research is needed to evaluate the effectiveness of these types of tailored interventions in reducing smoking and lung cancer rates in women.

Breast Cancer

The American Cancer Society estimated that approximately 182,000 new cases of breast cancer would be diagnosed in the United States in 1997, resulting in about 44,000 deaths (Parker *et al.*, 1997). Breast cancer accounts for about 30% of all incident cancer cases among women and approximately 17% of cancer deaths (Parker *et al.*, 1997). Although not uncommon in younger women, the incidence of breast cancer increases with age, with about 56% of mortality and 48% of new cases occurring in women aged 65 years and older (US Preventive Services Task Force, 1996). US women have an estimated 1 in 8 lifetime risk of developing breast cancer (Parker *et al.*, 1997), with a median age of onset of 64 years (American Cancer Society, 1995).

Ethnic differences in breast cancer rates have been identified. White women have the highest incidence rates, but African-American women have higher mortality (Moormeier, 1996; Walker, Figgs, & Zahm, 1995). In contrast, incidence and mortality rates are lower for Hispanic women than for whites. These differences have been variously related to differences in access to care, to cultural differences in lifestyle factors, and to genetics (e.g., American Cancer Society, 1997). Genetic factors also underlie ethnic variations in subpopulations of women. For example, Jewish women of Ashkenazi descent are at increased risk of breast cancer, probably due to the relatively high prevalence of an identified genetic mutation in this population (Berman *et al.*, 1996).

Geographic differences also may contribute to ethnic variations, since breast cancer rates vary by geographic location. For example, Japanese women have a very low rate of breast cancer, while women in England and Wales have the highest rates in the world (Travis, 1988). The United States ranked 13th in the world in breast cancer incidence for the years 1990 to 1993 (Parker *et al.*, 1997). Based on ecological studies, it has been suggested that the international variation seen in breast cancer rates is due primarily to environmental differences (Shimizu *et al.*, 1991), particularly diet (Matos, Parkin, Loris, & Vilensky, 1990; Wu *et al.*, 1996). For example, studies of Asian women who move to the United States have shown that incidence of breast cancer rises with length of residence in this country, as consumption of traditional foods decreases (Micozzi, 1985; Wu *et al.*, 1996).

The death rate from breast cancer similarly varies within the United States. Washington, DC, has a breast cancer mortality rate that is almost three times that of Utah (Travis, 1988), and the mortality rate in the New York City–Philadelphia, PA, metropolitan area is more than 7% higher than that for the rest of the northeastern United States (Kulldorff, Feuer, Miller, & Freedman, 1997). Again, the possibility of lifestyle differences is being investigated, although access to care may play a role as well.

Risk Factors for Breast Cancer

Breast cancer is a multifactorial disorder with a number of known risk factors. Recognized risk factors include sociodemographic, environmental, genetic/biological, and lifestyle determinants. None of the known risk factors for breast cancer invariably causes the disease; thus, it is likely that physiological and genetic factors make breast tissue susceptible to cancer, but that additional factors are important for actual cancer development. Risk factors are also likely to interact synergistically. For example, a genetic mutation may interact with lifestyle behaviors to increase breast cancer risk. As with CVD, some risk factors for breast cancer are nonmodifiable, while others can be influenced by changes in lifestyle behaviors. Knowledge of both types of risk factors is important to reduce risk. However, screening for early detection is also essential to decrease mortality from breast cancers that do develop.

Nonmodifiable Risk Factors. Nonmodifiable risk factors include genetic and biological factors, family history, and some environmental exposures. Although the risk associated with these factors usually cannot be altered, knowledge of them is important for assessing overall risk and may provide an impetus for changing other, modifiable risk behaviors.

Female gender is the primary nonmodifiable risk factor for breast cancer, and it carries the highest risk. While breast cancer is not unique to women, it occurs far less commonly in men (American Cancer Society, 1997). The excess risk attributable to female gender is primarily the result of female reproductive characteristics and is thought to be due to levels of endogenous reproductive hormones, including estrogen, progesterone, and possibly prolactin (Kelsey & Bernstein, 1996; Toniolo, 1997). Some of these reproductive factors tend to reduce risk, while others elevate it. Women who undergo an early menarche are more likely to develop breast cancer than women with later onset. The menarche effect exerts its strongest influence on premenopausal breast cancers (Kelsey & Bernstein, 1996). Age at menopause also affects breast cancer risk. Women who have natural menopause before age 45 have only about half the risk of breast cancer compared with women whose menopause occurs after age 55 (Rozenberg et al., 1996).

Age at first full-term pregnancy is significantly related to both pre- and post-menopausal onset of breast cancer. Risk is lowest for women who have a full-term pregnancy before age 20 and highest for nulliparous women and women with a first full-term pregnancy after age 35 or 37 (Helmrich et al., 1983; La Vecchia et al., 1987). There is also some evidence that lactation may reduce risk for breast cancer (Freuden-heim et al., 1997; Romieu, Hernandez-Avilla, Lazcano, Lopez, & Romero-Jaime, 1996), but the protective effect appears to be weak (Freudenheim et al., 1997).

After female gender and the associated reproductive characteristics, the strongest risk factor for breast cancer is increasing age. The increased risk for breast cancer and other cancers that is connected with the aging process is most likely due to factors such as environmental assaults on the body that may eventually lead to mutagenesis.

Women who have a mother or sister with breast cancer are at increased risk for developing the disease themselves (Kelsey & Bernstein, 1996), either because of genetics or shared environmental factors. Although genetically conferred susceptibility is responsible for only a small percentage of total cases (e.g., de Silva et al., 1995), genetic susceptibility carries a high probability of developing the disease and the risk is inversely related to age. About 33% of cases among women 19–29 years old can be attributed to genetics, compared with about 2% among women aged 70–79 years (Claus, Schildfraut, Thompson, & Risch,1996). Considerable research is ongoing in this area to determine the exact location and number of genes that might be involved and several specific genetic mutations have been identified (e.g., Andersen, 1996; Lerman, Seay, Balshem, & Audrain, 1995).

Other nonmodifiable factors have been found to elevate breast cancer risk. Having a previous diagnosis of breast cancer or some other form of breast disease can increase risk (US Preventive Task Force, 1996). Other studies suggest an association between adult stature and risk for breast cancer (Hunter & Willett, 1996; Palmer et al., 1995; Swanson et al., 1996; Trentham-Dietz et al., 1997). Certain types of environmental exposures also have been implicated, including some forms of ionizing radiation, electromagnetic fields (Kelsey & Bernstein, 1996), and environmental estrogenic compounds (Davis et al., 1993). The data in support of the risk associated with environmental exposures are sparse and sometimes contradictory (e.g., Kelsey & Bernstein, 1996; Krieger, Wolff, Hiatt, Rivers, & Vogelman, 1994; Wolff & Weston, 1997), but investigations of these types of relationships are continuing.

Modifiable Risk Factors. The modifiable risk factors for breast cancer are primarily related to lifestyle behaviors. As discussed in Chapter 13 in this volume, the evidence from ecological studies has provided strong support for a role for dietary factors in some cancers. Research on dietary intake and breast cancer has focused primarily on four factors: (1) high levels of consumption of saturated or unsaturated fats and cholesterol; (2) total energy intake; (3) elevated protein consumption; and (4) low intake of dietary fiber or specific nutrients, usually associated with low consumption of fruits and vegetables (Clavel-Chapelon, Niravong, & Joseph, 1997). Epidemiological studies of the relationship between dietary fat intake and breast cancer have yielded inconsistent results (Clavel-Chapelon et al., 1997). While most studies have reported a positive association between saturated fat and breast cancer risk, the effect appears to be small. However, Clavel-Chapelon and colleagues (1997) reported that fat intake was associated with increased risk in a majority of studies when menopausal status was taken into account. Kohlmeier and Mendez (1997) suggest that the inconsistent results regarding dietary fat and breast cancer may be due to lack of differentiation among various fatty acids, but fat may also exert a carcinogenic effect by contributing to excess energy intake and/or obesity.

Studies of protein consumption generally support a positive association with breast cancer, but, once again, the increased risk appears to be small and is supported primarily by case–control studies. Studies of fiber intake, fruit and vegetable consumption, and specific nutrients (vitamin C, vitamin A, beta-carotene and retinol, and vitamin E) also show contradictory results (Clavel-Chapelon et al., 1997; Hunter & Willett, 1996). At this time, the association between diet and breast cancer remains unclear despite considerable research. Studies are continuing to examine other dietary compounds such as phytoestrogens (naturally occurring plant estrogens), which early research suggests may be protective against breast cancer (Kohlmeier & Mendez, 1997).

The dietary factor that has shown the strongest and most consistent association with increased risk for breast cancer is alcohol consumption. A dose–response relationship has been observed, with a modest increase in risk associated with consumption of one drink per day, and higher levels of risk associated with intake of greater amounts of alcohol (Clavel-Chapelon et al., 1997; Hunter & Willett, 1996). Similar to the mechanisms underlying many of the other risk factors for breast cancer, the increased risk associated with alcohol consumption is believed to result from the influence of alcohol on estrogen metabolism (Kelsey & Bernstein, 1996).

A number of studies have found an association between body weight or body mass index and breast cancer (Hunter & Willett, 1996). Among premenopausal women, body weight is inversely associated with risk for breast cancer (Swanson et al., 1996), but the association is positive among postmenopausal women (Yong, Brown, Schatzkin, & Schairer, 1996). It is hypothesized that the positive association between obesity and breast cancer risk after menopause results from increased estrogen production promoted by excess body fat (Kelsey & Bernstein, 1996).

Physical activity has been associated with a reduced risk for breast cancer in a number of different study types, subject populations, and settings (Friedenreich & Rohan, 1995). This association has been reported for both occupational (Coogan et al., 1997) and leisure time activity (Thune, Brenn, Lund, & Gaard, 1997). Physical activity during adolescence does not appear to reduce risk for breast cancer later in life (Chen, White, Malone, & Daling, 1997; McTiernan, Stanford, Weiss, Darling, & Voigt, 1996), but at least one study reported decreased breast cancer rates among women who were physically active from menarche to one year prior to diagnosis (Bernstein, Henderson, Hanisch, Sullivan-Halley, & Ross, 1994). Physical activity has been hypothesized to reduce risk for breast cancer indirectly by influencing the amount or patterning of body fat, which may, in turn, influence other risk factors such as endogenous hormones (Friedenreich & Rohan, 1995).

A number of studies have indicated a link between use of exogenous hormones and breast cancer. Exogenous hormones are most commonly prescribed as oral contraceptives for premenopausal women or HRT for postmenopausal women. Early studies suggested a link between breast cancer and oral contraceptive use for some age groups of women (e.g., Helzlsouer & Couzi, 1995), and for women currently receiving HRT (Colditz et al., 1995). However, findings of no association between exogenous hormones and breast cancer have also been obtained (e.g., Persson, 1996). In early formulations for contraceptives and HRT, estrogen was given unopposed. Current estrogen preparations prescribed for women who still have a uterus are opposed with progesterone, a combination that has been postulated to reduce the increased risk for breast cancer associated with use of estrogen alone. However, at least one study reported no decrease in risk for women using combination estrogen and progesterone regimens (Colditz et al., 1995). Risk associated with use of exogenous hormones appears to be increased when other risk factors for breast cancer are present and when the exposure is long term or at high-dosage levels (Colditz et al., 1995; Travis, 1988). Endogenous estrogens appear to affect risk for breast cancer by altering tissue structure and cell growth and differentiation (Travis, 1988). Exogenous estrogens may operate in a similar manner and also may affect sensitivity to endogenous hormones, thus compounding the risk. Studies are continuing to evaluate the relationship between use of current exogenous estrogen preparations and breast cancer risk.

Prevention and Diagnosis of Breast Cancer

Efforts should be expended on primary prevention strategies such as dietary modification and regular physical activity, particularly for high-risk women. However, the strong contributions to breast cancer risk by nonmodifiable factors indicate that early detection through screening is essential for reducing breast cancer mortality. Overall 5-year survival rates for breast cancer among US women have increased dramatically in the past three decades (American Cancer Society, 1997), and much of this change can be attributed to increased use of screening techniques, resulting in earlier cancer detection and treatment.

Available screening procedures include breast self-exam (BSE), clinical breast exam (CBE), and mammography. The need for monthly BSE and annual CBE is generally accepted, although the accuracy of these screening techniques may be low (US Preventive Services Task Force, 1996). Mammograms are clearly beneficial for 50- 69-year-old women. However, there is considerable controversy over mammography screening for women under 50 (Miller, Baines, To, & Wall, 1992; Navarro & Kaplan, 1996; Tabar et al., 1995) and over 69 years old (US Preventive Services Task Force, 1996). As a result of the inconsistent findings regarding the efficacy of mammography for these age groups, organizations concerned with breast cancer detection and prevention have made different recommendations for screening guidelines. The American Cancer Society (1998) recommends yearly mammograms for all women aged 40 years and above. The report of the US Preventive Task Force (1996) recommends that women 50 to 69 years old have annual mammograms, but contends that the evidence is insufficient to advise routine screening for women outside of this age range. Recommendations from other concerned groups are similarly divided.

Despite the controversies, mammography use has increased significantly since 1987, even among groups that typically have had less access to preventive health care (Anderson & May, 1995). Overall screening rates almost doubled between 1987 and 1990, and the difference in mammography use between minority and white women was substantially reduced by 1992 (Rimer, 1994). Despite these gains, mammography screening rates are still low and subject to considerable geographic variation within the United States (Rimer, 1994). Women who are older (over age 75 years), have low education and income levels, and live in nonmetropolitan areas still have screening rates well below those of women who are younger (50–74 years), better educated, more affluent, and urban dwellers (Rimer, 1994). In addition to socioeconomic and access factors, mammography screening may be adversely influenced by psychological barriers such as fear or anxiety regarding the procedure or possible findings and by competing priorities. The major facilitators for getting a mammogram are physician recommendation, social support, perceived susceptibility to breast cancer, and access to care (Rimer, 1994). Interventions aimed at increasing provider referrals for routine mammographies can increase screening rates and subsequently reduce breast cancer mortality through early detection and treatment.

Behavioral interventions are needed to encourage and assist women in changing high-risk lifestyle behaviors, while motivating them to follow recommended screening guidelines for BSE, CBE, and mammography. Barriers to mammography screening must be removed to allow access for underserved women. Interventions aimed at both primary and secondary prevention are crucial to the goal of reducing the suffering and death associated with this disease.

Osteoporosis

Osteoporosis is a syndrome of silent bone loss and deterioration of bone quality resulting in increased bone fragility and risk for fracture (Dempster & Lindsay, 1993). The hip, wrist, and vertebrae are the most common fracture sites (USDHHS, 1991), and almost all fractures in the elderly are related in part to decreased bone mass (Johnston, Slemenda, & Melton, 1991). The health impact of osteoporotic fractures is enormous. Hip fracture is the most devastating complication of osteoporosis, occurring in one in every three women and one in every six men by extreme old age (Riggs, 1992). Within one year of hip fracture, 5 to 20% of patients die. Among those who survive, 50% are incapacitated by loss of functional independence and mobility (Consensus Development Conference, 1993). Unlike hip fractures, fractures of the vertebrae are not deadly, but they are much more common than hip fractures and they cause considerable pain and deformity. Unfortunately, osteoporosis is becoming more problematic because of both increases in longevity and in age-adjusted fracture rates.

Women and men of all ethnicities lose bone due to aging at all skeletal sites (Dempster & Lindsay, 1993); however, women are at much greater risk than men for developing osteoporosis. An estimated 50% of women over age 45 and 90% over age 75 have osteoporosis and more than half of these women will have fractures (USDHHS, 1990). In the decade preceding menopause, women lose bone mass more rapidly than men (Pollitzer & Anderson, 1989). In the 5- to 10-year period following menopause, bone loss accelerates and becomes more rapid than the normal loss due to aging (Ettinger & Grady, 1993). Thus, women are at greater risk than men due to the combined effects of menopausal and aging bone loss.

Osteoporosis occurs in every population and geographic area, but the incidence of fracture differs among populations and ethnic groups (Consensus Development Conference, 1993). Osteoporosis occurs more commonly in Caucasian and Asian women than in African-American or Hispanic women. The lifetime risk of hip fracture for the average 50-year-old white woman in the United States is 16–17% (Cummings & Black, 1995), exceeding the combined risk for cancers of the breast, ovary, and uterus. Prevalence of vertebral osteoporotic fractures is also high. For example, one study reported a prevalence of 60% for Japanese-American women (Ross, Davis, Epstein, & Wasnich, 1991). African-American and Hispanic women have one third to one half fewer fractures than white women (Riggs & Melton, 1992), but these women are still at risk for osteoporotic fracture.

Risk Factors for Osteoporosis

In addition to sex and ethnicity, other proposed risk factors for osteoporosis include: family history of osteoporosis, estrogen deficiency, inadequate calcium and vitamin D intake, physical inactivity, leanness, smoking, excessive alcohol intake, use of certain medications, and excessive protein intake (Chesnut, 1990; Kreiger, Kelsey, Holford, & O'Connor, 1982; USDHHS, 1991). Two powerful predictors of risk are a history of previous fracture not due to trauma and low bone mineral density or bone mass. Low bone mass may occur if insufficient bone is deposited during growth and/or if excess loss occurs (Dempster & Lindsay, 1993) and low bone mass increases the risk of fracture (Cummings & Black, 1995). Peak bone mass is in large part genetically determined; however, the capacity to fully achieve peak bone mass depends on other factors, such as dietary and physical activity habits.

Screening and Diagnosis of Osteoporosis

Screening techniques using X ray and other procedures to measure bone density are needed to correctly classify an individual woman's fracture risk (Cummings & Black, 1995). Standard X rays are not sensitive to bone loss and are not useful for osteoporosis screening. Currently, the most useful technique for measuring bone density is dual energy X ray absorptiometry (DXA).

In addition to measures of bone density, determining the rate of bone loss may be important in predicting risk of osteoporotic fractures (Christiansen, Riis, & Rodbro, 1987; Riis, 1991). Besides repeated bone density tests, certain biochemical markers of bone formation or bone destruction found in either blood or urine have been proposed as methods to assess rate of bone turnover at the time of an initial bone density test. This is an area of active research as more studies are needed to clarify the role of these tests in screening and diagnosis of osteoporosis.

Guidelines for osteoporosis screening have been proposed (Consensus Development Conference, 1997). These guidelines recommend screening in specific situations, not general screening of all postmenopausal women. Screening is recommended for women who are thought to be at risk for osteoporosis based on their age, ethnicity, family history, and other risk factors.

Prevention and Treatment of Osteoporosis

Primary Prevention and Treatment

Skeletal bone mass largely peaks by age 20, but bone mass may still be acquired up to age 30. Thereafter, bone mass begins to decline. This suggests that primary prevention strategies for osteoporosis vary with age. Childhood, adolescence, and young adulthood are the times to maximize bone mass; however, the long-term effectiveness of such strategies is unknown. Since bone mass begins to decline in the 30s, mid-life is the time to work to preserve mass. Later in life, those who develop osteoporosis can take measures to prevent further bone loss and fractures. The modifiable risk factors for osteoporosis should be targeted at all ages, including dietary factors, medications, physical activity, smoking, and alcohol use. After menopause, estrogen replacement therapy or other bone-preserving medications and fracture prevention also must be considered.

Public health measures should emphasize the importance of good nutrition and exercise and the osteoporotic effects of smoking and excess alcohol. Nutritional education must include a focus on obtaining adequate amounts of calcium and vitamin D. Adequate intakes of these nutrients are necessary for the young to achieve their maximum potential bone mass, but average calcium intakes in young women are below the presently recommended threshold (Consensus Development Conference, 1994). These same strategies may be helpful to older women who can still make changes to reduce bone loss. For elderly women, educational efforts also should focus on fall prevention, resources for information, evaluation for medication for those at risk, and support and assistance in coping with osteoporosis.

Secondary and Tertiary Prevention and Treatment

Medical prevention and treatment efforts have focused on postmenopausal women. Current drug treatments for osteoporosis include calcium, estrogen replacement therapy, synthetic estrogen receptor modulators, bisphosphonates, and calcitonin. These treatments prevent the resorption of bone (Riggs & Melton, 1992). Drugs to markedly increase bone formation are under investigation but are not yet available for treatment (Riggs, 1992).

Epidemiological studies (e.g., Cauley et al., 1995) and clinical trials (e.g., Prince et al., 1991) have shown that estrogen lowers the risk of wrist and hip fractures by about 50% (Lindsay, 1991). Hormone replacement therapy has been the mainstay of osteoporosis treatment and prevention regimens. However, the use of HRT for osteoporosis is controversial due to the association of long-term estrogen use with breast cancer (Colditz et al., 1995), as well as to adverse side effects such as vaginal bleeding and breast tenderness. Unfortunately, a woman's risk of fracture is decreased only as long as she continues to use HRT. Questions also remain about the optimum time to initiate estrogen therapy for fracture prevention, especially for prevention of hip fractures in very elderly women.

Studies of the associations of the relationships between dietary calcium intake, bone density, and risk of osteoporosis have been inconsistent. However, adequate intake of dietary calcium and vitamin D is likely to be important in the treatment of osteoporosis, as abnormalities in vitamin D metabolism and decreases in calcium absorption with age are important in the pathogenesis of osteoporosis. Unfortunately, vitamin D insufficiency and inadequate calcium intake are fairly common in women, especially elderly women, and supplementation is often necessary for adequate intake (Gloth, Gunderberg, Hollis, Haddad, & Tobin, 1995). Thus, efforts are needed to promote adequate calcium and vitamin D intake at all ages.

Calcitonin is a hormone involved in calcium metabolism that may work by suppressing bone loss and/or by increasing bone density (Avioli, 1992). It has few side effects and is available in nasal spray formulation and injectable forms. In addition, a recently FDA-approved bisphosphonate compound, alendronate, has been shown to increase bone density and reduce vertebral fractures in postmenopausal women (Liberman *et al.*, 1995). While potential adherence problems and rare side effects have been reported, alendronate represents an important advance in the treatment of osteoporosis and its availability may help promote awareness and treatment of the disease.

Drug treatment should be combined with preventive and other treatment strategies, and effective medical management of osteoporosis requires multidisciplinary evaluation and intervention. Maintenance and promotion of appropriate levels of physical activity in combination with effective pain control when needed are important in preventing further rapid bone loss. Physical therapy and specific orthopedic and rehabilitative interventions may also be required. Tertiary prevention efforts should focus on maintaining activity levels and preventing fracture, including reducing the patient's risk for falls by assessing and intervening on environmental risks (such as those in the home) to help prevent fracture (Tinetti & Speechley, 1989). Dietary assessment and counseling should aim to achieve adequate levels of calcium and vitamin D intake; with prescription of dietary supplements as needed to reach nutritional goals. The optimum exercise program for fracture prevention is an area of current research. The American College of Sports Medicine (1995) recommends regular weight-bearing exercise and activities to improve strength, flexibility, and coordination.

Nonadherence to osteoporosis regimens has received little research attention. For example, nonadherence is probably the major reason for continued bone loss among women prescribed HRT. In some cases, adherence problems occur because women are not convinced of the benefits of therapy (Rothert *et al.*, 1994) and/or because they underestimate their risk of osteoporotic fracture (Haynes & Knickerbocker, 1995). There are also differences in physicians' beliefs about the long-term benefits and risks of HRT (Hemminki, Topo, Malin, & Kangas, 1993) that likely affect acceptance and use of HRT among women. Barriers to adherence and acceptance of HRT include short-term side effects, fear of cancer, and lack of knowledge regarding benefits and risks of therapy. Additional research is needed to develop interventions that might enhance adherence to medication or lifestyle regimens in patients with osteoporosis.

Summary and Conclusions—Studies to Close the Knowledge Gap

As mentioned earlier in this chapter, increasing numbers of funded studies are beginning to narrow the gaps in our knowledge about women's health issues. The largest of these studies, the NIH-funded Women's Health Initiative (WHI), focuses on risk factors and prevention of cardiovascular disease, cancer, and osteoporosis. The 40 clinical centers involved in the Clinical Trial and Observational Studies components of WHI will follow a total of 164,500 postmenopausal women ages 50 to 79 for approximately 10 years to identify risk factors and assess the impact of promising interventions on CVD, breast and colorectal cancer, and osteoporosis. Women in the clinical trial participate in one or more of the three study arms: HRT, dietary modification, and calcium–vitamin D supplementation. Women in the observational study will be followed to identify predictors of diseases that affect postmenopausal women (Rossouw *et al.*, 1995).

The NIH has also joined forces with the Centers for Disease Control (CDC) to fund community studies at eight of the CDC's Prevention Research Centers. These studies focus on CVD prevention and/or on common risk factors for CVD, cancer, and osteoporosis. For example, studies at two centers are implementing and evaluating the effectiveness of community-based interventions for smoking cessation, nutrition, and physical activity in reducing CVD risk in African-American women aged 40 and older. Another group will design and evaluate an intervention to improve osteoporosis prevention behaviors in minority women. Other centers are developing and validating physical activity assessment instruments, conducting surveys to inform policy and environmental physical activity interventions, and testing interventions to improve diabetes care for minority and underserved women. A multicenter group has examined factors affecting women's attitudes and decisions regarding hysterectomy, oophorectomy, and HRT and will pilot test innovative interventions to assist women in their decision-making processes.

In addition to the WHI, many other studies funded by the NIH and CDC, as well as by private sources such as the Robert Wood Johnson and Kellogg foundations, are addressing reduction of risk for CVD, cancer, and osteoporosis in women. This explosion of women's health studies represents enormous progress toward closing the knowledge gap regarding the etiology and prevention of the big three killers and cripplers of women in this country. The rapid expansion of knowledge resulting from these prevention and treatment studies should fuel significant advancements during the first decades of the 21st century in the treatment and prevention of these chronic diseases in women.

References

Ades, P. A., Waldermann, M. L., Polk, D. M., & Coflesky, J. T. (1992). Referral patterns and exercise response in the rehabilitation of female coronary patients ages ≥162 years. *American Journal of Cardiology, 69,* 1422–1425.

Allan, R., & Scheidt, S. (1996). Stress, anger, and psychosocial factors for coronary heart disease. In J. E. Manson, P. M. Ridker, J. M. Gaziano, & C. H. Hennekens (Eds.), *Prevention and myocardial infarction* (pp. 274–307). New York: Oxford University Press.

Alonzo, A. A. (1986). The impact of the family and lay others on care-seeking during life-threatening episodes of suspected coronary artery disease. *Social Science Medicine, 22,* (12), 1297–1311.

American Cancer Society. (1995). *Cancer facts and figures—1995.* Atlanta, GA: Author.

American Cancer Society. (1997). *Cancer facts and figures—1997.* Atlanta, GA: Author.

American Cancer Society. (1998). *Cancer facts and figures—1998.* Atlanta, GA: Author.

American College of Sports Medicine. (1995). Position stand on osteoporosis and exercise. *Medical Science and Sports Exercise, 27,* i–vii.

American Heart Association. (1997). *1997 Heart and stroke statistical update.* Dallas, TX: American Heart Association.

American Heart Association. (1998). *Heart attack and stroke facts.* Dallas, TX: American Heart Association.

Andersen, T. I. (1996). Genetic heterogeneity in breast cancer susceptibility. *Acta Oncologica, 35*(4), 407–410.

Anderson, L. M., & May, D. S. (1995). Has the use of cervical, breast, and colorectal cancer screening increased in the United States? *American Journal of Public Health, 85*(6), 840–842.

Austin, M. A. (1988). Epidemiologic associations between hypertriglyceridemia and coronary heart disease. *Seminars in Thrombosis and Hemostasis, 14,* 137–142.

Avioli, L. V. (1992). Osteoporosis syndromes: Patient selection for calcitonin therapy. *Geriatrics, 47,* 61–64.

Baird, D. D., Tyroler, H. A., Heiss, G., Chambless, L. E., & Hames, C. G. (1985). Menopausal change in serum cholesterol: Black/white differences in Evans County, Georgia. *American Journal of Epidemiology, 122,* 982–993.

Balady, G. J., Fletcher, B. J., & Froelicher, E. S. (1994). Cardiac rehabilitation programs: A statement for healthcare professionals from the American Heart Association. *Circulation, 90,* 1602–1610.

Baldini, E. H., & Strauss, G. M. (1997). Women and lung cancer: Waiting to exhale. *Chest, 112* (Suppl. 4), 229S–234S.

Barrett-Connor, E., & Bush, T. (1989). Estrogen replacement therapy and coronary heart disease, In P. S. Douglas (Ed.), *Heart disease in women* (pp. 159–172). Philadelphia: Davis.

Berkman, L. F., & Syme, S. L. (1979). Social networks, host resistance, and mortality: A nine-year follow up study of Alameda County residents. *American Journal of Epidemiology, 109*(2), 186–204.

Berman, D. B., Costalas, J., Schultz, D. C., Grana, G., Daly, M., & Godwin, A. K. (1996). A common mutation in BRCA2 that predisposes to a variety of cancers is found in both Jewish Ashkenazi and non-Jewish individuals. *Cancer Research, 56*(15), 3409–3414.

Bernstein, L., Henderson, B. E., Hanisch, R., Sullivan-Halley, J., & Ross, R. K. (1994). Physical exercise and reduced risk of breast cancer in young women. *Journal of the National Cancer Institute, 86*(18), 1403–1408.

Brown, S. A., Hutchinson, R., Morrisett, J., Boerwinkle, E., Davis, C. E., Gotto, A. M., & Patsch, W. (1993). Plasma lipid, lipoprotein cholesterol, and apoprotein distributions in selected US communities: The Atherosclerosis Risk in Communities (ARIC) study. *Artherosclerosis and Thrombosis, 13,* 1139–1158.

Camp, D. E., Klesges, R. C., & Reylea, G. (1993). The relationship between body weight concerns and adolescent smoking. *Health Psychology, 12,* 24–32.

Cannistra, L. B., Balady, G. J., O'Malley, C. J., Weiner, D. A., & Ryan, T. J. (1992). Comparison of the clinical profile and outcome of women and men in cardiac rehabilitation. *American Journal of Cardiology, 69,* 1274–1279.

Caspersen, C. J., Christenson, G. M., & Pollard, R. A. (1986). Status of the 1990 physical fitness and exercise objectives: Evidence from NHIS 1995. *Public Health Report, 101,* 587–592.

Castelli, W. P. (1986). The triglyceride issue: A view from Framingham. *Amercan Heart Journal, 112,* 432–437.

Cauley, J. A., Seeley, D. G., Ensrud, K., Ettinger, B., Black, D., & Cummings, S. R. (1995). Estrogen replacement therapy and fractures in older women. *Annals of Internal Medicine, 122,* 9–16.

Cauley, J. A., Lucas, F. L., Kuller, L. H., Vogt, M. T., Browner, W. S., & Cummings, S. R., for the Study of Osteoportic Fractures Research Group. (1996). Bone mineral density and risk of breast cancer in older women: The study of osteoporotic fractures. *Journal of the American Medical Association, 276*(17), 1404–1408.

Centers for Disease Control. (1987). Cigarette smoking in the United States, 1986. *Morbidity and Mortality Weekly Report, 36,* 581–585.

Centers for Disease Control. (1991). Differences in the age of smoking initiation between blacks and whites. *Morbidity and Mortality Weekly Report, 40,* 755–756.

Cerqueira, M. D. (1995). Diagnostic testing strategies for coronary artery disease: special issues related to gender. *Journal of Cardiology, 75,* 52D–60D.

Chandra, V., Szklo, M., Goldberg, R., & Tonascia, J. (1983). The impact of marital status on survival after an acute myocardial infarction: A population based study. *American Journal of Epidemiology, 117,* 320–325.

Chen, C. L., White, E., Malone, K. E., & Daling, J. R.. (1997). Leisure-time physical activity in relation to breast cancer among young women (Washington, United States). *Cancer Causes and Control, 8*(1), 77–84.

Chesnut, C. H. (1990). Osteoporosis. In W.R. Hazzard, R. Andres, E. L. Bierman, & J. P. Blass (Eds.), *Principles of geriatric medicine and gerontology* (pp. 813–825). New York: McGraw-Hill.

Christiansen, C., Riis, B. J., & Rodbro, P. (1987). Prediction of rapid bone loss in postmenopausal women. *Lancet, 1,* 1105–1108.

Claus, E. B., Schildfraut, J. M., Thompson, W. E., & Risch, N. J. (1996) The genetic attributable risk of breast and ovarian cancer. *Cancer, 77*(11), 2318–2324.

Clavel-Chapelon, F., Niravong, M., & Joseph, R. R. (1997). Diet and breast cancer: Review of the epidemiologic literature. *Cancer Detection and Prevention, 21*(5), 426–440.

Cleary, P. D. (1987). Gender difference in stress-related disrders. In R. C. Barnett, L. Biener, & G. K. Baruch (Eds.), *Gender and stress* (pp. 39–72). New York: Free Press.

Colditz, G. A., Hankinson, S. E., Hunter, D. J., Willett, W. C., Manson, J. E., Stampfer, M. J., Hennekens, C., Rosner, B., & Speizer, F. E. (1995). The use of estrogens and progestins and the risk of breast cancer in postmenopausal women. *The New England Journal of Medicine, 332*(24), 1589–1593.

Colen, B. D. (1996). *Proceedings of the workshop on inherited breast cancer in Jewish women: Ethical, legal, and social implications.* Cleveland, OH: Center for Biomedical Ethics, Case Western Reserve University.

Consensus Development Conference. (1993). Diagnosis, prophylaxis, and treatment of osteoporosis. *American Journal of Medicine, 94,* 646–650.

Consensus Development Conference. (1994, Jun 6–8). Optimal calcium intake. *NIH Consensus Statement,* *12*(4), 1–31.

Consensus Development Conference. (1997). Who are candidates for prevention and treatment for osteoporosis? *Osteoporosis International, 7,* 1–6.

Coogan, P. F., Newcomb, P. A., Clapp, R. W., Trentham-Dietz, A., Baron, J. A., & Longnecker, M. P. (1997). Physical activity in usual occupation and risk of breast cancer (United States). *Cancer Causes and Control, 8*(4), 626–631.

Cornell, C. E., Norvell, N. K., Slater, S. J., Lindholm, L., & Limacher, M. C. (1994). Permorbid risk for CHD in women. *Annals of Behavioral Medicine, 16*(Suppl.), S123 (C001).

Cummings, S. R., & Black, D. (1995). Bone mass measurements and risk of fracture in Causasian women: A review of findings from prospective studies. *American Journal of Medicine, 98*(Suppl. 2A), 24S–27S.

Cummings, S. R., Black, D. M., & Rubin, S. M. (1989). Lifetime risks of hip, Colles', or vertebral fracture and coronary heart disease among white postmenopausal women. *Archives of Internal Medicine, 149,* 245–2448.

Davis, D. L., Bradlow, H. L., Wolff, M., Woodruff, T., Hoel, D. G., & Anton-Culver, H. (1993). Medical hypothesis: Xenoestrogens as preventable causes of breast cancer [Review]. *Environmental Health Perspectives, 101*(5), 372–377.

de Silva, D., Gilbert, F., Needham, G., Deans, H., Turnpenny, P., & Haites, N. (1995). Identification of women at high genetic risk of breast cancer through the National Health Service Breast Screening Programme (NHSBSP). *Journal of Medical Genetics, 32*(11), 862–866.

Demirovic, J., Sprafka, J. M., Folsom, A. R., Laitinen, D., & Blackburn, H. (1992). Menopause and serum cholesterol: Differences between blacks and whites. *American Journal of Epidemiology, 136,* 155–164.

Dempster, D. W., & Lindsay, R. (1993). Pathogenesis of osteoporosis. *Lancet, 341,* 797–801.

Eaker, E. D., & Castelli, W. P. (1987). Coronary heart disease and its risk factors among women in the Framingham Study. In E. D. Eaker, B. Packard, N. K. Wenger, T. B. Clarkson, & H. A. Tyroler (Eds.), *Coronary heart disease in women* (pp. 122–130). New York: Haymarket Doyma.

Ernster, V. L. (1996). Female lung cancer. *Annual Review of Public Health, 17,* 97–114.

Ettinger, B., & Grady, D. (1993). The waning effect of postmenopausal estrogen therapy on osteoporosis. *New England Journal of Medicine, 329,* 1192–1193.

Eysmann, S. B., & Douglas, P. S. (1993). Coronary heart disease: Therapeutic principles. In P. Douglas (Ed.), *Cardiovascular health and disease in women* (pp. 43–61). Philadelphia, PA: W.B. Saunders.

Folsom, Ar. R., Daye, S. S., Sellers, T. A., Hong, C. P., Cerhan, J. R., Potter, J. D., & Prineas, R. J. (1993). Body fat distribution and 5-year risk of death in older women. *Journal of the American Medical Association, 269,* 483–487.

French, S. A., Jeffery, R. W., Pirie, P. L., & McBride, C. M. (1992). Do weight concerns hinder smoking cessation efforts? *Addictive Behaviors, 17,* 219–226.

Freudenheim, J. L., Marshall, J. R., Veno, J. E., Moysich, K. B., Muti, P., Laughlin, R., Nemoto, J., & Graham, S. (1997). Lactation history and breast cancer risk. *American Journal of Epidemiology, 146*(11), 932–938.

Friedenreich, C. M., & Rohan, T. E. (1995). A review of physical activity and breast cancer. *Epidemiology, 6,* 311–317.

Geronimus, A. T., Neidert, L. J., & Bound, J. (1993). Age patterns of smoking in US black and white women of childbearing age. *American Journal of Public Health, 83,* 1258–1264.

Gibbson, R. J. (1993). Exercise ECG testing with and without radionuclide studies. In N. K. Wenger, L. Speroff, & B. Packard. (Eds.), *Cardiovascular health and disease in women. Proceedings of an NHLBI conference* (pp. 73–80). Greenwich, CT: Le Jacq Communications.

Glazer, M. D., & Hurst, J. W. (1987). Coronary atherosclerotic heart disease: Some important differences in men and women. *American Journal of Noninvasive Cardiology, 1,* 61–67.

Gloth, F. M. III, Gunderberg, C. M., Hollis, B. W., Haddad, J. G. Jr., & Tobin, J. D. (1995). Vitamin D deficiency in homebound elderly persons. *Journal of the Americn Medical Association, 274,* 1683–1686.

Gritz, E. R., Wellisch, D. K., Siau, J., & Wang, H. J. (1990). Long-term effects of testicular cancer on marital relationships. *Psychosomatics, 31,* 301–312.

Haynes, R. W., & Knickerbocker, R. K. (1995, September). Physician and patient views regarding the diagnosis and treatment of osteoporosis. Abstract presented at the 17th Annual Meeting of the American Society for Bone and Mineral Research.

Helmrich, S. P., Shapiro, S., Rosenberg, L., Kaufman, D. W., Slone, D., Bain, C., Miettinen, O. S., Stolley, P. D., Rosenshein, N. B., Knapp, R. C., Leavitt, T., Jr., Schottenfeld, D., Engle, R. L., Jr., & Levy, M. (1983). Risk factors for breast cancer. *American Journal of Epidemiology, 117*(1), 35–45.

Helzlsouer, K. J., & Couzi, R. (1995). Hormones and breast cancer. *Cancer, 76*(10 Suppl.), 2059–2063.

Hemminki, E., Topo, P., Malin, M., & Kangas, I. (1993). Physicians' views on hormone therapy around and after menopause. *Maturitas, 16*, 163–173.

Hjortland, M. C., McNamara, P. M., & Kannel, W. B. (1976). Some atherogenic concomitants of menopause: The Framingham Study. *American Journal of Epidemiology, 103*, 304–311.

Hunter, D. J., & Willett, W. C. (1996). Nutrition and breast cancer. *Cancer Causes and Control, 7*, 56–68.

Itri, L. (1987, July–August). Women and lung cancer. *Public Health Reports* (Suppl.), 92–96.

Johnston, C. C., Slemenda, C. W., & Melton, L. J. (1991). Clinical use of bone densitometry. *New England Journal of Medicine, 324*, 1105–1109.

Kelsey, J. L., & Bernstein, L. (1996). Epidemiology and prevention of breast cancer. *Annual Review of Public Health, 17*, 47–67.

Kennedy, J. W., Killip, T., Fisher, L. D., Alderman, E. L., Gillepie, M. J., & Mock, M. B. (1982). The clinical spectrum of coronary artery disease and its surgical and medical management. The Coronary Artery Surgery Study. *Circulation, 66*, 16–23.

Khan, S. S., Nessim, S., Gray, R., Czer, L. S., Chaux, A., & Matloff, J. (1990). Increased mortality of women in coronary artery bypass surgery: Evidence for referral bias. *Annals of Internal Medicine, 112*, 561–567.

Kohlmeier, L., & Mendez, M. (1997). Controversies surrounding diet and cancer. *Proceedings of the Nutrition Society, 56*, 369–382.

Kreiger, N., Kelsey, J. L., Holford, T. R., & O'Connor, T. (1982). An epidemiologic study of hip fracture in postmenopausal women. *American Journal of Epidemiology, 116*, 141–148.

Kreiger, N., Wolff, M.S., Hiatt, R. A., Rivers, M., & Vogelman, J. (1994). Breast cancer and serum organochlorines: A prospective study among white, black, and Asian women. *Journal of the National Cancer Institute, 86*(8), 589–599.

Kudenchuk, P., Maynard, C., Martin, J., Wirkus, M., & Weaver, W. D. (1996). Comparison of presentation, treatment, and outcome of acute myodardial infarction in men versus women (the Myocardial Infarction Triage and Intervention Registry). *American Journal of Cardiology, 78*, 9–14.

Kulldorff, M., Feuer, E. J., Miller, B. A., & Freedman, L. S. (1997). Breast cancer clusters in the northeast United States: A geographic analysis. *American Journal of Epidemiology, 146*(2), 161–170.

La Vecchia, C., DeCarli, A., Parazzini, F., Gentile, A., Negri, E., Cecchetti, G., & Franceschi, S. (1987). *International Journal of Epidemiology, 16*(3), 347–355.

Lavie, C. J., & Milani, R. V. (1995). Effects of cardiac rehabilitation and exercise training capacity, coronary risk factors, behavioral characteristics, and quality of life in women. *American Journal of Cardiology, 75*, 340–343.

Lerman, C., Seay, J., Balshem, A., & Audrain, J. (1995). Interest in genetic testing among fires-degree relatives of breast cancer patients. *American Journal of Medical Genetics, 57*, 385–392.

Lerner, D. J., & Kannel, W. B. (1986). Patterns of coronary heart disease morbidity and mortality in the sexes: A 26-year follow up of the Framingham population. *American Heart Journal, 111*, 383–390.

Levy, D., & Kannel, W. B. (1988). Cardiovascular risks: New insights from Framingham. *American Heart Journal, 116*, 2664–2667.

Liberman, U. A., Weiss, S. R., Broli, J., Minne, H. W., Quan, H., Bell, N. H., Rodriguez-Portales, J., Downs, R. W., Jr., Dequeker, J., Favus, M., Seeman, E., Recker, R. R., Capizzi, T., Santora, A. C. II, Lombardi, A., Shah, R. V., Hirsch, L. J., & Karpf, D. B. (1995). Effect of oral alendronate on bone mineral density and the incidence of fractures in postmenopausal osteoporosis. *New England Journal of Medicine, 333*, 1437–1443.

Lindheim, S. R., Legro, R. S., Bernstein, L., Stanczyk, F. Z., Vijod, M. A., Pressor, S. C., & Lobo, R. A. (1992). Behavioral stress responses in premenopausal and postmenopausal women and the effects of estrogen. *American Journal of Obstetrics & Gynecology, 167*, 1831–1836.

Lindquist, O. (1982). Intraindividual changes of blood pressure, serum lipids, and body weight in relation to menstrual status: Results from a prospective population study of women in Goteborg, Sweden. *Preventive Medicine, 11*, 162–172.

Lindquist, O., & Bengtsson, C. (1980). Serum lipids, arterial blood pressure and body weight in relation to the menopause: Results from a population study of women in Goteborg, Sweden. *Scandinavian Journal of Clinical & Laboratory Investigation, 40*, 629–636.

Lindsay, R. (1991). Estrogens, bone mass, and osteoporotic fracture. *American Journal of Medicine, 91*, 10S–13S.

Manson, J. E., Stampfer, M. J., Colditz, G. A., Willett, W. C., Rosner, B., Monson, R. R., Speizer, F. E., & Hennekens, C. H. (1990). A prospective study of obesity and risk of coronary heart disease in women. *New England Journal of Medicine, 322*, 822–889.

Marmor, A., & Zeira, M. (1993). Hormonal replacement therapy induces false-positive ST-segment depression in middle-aged women. *American Journal of Noninvasive Cardiology, 7,* 361–363.

Matos, E. L., Parkin, D. M., Loris, D. I., & Vilensky, M. (1990). Geographical patterns of cancer mortality in Argentina. *International Journal of Epidemiology, 19*(4), 860–870.

Matthews, K. A. (1992). Presidential address: Myths and realities of menopause. *Psychosomatic Medicine, 54,* 1–9.

Matthews, K. A., Siegel, J. M., Kuller, L. H., Thompson, M., & Varat, M. (1983). Determinants of decisions to seek medical treatment by patients with acute myocardial infarction symptoms. *Journal of Personality and Social Psychology, 44*(6), 1144–1156.

Matthews, K. A., Meilahn, E., Kuller, L. H., Kelsey, S. F., Caggiulla, A. W., & Wing, R. R. (1989). Menopause and risk factors for coronary heart disease. *New England Journal of Medicine, 321,* 641–646.

Matthews, K. A., Shumaker, S. A., Bowen, D. J., Langer, R. D., Hunt, J. R., Kaplan, R. M., Klesges, R. C., & Ritenbaugh, C. (1997). Women's Health Initiative: Why now? What is it? What's New? *American Psychologist, 52*(2), 101–116.

Maynard, C., Althouse, R., Olsufka, M., Ritchie, J. L., Davis, K. B., & Kennedy, J. W. (1989). Early versus late hospital arrival for acute myocardial infarction in the Western Washington Thrombolytic Therapy Trials. *American Journal of Cardiology, 63,* 1296–1300.

McTiernan, A., Stanford, J. L., Weiss, N. S., Darling, J. R., & Voigt, L. F. (1996). Occurrence of breast cancer in relation to recreational exercise in women age 50–64 years. *Epidemiology, 7*(6), 598–604.

Mermelstein, R. J., & Borrelli, B. (1995). Women and smoking. In A. L. Stanton & S. J. Gallant (Eds.), *The psychology of women's health: Progress and challenges in research and application* (pp. 309–348). Washington DC: American Psychological Association.

Micozzi, M. S. (1985). Nutrition, body size, and breast cancer. *Yearbook of Physical Anthropology, 28,* 175–206.

Miller, A. B., Baines, C. J., To, T., & Wall, C. (1992). Canadian National Breast Screening Study: 1. Breast cancer detection and death reates among women aged 40 to 49 years. *Canadian Medical Association Journal, 147*(10), 1459–1478.

Moore, S. M., & Kramer, F. M. (1996). Women's and men's preferences for cardiac rehabilitation program features. *Journal of Cardiopulmonary Rehabilitation, 16,* 163–168.

Moormeier, J. (1996). Breast cancer in black women. *Annals of Internal Medicine, 124*(10), 897–905.

Mosca, L., Manson, J. E., Sutherland, S. E., Langer, R. D., Manolio, T., & Barrett-Connor, E. (1997). Cardiovascular disease in women: A statement for healthcare professionals from the American Heart Association. *Circulation, 96,* 2468–2482.

National Heart, Lung, and Blood Institute (NHLBI). (1994). *Report of the Task Force on Research in Epidemiology and Prevention of Cardiovascular Diseases.* Washington, DC: US Department of Health and Human Services.

Navarro, A. M., & Kaplan, R. M. (1996). The mammography controversy: Current and future evidence. *Women's Health: Research on Gender, Behavior, and Policy, 2*(4), 261–266.

Palmer, J. R., Rosenberg, L., Harlap, S., Strom, B. L., Warshauer, M. E., Zauber, A. G., & Shapiro, S. (1995). Adult height and risk of breast cancer among US black women. *American Journal of Epidemiology, 141*(9), 845–849.

Parker, S. L., Tong, T., Bolden, S., & Wingo, P. A. (1996). Cancer statistics, 1996. *CA—A Cancer Journal for Clinicians, 65,* 5–27.

Parker, S. L., Tong, T., Bolden, S., & Wingo, P. A. (1997). Cancer statistics, 1997. *CA—A Cancer Journal for Clinicians, 47,* 5–27.

Pate, R. R., Pratt, M., Blair, S. N., Haskell, W. L., Macera, C. A., Bouchard, C., Buchard, D., Caspersen, C. J., Ettinger, W., Heath, G. W., King, A. C., Kriska, A., Leon, A. S., Marcus, B. H., Morris, J., Paffenbarger, R. S., Patrick, K., Pollock, M. L., Rippe, J. M., Sallis, J., & Wilmore, J. H. (1995). Physical activity and public health: A recommendation from the Centers for Disease Control and Prevention and the American College of Sports Medicine. *Journal of the American Medical Association, 273,* 402–407.

Persson, I. (1996). Cancer risk in women receiving estrogen–progestin replacement therapy. *Maturitas, 23* (Suppl.), 537–545.

Pierce, J. P., Fiore, M. C., Novotny, T. E., Hatziandreu, E. J., & Davis, R. M. (1989). Trends in cigarette smoking in the United States—Educational differences are increasing. *Journal of the American Medical Association, 261,* 56–60.

Pollitzer, W. S., & Anderson, J. J. B. (1989). Ethnic and genetic differences in bone mass: A review with a hereditary vs. environmental perspective. *American Journal of Clinical Nutrition, 50,* 1244–1259.

Prince, R. L., Smith, M., Dick, I. M., Price, R. I., Webb, P. G., Henderson, N. K., & Harris, M. M. (1991). Prevention of postmenopausal osteoporosis. A comparative study of exercise, calcium supplementation, and hormone-replacement therapy. *New England Journal of Medicine, 325*(17), 1190–1196.

Riggs, B. L. (1992). Osteoporosis. In J. B. Weingaarden, L. H. Smith, Jr., & J. C. Bennett (Eds.), *Cecil textbook of medicine* (pp. 1426–1431). Philadelphia, PA: WB Saunders.

Riggs, B. L., & Melton, L. J., III. (1992). The prevention and treatment of osteoporosis. *New England Journal of Medicine, 327*, 620–627.

Riis, B. J. (1991). Biochemical markers of bone turnover in diagnosis and assessment of therapy. *American Journal of Medicine, 91*, 64S–68S.

Rimer, B. K. (1994). Mammography use in the US: Trends and the impact of interventions. *Annals of Behavioral Medicine, 16*(4), 317–326.

Romieu, I., Hernandez-Avilla, M., Lazcano, E., Lopez, L., & Romero-Jaime, R. (1996). Breast cancer and lactation history in Mexican women. *American Journal of Epidemiology, 146*(6), 543–552.

Ross, P. D., Davis, J. W., Epstein, R. S., & Wasnich, R. D. (1991). Pre-existing fractures and bone mass predict vertebral fracture incidence in women. *Annals of Internal Medicine, 114*, 919–923.

Rossouw, J. E. (1996). Estrogens for prevention of coronary heart disease: Putting the brakes on the bandwagon. *Circulation, 94*(11), 2982–2985.

Rossouw, J. E., Finnegan, L. P., Harlan, W. R., Pinn, V. W., Clifford, C., & McGowan, J. A. (1995). The evolution of the Women's Health Initiative: Perspectives from the NIH. *Journal of the American Medical Women Association, 50*, 50–55.

Rothert, M., Padonu, G., Holmes-Rovner, M., Kroll, J., Talarczyk, G., Rovner, D., Schmitt, N., & Breer, L. (1994). Menopausal women as decision makers in health care. *Experimental Gerontology, 29*, 463–468.

Rozenberg, S., Liebens, F., Kroll, M., & Vandromme, J. (1996). Principal cancers among women: Breast, lung and colorectal. *International Journal of Fertility and Menopausal Studies, 41*(2), 166–171.

Schmidt, S. B., & Borsch, M. A. (1990). The prehospital phase of acute myocardial infarction in the era of thrombolysis. *American Journal of Cardiology, 65*, 1411–1415.

Seeman, T. E., & Syme, S. L. (1987). Social networks and coronary artery disease: A comparison of structure and function of social relations as predictors of the disease. *Psychosomatic Medicine, 49*, 340–353.

Shimizu, H., Ross, R. K., Bernstein, L., Yatani, R., Henderson, B. E., & Mack, T. M. (1991). Cancers of the prostate and breast among Japanese and white immigrants in Los Angeles County. *British Journal of Cancer, 63*(6), 963–966.

Shumaker, S.A., & Hill D.R. (1991). Gender differences in social support and physical health. *Health Psychology, 10*(2), 102–111

Smith, S. C., Blair, S. N., Criqui, M. H., Fletcher, G. F., Fuster, V., Gersh, B. J., Grotto, A. M., Gould, K. L., Greenland, P., Grundy, S. M., Hill, M. N., Hlatky, M. A., Miller, N. H., Krauss, R. M., Las Rossa, J., Ockene, I. S., Oparil, S., Pearson, T. A., Rapaport, E., & Starke, R. D., and the Secondary Prevention Panel, American Heart Association. (1995). Preventing heart attack and death in patients with coronary disease. *Circulation, 92*, 2–4.

Spelsberg, A., Ridker, P. M., & Manson, J. E. (1993). Carbohydrate metabolism, obesity, and diabetes. In P. Douglas (Ed.), *Cardiovascular health and disease in women* (pp. 191–216). Philadelphia: W.B. Saunders.

Stanton, A. L. (1995). Psychology of women's health: Barriers and pathways to knowledge. In A. L. Stanton & S. J. Gallant (Eds.), *The psychology of women's health: Progress and challenges in research and application* (pp. 3–21). Washington DC: American Psychological Association.

Steingart, R. M., Packer, M., Hamm, P., Coglianese, M. E., Gersh, B., Geltman, E. M., Sollano, J., Katz, S., Moye, L., & Basta, L. L., Lewis, S. J., Gottlieb, S. S., Bernstein, V., McEwan, P., Jacobson, K., Brown, E. J., Kukin, M. L., Kantrowitz, N. E., Pfeffer, M. A., for the Survival and Ventricular Enlargement Investigators. (1991). Sex differences in the management of coronary artery disease. *New England Journal of Medicine, 325*(4), 226–230.

Stone, P. H., Thompson, B., Anderson, H. V., Kronenberg, M. W., Gibson, R. S., Rogers, W. J., Diver, D. J., Theroux, P., Warnica, J. W., Nassmith, J. B., & Braunwald, E. (1996). Influence of race, sex, and age on management of unstable angina and non-Q-wave myocardial infarction: The TIMI III registry. *Journal of the American Medical Association, 275*, 1104–1112.

Swanson, C. A., Coates, R. J., Schoenberg, J. B., Malone, K. E., Gammon, M. D., Stanford, J. L., Shorr, I. J., Potischman, N. A., & Brintin, L. A. (1996). Body size and breast cancer risk among women under age 45 years. *American Journal of Epidemiology, 143*(7), 698–706.

Tabar, L., Fagerberg, G., Chen, H-H, Duffy, S. W., Smart, C. R., Gad, A., & Smith, R. A. (1995). Efficacy of breast cancer screening by age. *Cancer, 75*, 2507–2517.

Thomas, R. J., Miller, N. H., Lamendola, C., Berra, K.. Hedback, B., Durstin, J. L., & Haskell, W. (1996). National survey on gender differences in cardiac rehabilitation programs: patient characteristics and enrollment patterns. *Journal of Cardiopulmonary Rehabilitation, 16,* 402–412.

Thune, I., Brenn, T., Lund, E., & Gaard, M. (1997). Physical activity and the risk of breast cancer. *New England Journal of Medicine, 336*(18), 1269–1275.

Tinetti, M. E., & Speechley, M. (1989). Prevention of falls among the elderly. *New England Journal of Medicine, 320,* 1055–1059.

Toniolo, P. G. (1997). Endogenous estrogens and breast cancer risk: The case for prospective cohort studies. *Environmental Health Perspectives, 105* (Suppl. 3), 587–592.

Travis, C. B. (1988). Breast cancer: Risk factors. In *Women and health psychology: Biomedical issues* (pp. 203–228). Hillsdale, NJ: Lawrence Erlbaum.

Trentham-Dietz, A., Newcomb, P. A., Storer, B. E., Longnecker, M. P., Baron, J., Greenberg, E. R., & Willett, W. C. (1997). Body size and risk of breast cancer. *American Journal of Epidemiology, 145*(11), 1011–1019.

Turi, Z. G., Stone, P. H., Muller, J. E., Parker, C., Rude, R. E., Raabe, D. E., Jaffe, A. S., Hartwell, T. D., Robertson, T. L., Braunwalk, E., & the Milis Study Group. (1986). Implications for acute intervention related to time of hospital arrival in acute myocardial infarction. *American Journal of Cardiology, 58,* 203–209.

US Department of Health and Human Services (USDHHS). (1980). *The health consequences of smoking for women: A report of the Surgeon General* (pp. 133–136), Washington, DC: US Government Printing Office.

US Department of Health and Human Services (USDHHS). (1989). *Reducing the health consequences of smoking: 25 years of progress. A report of the Surgeon General.* DHHS Publication No. (CDC) 89-8411. Washington, DC: U.S: Government Printing Office.

US Department of Health and Human Services (USDHHS). (1990, September). *Healthy people 2000: National health promotion and disease prevention objectives.* DHHS publication #91-50212. Washington, DC: Public Health Service.

US Department of Health and Human Services (USDHHS). (1991, September). *Osteoporosis research, education and health promotion.* Public Health Service, National Institutes of Health publication # 91-3216. Washington, DC: US Government Printing Office.

US Preventive Services Task Force. (1996). *Guide to clinical preventive services* (2nd ed.). Baltimore: Williams & Wilkins.

Van Itallie, T. B. (1985). Health implications of overweight and obesity in the United States. *Annals of Internal Medicine, 1985,* 983–988.

Walker, B., Figgs, L. W., & Zahm, S. H. (1995). Differences in cancer incidence, mortality, and survival between African Americans and whites. *Environmental Health Perspectives, 103* (Suppl. 8), 275–281.

Weiss, W. (1997). Cigarette smoking and lung cancer trends: A light at the end of the tunnel? *Chest, 111,* 1414–1416.

Weissman, M. M., & Klerman, G. L. (1977). Sex differences in the epidemiology of depression. *Archives of General Psychiatry, 34,* 98–111.

Weitzman, S., Cooper, L., Chambless, L., Rosamond, W., Clegg, L., Marcucci, G., Romm, F., & White, A. (1997). Gender, racial, and geographic differences in the performance of cardiac diagnostic and therapeutic procedures for hospitalized acute myocardial infarction in four states. *American Journal of Cardiology, 79,* 722–726.

Williamson, D. F., Madans, J., Anda, R. F., Kleinman, J. C., Giovino, G. A., & Byers, T. (1991). Smoking cessation and severity of weight gain in a national cohort. *New England Journal of Medicine, 324,* 739–745.

Wolff, M. S., & Weston, A. (1997). Breast cancer risk and environmental exposures. *Environmental Health Perspectives, 105* (Suppl. 4), 491–496.

Wood, P. D., Stefanick, M. I., & Williams, P. T. (1991). The effects of plasma lipoproteins of a prudent weight reducing diet with or without exercise, in overweight men and women. *New England Journal of Medicine, 325,* 461–466.

Writing Group for the PEPI Trial. (1995). Effects of estrogen or estrogen/progestin regimens on heart disease risk factors in post-menopausal women. *Journal of the American Medical Association, 273,* 199–208.

Wu, A. H., Ziegler, R. G., Horn-Ross, P. L., Nomura, A. M., West, D. W., Kolonel, L. N., Rosenthal, J. F., Hoover, R. N., & Pike, M. C. (1996). Tofu and risk of breast cancer in Asian-Americans. *Cancer Epidemiology, Biomarkers and Prevention, 5*(11), 901–906.

Yong, L. C., Brown, C. C., Schatzkin, A., & Schairer, C. (1996). Prospective study of relative weight and risk of breast cancer: The Breast Cancer Detection Demonstration Project, follow-up study, 1979–1989. *American Journal of Epidemiology, 143*(10), 985–995.

CHAPTER 27

Sociocultural Factors and Prevention Programs Affecting the Health of Ethnic Minorities

Gina M. Wingood and Betty Keltner

Introduction

One of the most persistent and pressing public health problems in the United States today is the disparity in health between white and ethnic minority populations. Higher rates of disease, disability, and death for ethnic minorities compared to white populations have been documented for over a century. Epidemiological data have been informative with respect to quantifying the differential risk of disease conditions for ethnic minorities compared to whites; however, it provides less insight into the pervasive socioeconomic and cultural factors that are key determinants of health behavior. When conducting research with ethnic minority populations, it is important to understand the diversity of cultures and social forces that may differentially exert considerable influence on their health. Clearly, understanding the influences that shape health behavior is critical to the development and implementation of tailored and more efficacious programs designed to reinforce the adoption and maintenance of health preventive behaviors among ethnic minority populations.

Race, Ethnicity, and Culture

In public health the terms *race, ethnicity,* and *culture* are often used interchangeably. The implication appears to be that racial and ethnic categories define homogeneous populations in ways that are meaningful to their health status. However, the definition of a group as a race is not a function of biological or genetic differences between groups, but is dependent on the society's perception that differences exist and

Gina M. Wingood • Department of Behavioral Sciences and Health Education, Rollins School of Public Health, Emory University, and Emory/Atlanta Center for AIDS Research, Atlanta, Georgia 30322.   *Betty Keltner* • School of Nursing, University of Alabama at Birmingham, Birmingham, Alabama 35294.

Handbook of Health Promotion and Disease Prevention, edited by Raczynski and DiClemente. Kluwer Academic/Plenum Publishers, New York, 1999.

that they are important (Earls, 1993). Further, there is more genetic variation within races than between races. Ethnicity implies the existence of a distinct culture or subculture in which group members feel themselves bound together by common values and beliefs and are so regarded by other members of the society. When these beliefs, values, and behaviors are learned, shared, and homogeneous within an ethnic group, they may be cultural.

Diversity among Ethnic Minorities

White Americans account for 76.7% and the diverse ethnic minority groups constitute the remainder of the of the US population (US Bureau of the Census, 1984). Diversity among ethnic groups is evident in their countries of origin, region of residence in the United States, socioeconomic status, and degree of accommodation of mainstream American values and habits. The four major ethnic minority groups in the United States are African Americans, Hispanic Americans, Asian Americans, and Native Americans (American Indians, Alaskan Natives, and Native Hawaiians). African Americans account for 12% of the US population and are the largest ethnic minority group. Diversity among African Americans is most evident in the Afro-Caribbean population (i.e., Haitians and West Indians) (Earls, 1993). Under the current demographic transition occurring in the United States, Hispanics will soon be the largest ethnic minority group.

Hispanic Americans account for 7.2% of the US population and currently comprise the second largest ethnic minority group (Earls, 1993). While there are commonalities in language and religion among Hispanics, these characteristics only partially explain the more than two dozen Hispanic cultures present in the United States. Approximately one third of Hispanics are immigrants. The majority of Hispanic Americans are Mexican Americans; other major subgroups include Puerto Ricans and Cuban Americans.

Asian Americans account for 2.1% of the US population. Asian Americans represent another broad array of cultural groups that speak over 30 different languages and include Asian Indian, Chinese, Filipino, Japanese, Korean, Laotian, and Vietnamese. About 70% of Asian Americans are immigrants, mostly from Southeast Asia.

Native Americans account for 0.7% of the racial and ethnic population in the United States. Native Americans, including American Indians, Alaskan Natives, and Native Hawaiians, are also very diverse in terms of the number of different subethnic groups and constitute the widest degree of cultural diversity among all ethnic minorities in the United States. There are nearly 300 tribes, 278 reservations, and 209 native villages that are recognized by the federal government. Understanding the diversity among ethnic minority populations allows us to realize that members of racial and ethnic minority groups may be disproportionately at risk for disease; further, these differences may be a reflection of discriminatory practices directed against these populations.

Epidemiology of Health Conditions among Ethnic Minorities

Evidence on the relative risk of certain disease conditions such as infant mortality, cardiovascular disease, cancer, acquired immunodeficiency syndrome (AIDS), and drug use can be assessed. However, health statistics obtained from large-scale surveys are limited in their assessment of health preventive behaviors and sociocultural variables affecting these conditions. Furthermore, the epidemiological methods that are used to collect and analyze data from ethnic minority communities may be flawed, and thus bias how we interpret the data. The existing epidemiological data, however, do provide us a starting point from which to direct health prevention intervention efforts.

Diet-Related Health Conditions: Cancer and Cardiovascular Disease

Many aspects of diet and nutrition vary among racial and ethnic minority groups, this variation may contribute to interethnic differences in diet-related morbidity and mortality. Among adults, obesity and diabetes are problems for all ethnic minority populations. A high fat intake may contribute to the high prevalence rates of obesity among Hispanics, American Indians, and African Americans (Kumanyika, 1993). Furthermore, data indicate that African-American and Hispanic-American women have lower levels of physical activity compared with white women. African Americans have a higher prevalence of diet-related cancers, heart and vascular diseases, obesity, and diabetes compared to whites. Hispanics have a higher prevalence of pancreatic and stomach cancers compared to whites. Among Asian Americans, Japanese Americans have a higher prevalence of stroke; Japanese, Filipino, and Samoans have higher rates of hypertension, and Chinese Americans and Filipinos have higher rates of esophageal cancer compared with whites. Among Native Americans, stomach cancers and hypertension are more prevalent than among whites. Unfortunately, we do not yet have the knowledge or the tools to accurately access the role of diet among individuals. The diversity of ethnic minority populations and the lack of analytic tools to accurately assess the influence of diet in cardiovascular- and cancer-related conditions poses special challenges and promises new insights.

Smoking

The prevalence of smoking has been significantly higher in African Americans than in whites since 1966; however, a downward trend for smoking cessation has been observed (Chen, 1993). In 1987, 34.0% of African-American adults (both males and females) smoked compared to 28.8% of whites. Similarly, in 1985, young African Americans, 20–24 years of age, were less likely to smoke compared to their white peers. Moreover, African Americans are less likely to be heavier smokers and more likely to initiate smoking at a later age. Unfortunately, the smoking prevalence for other ethnic minority populations are not showing these downward trends.

The Hispanic Health and Nutrition Examination Survey (HHANES) reported a smoking prevalence of nearly 40% among Hispanic men and 26% among Hispanic women. There are no reliable national estimates of smoking among Asians; however, surveys have been conducted in several geographic regions, and smoking rates are highest among Vietnamese men (65%), Cambodian men (71%), and Laotian men (92%). Japanese and Filipino men living in Hawaii reported smoking rates of 29% and 25%, respectively. Rates of smoking among Asian women are relatively low. Smoking varies considerably among Native Americans. Smoking rates among Northern Plains Indians range from 42 to 70% of the population, and rates of smoking among Alaskan Natives have been reported at 56%, greatly exceeding the national average. Native Americans from the Southwest report much lower rates, ranging from 13 to 28% of the population. Cigarette smoking is the single-most important preventable cause of death and disease in the United States. Tobacco accounts for 87% of lung cancer deaths, 30% of all cancer deaths, 21% of deaths from heart diseases, and 18% of deaths from stroke. Progress in halting smoking must continue and accelerate if reductions in smoking related morbidity and mortality are a goal.

Acquired Immunodeficiency Syndrome

When acquired immunodeficiency syndrome (AIDS) first appeared in the United States in 1981, it was considered a disease of homosexual and injection-drug-using men. The impact on these male subgroups is still substantial. In 1994, according to the Division of HIV/AIDS at the Centers for Disease Control and Prevention, among males, 55% were white, 28% were African American, 16% were Hispanic, less than 1% were American Indian/Alaskan Native and Pacific Islanders, and less than 1% were Asian (Castro, 1993). The majority, 62%, of men who were infected with human immunodeficiency virus (HIV) through homosexual contact. Nearly 21% of men acquired human immunodeficiency virus (HIV) were infected through injecting drugs.

While most HIV infected individuals are men, 20% of all AIDS cases occur in women. The sociodemographics of HIV as well as the modes of exposure differ significantly in women compared with men. The majority of women, 54%, are African American, 25% are Hispanic, 20% are white, less than 1% are Asians, and less than 1% are American Indians/Alaskan Natives or Pacific Islanders. Unlike men, in which the majority of cases are attributed to homosexual contact, most cases of AIDS in women (45%) are attributed to injection drug use. However, the proportion of AIDS cases attributed to heterosexual contact has increased from 15% in 1983 to 39% in 1997. The HIV/AIDS epidemic continues to highlight the existing disparities in the health status of ethnic minorities in the United States. Identifying and intervening on sociocultural influences serves as a key to reducing the risk of HIV among ethnic minority populations.

Historically, epidemiologists have treated race and ethnicity as personal descriptors, such as age, however, without probing into the underlying social and cultural implications of these concepts. Today, it is more widely accepted that to understand the epidemiology of disease conditions among ethnic minorities requires a deeper understanding of the meaning of race.

Social Inequalities Affecting the Health of Ethnic Minorities

Historically, researchers have recognized the connection between an individual's social context and his or her health. Social variables such as income, education, and age are universally employed in an attempt to understand social factors affecting the health of ethnic minorities. In this section, we will briefly discuss the influence of socioeconomic class, social networks, racial discrimination, and targeted social marketing and their impact on the health of ethnic minority populations.

Socioeconomic Class

Social class is a theoretical concept indicating an individual's location in the social stratification system and their access to material resources, influence, and information (Mechanic, 1989). Socioeconomic status (SES) is a constellation of variables used as indicators for social class. Usually, SES includes measures of on educational level, income, and occupational rank (Haan & Kaplan, 1985). Further, social class can be assessed at different levels, including the individual, the family, and the community level. Numerous studies have demonstrated the inverse graded relationship between SES and health. Namely, the more advantaged groups, whether expressed in terms of education, income, or occupation, tend to have better health outcomes than members who are less advantaged. The distribution is not bipolar (i.e., advantaged vs. disadvantaged) but graded, so that each change in the level of advantage or disadvantage on any indices of SES in general is associated with a corresponding change in health.

Several studies have illustrated mechanisms by which social class inequities explain differences in health between whites and ethnic minorities. SES can affect the health of ethnic minorities by influencing access to preventive health care, exposure to occupational and environmental hazards, availability of health insurance, quality of care received, and type of treatment procedures utilized. Research attempting to explain the health disparity between whites and ethnic minority populations often adjusts for social class. Numerous studies have shown that adjusting for social class often substantially reduces (and at times eliminates) differences in health between white and ethnic minority populations. In many cases, however, differences in health still persists even after analyses are adjusted for social status. Differences in the health of ethnic minorities may then be explained by other social and psychological variables. One of these factors may be social networks.

Social Networks

Social networks are the sets of social linkages or interactions between individuals. The structure of social networks can be described in terms of dyadic characteristics (characteristics of the relationship between the focal individual and another person in the network) and in terms of the characteristics of the network as a whole (Berkman, 1984). Examples of dyadic characteristics include the extent to which resources and support are both given and received in a relationship (reciprocity), the extent to which a relationship is characterized by emotional closeness (intensity), and the extent to which a relationship serves a variety of functions (complexity). Examples of characteristics that describe a whole network include the extent to which network members are similar in terms of demographic characteristics, such as age, race, and SES; the extent to which network members live in close proximity to the focal person (geographical dispersion); and the extent to which network members know and interact with each other (density). There are a variety of channels through which social networks may have a positive impact on an individual's health. In a historic study, Marmot and Syme (1976) examined the buffering influence of social networks among Japanese men and its relationship to coronary heart disease.

Among men of Japanese ancestry, there is a gradient in the occurrence of coronary heart disease. Coronary heart disease (CHD) is lowest among men in Japan, moderately high among men in Hawaii, and highest among men in California. This gradient exists even when statistically adjusting for biological and behavioral factors including dietary intake, serum cholesterol levels, blood pressure, and smoking history. One study examined whether Japanese-American men with strong social networks had lower rates of CHD compared to Japanese-American men with weaker social networks (Marmot & Syme, 1976). The study reported that the most traditional group of Japanese-American men had the strongest social networks and a CHD prevalence as low as that observed among men in Japan. Conversely, Japanese-American men who were the most acculturated to Western culture had the weakest social networks and had a three- to fivefold excess in CHD prevalence. This difference in CHD rate between those men with the strongest and weakest social networks could not be accounted for by differences in the major coronary risk factors. This study illustrates that the availability of individual and community resources and enhanced social networks can increase the likelihood that stressors can be coped with in a way that reduces the adverse health consequences.

Racial Discrimination

Racial discrimination is an oppressive system of racial relations, justified by ideology, in which one racial group benefits from dominating another and defines itself and other through this domination (Krieger & Sydney, 1996). Racism is the expression of degrading beliefs and discriminatory behavior implemented by either institutions or individuals, as linked to their membership in racially defined groups. Hypertension research presents the most compelling evidence illustrating the association between racial discrimination and health.

One study conducted among African Americans in the South found that even after adjusting the analyses for age, basal metabolic levels, SES, and educational level, independent predictors of elevated blood pressure included racial discrimination at work, darker skin color, and high lifestyle incongruity (Dressler, 1990). This last construct assesses whether an individuals' lifestyle exceeds their educational level. The authors summized that the constant frustration that African Americans experience in seeking to claim a certain social status in the world but persistently being denied this status may result from low economic resources and racial discrimination.

Targeted Social Marketing

Social marketing has been described as the application of commercial marketing technologies to the analysis, planning, execution, and evaluation of programs designed to influence the voluntary behavior of target audiences in order to improve their personal welfare and that of their society (Moore, Williams, & Qualls, 1996). One question that has been raised is what if targeted marketing of ethnic minorities is not motivated by a health promotion rational but by more discriminatory and racist motives.

A recent study conducted by Moore et al. (1996) examined whether the increased consumption of alcohol and tobacco products by African Americans and Latinos was correlated with the targeted marketing practices of product distributors. The sample included white, Latino, and African-American tobacco and alcohol users of all ages, as from census track data. The results illustrated that differential consumption patterns of alcohol and tobacco products existed for African American, Latino, and white populations. Younger African Americans had lower consumption rates than their white peers; however, as they get older, this rate increased and surpassed that of their white peers. Additionally, African Americans had a lower smoking cessation rate among African Americans, were more likely to use mentholated brands of cigarettes that contain more nicotine and tar, and were more likely to consume malt liquors that had a greater alcohol content.

Concomitantly, African Americans who consumed more alcohol and tobacco also resided in areas in which there were significantly higher rates of targeted marketing of tobacco and alcohol products to ethnic minority groups. This was indicated by the a greater number of outdoor billboard advertisements in predominantly African-American urban neighborhoods and increased advertising in print media directed at African-American audiences. The correlational study design precludes any determination of whether the target marketing is racially motivated. Marketers claim that they are merely fulfilling the needs of a certain segment. It is difficult to know which came first, the demand for the product or the promotion of the product. More research is needed to answer this question to determine conclusively if there is a racist motive.

Critical Variables that Define Culture for Ethnic Minorities

Family Structure

Family structure is typically characterized by the configuration of adults in a household. However, the concept of household varies from culture to culture. Often, household is defined in terms of who resides in the home, but many cultural groups extend the definition to include people who reside beyond its walls. Nuclear families, consisting of two biological parents and their children, traditionally emphasize educational achievement and maximizing individual success in society. Extended families, consisting of relatives and near relatives, place more emphasis on group sharing and less on individual achievement. Extended families have more generations and larger numbers of children; therefore, the traditional culture can be transmitted with greater intensity. In these multigenerational families, the family unit structure becomes more effective in transferring to the local community the values of cooperation and group sharing that it espouses.

People who have strong ethnic identity will inevitably have strong family ties, since transmission of culture typically occurs within intimate family units. Extended family structures are normative among many minority cultures. Family members in this network of natural support relate to each other in ways similar to that found in the nuclear family of the dominant culture. Multigenerational bonds are strong and reinforced by family, community, and culture. Often, extended family live together or very close to each other so that daily family routines include interactions with grandparents, cousins, aunts, and uncles (Keltner, 1992; Keltner & Ramey, 1992, 1993). The extended family may be further organized into clans or other kinship units.

Another salient aspect of family structure is the increasing phenomenon of multi-ethnic families in which different cultural traditions are blended. Children with multi-ethnic heritage may have the physical appearance of one parent while embracing the traditions, values, and beliefs of the other. For example, a child of Japanese and Jewish parents could appear Asian yet practice the Hebrew faith. A person born to a Hispanic father and Hopi mother could have a Hispanic surname yet be reared exclusively with American Indian traditions. Although unions such as these may combine traditions, many times either family choice or parental separation leads to transmission of a dominant culture.

The family is important to health promotion efforts because basic health behaviors are learned in childhood. Health behaviors are practiced and reinforced in the context of daily routine, which is facilitated by common values and habits. Furthermore, it has been well documented that minority families have experienced marginalized health and education services. Because of this marginalization, there are legitimate suspicions about the credibility of health information from formal sources. A family member, generally an older woman with considerable life experience, is often the health authority for minority families. Folk healers, such as *curanderas* or medicine men, are members of the community and may pass healing skills and traditions through their own family lines. Among people who have not had extensive formal education, elders are keepers of knowledge. Scientists have identified two broad categories of people in terms of health education: information seekers and information avoiders. For minority populations, it can be a misrepresentation to refer to people as "information avoiders" merely because they do not actively participate in health education programs. Many people with ethnic minority heritage invest considerable trust in informal systems. Information about how to live a healthy life is sought daily in this country from medicine men, *curanderas*, and grandmothers.

Religion

Ethnic culture is not the only source of values, beliefs, and practices that affect health behavior. Religious faith can also be a potent influence on health behaviors. Religion gives meaning and serves as a protective force for behaviors that resist engagement with tobacco, alcohol, and drug use, high-risk sex, and violence. While certain ethnic groups have historical religious ties, this is not entirely uniform. For example, while the Baptist faith is known to be common among African Americans, along with Catholicism among Hispanics and Native Indian beliefs among American Indians, there are a variety of other common alliances such as African Americans who are Muslim, Hispanics who are Pentecostal, and American Indians families who have embraced the Christian faith for generations. In addition to principles of belief, people who are involved in any organized religion engage in rituals, traditions, and fellowship that continually reinforce behavioral standards. Alcohol is strictly forbidden by some faiths, such as Muslim and Pentecostal, and tobacco is used routinely in spiritual ceremonies by some American Indian tribes. Fundamental religious values such as these are not generally considered in the development of health promotion interventions. The dominant US cultural attitude that social drinking is typical for all people except recovering alcoholics or that tobacco is inherently bad disregards certain religious teachings. This dominant attitude is common among health behavior scientists and service providers, yet is in direct conflict with the religious values of large groups of people, particularly among ethnic minorities. When research and practice is based solely on dominant cultural values, deeply held religious beliefs not only have been disregarded but also disparaged. Insensitivity to basic cultural values further alienates minorities who have suffered historic abuses from public programs. Interventions that are culturally competent consider traditional health practices and respect cultural values in both design and implementation.

Language

Communication is common to the human species, yet considerable variation exists in language and communication styles. Hispanics in the United States, for example, represent diverse subgroups who share one prominent characteristic in common: the Spanish language. Even though the language is the same, dialects, terms, and referents are unique to regions. People with ancestry from Puerto Rico, Columbia, and

Mexico speak a common language with subgroup distinctions. Among the 500 American Indian tribes there are hundreds of languages, some that are nearly extinct and others that serve as the primary or exclusive language for individuals within tribes. Translators are sometimes employed in the development of health promotion interventions or materials. Techniques involved in translation have received inadequate attention considering the essential role that language plays in health education. Because nuances are characteristic of all languages, it is essential to use the strategy of back translation to assure that the intended meaning is communicated. Back translation involves translation back into English by a different person, independent of the original translation. Such a process is time consuming but provides confidence that fundamental meaning is retained in important health promotion messages. On a trip to Japan a popular American novel was discovered in a bookstore which the bookstore owner called *Angry Raisins*. The book was *The Grapes of Wrath*. This is an obvious example about how a literally accurate translation words can completely miss the intended meaning. Similarly, understanding the meaning of words used in English can be misconstrued. In Keltner's research (1993) among American Indian families who have children with disabilities, a computer program identified the theme of "burned out" as prominent in one of the participating tribes. However, in reviewing the interviews in closer detail it was discovered that families were referring to the experience of house fires—being burned out of their homes—which was relatively frequent on this particular reservation. Without careful attention to the intended meaning inherent in language, essential knowledge is missed or misunderstood.

Language has particular meaning associated within cultures as well. For some people, "aunt" or "grandmother" is an honorary title, not one that always indicates familial relationship. Likewise, "sister" may be a cousin who was raised in an extended family siblinglike relationship. It is important to determine at the outset of a project if the key factor to be learned is biological or interpersonal characteristics. This decision can guide training efforts and add clarity to health histories or data that are obtained by report. Training is one of the most important activities to assure quality programmatic and research results. Understanding of certain terms or concepts is based on experience. When lay outreach workers are asked to identify people who "best represent" a community, it is likely to result in a search for model citizens rather than residents who have typical health behaviors. As culturally sensitive health promotion interventions increasingly involve members of the community, especially in direct delivery of programs, special attention should be paid to how words are used and commonly understood within the culture.

Health Beliefs

Cultures have been sustained for centuries based on shared wisdom related to many aspects of behavior. Indeed, if reliability is defined in terms of consistency, it would seem that those who follow the scientific model have the less reliable source of health information. Consider, for example, the dramatic variations related to infant-feeding practices or prenatal care that have occurred for the past 30 years: feeding schedules, immunizations, recommended weight gain, and activities. While it is certainly not the case that folk practices are universally superior to the scientific approach, it is obvious that some of the most favored scientific theories will be refined or repudiated over the years. Empiricism is an enormous advance for prediction and control, but the search for knowledge will continue. A natural "fit" in philosophy is one that respects both models of health belief. When conflict exists between tradition and science, professionals should provide community leaders with the best evidence for their consideration as to how such a fit could occur. Such accommodations are facilitated when professionals become acquainted with community leaders and initiate communication as common interests are encountered. In one Hispanic community, a clergyman was consulted because infants were experiencing skin problems as a result of being "anointed with oil." After becoming aware of the problem and "prayerful deliberating," it was determined by the denomination that a drop of oil fulfilled the spiritual purpose of this ritual. At other times, health professionals will be challenged to accommodate cultural values and make changes in protocols or at least account for divergent values.

Ethnic cultures perpetuate fundamental values across generations. Therefore, most health beliefs are culturally embedded. Unlike people who become jogging enthusiasts or adopt a new vegetarian diet, persons who adhere to embedded health beliefs do not easily articulate what these health beliefs are because they are so much a part of unconscious routine. The values that underlie health behavior can reflect traditions that hold particular meaning for a culture. Adopting healthy behavior often involves some change in daily habit or routine. For some people, the change also must be congruent with cultural values and beliefs.

American Indian values associated with living in harmony promote positive health behaviors. Nevertheless, tribal variations cause different expressions. In the Northwest, many Indian tribes rely on fish as both dietary and economic staple, while to some tribes in the desert, fish are sacred and would never be eaten. As a dietary source, fish would be acceptable for some Indian tribes and not for others. The Hispanic disorder of "susto" or fright sickness attributed to ill-will is treated with methods in which serenity and social support is featured. Many African Americans embrace a religious faith that is personal and interactive, with divine guidance continually prompting a better lifestyle and obligating believers to help others. These examples of ethnic traditions are expressed in healthy behaviors but are motivated through cultural beliefs.

A particular benefit of the medical model is its consideration of unintended side effects. Little attention has been paid to the fact that behavioral interventions also can have side effects. Some health practices embedded in cultural traditions, such as dietary staples of Mexican meals or the original nomadic lifestyle of the Plains Indians, provided nutrition and activity patterns that were undermined when these ethnic minority groups were "helped" to become engaged with service systems of the dominant culture. As a result, while some problems may have been solved for Mexican Americans and American Indians, rates of dental caries and obesity leading to diabetes have soared. Housing projects that originally brought important improvements in the areas of sanitation and space caused the dispersement of extended families and the bulldozing of community churches. Positive health behaviors can be interrupted, as well as facilitated, by major social forces, including health education interventions.

Acculturation–Assimilation

Adherence to cultural values vary individually according to the level of acculturation. Acculturation involves the acceptance, in different degrees, of values, beliefs, and practices of the dominant culture. Involvement in cultural routines, practices, and rituals depends on the extent of acculturation. Education, SES, and even peer pressure are acculturating agents. *Bicultural* is a term used to identify people who can function within two cultures, perhaps knowing not only the language but also having practiced routines and rituals from the culture of their birth and the dominant culture. However, even among people who consider themselves acculturated, certain events such as the birth of a child or a life-threatening illness can prompt them to rely on health beliefs they might have previously felt were discarded. It is not unusual for a new Hispanic mother to want only family members to "babysit" her child or a health professional who grew up in a fundamentalist religion to turn to faith healing in a crisis. As a minority group becomes more highly acculturated into the mainstream of American values and customs, changes in health-related attitudes and behaviors may also occur. Conversely, acceptance of the predominant values may confer a risk for ethnic minority groups. Consequently, among more acculturated individuals the pattern of disease may mimic that experienced in the majority culture. For example, first-generation Mexican Americans experience lower rates of infant mortality and low birth weight than other groups. Later generations often either adopt unhealthy lifestyle behaviors of the dominant culture, such as smoking, or fail to engage in the protective factors practiced in their culture of origin, such as maintaining supportive social networks to mitigate stressors.

Assimilation is a sociological term that implies an abandonment of cultural ties to such an extent that people of color are indistinguishable in their values, beliefs, and practices from the dominant culture. Assimilation can be the result of generations of progressive acculturation. For American Indians, however, it is a marker of a federal program of the 1950s that moved thousands of families from reservations into cities as part of a massive assimilation effort. The boarding school legacies in which children were not allowed to speak their native language and were separated not only from parents but also from near-age siblings was another program of assimilation. Therefore, assimilation is a sensitive issue for many Indian people who have felt the threat of extermination from such policies. Indeed, some tribes have been formally "terminated" over the past few decades. Ethnic minorities also have created strategies to maintain cultural integrity within mainstream society. For example, concepts such as Afrocentricity, the degree to which traditional African values are conscientiously used by parents, reflects an effort to maintain the aspects of a culture. Cultural identity provides not only a framework of self-esteem and belonging but also a complex system of values, beliefs, and practices that have considerable influence on health status.

Examples of Culturally Sensitive Interventions

A Culturally Congruent Intervention for Weight Control among American Indians

There are extraordinarily high rates of non–insulin-dependent diabetes mellitus (NIDDM) among many American Indian tribes. Obesity is a major risk factor for NIDDM as well as coronary heart disease. The Zuni Diabetes Project was initiated in the 1980s to address an adult prevalence rate for NIDDM of 28.2%. Conventional health education approaches had resulted in limited interest and impact in the Zuni tribe. The counseling and health information approach had little appeal. It was determined that a systematic effort through a culturally congruent intervention would be more attractive to the Zuni. Key to the foundation of this program, which has permeated future interventions among the Zuni, has been tribal involvement in planning and executing the program (Attneave, 1989).

The Zuni were historically involved in walking and running as forms of transportation and recreation. Foot racing, for example, was a prominent activity among many adults and an activity to which children would aspire (Wilson, 1993). As acculturation occurred, Indian adults have become increasingly sedentary and the traditions of walking and running declined. This was also the case among the Zuni. The Zuni Diabetes Project used a community-based exercise intervention to promote health behavior that was culturally congruent and appealing to many members of the tribe. Weight, fasting blood glucose values, and the need for hypoglycemic medication were all significantly reduced for participants in this program (Heath, Wilson, Smith, & Leonard, 1991). The program has experienced some criticism, including concern that the current dominant culture fad and fascination with running was superimposed on the tribe (Walden, 1987). Such a critique serves as an important reminder that topics and ideas for research and programs are often culturally inspired and driven.

The issue of sustainability has become increasingly imperative as recent decades of programs, especially those in minority communities, demonstrate significant findings during a research study or demonstration project, then return to earlier, loss-positive health behaviors when resources and infrastructure are withdrawn. While sustainability is a concern for all health promotion programs, the limited economic and professional resources within minority communities, coupled with high risk and lower access to health services, makes the adoption of health programs by participants and communities paramount in the evaluation of health promotion programs. An important marker of success for the Zuni Diabetes Project has been its sustainability. As the key professionals have moved out of the community and funding has been terminated for nearly a decade, the continuation of the program by the tribe itself shows that the intervention and effects have been sustained (G. W. Heath, personal communication, April, 1997). Although certain elements and characteristics have changed, the community-based exercise program continues to be operated by the Zuni tribe. The spiritual meaning Indians ascribe to diabetes and health behavior involved in prevention and treatment of diabetes is often overlooked in health promotion interventions (Hill, 1996). When cultural traditions are incorporated in health promotion plans, spirituality will figure prominently for most Indian people. There may be varied reasons contributing to this critical result of the Zuni Diabetes Project but the participation and ownership of the program by the tribal leadership itself, as well as infrastructure and training of tribal members to continue the program, profiles large in the success of this program.

A Cancer Prevention Program for Hispanic Families

A broad community-based program for health promotion, *Programa a Su Salud* (To Your Health), was designed to demonstrate and study the effectiveness of mass media messages using culturally relevant models selected from the local community. This program serves a low-income Southwestern town that is 93% Hispanic. Baseline data indicated poor participation in health-promoting behaviors. *Programa a Su Salud* specifically addressed smoking reduction, diet, use of preventive services and practices, reduction of alcohol abuse, and increase of physical activity. These goals are standards known to enhance overall health and resilience as well as preventing specific disorders correlated with behaviors such as smoking and alcohol abuse. A lead agency was charged with improving the population participation in health promoting behaviors.

Experience with conventional models of health promotion have demonstrated little effectiveness among minorities who are at high risk for preventable disease, including many types of cancer. In developing a culturally sensitive program for this community, Amerzcua, McAlister, Ramirez, and Espinoza (1990) report that the main features of the community were (1) a predominantly Roman Catholic population that respects the Virgin of Guadalupe as both a religious and ethnic symbol, (2) a strong family orientation, (3) reliance on home remedies and "folk medicine," (4) high fat intake, and (5) heavy drinking patterns. Focus groups were conducted with residents to obtain community involvement in validating health needs, identifying culture-specific meanings of health, and planning culturally congruent interventions. Bandura's self-efficacy model provided the theoretical framework for this study. It was used because it accommodated the cultural values and preferences of the community.

The *A Su Salud* intervention used the concept of social reinforcement for paying attention to and imitating positive role models featured in mass media messages. One-page printed flyers titled " Seis Asesinos Importantes Andan Sueltos en el Condado de Maverick" (Six Important Assassins are Loose in Maverick County) described six avoidable risk factors associated with premature death in the county. The flyer announced coming broadcasts on the topic. It contained a checklist for preventive behaviors as well. Copies were inserted in local newspapers and distributed to thousands of homes. Two sets of television programs were produced for the intervention. The first consisted of 15 programs ranging in length from 5 to 10 minutes. These programs used role models and health information in a news format. A set of four 30-minute documentary-style programs followed. The 30-minute programs featured local role models who had started new health promotion behaviors. These community members told how they were successful in making changes, evoking the community and cultural characteristics such as family and spiritual supports. In the second year, social networks were mobilized to disseminate the intervention. There were 874 volunteers among the community who were involved in follow-up reenforcement "fighting the six killers." These people were distributed across multiple settings including neighborhoods, business, government, social clubs, health care providers, education, and religious organizations (Amerzcua *et al.*,1990).

Findings from the study showed that the intervention was well received by community residents. Interviews with 7860 residents showed that they had viewed an average of 10 television programs featuring roles models. Hundreds of residents had changed their behavior and were now incorporating one or more of the preventive health behaviors they had learned. Components of the *A Su Salud* intervention have been used in Hispanic communities in other locations. A peer education model, videotapes (Yancey & Walden, 1994), and a church-based health promotion program (Castro, 1993) targeted cancer prevention behaviors. Each demonstrated positive response to culturally sensitive interventions and behavioral change. Hispanic communities once considered resistant to health education models demonstrated that with culturally relevant tools and messages, health knowledge and health behavior can be improved. The purpose of health education is predicated on these substantive changes rather than participation in conventional health education programs.

A Culturally Sensitive HIV Prevention Intervention for African-American Women

The SISTA project (Sisters Informing Sisters about Topics on AIDS) is an HIV prevention intervention for African-American young adult women (DiClemente & Wingood, 1995). Women who participated in the five-session intervention received free child care and free transportation to the SISTA project, were financially reimbursed for their time, and were encouraged to discuss the project with their sexual partners. At the beginning of every session, women read a poem by an African-American female artist and discussed its relevance to the session. Prior to educating women regarding HIV prevention activities women in the intervention condition engaged in activities that fostered their self-esteem, built their self-respect, acknowledged their positive contributions to society, and allowed them to assert their self-worth as African-American women. From this perspective, women were able to develop a critical awareness of how maintaining a healthy sexual lifestyle was consistent with the norms and values of African-American communities.

Specifically, the first session focused on the importance of the African-American family and pride in oneself as an African-American female. The second session sought to enhance women's knowledge about HIV, emphasized the risks and consequences of engaging in HIV-associated behaviors, and discussed why African-American women are disproportionately represented among women with AIDS. The third session taught women to take personal responsibility for controlling their life, to foster equality within their relationships, and to assertively negotiate safer sex with their sexual partners. During this session, women discussed communicating with their partner as a strategy to break the silence that African-American women often harbor within themselves. This allowed women to act outside the passive–submissive roles that our culture has forced on them, but not to act demeaning or be demanding toward their partner. Women were then taught to take more control over their bodies by developing skills in properly and consistently using condoms. Additionally, this session stressed that safer sex among young adults was becoming more of a norm and exercises were employed that emphasized the normative nature of condom use. Finally, in the fifth session women were taught coping strategies and alternatives to unsafe sex.

The analyses revealed that compared with women in a delayed education control condition, women in the five-session intervention significantly increased consistent condom use, sexual self-control, sexual communication, sexual assertiveness, and partners' adoption of norms supporting consistent condom use. Women in the one-session HIV education condition failed to show any increase in knowledge, attitude, skills, norms, or behaviors supportive of safer sex.

This program is notable because it is the first community-based randomized controlled HIV prevention intervention to significantly enhance consistent condom use. The success of the intervention may be attributed to the application of the theory of gender and power to provide a gender-specific framework that focused on African-American male–female relationships in developing and implementing the social skills intervention. Furthermore, the intervention employed African-American female peers to implement the intervention. Peer educators served as excellent role models because they were comfortable in asserting their self-worth and endorsed the nontraditional practices of requesting their partners to use condoms and refusing sexual advances for unsafe sex.

A Culturally Sensitive HIV Prevention Program for Asian and Pacific Island Men

Previous research has shown that homosexual Asian and Pacific Island men confront unique challenges in coping with their identity and HIV preventive practices. In many Asian cultures where male children have obligations to marry and perpetuate the family and its name, homosexuality is socially deviant and brings family dishonor (Choi *et al.*, 1996). Many homosexual Asian and Pacific Island men are unable to accept their sexual identity due to the fear that they may dishonor the family name and be ostracized by their family and other community members. Consequently, many Asian and Pacific Island men minimize their personal vulnerability for HIV and are more likely to engage in unsafe sexual practices. Further increasing their risk for HIV is the internalized negative sexual images of homosexual Asian and Pacific Island men (i.e., asexual, passive) frequently held by many white homosexual men, resulting in a lowered self-esteem and inability to assert themselves in sexual relationships.

A culturally sensitive HIV risk reduction intervention was designed to address the specific needs of homosexual Asian and Pacific Island men. This intervention was conducted at the Living Well Project, a community-based agency providing social support services to homosexual Asian Pacific Islanders (API) in the San Francisco Bay area. All intervention materials were extensively pilot-tested for their cultural relevance with members of the API homosexual community. The one-session, 3-hour intervention consisted of four components. The first component focused on fostering positive ethnic and sexual identities through sharing negative experiences of being an API and homosexual and building support around self-image. The second component emphasized safer sex education, by discussing the negative and positive reasons for practicing safer sex, by providing facts about HIV transmission, and by role-playing a safer-sex vignette that addressed HIV risk with different types of partners (i.e., with a casual or regular partner, with a person living with HIV/AIDS). The third component emphasized factual information on condoms, proper condom use skills, and ways to eroticize condoms. The final component of the intervention focused on enhancing skills to negotiate safer sex with a resistant partner and refusing an unsafe sexual encounter.

Compared to men in the control condition, men in the intervention condition reported a significant reduction in the number of sexual partners at 3-month follow-up ($P = 0.003$). Additionally, Chinese and Filipino men who were randomly assigned to the intervention reduced their frequency of unprotected anal intercourse at 3-months follow-up by more than half when compared to their counterparts in the control condition (OR = 0.41; 95% CI, 0.19–0.89; $P = 0.024$). The authors concluded that efficacious HIV prevention interventions for API homosexual men must be culturally sensitive, focus on condom use, and sexual negotiation and sexual refusal skills.

Summary and Conclusions: Designing, Implementing, and Evaluating Effective Interventions Targeting Ethnic Minority Populations

In reviewing the literature on effective interventions conducted among ethnic minorities, interventions that achieve behavior change seem to possess several important criteria. Foremost, effective health behavior interventions often target a population. Targeting is the process of identifying the population subgroup by parameters relevant to the program objectives. Once the population is identified, the health intervention needs to be tailored or adapted to best fit the relevant needs and characteristics of the specified target population. Simply having an intervention that uses ethnically similar peers to implement a program or using educational brochures illustrating peers the same race as the target population would not constitute a tailored program. The intervention should contextualize the health topic within a framework that address ethnic pride, cultural awareness, and values prioritized by the ethnic population being targeted.

Second, behavioral interventions that are guided by psychological theories, in particular, social cognitive theory, diffusion theory, and the transtheoretical model of behavior change, enhance knowledge, provide skills, emphasize social support for behavior change, and are effective at promoting the adoption and maintenance of health protective behavior (DiClemente & Peterson, 1994). However, effective interventions for ethnic minority populations also often include social structural frameworks to address issues such as acculturation, familial influences, empowerment, and religious beliefs and practices. While skills building is clearly important, engaging in unhealthy behaviors is not only the result of a deficit of knowledge, motivation, or skills, but also has meaning within an individuals sociocultural context.

Additionally, many effective behavioral interventions for ethnic minorities are peer-led (DiClemente & Petersen, 1994). Theoretically, peer involvement offers a number of advantages over traditional, didactic prevention interventions. Derived from social cognitive theory and based in development theory, peer-facilitated interventions recruit and train peers indigenous to a large target population to serve as leaders, educators, and counselors. Peer interventions offer a number of advantages over professional or adult-led programs when working with young adults. Peers may be more effective teachers of social skills and more influential models of health-promoting behavior and can serve as credible role models because they are members of the young adults' social milieu. Peers can also help to change normative expectations about the frequency of the targeted behavior in the peer group. Finally, peers can offer social support for performance of desired behaviors and for avoidance of health-damaging behaviors.

Effective prevention interventions designed to reduce the risk of unhealthy behaviors are urgently needed to avert further escalation of disease and disability among ethnic minorities. Ultimately, however, reducing unhealthy risk behaviors is dependent not only on the development, implementation, and evaluation of culturally sensitive prevention interventions, but also on how effectively these interventions can be translated into existing community prevention activities and how rapidly they can be disseminated and maintained within communities.

References

Attneave, C. (1989). Who has the responsibility? An evolving model to resolve ethical problems in intercultural research. *American Indian and Alaska Native Mental Health Research, 2*(3), 18–24.
Berkman, L. F. (1984). Assessing the physical health effects of social networks and social support. *Annual Review of Public Health, 5*, 413–432.
Castro, K. G. (1993). Distribution of acquired immunodeficiency syndrome and other sexually transmitted diseases in racial and ethnic populations, United States, influence of life-style and socioeconomic status. *Annals of Epidemiology, 3*, 181–184.

Chen, V. W. (1993). Smoking and the health gap in minorities. *Annals of Epidemiology, 3,* 159–164.

Choi, K., Lew S., Vittinghoff, E., Catania, J. A., Barrett, D. C., & Coates, T. J. (1996). The efficacy of brief group counseling in HIV risk reduction among homosexual Asian and Pacific Islander men. *AIDS, 10,* 81–87.

DiClemente R. J., Peterson, J. (1994). Changing HIV/AIDS risk behaviors: The role of behavioral interventions. In R. J. DiClemente & J. Peterson (Eds.), *Preventing AIDS: Theories and methods of behavioral interventions* (pp. 1–4). New York: Plenum Press.

DiClemente, R. J., & Wingood, G. M. (1995). A randomized controlled social skills trial: An HIV sexual risk-reduction intervention among young adult African-American women. *Journal of the American Medical Association, 274,* 1271–1276.

Dressler, W. W. (1990). Lifestyle, stress and blood pressure in a southern black community. *Psychosomatic Medicine, 52,* 182–198.

Earls, F. (1993). Health promotion for minority adolescents: Cultural considerations. In S. G. Millstein, A. C. Petersen, & E. O. Nightingale (Eds.), *Promoting the health of adolescents* (pp. 58–72). New York: Oxford University Press.

Faer, M. (1995). The intergenerational life history project. *Public Health Reports, 110*(2), 194–197.

Haan, M., & Kaplan, G. A. (1985). The contribution of socioeconomic position to minority health. In *Report of the Secretary's Task Force on Black and Minority Health, Vol II: Cross-cutting issues in minority health* (pp. 67–103). Washington, DC: US Department of Health and Human Services, US Government Printing Office.

Heath, G. W., Wilson, R. H., Smith, J., & Leonard, B. E. (1991). Community-based exercise and weight control: Diabetes risk reduction and glycemic control in Zuni Indians. *American Journal of Clinical Nutrition, 53*(6), 1642–1646.

Hill, M. (1996). Science should serve the community. *Tribal College, 7*(4), 12–44

Keltner, B. (1992). Family influences on child health. *Pediatric Nursing, 18*(2), 128–131.

Keltner, B., & Ramey, S. (1992). The family. *Current Opinion in Psychiatry, 5,* 638–644.

Keltner, B., & Ramey, S. (1993). Family issues. *Current Opinion in Psychiatry, 6*(5), 629–634.

Krieger, N., Sidney, S. (1996). Racial discrimination and blood pressure: The CARDIA study of young black and white adults. *American Journal of Public Health, 86,* 1370–1378.

Kumanyika, S. K. (1993). Diet and nutrition as influences on the morbidity/mortality gap. *Annals of Epidemiology, 3,* 154–158.

Marmot, M. G., & Syme, L. (1976). Acculturation and coronary heart disease in Japanese Americans. *American Journal of Epidemiology, 104,* 225–247.

Moore, D. J., Williams, J. D., & Qualls, J. W. (1996). Target marketing of tobacco and alcohol-related products to ethnic minority groups in the United States. *Ethnicity and Disease, 6,* 83–98.

Novello, A., & Soto-Torres, L. (1993). One voice, one vision—Uniting to improve Hispanic–Latino health. *Public Health Reports, 108*(5), 529–533.

US Bureau of the Census. (1984). *A statistical profile of the American Indian population: 1980 census.* Washington, DC: US Government Printing Office.

Walden, H. (1987). A second opinion on Zuni diabetes. *Public Health Reports, 102*(2), 123–125.

Wilson, R., & Horton, D. (1993). Prevention and early treatment of NIDDM. *Diabetes Care, 16*(1), 376–377.

Wyche, K. F., & Rotheram-Borus, M. J. (1990). Suicidal behavior among minority youth in the United States. In A. R. Stiffman & L. E. Davis (Eds.), *Ethnic issues in adolescent mental health* (pp. 323–338). Newbury Park, CA: Sage.

Yaancy, A., & Walden, L. (1994). Stimulating cancer screening among Latinas and African American women. *Journal of Cancer Education, 9*(1), 46–52.

CHAPTER *28*

Health Promotion and Disease Prevention in Developing Countries

David Coombs and Walter Mason

Introduction

This chapter is divided into three parts. The first begins with an overview of contemporary health conditions and trends in developing countries, as well as their socioeconomic correlates and the problem of measuring the impact of disease. The second part provides a description of four contemporary behavior change models successfully used with individuals and communities, mainly in the United States and other established market economies. These models have been applied to some degree in developing countries that, given appropriate adaptation to local cultures and socioeconomic conditions, merit additional applications, especially in situations where other remedies have reached their limits or cannot be used. Ideas of how these models may be usefully applied to specific health-related issues in developing countries are presented. Finally, new policies and programs to improve the health and well-being of the poor and disadvantaged in developing countries are discussed. This overview demonstrates that behavioral change is, at present, the only practical means for preventing disease and ill health in many countries.

Disease, Health, and the Quality of Life

As the 20th century comes to a close, the gap between health and quality of life in the established market economies of Europe, North America, Japan, and other industrially developed and the poorer countries of the world continues to widen despite determined efforts to attenuate this gap (Basch, 1990). The world population

David Coombs • Department of Health Behavior, School of Public Health, UAB Center for Health Promotion, University of Alabama at Birmingham, Birmingham, Alabama 35294.   *Walter Mason* • Department of Epidemiology and International Health, School of Public Health, UAB Center for Health Promotion, University of Alabama at Birmingham, Birmingham, Alabama 35294.

Handbook of Health Promotion and Disease Prevention, edited by Raczynski and DiClemente.
Kluwer Academic/Plenum Publishers, New York, 1999.

now exceeds 5.7 billion and is projected to reach 8.3 billion by the year 2025, of whom approximately 85% will live in the less developed countries, including China (Haub & Yanagishita, 1995). In spite of many advances, including an increase in life expectancy at birth to a worldwide average of 65 years, in the less developed countries old problems remain. Differences in gross national product (GNP) and purchasing power, reported in US dollars, shows that on a per capita basis, purchasing power in Switzerland, Japan, the United States, and the United Kingdom still exceeds that of the poorest countries by 50-fold (Haub & Yanagishita, 1995). The World Health Organization (WHO) suggests that, at the present time, the accumulated wealth of the richest 385 individuals in the world exceeds the annual income of the lowest 2,700,000 (Pfister, 1997). In practical terms, few fiscal resources are available for investment in health or health infrastructure. Among the lowest income peoples living under conditions of "absolute poverty," 80% or more of income is spent on food, leaving little for shelter, clothing, education, and other needs, including health (Basch, 1990). Education of children and women continues to be neglected in many places. In the least developed countries, adult female literacy in 1995 lagged behind men, at 38% compared to nearly 60% for males. This is again reflected in the percentage of females (45%) enrolled in primary school after adjustment for age and educational level, during the period 1990–1995. Although still lagging behind males, there has been a major increase in enrollment since 1960 (UNICEF, 1997). Considering that females are the major family caregivers, maternal education is an important factor in the determination of health and prevention of disease (King, 1990). Research to date has shown that in addition to obtaining specific knowledge related to health, the education of primary caregivers increases the acceptance of new ideas and acceptance of responsibility for health outcomes in the family (Rasmuson et al., 1988).

Access to medical care and knowledge needed for self-care and disease prevention continues to be limited in developing countries. Although the total number of medical practitioners continues to rise, major disparities in their location and accessibility to poorer individuals has not caught up. In 1993, many countries were estimated to have fewer than 80 physicians per 100,000 population compared to the corresponding US figure of 245. (WHO Estimates of Health Personnel—physicians, dentists, and nurses/midwives around 1993: http://www.who.int/whosis). At the same time, medical knowledge has continued to advance, especially in the treatment for major causes of mortality, such as cholera, as seen in the 1991 outbreak in Latin America in which mortality was reduced to less than 1% (Pan American Health Organization, 1991). Improvements in the management of pediatric diarrhea through oral rehydration therapy by mothers and local health workers has contributed to the reduction in child deaths attributable to diarrhea from approximately 4.5 million per year in 1990 to just over 2.5 million in 1995 (UNICEF, 1997). Often simple measures, such as replenishment of critical electrolytes lost in diarrhea by oral administration of sugar–salt solutions, have led to major inroads against mortality from childhood diarrhea. Still, the Water Supply and Sanitation Working Group on Sanitation estimates that nearly 2 billion people lack safe means of managing their own excreta, and that this number will not diminish appreciably over the next 40 years (Simpson-Hebert, 1996). Thus, low-income populations of developing countries will remain at high risk for enteric infections in the foreseeable future. Not surprisingly, infectious diseases, especially those of childhood, are still the leading cause of death in the world (WHO, 1996a).

Disease in the Developing World

Understanding disease in the developed regions of the world is difficult; in the underdeveloped it is even more problematical. In addition to the multiplicity of causes, inaccurate data collection and poor recording and reporting of death may exaggerate or minimize existing situations. Even basic information on cause of death and numbers of deaths may be difficult to assemble. This is exacerbated by interactions between conditions affecting disease outcomes (e.g., nutritional status) that also may be responsible for morbidity and mortality in their own right. Diseases are not uniformly distributed in the population by age, sex, or race, as well as other predisposing conditions. Thus, it is difficult to gain a broad perspective on the problem. Diseases and conditions may be broken down in a variety of ways, including rank as a cause of death (e.g., 10 leading causes of death); place (endemicity); association with specific conditions (e.g., environment); special groups (childhood–mothers); interventions (vaccine preventable); and status (emerging/increasing/decreasing). This has resulted in a somewhat confused picture as to the causes of morbidity and mortality. Morbidity and mortality figures may not give the true picture of disease impact. It does not reflect loss of productivity or suffering associated with disease nor does it reflect strategies needed to improve conditions. To obtain a new perspective, Murray and Lopez (1996) have suggested focusing on disability and the loss of productivity associated with diseases and conditions arranged in three broad groups.

Disability notwithstanding, simple ranking by cause of death shows that communicable diseases accompanied by maternal, perinatal, and nutritional conditions accounted for one third of all deaths in the world for 1990 (Murray & Lopez, 1996). In underdeveloped areas, the proportion of deaths attributable to communicable disease increases in proportion to the lack of economic development and level of poverty. These are, in a sense, the causes of death associated with poverty. However, noncommunicable diseases and accidents have increased and are increasing as causes of death in underdeveloped areas (and not necessarily as a result of increasing association with affluence) (Murray & Lopez, 1996).

The contrast between the leading causes of death in developed and developing regions of the world is shown in Table 1. Despite much of the world having gone through a shift in the principal causes of death, communicable diseases, maternal, neonatal, and nutritional conditions still account for a high proportion of all deaths each year. Of some 17.3 million deaths from communicable diseases, during 1990, 16.5 million of them were in developing countries (Murray & Lopez, 1996). Many of these diseases are associated with childhood, limited access to medical care, and poor sanitary conditions that poverty creates. Despite much success in achieving improvements, this group of diseases and conditions remains at the forefront of problems in the developing world.

The numbers of deaths and illnesses, however, do not give a true picture of the impact of disease and disability that results. It has long been understood that poor health leads to low productivity and low productivity to poor health as resources become even more limited. Thus, a vicious circle exists, contributing to the problem of socioeconomic development. Murray and Lopez (1996) recommend the reporting of disease impact in terms of disability-adjusted life years (DALYS) with attribution of risk factors as a better approach to estimating the impact or burden of diseases than

Table 1. The Ten Leading Causes of Death, 1990[a]

Developed regions			Developing regions		
	Deaths ('000s)	Cumu-lative %		Deaths ('000s)	Cumu-lative %
All causes	10,912		All causes	39,554	
1 Ischemic heart disease	2,695	24.7	1 Lower respiratory infections	3,915	9.9
2 Cerebrovascular disease	1,427	37.8	2 Ischemic heart disease	3,565	18.9
3 Trachea, bronchus, and lung cancer	523	42.6	3 Cerebrovascular disease	2,954	26.4
4 Lower respiratory infections	385	46.1	4 Diarrheal diseases	2,940	33.8
5 Chronic obstructive pulmonary disease	324	49.1	5 Conditions arising during the perinatal period	2,361	38.7
6 Colon and rectum cancers	277	51.6	6 Tuberculosis	1,922	43.4
7 Stomach cancer	241	53.8	7 Chronic obstructive pulmonary disease	1,887	46.1
8 Road traffic accidents	222	55.8	8 Measles	1,058	48.7
9 Self-inflicted injuries	193	57.6	9 Malaria	856	50.9
10 Diabetes mellitus	176	59.2	10 Road traffic accidents	777	52.8

[a] From Murray & Lopez, 1996, Table 3.12 (pp. 179–80).

simple morbidity and mortality data. This adjustment weights diseases and conditions that have greater impact on potential economic development, for example, those attacking early in life or those that produce disability that may continue, as having an increased impact on productivity. Attributable risks for this approach and for any disease for which there is no simple, single cause are more complicated and may include risk factors from multiple areas, such as occupation, socioeconomic status, behavior (e.g., unsafe sex, smoking, use of illicit drugs), genetics and environment (hypertension, air pollution), and so forth (Murray & Lopez, 1996).

Although the situation is not new, the result of summarizing disease impacts shifts the order of disease rankings, which allows prioritization by burden. Table 2 shows the impact of poor water supply, sanitation, and hygiene on health measured

Table 2. Global Burden of Disease and Injury Attributable to Selected Risk Factors, 1990[a]

Risk factor	Deaths ('000s)	As % of total deaths	YLLs ('000s)	As % of total YLLs	YLDs ('000s)	As % of total YLDs	DALYs ('000s)	As % of total DALYs
Malnutrition	5,881	11.7	199,486	22.0	20,089	4.2	219,575	15.9
Poor water supply sanitation and personal and domestic hygiene	2,668	5.3	85,520	9.4	7,872	1.7	93,392	6.8
Unsafe sex	1,095	2.2	27,602	3.0	21,000	4.5	48,702	3.5
Tobacco	3,038	6.0	26,217	2.9	9,965	2.1	36,182	2.6
Alcohol	774	1.5	19,287	2.1	28,400	6.0	47,687	3.5
Occupation	1,129	2.2	22,493	2.5	15,394	3.3	37,887	2.7
Hypertension	2,918	5.8	17,665	1.9	1,411	0.3	19,076	1.4
Physical inactivity	1,991	3.9	11,353	1.3	2,300	0.5	13,653	1.0
Illicit drugs	100	0.2	2,634	0.3	5,834	1.2	8,467	0.6
Air pollution	568	1.1	5,625	0.6	1,630	0.3	7,254	0.5

[a] From Murray & Lopez, 1996, Table 6.2 (pp. 311).

by years of life lost (YYLs) and disability-adjusted years (DALYs). After malnutrition, to which it is linked, poor sanitation is still the single largest contributor to ill health. Importantly, the approach shows that worldwide unsafe sex, tobacco, and alcohol abuse are already major risk factors. According to the authors, the ten risk factors shown in Table 3 accounted for over one third of the burden associated with disease in 1990 (Murray & Lopez, 1996). This is especially interesting in comparison to the established market economies of what was previously thought to be largely a problem of their own affluence, such as use of tobacco. Use of tobacco is now the major cause of DALYs in the developed world, and is expected to grow to roughly twice the DALY level attributable to diarrhea and human immunodeficiency virus (HIV) by the year 2020 (Murray & Lopez, 1996).

Medical Knowledge

Dissemination of medical information seems to be less of a problem within the medical community than between practitioners and their patients. This is borne out by the large number of physicians and other practitioners who seek education in the developed world and by rapid communication techniques of electronic mail and development of "virtual" journals, which are available wherever telecommunications exist. The movement of information at this level is very rapid. However, there continues to be a lag in getting information into the hands of the people most needing it, such as female heads of households. Thus, in the case of simple therapy for diarrheal disease developed at the International Center for Diarrheal Disease Research-Bangladesh (ICDDR-B) in Dhaka, it has taken the consistent effort of UNICEF, WHO, and other multilateral, national and nongovernmental organizations 10 years to make progress in the acceptance and use of oral rehydration solutions for electrolyte replacement. Data do show that the number of deaths from dehydration associated with diarrhea have declined from 1990 to 1995, from approximately 4 million to $2\frac{1}{2}$ million (WHO, 1996a; UNICEF, 1997). This is thought to result largely from improvements in home management of diarrhea, as improvements in sanitation and water supply, while up, continue to lag behind (WHO, 1996b, 1998a).

Table 3. The Leading Causes of Disability, World, 1990[a]

		Total (millions)	Percent of total
	All causes	472.7[b]	
1	Unipolar major depression	50.8	10.7
2	Iron-deficiency anemia	22.0	4.7
3	Falls	22.0	4.6
4	Alcohol use	15.8	3.3
5	Chronic obstructive pulmonary disease	14.7	3.1
6	Bipolar disorder	14.1	3.0
7	Congenital anomalies	13.5	2.9
8	Osteoarthritis	13.3	2.8
9	Schizophrenia	12.1	2.6
10	Obsessive–compulsive disorders	10.2	2.2

[a] From Murray & Lopez, 1996, from Table 4.13 (p. 236).
[b] Disability is in YLDs, years lived with a disability. For a detailed explanation of this measure see Murrary & Lopez, 1996 (pp. 33–45).

Development and Disease

Economic development has led to unforeseen increases in specific diseases as well as improvements in health. Under conditions of poverty, scarce resources are dedicated to meeting survival needs of food and shelter. Thus, improvements in economic well-being are usually associated with improvements in health, produced by better housing, better nutrition, availability of sanitary infrastructure, access to medical services and education, and availability of knowledge about disease causation and treatment in the community. Economic development may result in changed practices and conditions affecting the lowest income levels, such as subsistence farmers. Introduction of new agricultural practices and damming of rivers for flood control, irrigation, or power generation have historically caused dislocations or changes which affect health. These have resulted from environmental change, producing ecological disruptions that favor the introduction or expansion of endemic disease into new areas. The classic example is the construction of the Aswan High Dam on the upper Nile River. This resulted in conditions that favored the growth of snails that served as an intermediate host in the life cycle of human schistosomiasis and eventually extending the range of disease into areas previously unaffected.

Alternatively, economic development may result in cultural conflict between the old ways of doing things and new processes or resource exploitation. Deforestation, with resulting effects on water quality due to increased soil erosion and the shifting of habitats that may favor vector species over nonvectors, has also been identified. Deforestation to permit new agricultural developments also may bring increased numbers of people into contact with disease vectors such as those responsible for the transmission of malaria. Preliminary analysis of malaria data for the 1996–1997 malaria season in Chantaburi province, Thailand, indicates that one third of new cases of malaria are in newly created plantations (Tropical Disease Research News, 1997). Change in usage patterns for pharmaceuticals, foods, household chemicals, pesticides, and their containers also may affect health as access occurs. Culture in conflict has been a consistent theme in economic development, creating new problems out of old ones. Dietary changes associated with changing income, pressures of time, and the drive to be *a la mode* have created for the first time obesity in populations where it did not heretofore exist. The disposal of human waste(s), which is relatively simple at the individual level, becomes progressively more complex and expensive in urban developments, making it difficult to produce the needed infrastructure for the collection and treatment of human wastes at a rate compatible with urban growth. Witness the fact that much of the world's sewage is discharged untreated or undertreated as a result of the high cost of treatment plants and their operation (WHO, 1998a). Technology is inextricably intertwined with culture; thus, technology-based solutions often have limits imposed not by the technology per se, but by the ability of diverse groups to utilize specific technologies, including maintenance. Abandoned wells bear testimony to the inability of many rural villages to maintain them once installed by governments or nongovernmental organizations. Counteracting this through the education and involvement (vestment) of the beneficiaries in selecting strategies and technologies has become the watchword in international development. It is an underlying principle in the "reverse technology transfer" of disease prevention strategies from the developing world to rural programs in developed countries (Mason *et al*, 1993).

The principal barrier to improvements in health in the developing world is poverty and the lack of resources to address the problems it causes. This often results in the proverbial condition of having to lift oneself by one's own "bootstraps," a nonviable solution that has long-standing recognition. There are other complicating factors as well. First, population growth is accompanied by increased urbanization as people seek a better life. This places additional stress on tottering infrastructures for water supply and sanitation, as well as health care. The megacities of the next millennium will not be in the countries with established market economies, but in the developing world (Otten, 1992). At present, some 100 million people live in absolute poverty and for whom the purchase of essential medicines and health care services is impossible.

Given the chronic shortages of material resources, there is increasing interest in using behavioral change strategies to speed up the health transition in developing countries. Biomedical and environmental change technologies have not been able to achieve this transition in most developing societies. The efficacy of behavioral methods has been increased by better educational techniques, improved worldwide educational and economic conditions, related improvements in communication/transportation infrastructure, proliferation of donor agencies, and interest in developing the "global village" of markets and consumers. The following section describes selected behavioral change models and techniques now being used or tested in developing countries.

Behavior Change in Developing Countries

The models described are the outgrowth of collaborative work by scholars and practitioners. To change the behavior of individuals, they focus on changing beliefs, attitudes, motives, and behavioral intentions. To bring about behavior change in large groups or populations, the focus is on mass media persuasion and governmental mechanisms such as laws, regulations, and taxes. Change agents in the field look for any usable pressure point or opportunity for achieving behavior change. These may be, for example, a mother's desire to protect the health of her family, personal feelings of vulnerability or susceptibility to specific diseases, peer pressure to conform to new social norms, enhancing self-efficacy (self-confidence) in one's ability to adequately perform new behaviors, or the use of policies and regulations to control behaviors.

The traditional approach of change agencies has been to emphasize institutional changes, independently of individual beliefs, attitudes, or intentions. This approach applied to smoking cessation or prevention involves policies and official laws/regulations to reduce access to tobacco products through sales restrictions, higher taxes/prices, no smoking policies, or all of these. Such macro-level strategies are often successful in the United States but are more difficult to achieve in developing countries due to greater opposition from powerful commercial and governmental interest groups and greater difficulties with enforcement of laws and regulations.

Voluntary change through the health education approach has its own problems. It is time consuming, labor intensive, and often slow to produce behavior changes. Albee and Gulotta (1997) comment that "Education (by itself) increases knowledge; occasionally, it changes attitudes; rarely does it alter behavior" (p. 17). They believe education must be combined with an effective system of laws and regulations, social support from "honest, trusting, empathetic, caring" friends, and from opportunities to learn personal skills that improve problem-solving competencies.

A number of projects to produce behavior change have been tested in developing countries. Some have been done on a population basis like the Academy for Educational Development programs to promote oral rehydration therapy to prevent dehydration from diarrheal diseases (Hernandez, de Guzman, Cabanero-Verzosa, & Seidel, 1993; Mantra, Davies, Sutisnaputra, & Louis, 1993; Ramah & DeBus, 1993; Saunders et al., 1993; Sutisnaputra et al., 1993; Zimicki, 1993). The academy has combined elements from different behavioral models, such as social learning theory, social marketing, and diffusion of innovations at both the individual and population levels, into single behavior change programs (for example, see Seidel, 1993 and other publications in the Healthcom series by the Academy for Educational Development in Washington, DC).

Other projects have tried interactive educational techniques at the grassroots level that also combine elements from different models. The learner-centered, problem-posing, self-discovery, action-oriented (LePSA) technique, developed in Kenya, utilizes observational learning, improved self-efficacy, greater awareness of the consequences of untreated disease conditions with other elements from social learning theory and the health belief model to elicit positive change at the village level (see Shaffer, n.d.).

It is important to note that even highly successful, resource-intensive pilot educational programs cannot usually obtain support for replication due to a lack of resources and inadequate service delivery in poor countries. The simpler and less resource-intensive a program is, the better its chances for survival. A focused program to persuade and motivate mothers to bring children to a health post for immunization is often more feasible than one to make vaccines widely accessible across a large area.

Selected Strategies for Behavior Change

Selected behavior change strategies are described below. Selection was based on their potential utility in developing countries. A good overview of these and other behavioral strategies is found in Chapter 3, this volume, as well as in Glanz, Lewis, and Rimer (1991). For each strategy an overview is presented followed by a description of principal components and examples of applications in developing countries. It is important to realize that a successful change program may utilize a variety of strategies; change agents should use whatever "works," irrespective of the source.

The Health Belief Model

The health belief model (HBM) explains why individuals do (or do not) behave appropriately to prevent illness/disability or remedy the effects of existing illness/disability. The HBM provides a framework for health promotion programs that increase: (1) screening behaviors to detect health-related problems such as malnutrition, that is, growth monitoring; (2) preventive behaviors such as immunization, smoking cessation, appropriate use of oral rehydration therapy, and antibiotics; (3) the use of reproductive health methods to prevent pregnancy, HIV, or STDs; and (4) community-based activities for change, that is, obtaining potable water and sanitation.

The HBM specifies the following explanatory factors for health-related behaviors: (1) an individual's beliefs about the seriousness of a specific health problem (in terms of consequences); (2) the individual's beliefs about her or his personal susceptibility or exposure to the problem; (3) the individual's perceptions of personal barriers to reducing susceptibility–exposure; and (4) the individual's feelings of self-efficacy (self-confidence) for making changes needed to reduce susceptibility–exposure; and (5) the individual's beliefs about benefits to be gained from taking action. The HBM can also be applied to beliefs about another's susceptibility to a disease, that is, a mother's beliefs about her children.

In the United States, influenza vaccination coverage has been greatly widened by targeting high-risk groups with educational programs that increased feelings of susceptibility and fear of the consequences of influenza (see, for example, Larson *et al.*, 1979). "Fear" arousal strategies also have been incorporated into another theoretical model called protection motivation theory (Rogers, 1983).

HBM components are defined as follows:

1. *Perceived personal susceptibility* to a specific health problem such as dehydration from diarrhea, or malaria; involves beliefs about the probability that oneself or significant others will experience a given problem.
2. *Perceived seriousness* of a specific health problem involves beliefs about its consequences, that is, the amount and impact of pain, the likelihood of permanent damage/disability or death, time lost, dependency on others, and cost of necessary remedies.
3. *Perceived benefits* from specific actions that may be taken to prevent or remedy a problem. This may include beliefs about the effectiveness of vaccines in preventing tetanus, beliefs that oral rehydration therapy will prevent dehydration and death, or beliefs that clean water/sanitation reduces the incidence of diarrheal diseases. Perceived benefits also include evaluations of the importance of disease reduction/prevention outcomes to individuals, that is, the value of significantly less diarrheal disease in households where residents are accustomed to diarrheal disease and parasites).
4. *Perceived barriers* or costs of specific preventive actions. These encompass beliefs about the time, effort, and monetary costs required. They depend on a host of objective and subjective factors like distance to health posts, access to transportation, time and effort required to obtain clean water/sanitation, passive acceptance of waterborne disease and its consequences, and spousal resistance to the use of reproductive health methods.
5. *Self-efficacy* is the belief that one is personally able to prevent or remedy a serious health-related problem, that is, a woman's confidence that she can persuade a reluctant husband to use a pregnancy prevention method.

In any decision-making situation, the HBM components balance and compensate for each other. If a health service or preventive program is not available or is of poor quality, then perceived personal susceptibility is not likely to result in action. Conversely, availability of good preventive and remedial services alone will not motivate action if a condition is perceived as irrelevant, trivial, or not preventible.

The HBM has proven especially useful in identifying psychosocial barriers to change as well as psychosocial factors that can stimulate change processes. The following are suggested applications. *Applications* of the HBM in developing countries may include:

1. *Assessment of a community's readiness to adopt new behaviors to prevent illness/disability.* To an outsider, the objective need to remedy endemic disease conditions may be evident especially when feasible, culturally appropriate solutions are at hand. However, the need for action may not be evident to the members of the community. The HBM can frame questions so that people become aware of and prioritize: (1) problems they believe to be most serious; (2) feasible solutions (with respect to time and effort required); and (3) potential barriers to action and problem-solving including, the ability to sustain new behaviors required for problem solving. Answers indicate a priori realistic behavioral change programs that are acceptable.

2. *Development of specific health promotion programs to teach, motivate, and enable new behaviors.* If assessment data show that mothers will lengthen breast-feeding and wean appropriately, then information on specific barriers can help develop a realistic intervention. If mothers express little self-efficacy to prolong breast-feeding due to household conditions and/or pressures by powerful mothers-in-law to wean early, then any intervention would have to work around these barriers.

3. *Evaluation of the effectiveness of health promotion programs.* The HBM can identify the limitations of an intervention, that is, perceptions of mothers that the effort required to correctly prepare and use oral rehydration solutions (ORS) is not worth the time and trouble. The HBM can suggest methods to better educate mothers about the seriousness of dehydration or the benefits of ORS and increase feelings of self-efficacy about preparing ORS on a day-to-day basis.

Two good empirical examples of the application of the HBM to health-related issues in developing countries can be found in Stanton, Black, Engle, and Pelto, (1992) and in Kloos (1995). We emphasize again that planning, implementation, and evaluation of any behavioral intervention often requires multiple strategies. Seemingly simple behaviors such as the correct preparation of ORS involve numerous steps. A behavioral profile for ORS in a Honduran diarrhea control program lists 38 cognitive and behavioral steps to be understood and followed by a child's caregiver (Rasmuson *et al.*, 1988a). The same publication lists 39 specific "prevention behaviors" to prevent the occurrence of diarrheal diseases.

Social Learning Theory

Social learning theory (SLT) posits that individual behavior is the result of complex interactions between three basic psychosocial forces: (1) thought processes (cognitions), such as anticipated outcomes of specific behaviors (and their value to oneself or significant others); (2) lessons learned from one's own and others successes/failures; (3) the immediate physical and social environments including media information and the behaviors of one's peers, family members, and friends; and (4) the behavior itself, that is, behavior as a process with feedback from others leading to behavioral adjustments and feelings of greater self-efficacy. According to Albert Bandura (1986), these three forces continuously change and reinforce each other.

To illustrate these processes, assume that a couple in a developing country use periodic abstinence to avoid pregnancy because information about other methods is minimal and because they believe it is the only pregnancy prevention method approved by family, friends, and peers. Further, suppose that a full range of reproductive health services becomes available, while information on these services is disseminated and reinforced by positive opinions from respected peers. In this case, change agents may motivate the couple to consider a modern method of contraception. If the woman visits the new service and her positive attitudes toward a specific method(s) are reinforced, she may choose one and learn the necessary skills for using it. Personal experimentation then increase feelings of self-efficacy and the belief that the method prevents unwanted pregnancy. By this process, a new contraceptive behavior is established and reinforced by pregnancy avoidance and spouse approval. Finally, growth in community acceptance establishes a social norm that can sustain the new behavior. This oversimplified hypothetical example also shows that complex, value-laden new behaviors are not derived from a single prior cause.

To effectively implement the SLT on a large scale is difficult in a developing country. However, specific aspects of the model may be feasible. An agency could effectively use SLT teaching principles to increase the learning and practice of a new health behavior. Thus, for example, change agents could use tangible, highly valued but inexpensive incentives to reward mothers for mastery of a specific skill such as growth monitoring for detection of child malnutrition. Another technique is to involve community role-models in the program and persuade them to "model" the proper use of growth monitoring.

Major *SLT components* include:

1. The *personal environment* or anything physically external to an individual which could affect performance of a specific behavior. This construct includes what is objectively "out there," such as ability to use health services and positive or negative social support, as well as one's perception of the environment, that is, beliefs about the availability and utility of social support and perceptions of social norms.

2. Individual *behavioral skills* needed to perform a new behavior.

3. *Expectations* or outcomes expected from performance of a new behavior. The immediate outcome expected of a reproductive health method is usually pregnancy prevention. However, longer-term expectations might include an easier work load for mothers or more time for income producing activities. Awareness of expectations like these is very important. Because all expected outcomes are incentives or disincentives for a given behavior, they must be identified early. Tangible incentives with a relatively rapid "payoff" are more immediately effective in persuading individuals to change than abstract, nonspecific incentives such as "higher living standards" and longer, healthier lives.

When expectations are negative or mixed, a change agent should reduce negative expectations, if possible, and/or emphasize positive outcomes. In some cases this requires reducing the perceived probability of negative outcomes (like side effects of given contraceptives). It should also be noted that highly valued outcomes/incentives will not work if an individual believes she/he is not competent to change behaviors. This important aspect is explained under "self-efficacy" below.

4. *Expectancies* are the importance that individuals place on specific outcomes/incentives to change behavior, in which a higher value is usually placed on immediate, tangible benefits. In cases where multiple expected outcomes are present, it is crucial to determine which are most important to individuals whether these be positive or negative.

5. *Behavioral self-control* or setting specific, realistic behavioral goals to achieve valued outcomes. Effective pregnancy prevention requires learning to use a reliable reproductive health method. Individuals best learn new skills when they are broken into small, specific, and sequential "steps" that can be "rewarded" either by the teacher or the self. This also motivates the learning process because progress is visible.

6. *Observational learning from role models* or observing others perform a specific behavior of interest. Individuals also learn vicariously from seeing others fail. Observational learning from "role models" is a powerful and efficient learning technique and is usually incorporated into interactive education methods. Clearly, the TV, radio, and print media make skillful use of role models to sell everything from cigarettes to condoms.

7. *Behavioral reinforcements/rewards* come from many sources including fulfillment of expected outcomes, positive feelings about doing the "right" thing, and anticipation of future rewards.

8. *Self-efficacy* is the perceived probability that one can successfully learn and carry out a new behavior (including the overcoming of personal and environmental obstacles). Bandura (1986) believes people will not attempt a new behavior, no matter how important, if failure is anticipated. Self-efficacy is enhanced when new behaviors are broken into simple, concrete, easily learned steps and then practiced in a non-threatening environment. Maibach (1995) points out that self-efficacy is complex and includes: (1) perceptions of one's competence to apply sufficient effort and persistence to overcome barriers/master a new behavior; and (2) a generally optimistic outlook that success will follow effort.

The SLT is relevant to these three basic stages in program development: (1) evaluation or assessment of the need for and utility/feasibility of a new program; (2) providing a structure for implementing a new program; and (3) evaluating program effectiveness. *Applications* of the SLT in developing countries may include:

1. *Assessment* of the readiness of a community, family, or individual to adopt new behaviors. The SLT can be used to develop measures of how receptive individuals and groups are to changing behaviors. Examples include: (1) levels of positive or negative community support for behavior change; (2) the value attached to expected results of new behaviors (in which values act as incentives for their adoption); (3) the degree to which role models in the community (and media) motivate learning and change; (4) the relevance of currently held knowledge and skills for accepting and learning new behaviors; and (5) the optimal number of steps per skill to maximize the learning of that skill. Answers indicate whether a program or intervention to promote a new behavior is feasible and, if so, changes needed in the environment, knowledge, attitudes, and skill levels to gain acceptance of the new behavior.

2. *Development* of focused health promotion programs to teach, motivate, and facilitate adoption of new behaviors. If assessment data show that people in a community are ready, willing, and able to develop a source of potable water, then SLT can indicate measures to determine types of potable water source/systems with the greatest potential for adoption. Measures should show: (1) time and energy people will spend on installing different potable water sources and systems; (2) time/energy they will expend on carrying potable water at varying distances from home; (3) the value of potable water compared to "costs" of money, time, and effort to utilize and main-

tain different potable water systems; (4) specific knowledge and skills needed to develop and maintain different water sources; (5) feelings of competence to master skills including those required to work together; and (6) best collective mechanisms to maximize accountability of designated individuals to maintain a potable water system.

3. *Evaluation* of the effectiveness of a health promotion program in teaching, motivating, and enabling new behaviors. In common with the HBM, SLT can be used to measure the effects of an intervention at different levels, that is, how effective was the local organization in developing a new water source, how effective were educational methods in communicating needed skills and motivating behavior changes, what barriers if any were encountered, and to what degree did the new system affect the prevalence of waterborne diseases in the community. A good comparison of the HBM and SLT may be found in Rosenstock and Kirscht (1988).

Diffusion of Innovations Theory

Diffusion theory is used to explain how and why innovations (new behaviors–practices–products) are adopted (or not) in communities and populations. Explanations include how differences in the characteristics of the innovation itself and its potential adopters predict successful adoption. This information shows how an innovation can be modified to make it more acceptable and how to identify "early adopters" of the innovation who will introduce it to the community.

Contemporary diffusion theory was developed in the 1950s by rural sociologists studying the adoption of new agricultural practices in developing countries (Rogers, 1962, 1995). Subsequently, it has been applied to health-related issues such as family planning, antibiotic drug use, and health education. Social marketing experts use diffusion theory to make condoms more attractive and acceptable through changes in shape, color, and packaging (see Bond and Dover, 1997, for a comprehensive review of condom diffusion programs in Zambia). Social marketers also use diffusion principles in designing media messages to raise awareness and create positive attitudes toward condom use. Diffusion theory includes many other elements, and the reader is referred to Everett Rogers' (1995) latest edition of *Diffusion of Innovations* for more information.

Diffusion theory postulates that the following characteristics enhance the probability of an innovation's adoption.

1. The *compatibility* of an innovation with the sociocultural values, economy, and current technology of a population into which it is introduced. A new potable water system is more acceptable if it is superior to the present system with respect to physical access for users, ease or simplicity of use, provision of adequate amounts of good quality water, cost, and ease of maintenance. A contrary example would be proposing a water system that depended on a relatively complex pump that depended on skilled maintenance and imported replacement parts. A contrary example would be attempting to gain acceptance of condoms in a culture hostile to reproductive health *per se* and especially to barrier methods.

2. *Flexibility* of innovations to fit local conditions. Successful recipes for homemade oral rehydration solutions have been developed with local participation to substitute for expensive or inaccessible commercial solutions. However, educating community health workers and mothers to mix and administer the solution correctly

requires an intensive, localized, hands-on teaching approach with careful follow-up (Northrup, 1993).

Conversely, "high-tech" products or services introduced by bureaucratic organizations without local adaptation/simplification have failed or produced negative outcomes. Examples of the latter include the introduction of infant formula into poor areas where good quality water is not available; the introduction of wrong-gender community health workers who are improperly trained for grassroots work or not accountable to the community for their performance.

3. *Reversibility* of innovations for the resumption of previous practices. Innovations that cannot be terminated without leaving a vacuum and significant problems should not be introduced. Thus, infant formula should not be introduced where the negative consequences of termination cannot be quickly reversed by resumption of breast-feeding.

4. *Relative advantage* of innovations over previous practices. A new potable water source closer to households, providing good quality water (by local standards), should be readily adopted unless an important problem is overlooked. If the system also reduces the incidence of disease, so much the better. This would probably *not* be a system of pumping that is relatively complex, breaks down frequently, and cannot be easily repaired by local people with available parts; or a system easily maintained but located where there is no tradition or structure for community maintenance such that no one takes responsibility for the system.

Another illustration of relative advantage is found in the spontaneous acceptance of antibiotics in developing countries. This is likely because of the visible superiority of their effect(s) on disease combined with easy access (over-the-counter) and low cost in packets of one or two capsules (Whyte, 1992; Goel, Ross-Degnan, Berman, & Soumerai, 1996). Technological innovations requiring little behavior change may demonstrate big advantages that hasten adoption. Comparisons of the rapid spread of antibiotics to the much slower adoption of reproductive health services and methods are a case in point. However, many technological innovations have gone through rapid cycles of adoption and failure because subtle and necessary behavioral changes or infrastructure support were overlooked. Examples include infant formula, village pumps that could not be maintained, and pour-flush toilets that people would not clean or maintain.

5. *Complexity* or innovations difficult to understand, operate, or maintain. Early methods for home-based monitoring of infant and child growth were too complicated for effective use. Yet, initial failures pointed the way to simpler methods effectively used by mothers with low literacy skills.

6. *Cost-efficiency* or "cost-benefit" of an innovation. Innovations are evaluated informally by individuals with respect to benefits anticipated (or promised) versus expected costs. Costs involve expenditures of money, time, energy, or other resources for individuals to learn to use the innovation and the potential loss of money, time energy, or reputation if it fails. The more perceived benefits outweigh costs, the greater the likelihood of adoption.

There may be hidden, unexpressed benefits, real or imagined, that are used in making decisions. Some innovations are heavily pressed on communities, irrespective of their potential utility, because first-world donors, politicians, bureaucrats, or even community health workers receive side benefits or hidden rewards ranging from patronage and payoffs to enhanced prestige, power, and self-esteem. Judith Justice (1986) relates how a poorly planned, culturally inappropriate, and ultimately dysfunctional community health worker model was imposed on rural communities in Nepal because of "hidden agendas" of the donor agency and government ministry.

Within any community, it is usually the case that some people perceive more benefits, while others believe that, for them personally, costs outweigh benefits. Thus, a village leader or shaman may believe that an innovation, however beneficial for the community, will reduce her or his influence if it is controlled by others. Overcoming obstacles of this kind requires convincing opponents that personal cost-benefit calculations are mistaken or unduly negative. They need to perceive benefits they personally will receive and, if appropriate (and feasible), additional benefits may be "created" to co-opt them. The village leader who feels threatened by an innovation might be given a role and stake in its planning and implementation processes. These kinds of adaptations or solutions require cultural sensitivity, good sociopolitical skills, judgment, and leverage.

7. *Risk* refers to the perceived uncertainty that accompanies an innovation. The lower the perceived risk, the greater the likelihood of adoption. Agricultural extension agents introducing a new seed or fertilizer often confront this issue with subsistence farmers who cannot afford to lose any of their crop. Community demonstration projects to pilot test new seed (using local skills and methods of cultivation) can induce "early adopters" to experiment with new seed in small batches. An analogous example in public health is the introduction of a technically proven new reproductive health method. In this case, *perceived* risks for trying the method may be community disapproval, undesirable side effects, and unwanted pregnancy. Persuading community role models to use and "model" the new method might work if pregnancies are indeed reduced with minimal side effects. Again, it is important to know all the significant perceived risks, real or imagined, that may be present and not readily expressed.

Finally, it is important to note that these characteristics are interrelated and compensate for each other. An innovation such as a sanitary pit latrine may have great relative advantage in terms of keeping water clean, reducing exposure to feces, and eliminating odor, providing privacy, and so forth, but may be "costly" in terms of installation, maintenance, and access. The key to acceptance is to know the issues going in so as to adapt the innovation and, if possible, minimize disadvantages while providing valued incentives or side benefits to increase adoption rates.

Each community will have individuals who are at different stages of readiness to adopt an innovation. Change agents should identify these persons, especially potential early adopters. Characteristics of *adopters* that predict adoption of innovation include:

1. *Innovators* who are first in a community to adopt an innovation. As a rule, they constitute a small percentage of potential adopters. They are relatively well-educated, have consistent exposure to new ideas through mass media, actively seek new information, enjoy experimenting with new practices or products, and possess the social and financial resources to take risks and absorb failures. They are high enough in the social hierarchy to be indifferent to or unhurt by criticism. This group "breaks the ice," by making innovations visible and concrete.

2. *Early adopters* are well integrated into the local social system. Early adopters are usually respected and trusted opinion leaders with high rates of participation in

community affairs. Thus, they make good role models and advocates for an innovation; even when they do not adopt it, others may ask their opinion. They are often well-educated persons such as physicians, other health workers, school teachers, and religious leaders who have consistent exposure to mass media and positive attitudes toward change.

3. *Early majority* persons are usually not leaders but are well integrated into their community. They are open to communication channels and early adopters as role models. If persuaded, they adopt an innovation before the typical community member and "bridge" early adopters with the rest. In a village setting, these might be mothers of small children who are well connected to local leaders and/or community health workers interested in health issues and ready to take calculated risks.

4. *Late majority* members are skeptical and cautious about something new even if the advantages are understood. Their slow approach may be due to innate conservatism, previous bad experiences, lower risk-taking margins, peer pressure from family and friends, or beliefs they cannot learn to use an innovation or that it will not confer important benefits.

5. *Laggards* are last to adopt an innovation. They are usually the most conservative and least educated, highly skeptical of receiving significant benefits, worried about personal losses from an innovation's failure (including embarrassment at being unable to master it), suspicious of the innovation's advocates, and possessed of very low margins for risk taking. They also may be subject to heavy peer or family pressure not to adopt. Some members of this category may never adopt the innovation.

Diffusion theory involves many more details including optimum types of diffusion networks, differential roles of opinion leaders, the roles and characteristics of change agents, and the direct/indirect (unforseen) consequences of innovations (Rogers, 1995) (see also "Diffusion of Health Promotion Innovations" by Orlandi, Landers, Weston, and Haley, 1990).

As with the HBM or SLT, diffusion theory can be used in whole or in part to enhance the speed and scope of an innovation's adoption. It can show in advance how an innovation should be modified for better acceptance in a specific population. *Applications* of diffusion theory to developing countries may include:

1. *Assessment* and comparison of a proposed new product/practice with that which it may replace. Ideally, this should be done with local "innovators" and early adopters whose acceptance are crucial to convincing others. A good assessment shows whether or not a proposed innovation is likely to be adopted and useful. It indicates that modifications needed to enhance the innovation's acceptability and utilization. When alternative innovations are considered at the same time, comparisons indicate which one(s) fits best into the local context. Therefore, different contraceptive methods or different versions of the same method can be compared in order to select those most likely to be adopted.

In some cases, good assessments simply involve illustrating the innovation to local informants. As a Peace Corps volunteer in rural Chile, one of the authors noticed that the laying hens of small farmers wandered at will, resulting in frequent mortality from passing motor vehicles and a high proportion of lost eggs. At an informal village meeting he proposed that the farmers construct chicken coops. Farmers present knew the advantages of coops but rejected the "innovation" because they could not afford to vaccinate the hens to prevent the occurrence and rapid spread of diseases that result from crowding. They suggested that it would be better to devise a practical means for obtaining necessary vaccines and related supports for chicken breeding in coops. They strongly emphasized that little persuasion would then be required for chicken coop adoption.

New products or practices may also possess "barrier" characteristics that are undetected until a sample of potential adopters have implemented steps in their everyday use. Agricultural extension work provides numerous examples of innovations that failed or required extensive modifications because of covert barriers, that is, high-yield seeds or cultivation techniques requiring management skills/behaviors and/or resources that were not apparent until small farmers actually tried to use the innovations. A good assessment of relative advantage and compatibility with existing conditions and so forth may show that a new product/practice is not likely to be accepted. This conclusion is disappointing but saves a great deal of time, energy, frustration, and disillusionment on the part of change agents and target group members.

2. *Diffusion* or dissemination (and adoption) of a new product/practice in a population. At this stage, diffusion theory provides a framework for identifying different categories of adopters. Acceptance by "early adopters" is important in order to utilize them as role models for the majority. Respected mothers who adopt a homemade oral rehydration solution or a new growth monitoring technique make a powerful selling tool for other changes as well.

After the innovation has become widely diffused, it should be promoted among nonadopters. Change agents may then reexamine the innovation to determine if it is too complex or lacks relative advantage for nonadopters. Barriers may be simple as in the lack of transportation to geographically isolated "laggards" or difficult as in overcoming peer/family and religious opposition to reproductive health methods. It is possible that a given innovation cannot be made acceptable to this group. More appropriate alternatives may be feasible.

3. *Evaluations* of strategies used to gain adoption. Adopter categories can be subdivided to estimate the effectiveness of different promotional messages and media. Thus, messages via selected mass media may be sufficient to achieve adoption by "innovators," whereas mass media, reinforced by contacts with health workers, are necessary for "early adopters" and personal demonstrations/role modeling (by health workers) and local opinion leaders may be required for "early majorities" of adopters.

Health-related outcomes also can be evaluated. If a new potable water system significantly lowers intestinal disease for early adopters but not others, then diffusion theory can help determine why. If others are actually using the new source along with contaminated water from other sources, then the new water system may not be sufficiently accessible for everyday use.

Social Marketing

Kotler and Andreasen (1991) defines social marketing as a methodology for "designing, implementing and controlling programs seeking to increase the acceptability of a social idea or practice in a target group" (p. 434). Social marketing has been derived from theories in consumer behavior and the social sciences. Specific social marketing techniques mimic commercial marketing by thoroughly pretesting a new product among target consumers to determine product benefits, acceptable prices, how product access can be maximized, and the most effective promotional media.

Unlike commercial marketing, social marketing is designed to promote products and practices that may not require the exchange of money. It is often directed at people who lack time, energy, and money (Novelli, 1990). Marketing new water/sanitation systems or new reproductive health methods in developing countries is more challenging than promoting new music compact disks, designer running shoes, or other consumer goods.

Social marketing methods have been used in developing countries since the 1970s (for example, see Rasmuson *et al.*, 1988; Seidel, 1993). It is most effective with innovations that are straightforward in terms of new behaviors and that demonstrate visible benefits. Concrete examples include immunization of infants and children and oral rehydration therapy. Its effectiveness with more complex, value-laden practices, requiring long-term use, such as new reproductive health behaviors, is less obvious. Recently, social marketing methods have proved effective in promoting condom use among males at high risk for HIV infection in parts of Africa; however, critics insist that empowering women to "persuade" men to use them would be considerably more effective (Heise & Elias, 1995).

Social marketing components involved in the design of social marketing campaigns include:

1. *Marketplace research and analyses* to gather information about a target population in order to tailor marketing campaigns to the needs/wants of that population. The target population has to be defined, that is, who are potential early adopters/users of a child health innovation? Are they natural helpers/informal leaders in a population of low-income mothers of infants and children under 13 years of age? Information needed is demographic and psychosocial (lifestyles, current behaviors/wants/needs relative to the innovation, values, stages of readiness to adopt an innovation). Separate information is needed to identify the best promotional media and the best distribution mechanisms. To raise awareness and create a need for oral rehydration therapy, middle-class women in radio soap operas may be the best vehicle for one group versus television public service announcements for another, or radio diffusion combined with comic books for a third group.

2. *Pretest of the innovation* in a representative sample of the target population is the next step. Commercial marketers carefully and scientifically select pretest population samples. However, a reasonably good approximation of intended users is often adequate to estimate product acceptability, patterns of use, perceived benefits, and needed changes in marketing strategies or the product itself. A new type of pit latrine could be pretested in a sample of villages with respect to locations, frequency of use, features that should be changed, the maximum and average amounts of time, money and effort villagers will expend on obtaining, locating, and maintaining the latrine, and the most effective media/messages for persuading early adopters to install and use it. This example involves acquisition of a new material product along with new practices or behaviors. If current practices entail the simple use of nearby fields or streams, then substituting a time-consuming, complex new product and set of behaviors to provide "better health" or enhance the survival of infants and children may not seem worthwhile. If the pretest suggests that problems cannot be resolved, then an alternative product is necessary or perhaps limited modifications such as

more attractive packaging for a new condom, or a simpler access/pricing strategy for pit latrines or water pumps. After modifications, another pretest is desirable.

3. *Introduction of the innovation* in the target population(s). If pretesting was well done, this step will mostly demonstrate the effectiveness of promotional strategies, the adequacy of distribution channels, and acceptable adoption rates.

4. *Evaluation of the social marketing campaign* including: (1) gathering "process" data to detect flaws in campaign mechanisms; and (2) collecting impact data to measure adoption rates by target subgroups. Impact data can also provide for corrective feedback to any aspect of the system, that is, repackaging condoms, making a new pit latrine more affordable/easier to build and maintain, reformulating a food recipe to local taste and appearance, or using different media at different times with different messages. A lack of sophisticated evaluation tools can be overcome by directly observing the marketing/adoption process and using focus groups to elicit the details and problems.

Social marketing methods have been used in developing countries for 20 years across many health problems. Below are a few examples of its many uses:

1. A 1979 pilot project to promote the use of ORT in Honduras and Egypt illustrates an early and successful application. Carefully developed and pretested marketing campaigns were aimed at mothers via radio, television, and print media. Both campaigns had significant, short-term effects. Within 2 years, the proportion of Honduran mothers able to identify and use ORT increased from 1.5 to 95%, while infant and child deaths from diarrhea dropped significantly in both countries. These effects were attributed primarily to the social marketing campaigns. Subsequent applications in Ecuador, Peru, and Swaziland were also successful extending to marketing campaigns for tuberculosis and malaria self-care and to Colombia, where a social marketing campaign to improve childhood immunization increased coverage from 40 to 90% in 1984 (Rasmuson *et al.*, 1988; HEALTHCOM Project, 1985; Seidel. 1992).

2. In Indonesia, a pilot marketing project to persuade rural mothers to adopt more nutritious, locally available foods used "concept verification" to develop acceptable new food combinations (McDivitt, McDowell, & Zhou, 1991). Ethnographic research identified local foods that could be combined to achieve higher nutritional content. Then, specially trained "Kaders" (community health workers) worked with a sample of mothers to develop and pretest new food combinations. This produced acceptable, highly nutritious foodstuffs made from cheap local ingredients that were easily and quickly prepared.

Social marketing has been widely criticized for using commercial advertising methods to "sell" socially desirable innovations. Other critics insist that without continuous mass media promotion, adoption rates fall as early adopters stop using the innovation and their knowledge and skills deteriorate. Continuous mass media promotion is generally too expensive for developing countries to maintain without foreign aid.

For change agents working at the grass roots, media-based social marketing may not be feasible. Nevertheless, social marketing methods can be adapted to evaluate the acceptability and utility of an innovation at the local level. Adaptations include gathering background data on current products/practices and pretesting an innovation with representative groups for compatibility with existing lifestyles, perceived benefits, the "price" (broadly defined) adoptees will pay, and the efficacy of educational messages. Focus groups of pretest adopters are especially good for identifying and clarifying issues.

Varieties of social marketing are constantly being developed to fit specific situations and products. An earlier version was used in Canada during the 1940s to provide more effective agricultural extension education through the Radio Farm Forum. That strategy basically involves communicating an educational or promotional message through radio, television, videotape, and so forth to a relatively small interest group with a facilitator present. After the message is delivered, the facilitator guides a discussion focused on the potential utility of the innovation. The discussion is a critique of the proposed innovation that leads to outright rejection or acceptance with modifications. After discussion, a concrete decision is made regarding further action needed, if any, that is, obtain more information, suggest modifications for local adoption, or experiment with the innovation. The facilitator then must coordinate follow-up. The facilitator structures the discussions with an interactive learning strategy such as the LePSA (learner-centered, problem-posing, self-discovery, action-oriented).

Hornik (1988) provides a good critique for applications of this technique in developing countries. Effective implementation on a national scale requires a high degree of coordination and cooperation between local community health workers and media-savvy technical experts. Obviously, this would be difficult for many developing countries. However, the technique could be utilized at any level with audio- or videotape by a community health worker relatively expert with an issue and skilled at group discussions.

Other Aspects of Disease Prevention Strategies

Strategies to improve health have taken both vertical and horizontal approaches. In the vertical or top down approach, interventions have been targeted largely at individual diseases or conditions, often on a global scale. Under the Tropical Disease Research Program of the WHO, these have focused on diseases associated with poverty, including malaria, schistosomiasis, lymphatic filariasis, onchocerciasis, leprosy, African trypanosomiasis, Chagas disease, and leishmaniasis. Success has been varied. Successful eradication of smallpox was brought about in 1978, and it appears that dracunculiasis (guinea worm disease), a painful and debilitating disease with complications of frequent crippling and pain, will soon follow. Efforts to eliminate other infectious diseases, some of which appear to be reemerging, for example, cholera, in the Western hemisphere have been less successful. Efforts to control others with global distributions have not fared as well, for example, malaria, dengue, and Chagas disease. It has become clear that "magic bullets" are few and far between in spite of advances in vaccinations and pharmacotherapy. Control and eradication require that the disease or condition be attacked in such a way that the spread of the agent or risk factors associated with the condition are reduced to the level where propagation fails and finally the cause eliminated. In the case of smallpox (and soon polio), the infectious agent was removed from circulation because of long-lasting immunity granted by immunization and a worldwide effort to obtain the needed degree of coverage. Guinea worm also may be eradicated soon based on amelioration of conditions required for its spread and the relatively short life of the agent, which allows it to die out on its own once transmission is slowed.

Regardless of program structure, the field of international health has long recognized the role of behavior in both transmission and control of disease. Lack of success in interventions previously thought to be largely outside of the scope of behavior (e.g., water supply and sanitation) have been tied intimately to fundamental human behavior in the selection of practices for waste disposal, obtaining and protecting safe water supplies, and control of hygiene-based diseases such as diarrhea, scabies, and trachoma. This has led to involvement of women in decision making with regard to water and sanitation, as the primary care providers in the family and the ones most likely to be involved in securing water or promoting sanitation (Van Wijk, 1985; Elmendorf & Kruiderink, 1983; WHO, 1998b). The incorporation of behavior in strategies to promote sanitation has become the basis for transforming low-income, often illiterate people and communities. The time in which control strategies might be implemented through improvements in infrastructure, environmental quality, or food supply and nutrition without taking into account behavior at the individual and community levels is past. This is reflected in international efforts directed against a long list of current threats, including the three groups of diseases and conditions identified by Murray and Lopez (1996). Today, it is difficult to imagine diseases or conditions in which behavior does not play a major part.

The availability of strategies and interventions, or "tools," to prevent and reduce the burden of disease does not equate with their proper use; thus, further research is needed in this area (WHO, 1996c). The report of the ad hoc Committee on Health Research Relating to Future Intervention Options identifies "three broad reasons to explain the persistence of a disease in a population: "(a) lack of knowledge about the disease and its prevention, (b) a lack of tools and (c) failure to use the existing tools efficiently" (Box S.2). Improved use of existing tools can be obtained through increased technical efficiency, better resource allocations, and application of needed resources to behavioral research.

In low- and middle-income countries, programs that attack STD transmission through behavioral change, and promote measles intervention, breast-feeding, smoking prevention and cessation are especially attractive. The report states that the primary reason for persistence of the burden of pneumonia lies in the failure of medical care service providers and patients to use existing tools efficiently, for example, proper use of antibiotics by health care providers and patients, not a lack of knowledge about the disease.

In the case of "sanitary diseases" associated with sanitation and hygiene, the Water Supply and Sanitation Collaborative Council (WS&SCC) Working Group on the Promotion of Sanitation has identified ten barriers to progress in sanitary improvements (WHO, 1998a). These include behaviorally linked components that affect political will, professional prestige, policy and institutional frameworks, resource utilization, approaches, consumer preferences, promotion and public awareness, and gender roles (WHO, 1998a). These are affected by cross-cutting issues such as taboos and beliefs that may be held by individuals or exist with cultures, thereby limiting strategies and interventions to those with which they fit.

Behavior is an intimate part not only of the problem of transmission in this category, but also in the acceptance of interventions. Such basic behaviors as those involved in establishing toilet preferences and practices and hygiene are deeply rooted in cultural traditions and often difficult to change.

The increasing "globalization" of economies has, without doubt, both positive and negative affects on health and public health law (Yach & Bettcher, 1998a). As outbreaks such as the recent Bovine Spongiform Encephalitis (BSE or "mad cow disease") have demonstrated, the movement of materials, such as feed stuffs, may affect herds and populations beyond the area of immediate concern. Such possibilities exist among all diseases, both known and emerging, but are especially important in the latter where routine surveillance may not exist. Globalization is not an entirely new trend (Navarro, 1998), and the potential effect on increased trade and the movement of "emerging infectious diseases," especially into developed market economies, has been noted earlier. Within the international community, concern exists as to its long-range effect on policy supporting health, primarily in the developing economies, where health concerns may be placed on the back-burner to more pressing concerns of economic crises (Navarro, 1998).

At this time, WHO, the World Health Assembly, and FAO coordinate the bulk of international agreements affecting health. These are accomplished under international law, largely through binding and voluntary (nonbinding) recommendations of the organizations (Yach & Bettcher, 1998b). This in effect creates a behavioral environment where economic policymakers need be aware of the consequences of their decisions on health, as well as economics.

Summary: Primary Prevention in Practice

Health programs affecting the developing world are as varied as the governments, agencies and organizations supporting them. The most concerted effort is linked to the United Nations through multilateral organizations addressing health, food security, children, science and culture, development, and security. The primary multilateral agencies operate under mandates set out in the charter of the United Nations. These include the WHO, which is arguably the lead agency in international health. Under its charter, the WHO, located in Geneva, with regional offices in Europe, Africa, the Middle East, Asia, the Western Pacific, and the Americas, addresses diseases in broad categories: infectious agents, food; waterborne and soilborne diseases; vector-borne disease; diseases of infants, children, and adolescents, adults and the elderly; environment; and lifestyles. It also invests in the development of health infrastructure via medical education and dissemination of health information (WHO, 1996a). Beginning with the declaration of Alma Ata in which member nations pledged support for Health for All, a primary health care plan was conceived that would bring prevention and medical services to a greatly increased segment of the population. The WHO has worked to improve health of women and children through programs aimed at reducing risks associated with pregnancy and promotion of birth spacing, breast-feeding, immunization against vaccine-preventable diseases of childhood, nutrition and growth monitoring, and home management of diarrhea (Basch, 1990). The WHO interacts with member nations in an advisory and consultative capacity both to support the collection of health and population data on a worldwide basis, and to coordinate support of programs addressing specific diseases and conditions. This is in addition to working with targeted groups in each of the areas outlined above. The International Bank for Reconstruction (World Bank), UNICEF (United Nations Children's Fund), United Nations Development Program (UNDP), United Nations Scientific Educational and Cultural Organization (UNESCO), and Food and Agricultural Organization (FAO) overlap in areas of health, environment, and development, in many areas that involve behavior as the primary element in prevention and control.

The WHO has divided priorities for action into three groups. "Old diseases–old problems," includes diseases for which considerable experience exists but which have not been eradicated or brought to an acceptable level of control. Diseases in this category have well-established cost-effective interventions (e.g., immunization, improved sanitation) but remain problems in spite of this knowledge, often because of behavioral issues and resistance to change. Diseases and conditions in this category include vaccine-preventable diseases of childhood (diphtheria, whooping cough, tetanus, poliomyelitis, measles, tuberculosis, hepatitis B, yellow fever, and vitamin A supplementation), acute respiratory infections, water- and food-borne diseases (largely fecal–oral transmitted diseases and those involving poor sanitation), soil-transmitted helminths, and STDs.

The category, "old disease–new problems," is made up of diseases that have been recognized for a long time but which are once again on the rise. These include tuberculosis and vector-borne diseases such as malaria and dengue. In many cases, effective medical interventions are known as well, but are increasingly compromised by development of antimicrobial and pesticide resistance of the agents and their vectors.

"New diseases–new problems" include those disease that have been identified since the 1970s and/or those that are emerging in populations where they did not previously exist. These include diseases such as the recently recognized Ebola and Marburg viruses, other viral hemorrhagic fevers (Hantavirus), and HIV/AIDS, about which the role of behavior is being defined.

The WHO places first priority on eradicating selected diseases in the first category. The first tier includes poliomyelitis, guinea worm, leprosy, neonatal tetanus, and Chagas disease (American trypanosomiasis), followed by measles and river blindness (onchocerciasis). Second priority has been given to diseases such as tuberculosis and malaria that are on the rise in spite of being well known, and third priority to attacking newly emerging diseases.

Many of the current diseases and conditions in the developing world are amenable to control by cost-effective measures that integrate behavioral change with vaccines and infrastructure for sanitation and water supply. The World Bank notes that behavior is linked to economic development and that improvements in income may be accompanied by adoption of practices that are detrimental to health as well as beneficial (Jamison, Mosley, Measham, & Bobadilla, 1993). Behavioral areas targeted for action by the World Bank include improved hygiene, breast-feeding, sexual comportment, use of tobacco and alcohol, overeating, and sedentary living (Jamison et al., 1993). The international experience has proved that social marketing, behavior analysis and promotion, and increased utilization of health care service improve health status (Ramuson et al., 1988; UNICEF, 1997).

Advances in medical knowledge have contributed much to our understanding of disease and disease processes in the poorer nations of the world. However, use of this knowledge is limited by a lack of resources. Many of the poorer nations, such as the former nation of Zaire, often have minuscule budgets for health. These nations necessarily need to focus on prevention by population-based, low-cost means. Thus, education for behavior change is becoming increasingly valuable.

A large portion of the burden attributable to ill health is amenable to behavioral interventions. These include infectious diseases and conditions traditionally associated with poverty as well as those of affluence including vector-borne disease such as dengue and malaria. Modifiable risk factors of note include malnutrition, poor sanitation and personal and domestic hygiene, unsafe sex, tobacco and alcohol use, occupational hazards, hypertension, physical inactivity, use of illicit drugs, and polluted air (Murray & Lopez, 1996). These are diseases for which there is a strong element of human behavior in both transmission and the unavailability of low-cost interventions such as immunization and public water supply. Experience has shown that even where low-cost "physical" strategies such as clean water exist, behavior plays a major role in the dissemination and acceptance of those interventions. Thus, behavior change interventions will continue to play an integral role in improving the health of people in developing countries.

References

Albee, G. W., & Gulotta, T. P. (1997). Primary prevention's evolution. In G. W. Albee & T. P. Gulotta (Eds.), *Primary prevention works* (pp. 3–22). Thousand Oaks, CA: Sage.

Bandura, A. (1986). *Social foundations of thought and action.* Englewood Cliffs, NJ: Prentice Hall.

Basch, P. F. (1990). *Textbook of international health.* New York: Oxford University Press.

Blackman, J. M., Goodwillie, R. N., & Webb, R., (1991). *Environment and development in Africa: Selected case studies.* EDI Development Policy Case Series; Analytical Case Studies. No. 6. Washington, DC: World Bank.

Bond, V. & Dover, P. (1997). Men, women and the trouble with condoms: Problems associated with condom use by migrant workers in rural Zambia. *Health Transition Review, 7* (Suppl.), 377–392.

Brides and Abel Project Summary. (1990). *Female education and infant mortality.* Chapel Hill, NC: Research Triangle Institute.

Elmendorf, M., & Kruiderink, A. (1983). *Promotion and support for women's participation in the IDDSWSSD. Report on Mission to Honduras.* New York: PROWESS/UNDP.

Glanz, K., Lewis, F. M., & Rimer, K. (Eds.). (1991). *Health behavior and helath education: Theory, research and practice.* San Francisco: Jossey-Bass.

Goel, P., Ross-Degnan, D., Berman, P., & Soumerai, S. (1996). Retail pharmacies in developing countries: A behavior and intervention framework. *Social Science and Medicine, 42,* 1155–1161.

Haub, C., & Yanagishita, M. (1995). *World population data sheet.* Washington, DC: Population Reference Bureau.

HEALTHCOM Project. (1985). *Lessons from five countries.* Washington, DC: Academy for Educational Development.

Heise, L. L., & Elias, C. (1995). Transforming AIDS prevention to meet women's needs: A focus on developing countries. *Social Science and Medicine, 40,* 931–943.

Hernandez, J. R. S., de Guzman, E. M., Cabanero-Verzosa, C., & Seidel, R. (1993). From idea to mass media: Teaching mothers the concept of dehydration. In R. Seidel (Ed.), *Notes from the field in communication for child survival* (pp. 69–78). Washington, DC: Academy for Educational Development.

Hornik R. C. (1988). *Development communication: Information, agriculture, and nutrition in the third world.* Philadelphia: Annenberg School of Communication, University of Pennsylvania.

Jamison, D. T., Mosley, W. H., Measham, A. R., & Bobadilla, J. L. (1993). *Summary: Disease control priorities in developing countries.* Washington, DC: World Bank/Oxford University Press.

King, E. M. (1990). Educating girls and women: Investing in development. Washington, DC: World Bank.

Justice, J. (1986). *Policies, plans and people: Culture and health development in Nepal.* Berkeley: University of California Press.

Kloos, H. (1995). Human behavior, health education and schistosomiasis control. *Social Science and Medicine, 40,* 1497–1511.

Kotler, P., & Andreasen, A. R. (1991). *Strategic marketing for non-profit organizations* (4th ed.). Englewood Cliffs, NJ: Prentice Hall.

Larson, E. B., Olsen, E., Cole, W., & Shortell, S. (1979). The relationship of health beliefs and a postcard reminder to influenza vaccination. *Journal of Family Practice, 8,* 1207–1211.

Maibach, E. W. (1995). Moving people to behavior change: A staged social cognitive approach to message design. In E. M. Maibach & R. L. Parrott (Eds.), *Designing health messages: Approaches from communication theory and public health practice* (pp. 41–64). Thousand Oaks, CA: Sage.

Mantra, I. B., Davies, J., Sutisnaputra, O. M., & Louis, T. (1993). Effective training for community health workers: diarrhea case management in rural Indonesia. In R. Seidel (Ed.), *Notes from the field in communication for child survival* (pp. 147–156). Washington, DC: Academy for Educational Development.

Mason, J. W., Coombs, D. C., Stalker, V., Branigan, E. S., Badham, A., Stephensen, C. B., & Jolly, P. (1993). Bringing appropriate technology home: Rural Alabama as a site for field training in international health. San Francisco, APHA Session No. 3212: Global Approaches to Manpower Development in Public Health: International Perspectives, October 24–28, 1993.

McDivitt, J., McDowell, J., & Zhou. F. (1991). *Evaluation of the Healthcom Project in West Java, Indonesia: Results from surveys of mothers and volunteer health workers.* Philadelphia: CIHDC, Annenberg School for Communication, University of Pennsylvania.

Murray, C. J. L., & Lopez, A. D. (1996) Quantifying the burden of disease and injury attributable to ten major risk factors. In C. J. L. Murray & A. D. Lopez (Eds.), *The global burden of disease: A comprehensive assessment of mortality and disability from diseases, injuries, and risk factors in 1990 and projected to 2020* (pp. 295–394). Cambridge, MA: Harvard University Press for the World Health Organization and World Bank.

Navarro, V., (1988). Comment: Whose globalization? *American Journal of Public Health, 88,* 742–743.

Northrup, R. (1993). Oral rehydration therapy: From principle to practice. In J. Rohde, M. Chatterjee, & D. Morley (Eds.), *Reaching health for all* (pp. 423–456). Delhi, India: Oxford University Press.

Novelli, W. D. (1990). Applying social marketing to health promotion and disease prevention. In K. Glanz, F. M. Lewis, & K. Rimer (Eds.), *Health behavior and health education: Theory, research and practice* (pp. 342–369). San Francisco: Jossey-Bass.

Orlandi, M. A., Landers, C., Weston, R., & Haley, N. (1990). Diffusion of health promotion innovations. In K. Glanz, F. M. Lewis, & K. Rimer (Eds.), *Health behavior and health education: Theory, research and practice* (pp. 288–313). San Francisco: Jossey-Bass.

Otten, A. L. (1992, April 28). People patterns. *Wall Street Journal,* p. B1.

Pan American Health Organization. (1991). Cholera situation in the Americas. An update. *Epidemiological Bulletin, 12*(4), 11–13.

Ramah, M., & DeBus, M. (1993). Development of a new ORS product identity in Mexico. In R. Seidel (Ed.), *Notes from the field in communication for child survival* (pp. 189–200). Washington, DC: Academy for Educational Development.

Rasmuson, M. R., Seidel, R. E., Smith, W. A., & Booth, E. M. (1988). *Communication for child survival.* Philadelphia, PA: HEALTHCOM Project, Annenburg School of Communications, University of Pennsylvania.

Rogers, E. M. (1962). *Diffusion of innovations* (1st ed.). New York: Free Press.

Rogers, E. M. (1995). *Diffusion of innovations* (4th ed.). New York: Free Press.

Rogers, R. (1983). Cognitive and physiological fear appeals and attitude change. In J. Cacioppo & R. Petty (Eds.), *Social psychophisiology* (pp. 153–176). New York: Guilford Press.

Rosenstock I. M., & Kirscht, J. P. (1988). Social learning theory and the health belief model. *Health Education Quarterly, 15,* 175–183.

Saunders, S. G., Escoto, C., Barahona, M. R., Fiallos, C. E., Corrales, G., Rosenbaum, G., & Seidel, R. (1993). Public and private sector collaboration for the commercial marketing of ORS in Honduras. In R. Seidel (Ed.), *Notes from the field in communication for child survival* (pp. 177–188). Washington, DC: Academy for Educational Development.

Seidel, R. (1992). *Results and realities: A decade of experience in communication for child survival.* Washington, DC: Academy for Educational Development.

Seidel, R. (1993). (Ed.), *Notes from the Field in Communication for Child Survival.* Washington, DC: Academy for Educational Development.

Shaffer, R. (n.d.). *Community-balanced development.* MAP Monograph No. 1, East Africa Series. Nairobi, Kenya: MAP International.

Simpson-Hebert, M. (1996). *Sanitation myths: Obstacles to progress?* Stockholm, Sweden. Paper presented at the Stockholm Water Conference, August 7, 1996.

Stanton, B., Black, R., Engle, P., & Pelto, G. (1992). Theory-driven behavioral intervention. Research for the control of diarrheal diseases. *Social Science and Medicine, 35,* 1405–1420.

Sutisnaputra, O. M., Sulaiman, N. S., Noerjandari, A., Louis, T., & Seidel, R. (1993). The development of counseling cards for community health workers: An aid to teaching mothers proper diarrheal case management in West Java Province, Indonesia. In R. Seidel (Ed.), *Notes from the field in communication for child survival* (pp. 111–118). Washington, DC: Academy for Educational Development.

Tropical Disease Research News. (1997). Environment and disease. Geneva, CH. UNDP/World Bank/WHO Special Programme for Research and Training in Tropical Diseases, No. 53, pp. 1–3.

UNICEF. (1997). *The state of the world's children.* New York: Oxford University Press.

van Wijk, C. (1985). Participation of women in water supply and sanitation: Roles and realities. (Technical paper, No. 22). The Hague, The Netherlands: IRC and PROWESS/UNDP.

Whyte, S. R. (1992). Pharmaceuticals as folk medecine: Transformations in the social relations of health care in Uganda. *Culture, Medicine, and Psychiatry, 16,* 163–186.

World Health Organization (WHO). (1996a). Executive summary. *The World Health Report for 1996: Fighting disease, fostering development.* http:/www. who. ch/whr/1996/exsume. htm.

World Health Organization (WHO). (1996b). Water supply and sanitation sector monitoring report. Geneva, CH. WHO/EOS/96. 15.

World Health Organization (WHO). (1996c). *Investing in health research and development.* Geneva, CH. Report of the ad hoc Committee on Health Research Relating to Future Intervention Options. TDR/Gen/96. 1.

World Health Organization (WHO). (1998a). *Sanitation promotion toolkit.* Geneva, CH. Working Group on the Promotion of Sanitation.

World Health Organization (WHO). (1998b). *PHAST step-by-step guide: A participatory approach for the control of diarrhoeal disease.* Geneva, CH. Participatory Hygiene and Sanitation Transformation Series WHO/EOS/98. 3.

Yach, D., & Bettcher, D. (1998a). The globalization of public health, I: Threats and opportunities. *American Journal of Public Health, 88,* 735–738.

Yach, D., &Bettcher, D. (1998b). The globalization of public health, II: The convergence of self-interest and altruism. *American Journal of Public Health, 88,* 735–741.

Zimicki, S. (1993). Understanding the diarrhea problem in the Philipines: Research as a basis for message design. In R. Seidel (Ed.), *Notes from the fields in communication for child survival* (pp. 7–16). Washington, DC: Academy for Educational Development.

PART VIII

Policy Perspectives

CHAPTER 29

The Role of Health Care Organization in Health Promotion and Disease Prevention

Janet M. Bronstein

Introduction

The 1990s have seen a rapid increase in the portion of the US population whose health care costs are paid for by managed care organizations. Managed care organizations take various forms, but all involve arrangements that combine the financing of health services with efforts to coordinate, integrate, and manage service provision so that patients receive only the care that is necessary to improve their health status. By 1995, the managed care approach to paying and coordinating health care affected 73% of the privately insured population (Jensen, Morrisey, Gaffney, & Liston, 1997), with 29% of those covered by Medicaid (US Health Care Financing Administration, 1997) and 7% of those over 65 and covered by Medicare (US General Accounting Office, 1996).

Many professionals in the provider, patient, policy, and public health communities have expressed concerns about potential negative impacts of managed care. Concerns are expressed that autonomous clinical decisions made by providers are being rejected by cost-conscious, rule-oriented organizations; that managed care organizations will attempt to lower costs by creating barriers to access for necessary services; and that the lower volume and prices for services paid to physicians and hospitals by managed care organizations will reduce their revenue to such an extent that they will be forced to limit the amount of free or below-cost medical care they provide to uninsured or poorly insured populations. However, one aspect of the increasing dominance of the managed care approach to health services delivery has been the source of much optimism: Managed care will raise awareness and increase utilization of health promotion and disease prevention services in health care organizations.

Janet M. Bronstein • Department of Health Care Organization and Policy, School of Public Health, University of Alabama at Birmingham, Birmingham, Alabama 35294.

Handbook of Health Promotion and Disease Prevention, edited by Raczynski and DiClemente. Kluwer Academic/Plenum Publishers, New York, 1999.

Both the American Public Health Association and the Centers for Disease Control and Prevention (CDC) have active task forces examining opportunities for cooperation between managed care organizations and organizations focused on disease prevention and health promotion (*The Nation's Health*, 1997; Harris, Gordon, White, Strange, & Harper 1995). The sense of optimism is expressed in statements such as the following in the *Journal of Occupational and Environmental Medicine*:

> As we stand at the doorway to the twenty-first century, we are witnessing the restructuring of American health care from a fragmented cottage industry to an actual health care system. This new system is emerging from a foundation of managed care and will be built upon the pillars of prevention. (Loeppke, 1995, p. 558)

Will managed care actually deliver on these promises of delivering health promotion and disease prevention programs? The sense of elation so widely expressed about managed care supporting disease prevention and health promotion is in contrast to the many doubts expressed about the impact of the new financing arrangements on other important health care delivery issues. Further, the promise of a health promotion and disease prevention emphasis in managed care highlights sharply the barriers to an orientation on health promotion and disease prevention orientation in the traditional US health care system. This chapter first examines the traditional health care organizational settings for the extent to which disease prevention and health promotion services have been distributed to the population. An understanding of the established structure helps to reveal why these activities are often marginalized within health care organizations and consequently why they are often provided in a less-than-ideal manner to only selected segments of the population at risk.

The chapter then explores the premises of managed care and the reasons why these new organizational forms and financing arrangements are thought to be more conducive to the provision of disease prevention and health promotion services to the population. Finally, the chapter explores the real barriers that face managed care organizations as they attempt to increase the provision of disease prevention and health promotion services. This leads to a discussion of the types of information and the complementary organizational forms that will be required to ensure that increased managed care penetration fulfills its promise to increase the availability and delivery of disease prevention and health promotion to the population.

The Established Health Care System

The professionalization of health care in the United States that took place in the late 19th and early 20th centuries resulted in the rise of the cultural authority of the physician and coincided with a paradigm shift in the understanding of the nature of ill health. The "germ theory" of disease replaced earlier notions that illness was caused by generally negative environments or by the failure of individuals to take actions to preserve their internal healthful balance. Rather, ill health was thought to be caused by specific external agents that indiscriminantly infected those who were exposed. The primary emphasis in health care shifted to activities oriented to cure illnesses, not prevent them. Physicians positioned themselves as the health professionals whose expertise was in curative techniques, and they increasingly replaced midwives, homeopaths, and other health care providers as the care providers of choice for those with resources (Starr, 1982). Even public health professionals began to emphasize examining and curing individual illnesses as the primary approach to improving population health, replacing large-scale sanitation efforts (Fee, 1997).

Physicians developed as the provider of medical services. Physicians prescribe medications, authorize hospital admissions, provide surgical treatments, and authorize the use of physical therapy and other types of treatments. In the United States, the vast majority of physicians have practiced alone or in small groups, essentially comprising thousands of small businesses or a cottage industry. Each physician small business must bear the cost of facilities and support staff in addition to meeting physician salary expectations. Thus, each physician business has substantial revenue requirements in order to remain financially viable.

For financial reasons, these physician small businesses are not geographically distributed in proportion to the medical needs of the population but in proportion to the location of customers most able to purchase their services. Physician density has increased dramatically in the United States as a whole in the past several decades, increasing from 144 per 100,000 population in 1950 to 159 per 100,000 in 1970, and then to 236 per 100,000 by 1990, but physicians have still moved only gradually to more rural areas of the country, while some facilities that supported physician practices in inner-city areas have closed or relocated to more prosperous areas (Anderson, 1995).

The enormous increase in the number of physician businesses operating in the United States has been made possible by the increase in the proportion of the population covered by third-party health insurance. Private health insurance covers 71% of the population, with 90% of those individuals receiving coverage through employment-based plans. Government-sponsored health insurance covers 17% of the population, including nearly all individuals over age 65, all children under age 12 with family incomes below the poverty level, and some low income and disabled adults (Employee Benefits Research Institute, 1996). Because most individuals do not pay personally for health services, they tend not to consider costs when they decide whether to seek services, how many services to use, or which physicians to select for care. Because consumers are not price-sensitive, physician small businesses have not competed with one another based on price and have not concerned themselves with limiting the total costs of the care they provide. Thus, they have avoided the downward pressure on prices that might be expected with the increased availability of service providers. This has enabled more physician small businesses to meet their revenue expectations, but it also has meant that direct medical service prices for consumers without health insurance are high.

Thus, most people without health insurance, along with those whose health insurance is not totally comprehensive, find health care services needed for any serious illness and certainly for any hospitalization basically unaffordable (Blendon et al., 1994). An entire additional secondary structure, often referred to as the health care safety net, has grown up to meet, at least partially, the health care needs of those who cannot afford to purchase services from physician small businesses. The nature of these safety nets varies markedly across communities, but they are dominated for the most part by government-subsidized providers, including federally sponsored community health centers, state-sponsored public health departments, and state- and locally sponsored hospitals (Baxter & Mechanic, 1997).

Because physician offices are not distributed geographically in proportion to the population, because medical services are so personally costly for those without insurance, and because safety nets are so varied in availability and capacity across communities, some important segments of the population have limited access to medical services. Health promotion and disease prevention services distributed through physician offices are similarly unevenly available to the general population and may be least available to the highest-risk populations.

Even those segments of the population with access to medical services may fail to receive disease prevention and health promotion services in these settings. Table 1 compares self-reported rates of receipt of selected screening services for adults with and without health insurance. While it is clear that those with health insurance and with a usual source of care are more likely to use clinical preventive services, the table also shows that disease prevention services are underused, even by individuals with insurance and a usual source of medical care. Underuse of preventive care has been documented in several national studies (Salem, 1995; Davis, Bialek, Parkinson, Smith, & Vellozi, 1990). Physician training, the nature of the doctor–patient relationship, and economic constraints are factors that help to explain this situation.

Many physicians have not been trained in key aspects of preventive care and are not well informed about current recommendations for prevention services (Finocchio *et al.*, 1995). Lack of training in health promotion and disease prevention is related to the general expectation that the physician's role is to provide an immediate effective therapy for the cure of illnesses. The positive impact of preventive and health promotion services is not documented and communicated to clinicians in the same manner as the positive impact of therapeutic techniques. In fact, the multiple guidelines or recommendations for preventive care sometimes conflict with each other, leaving physicians unsure about which services to provide (Bailey & Womeodu, 1996). In addition, the pressure toward specialization, both during medical education and later in practice, encourages physicians to specialize in diagnosing and treating ailments of a specific type; this model of medical care is not particularly supportive of a generalist or comprehensive view of patient health.

Although continuity of care between patients and physicians over long time periods is a cultural ideal within medical practice, the structure of the market for physician services is such that patients can freely choose new physicians at any time for

Table 1. Rates of Receipt of Selected Prevention Services[a]

	With health insurance	Without health insurance
Males, 18–64		
Has usual source of medical care	82%	59%
Had cholesterol level checked in previous 2 years	65%	36%
Had digital rectal exam in previous 2 years	51%	27%
Ever had proctoscopy exam	38%	20%
Females, 18–64		
Has usual source of medical care	90%	82%
Had mammogram and clinical breast exam in previous 2 years	69%	35%
Had digital rectal exam in previous 2 years	51%	29%
Ever had proctoscopy exam	32%	22%

[a]Based on the 1993 Behavioral Risk Factor Surveillance System, a nationally representative telephone survey of adults, as reported by the CDC (Salem, 1995).

any type of health problem. Safety net institutions, in particular, are oriented toward the treatment of immediate acute problems by whatever medical staff is available. They are meant to serve as temporary substitutes for physician business-based care, and thus they have no expectation of maintaining long-term relationships with patients. Because physician–patient relationships in both the physician small business and the safety net sectors are assumed by both parties to be time-limited and problem focused, they provide limited opportunities for early intervention or for long-term preventive counseling and follow-up concerning reducing health risks.

In addition, most physicians, practicing alone or in very small groups with a need to control overhead costs in order to maximize their personal income, elect to not employ health educators, nutritionists, or behavioral specialists who are trained to provide disease prevention and health promotion services. Safety net institutions have greater organizational capacity but also may be reluctant to commit public funds that may vary in amount from year-to-year toward developing capacity in preventive services. Thus, even physicians who are knowledgeable enough and have strong enough relationships with their patients to be able to recommend a health promotion service, such as a smoking cessation program, for example, may be unable to provide or unwilling to directly refer their patients to such a service.

Finally, but probably most significantly, the fee-for-service financing system that supports the traditional US health care system is organized to reimburse physicians for discrete, technical services provided. The more services provided and the more technical the nature of these services, the greater the revenue generated from a physician encounter. Furthermore, most preventive services, even the more technical ones such as screening tests, have generally not been covered by third-party health insurance. From an insurer's point of view, the refusal to cover preventive services is logical. Insurance is designed to collect a pool of money to cover unexpected events such as illness in a population, with the assumption that only some proportion of the covered population will need to use care over a given period of time. Preventive services provided to everyone in a population are a predictable expense; including these services in insurance coverage only raises the price of the premium for everyone in the population. Mandates to provide insurance coverage for preventive services have been resisted both by insurers and employers purchasing insurance on this basis, and organized policy efforts to encourage such coverage, even within the Medicare program, have been lacking (Davis *et al.*, 1990).

Both patients and physicians have grown accustomed over time to having all health services covered by third-party reimbursement. The out-of-pocket costs encountered by patients receiving preventive services and/or the unreimbursed time and resources expended by physicians in providing services that cannot be billed create additional significant barriers to the provision of disease prevention and health promotion services in physician offices. Therapeutic encounters face no such barriers to use, and in terms of revenue generation are a far better use of physician time.

In sum, medical care organizations, as traditionally arranged in the United States, have been very poor settings for the widespread provision of disease prevention and health promotion services. The dominant mode of organization—the physician office practice—is not readily available to all segments of the population and is particularly less available to some of the highest-risk populations. Even within physician practices, preventive services are marginalized. Physicians are not well trained in their provision. They are very limited, both organizationally and economically, in their ability to employ the types of professionals who are trained in the provision of preventive care. The majority of disease prevention and health promotion services are not covered by health insurance, and patient out-of-pocket costs combined with physicians' unreimbursed resource expenditures additionally limit the extent of such care that is available in medical care settings.

The Promise of Managed Care

The historical roots of contemporary managed care lie in the prepaid group practices of the early 20th century. These were industry or community-based contractual arrangements through which physicians were paid a monthly amount per enrolled individual, and they agreed to provide all needed medical care for this payment. These arrangements were fiercely opposed by independent small business physicians and their professional associations, primarily because they allowed payers for a large group of patients to negotiate favorable prices for services. Physicians who participated in prepaid group practices faced social sanctions from the professional community (including threats to licensure), while many states enacted restrictive regulations, such as physician freedom-of-choice rules, that limited the nature of the contracts that could be legally written (Starr, 1982).

The political climate for prepaid health plans began to change in 1970. The amount being paid for medical services, primarily by corporate and government-sponsored health insurance plans, had begun to escalate rapidly. Addressing this issue, but also addressing social concerns about the availability of medical care for those without health insurance, Democratic Senator Edward Kennedy launched a political initiative in support of national health insurance. The Republican Nixon Administration felt forced to respond with an effort that also addressed care access and cost, but which avoided involving the government in a massive social benefit program. With the assistance of Paul Ellwood, a health policy leader with an interest in reforming the established, physician small business health care system, the Administration developed a strategy to support the expansion of private sector prepaid health plans, which Ellwood renamed "health maintenance organizations (HMOs)" (Starr, 1982).

While the effort to promote prepaid health plans was opposed by the American Medical Association, political circumstances of the time limited the profession's ability to block the effort. Some loans were made available for start-up of prepaid organizations in medically underserved areas. HMOs that met certain federal standards were allowed to offer their services to Medicare beneficiaries, and large employers were required to offer them as a health insurance option for employees. While these policy supports were helpful, the young HMO industry probably benefited most from the publicity and the legitimacy conferred by this interest expressed by a conservative, Republican president in the business community (Brown, 1983). Enrollment in HMOs and the various other forms of managed care increased from 2 to 50% of the insured population between 1980 and 1993 (Silverman et al., 1995).

Both the federal government and private employers have been most interested in the managed care alternative, because it promises to stabilize and lower health care costs. However, because the structure that has developed for lowering costs contrasts directly with many of the features of the physician small-business-based health care system described earlier in this chapter, managed care is also more conducive than the traditional system for the provision of disease prevention and health promotion services.

In their original and most comprehensive form, managed care arrangements finance medical care through prepayment or capitation. Under such arrangements, either an organization that employs physicians or the physicians themselves receive a set amount of money in advance for each patient whose medical care they are contracted to provide. All medical care that is determined to be necessary is then provided, with the costs absorbed by the organization or the physicians. The difference between the prepaid amount and the cost of the resources expended is the profit retained by the providers. While providers will lose money on some patients if the costs of meeting their need for care exceed the prepaid amount received, on a population basis they should retain enough money to remain financially viable. The better they are able to control the medical costs of the covered population, the more money the organization or the physicians themselves will make.

Capitation reverses the typical incentives built into the traditional fee-for-service system. Under fee for service, providers benefit financially by providing more services to patients. Under capitation, providers benefit financially by providing fewer services to patients, since that lowers their costs and allows them to retain more of the prepayment as profit.

One way to provide fewer medical services to a population is to prevent the occurrence of diseases. Unlike traditional physician small businesses then, managed care organizations benefit the most if the patients for whom they are contracted to provide care never actually need their services. Thus, under capitated managed care systems, disease prevention and health promotion services take on a direct financial value. To the extent that disease prevention and health promotion services are less costly to provide than therapeutic services, managed care organizations actually benefit financially from substituting preventive for curative services. In contrast to traditional indemnity insurers, most HMOs cover the costs of preventive care (Davis *et al.*, 1990).

Besides reversing the traditional financial disincentives to the provision of preventive services in medical care organizations, managed care arrangements help to facilitate the type of physician–patient relationships that are more conducive to disease prevention and health promotion. First, managed care organizations and their physician contractors know in advance who their patients will be, and thus have the opportunity to provide disease prevention and health promotion services at the point when they can be most effective, before individuals get sick. Second, in order to pay on a capitation basis, to manage costs and to coordinate services, most managed care organizations find it most effective to designate one physician as a "gatekeeper" who reviews and arranges for each patient's care. This gatekeeper physician is usually an internist or a family physician who is trained or at least prepared to provide primary rather than specialty-oriented care, to monitor resource expenditures, to emphasize prevention and early intervention, and to take responsibility for the health status of a whole population, including individuals who are not actively seeking health care (Greenlick, 1995). Patients must receive referrals from these physicians in order to use the services of other providers. Thus, there is a mutual expectation that the managed care physician–patient relationship is oriented toward primary care, proactive and continuous over a period of time. In theory at least, this shared expectation should be more conducive than the traditional, episodic, problem-based approach to the provision of disease prevention and health promotion strategies that work over long periods of time and require continuous monitoring and patient education and counseling.

Because managed care organizations create an intermediate institution between a large group of patients and a large group of physicians, they can compensate for some of the other barriers to the provision of preventive services that are related to the cottage industry structure of the physician small-business-based system. Managed care organizations have the ability to track service use across a whole population. They can identify patients who may be potentially at risk for certain conditions, as well as patients who should receive screening tests, and communicate with them directly, encouraging them to seek preventive care. Managed care organizations can afford to employ or contract with disease prevention and health promotion specialists so that smoking cessation programs, nutrition counseling, and other risk reduction interventions are readily available to the enrollees of managed care plans and to referring physicians. Also, managed care organizations are able to provide contracting physicians with information and advice on the value of preventive services to their patients, compensating for the uneven knowledge and skill that many physicians have in the area of prevention (Morrow, Golding, & Clark, 1995; Solberg *et al.*, 1996).

In fact, because of the contractual relationship between managed care organizations and physicians, these organizations can actually mandate the provision of specified preventive services to their enrolled patients. Thus, they do not have to depend on physicians' uneven knowledge or preferences for providing disease prevention and health promotion care. Managed care organizations are increasingly being encouraged or required to report the rates at which their enrollees receive preventive services such as mammographies, Pap smears, and immunizations. These utilization rates are used to score and compare organizations on the basis of the quality of health care provided to enrollees. This provides a significant incentive for managed care organizations to influence physicians to provide these services to enrollees.

By reversing the financial incentives, altering the expectations and constraints on the patient–physician relationship, making appropriate resources available, and reducing the impact of variable physician and patient knowledge about disease prevention and health promotion, managed care organizations can potentially eliminate many of the barriers toward the provision of disease prevention and health promotion services that characterize the traditional medical care system. Comparisons made since the early 1980s suggest that preventive services tend to be provided more frequently in managed care contexts than in the traditional fee-for-service system (Newhouse, 1993; Bailey & Womeodu, 1996).

Many managed care organizations have encouraged the provision of preventive and health promotion services because it makes good medical and financial sense. In addition, the provision of no-cost preventive and health promotion services to enrollees of managed care organizations has proved to be a sound marketing tactic for these organizations, as they compete with traditional indemnity insurers for enrollees in the workplace (Feldman, Finch, Dowd, & Cassou, 1989). Coverage of prevention services is particularly attractive to healthier enrollees with an orientation toward reducing their risk of illness. To the extent that these individuals disproportionately choose to enroll in managed care organizations rather than competing insurance plans, these organizations will have lower costs of care than their competitors. Lower costs of care enable them to keep their prices for coverage relatively low and enable them to retain more of their prepaid premiums as profits.

Can Managed Care Fulfill the Promise of Providing Health Promotion and Disease Prevention Services?

It is clear why advocates of increased utilization of preventive services are excited about the recent rapid growth of managed care. Not only do many aspects of the managed care approach counteract traditional barriers to the provision of these services, but managed care organizations have several positive incentives to encourage disease prevention and health promotion in their covered populations. However, several caveats concerning the nature of managed care, as it is actually evolving in the United States, temper some of this enthusiasm.

The form of managed care that is spreading most rapidly in the insured population is the form that looks least like the original prepaid group practices or HMOs. Staff-model HMOs, in which physicians are paid a salary while the organization itself takes in a capitation payment for each enrollee and covers the costs of providing care, are the form of managed care that most thoroughly reverse the incentives for providing high-volume curative services which are inherent in the fee-for-service system. As of 1993, staff-model HMOs provided care for only 4% of all managed care enrollees (Silverman *et al.*, 1995). Although they are frequently the most reasonably priced managed care alternative competing for enrollment from employers, they are less popular with enrollees because they restrict people's choice of physicians. Their relative lack of popularity creates pressure on employers who purchase insurance to offer alternative forms of managed care.

More popular forms of managed care are actually contractual arrangements between an insurance entity and a set of independent physician practices. Primary care physicians in these arrangements seldom bear the full risk of capitation, and thus have less incentive to control costs (Hillman, Welch, & Pauly, 1992). More commonly, they are paid fees for services provided, usually at a rate discounted from the fees paid by indemnity insurers, but they receive a financial bonus if the overall costs paid for their assigned patients is less than anticipated by the capitation payment. Specialist physicians providing care for managed care patients on a referral basis are nearly always paid on a fee-for-service basis.

So, most managed care arrangements are still built on the traditional physician small business system, and most physician small businesses participate contractually in multiple managed care arrangements as well as continue to operate a traditional fee-for-service practice. This means that few physicians are fully subject to the reverse incentives of capitation payment across all of their patients. This weakens the impact that capitation has on the treatment of any patients, since it is unreasonable to expect physicians to selectively alter their entire mode of practice, depending on the nature of each patient's insurance. These independent practice arrangements also may limit the extent to which a managed care organization has the infrastructure to support elaborate tracking and protocol systems or employ health promotion–disease prevention specialists who can be used to see patients on physician referral.

The preference of many patients to freely choose providers and to leave the network as they desire in exchange for paying a larger out-of-pocket fee also weakens the expectation that the relationship between gatekeeper physician and patient is all-encompassing and continuous. At the same time, physicians acting as gatekeepers may experience acute time pressures as they take on responsibility for the care of increasing numbers of patients. Lowered revenues from their practice add to the pressure to see as many patients as possible in a short amount of time. New financing arrangements make physicians more aware of the costs of tests and other treatments they provide and may lead to decisions to forego tests and treatments that are not related to immediate therapeutic needs. Thus, the managed care environment, as it is currently playing out in the health care system, may actually create new barriers to the provision of preventive care (Bailey & Womeodu, 1996).

The market for insurance has grown much more price competitive with the entry of a large number of managed care firms into most communities. For the most part, these insurers are competing with each other for contracts with employers to offer services to employees, and then competing again with a smaller number of firms to enroll large numbers of these enrollees. Most employers review their selection of insurance options annually and also allow their employees to change insurers annually. This shortened time horizon reduces the financial value that many disease prevention and health promotion activities have for managed care organizations, because they do not expect to cover enrollees on a long-term basis. Those risk reduction activities that produce health benefits over the lifetime may produce financial savings for subsequent insurers, while representing only a cost to the covering managed care organization.

The whole concept of encouraging investments in disease prevention and health promotion activities primarily because they will reduce by an equivalent or greater amount the costs of treating diseases is a double-edged sword for current preventive practices. Certainly, many screening tests and preventive interventions can save money for high-risk or affected individuals through early disease detection or prevention of adverse health outcomes, but it is extremely difficult to target the appropriate individuals in advance. Interventions applied too broadly, particularly costly interventions such as mammographies, are likely to generate more costs than they save, particularly for relatively small groups of insured individuals over a relatively short time period. Health promotion interventions such as smoking cessation or weight reduction are easier to target to at-risk individuals, but without appropriate administration of the intervention are often not effective in reducing risks. Evaluated economically, these preventive activities also may not be a good financial investment for a managed care company. Thus, while disease prevention and health promotion as concepts have a new financial value under managed care, current preventive practices often do not measure up to cost effectiveness standards (Davis *et al.*, 1990). Unfortunately, the cost pressures that managed care organizations experience as they try to remain financially viable in a competitive marketplace make it difficult for them to promote the provision of services that do not have a clear financial benefit, even when they do have an identifiable potential health benefit (Bailey & Womeodu, 1996).

A final caveat concerns the size and the selective nature of the population segments who are actually affected by managed care. The first section of this chapter noted that the physician small business sector of health care delivery often fails to reach high-risk segments of the population, particularly those who live in rural and inner-city locations and those without health insurance. It was then noted that disease prevention and health promotion services are often marginalized within medical care settings because of the incentives of the fee-for-service system; the expectations and constraints on physician–patient relationships; limited economies of scale for the provision of preventive and health promotion services; and an uneven knowledge base about these services by physicians. The promise of managed care for prevention rests essentially in the reversal of this second set of factors, changing financial incentives, providing better information on prevention protocols, facilitating early access to a population, and promoting comprehensive primary care.

However, an increased value placed on prevention by one set of options available under employer-purchased insurance does not effect the segment of the population with no health insurance. This segment grew from 15.2 to 17.4% of the population between 1988 and 1992 (Employee Benefits Research Institute, 1996). The increased prevalence of managed care does not increase the availability of medical care settings in rural and inner-city areas. In fact, to the extent that increases in managed care contracts create cost pressures on physician small businesses and safety net providers, they become less able to provide any kind of medical services to underserved population segments. Thus, the health promotion and disease prevention benefits that are supposed to flow from the increased participation of the population in managed care organizations will not accrue equally across all population segments and again may remain least available to some of the highest-risk individuals.

What Other Actions Are Needed?

The restructuring of the traditional small business physician system for delivering care clearly provides an opportunity for increasing the availability of disease prevention and health promotion services. Larger organizations with advanced contact with a specific group of people can support specialized disease prevention and health promotion services and can provide tracking and advance contact with individuals before they get sick The reversal of financial incentives so that providers benefit from helping patients stay healthy as much as they benefit from treating them when they are sick, with accompanying revised training for physicians so that they are aware of and committed to the value of providing this care, is also a significant change that will benefit prevention and promotion activities.

To make these promises a reality, it is critically important that the cost-effectiveness of current disease prevention and health promotion practices be documented and wherever possible improved. This means finding ways to accurately target individuals at-risk, rather than making blanket recommendations for the provision of prevention and screening interventions to whole populations. It also means lowering the costs and improving the effectiveness of interventions for meeting specific, health-related goals. As the cost-effectiveness of the interventions themselves improve, the value of disease prevention and health promotion can be communicated more persuasively to the managed care organizations and to the medical and broader health care community. As the practicing health care community becomes more convinced about the value of specific disease prevention and health promotion services, training programs for physicians and other health personnel can respond by preparing graduates for more prevention-oriented care provision.

As encouraging as this scenario may be, managed care is clearly not the panacea that will support the delivery of a wide range of disease prevention and health promotion services to the entire population. Some interventions will only be cost-effective when they are applied to an entire population over many years. Given the current structure of a mixed private and public and competitive insurance market, no insurance arrangement in the foreseeable future is going to cover that many people predictable over that long a time period. Because not all the interventions that are potentially beneficial can be shown to be cost-effective under these constraints, they will not all be paid for or provided within managed care organizations. Furthermore, the benefits of health care delivery restructuring and medical personnel retraining will remain unavailable to those who are distant from or cannot afford to use medical care, except from safety net providers on an acute, episodic basis. There remains a need for a community-based vehicle or set of vehicles, such as public health departments, school systems, and nonprofit community agencies, that can make disease prevention and health promotion services available to the general public outside of medical care organizations. To the extent that managed care organizations, hospitals, and other health care organizations support the provision of prevention and promotion services in community-based settings as well as internally, both by providing resources for community programs and by supporting them in the political arena, the promise of managed care and other health care restructuring trends for increasing the use of these services can be fulfilled (Gordon, Baker, Roper, & Omenn, 1996).

ACKNOWLEDGMENTS. Dr. Michael A. Morrisey provided very helpful background materials for the completion of this chapter.

References

Anderson, O. W. (1995). The health services establishment is becoming an independent variable: A life of its own. *Medical Care Research and Review, 52*(1), 6–33.

Bailey, J. E., & Womeodu, R. J. (1996). Prevention in managed care: Obstacles and opportunities. *Journal of the Tennessee Medical Association, 89*(4), 122–125.

Baxter, R. J., & Mechanic, R. E. (1997). The status of local health care safety nets. *Health Affairs, 16*(4), 7–23.

Blendon, R. J., Donelan, K., Hill, C. A., Carter, V., Beatrice, D., & Altman, D. (1994). Paying medical bills in the United States. Why health insurance isn't enough. *Journal of the American Medical Association, 271*(12), 949–951.

Brown, L. D. (1983). *Politics and health care organization: HMOs as federal policy.* Washington DC: The Brookings Institution.

Davis, K., Bialek, R., Parkinson, M., Smith, J., & Vellozi, C. (1990). Paying for preventive care: Moving the debate forward. *American Journal of Preventive Care, 6*(S2),1–32.

Employee Benefits Research Institute. (1996). Sources of health insurance and characteristics of the uninsured. *EBRI Issues Brief, No. 179.*

Fee, E. (1997). The origins and development of public health in the United States. In R. Detels, W. W. Holland, J. McEwen, & G. S. Omenn (Eds.), *Oxford textbook of public health,* Vol. I. *The scope of public health* (pp. 35–54). New York: Oxford University Press.

Feldman, R., Finch, M., Dowd, B., & Cassou, S. (1989). The demand for employment-based health insurance. *The Journal of Human Resources, 24*(1), 115–142.

Finnochio, L. J., Bailiff, P. J., Grant, R. W., & O'Neil, E. H. (1995). Professional competencies in the changing health care system: Physicians' views on the importance and adequacy of formal training in medical school. *Academic Medicine, 70*(11), 1023–1028.

Greenlick, M. R. (1995). Educating physicians for the twenty-first century. *Academic Medicine, 70*(3), 179–185.

Gordon, R. L., Baker, E. L., Roper, W. L., & Omenn, G. S. (1996). Prevention and the reforming U.S. health care system: Changing roles and responsibilities for public health. *Annual Review of Public Health, 17,* 489–509.

Harris, J. R., Gordon, R. L., White, K. E., Strange, P. V., & Harper, S. M. (1995). Prevention and managed care: Opportunities for managed care organizations, purchasers of health care, and public health agencies. *Morbidity and Mortality Weekly Report, 14,* 1–10.

Hillman, A. L., Welch, W. P., & Pauly, M. V. (1992). Contractual arrangements between HMOs and primary care physicians: Three-tiered HMOs and risk pools. *Medical Care, 30*(2), 136–148.

Jensen, G. E., Morrisey, M. A., Gaffney, S., & Liston, D. K. (1997). The new dominance of managed care: Insurance trends in the 1990s. *Health Affairs, 16*(1), 125–136.

Loeppke, R. R. (1995). Prevention and managed care: The next generation. *Journal of Occupational and Environmental Medicine, 37*(5), 558–562.

Morrow, R. W., Gooding, A. D., & Clark, C. (1995). Improving physicians' preventive health care behavior through peer review and financial incentives. *Archives of Family Medicine, 4*(2), 165–169.

Newhouse, J. P., and the Insurance Experiment Group. (1993). *Free for all? Lessons from the RAND Health Insurance Experiment.* Cambridge: Harvard University Press.

Salem, N. (1995). Health insurance coverage and receipt of preventive health services—United States, 1993. *Journal of the American Medical Association, 273*(14), 1083–1084.

Silverman, C., Anzick, M. Boyce, S., Campbell, S., McDonnell, K., Reilly, A., & Snider, S. (1995). *EBRI databook on employee benefits.* Washington DC: Employee Benefits Research Institute.

Solberg, L. F., Kottke, T. E., Brekke, M. L., Calomeni, C. A., Conn, S. A., & Davidson, G. (1996). Using continuous quality improvement to increase preventive services in clinical practice—Going beyond guidelines. *Preventive Medicine, 25,* 259–267.

Starr, P. (1982). *The social transformation of American medicine.* New York: Basic Books.

The Nation's Health. (1997, May/June). APHA board adopts managed care plan, extends task force. *The Nation's Health, XXVII,* 5, 1.

US General Accounting Office. (1996). *Medicare HMOs. Rapid enrollment growth concentrated in selected states.* GAO/HEHS-96-63. Washington, DC: Government Printing Office.

U.S. Health Care Financing Administration. (1997). National summary of Medicaid managed care programs and enrollment. HCFA.Gov home page, World Wide Web.

CHAPTER *30*

The Role of Governmental Public Health Agencies

Stuart A. Capper

Introduction

It is likely that some form of community-oriented public health practice has existed since the beginning of human communities. Early written records suggest that "community organization" dealt with issues of hygiene, and archeological records that predate recorded history suggest some community orderliness to the basic tasks of daily living. The education of community members in the substance of these practices and the importance of compliance for the sake of the community and self are also rooted in antiquity. The Old Testament contains rules for food handling and preparation as well as consumption practices. Members of biblical communities were continuously educated in these practices. [It should be noted that there is no evidence that the biblical prescriptions on food preparation and consumption were rooted in health concerns. It was 1000 years after the origins of the Old Testament before any reference is made to the possible salutary health effects of these practices (Plaut, Bamberger, & Hallo, 1981).] Clearly, community organization for hygiene and the promotion of hygiene through education coexisted well before the era of modern public health.

The purpose of this chapter is to examine this coexistence today by discussing the role of governmental public health organizations in health promotion activities. Specifically, this chapter will address three subjects: (1) the current structure and functions of the United States public health system as represented by federal, state, and local governmental public health agencies; with an emphasis on (2) the history and current status of health promotion activities conducted by governmental public heath agencies; and (3) the legal basis and ethical framework for health promotion through governmental authority.

Stuart A. Capper • Department of Health Care Organization and Policy, School of Public Health, University of Alabama at Birmingham, Birmingham, Alabama 35294.

Handbook of Health Promotion and Disease Prevention, edited by Raczynski and DiClemente. Kluwer Academic/Plenum Publishers, New York, 1999.

Structure and Functions of the United States Public Health System

This analysis deals with the public health system as government enterprise. Although many consider the "public health system" to go well beyond government organizations, our purpose is to discuss community organization through government and health promotion. Therefore, we will describe the current system in terms of the agencies and organizations that have significant responsibility for public health activity at the federal, state, and local government levels.

Even though we will attempt to limit our discussion to government enterprise, there will be difficulties in confining our sphere of interest. As will be discussed further in this chapter, health departments vary widely in the types of services they provide. While many provide substantial personal therapeutic and preventive health services, others provide little or no individualized service. Some public health agencies provide only population-based prevention interventions, while others provide essentially preventive medicine in the form of individualized screening and risk reduction interventions. Therefore, even though the goal of this chapter is to discuss government roles in population-based health promotion and health education, we will likely stray into the arena of preventive medicine and activities of individual practitioners in health promotion.

Federal Public Health Activity

Although it is relatively easy to identify the agencies at the state and local levels that have responsibility for public health activity, this task is not as straightforward when one considers the federal government. The size and diversity of federal organizations and the numerous constituencies directly affected by public health regulation often have led to a confusing allocation of public health responsibility within several different agencies of the executive branch of government. This lack of organizational focus encompasses the major activities of public health including health promotion. There is no single agency charged with the federal leadership role in health promotion.

Significant public health responsibility exists within agencies such as the Department of Agriculture and the Environmental Protection Agency. However, the Department of Health and Human Services appears to be the federal organization with the most significant involvement in health promotion.

The Department of Health and Human Services (DHHS) was originally established by Congress in 1953 as the Department of Health, Education and Welfare. It has undergone many programmatic changes since that time, one of the most recent and most significant being the removal of the Social Security Administration from DHHS in March 1995. At this time, the Office of the Secretary of Health and Human Services has 12 major program organizations, as shown in Fig. 1. Although it is possible to identify some type of public health activity in each of these program organizations, some of the agencies are much more clearly involved in public health and to varying degrees health promotion than others.

The public health activities undertaken within the DHHS generally fall into the four categories of (1) providing funding for prevention and promotion activities at the state and local levels, (2) conducting research in a broad array of health related areas, (3) conducting data gathering, surveillance activities, and information dissemination on a wide range of health topics, and (4) health-related regulatory activities

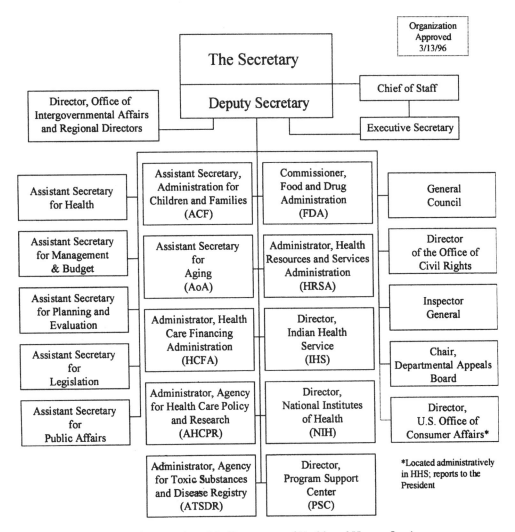

Figure 1. Organization of the Department of Health and Human Services.

(Public Health Service, 1995). What follows are brief examples from several of the 12 DHHS programmatic divisions that were chosen to illustrate the variability in the functions and health promotion activities carried out within DHHS.

In 1980, Congress created the Agency for Toxic Substances and Disease Registry (ATSDR) to implement the health-related sections of laws that protect the public from hazardous wastes and hazardous environmental spills. The Comprehensive Environmental Response, Compensation, and Liability Act of 1980 (CERCLA), commonly known as the "Superfund" Act, provided the Congressional mandate to remove or clean up abandoned and inactive hazardous waste sites and to provide federal assistance in toxic emergencies. ATSDR is charged (1) to assess the presence and nature of health hazards at specific Superfund sites, (2) to help prevent or reduce further exposure and the illnesses that result from such exposures, (3) to expand the knowledge base about health effects from exposure to hazardous substances, (4) to conduct public health assessments at legitimate hazardous waste facilities as requested by the Environmental Protection Agency (EPA), states, or individuals, and (5) to assist EPA in determining which substances should be regulated and the levels at which substances may pose a threat to human health. Clearly, charge number two places this agency firmly in the arena of prevention and health promotion, especially through risk communication. Primarily through its Division of Health Education and Communication, the ASTDR has a variety of health promotion activities. These include newsletters such as "Hazardous Substances and Public Health" and educational case studies on environmental hazards and environmental medicine. Recognizing the importance of its health risk communications the agency has produced an extensive document entitled, "A Primer on Health Risk Communication Principles and Practices," to improve the effectiveness of its promotion activities (Agency for Toxic Substances and Disease Registry, n.d.).

The Centers for Disease Control and Prevention (CDC) describes its programs as preventing unnecessary disease, disability, and premature death and promoting healthy lifestyles. The CDC programs are based on epidemiology, disease surveillance, and laboratory research. Program and research findings are communicated through publications and training to state, local, and international health professionals, public health practitioners and private sector groups. Although the CDC provides little ongoing risk communication or health promotion to individuals, it does provide funding for an extensive program of health promotion and disease prevention research. This agency also provides substantial support and information to state and local public health agencies in their health promotion and health education activities.

The Food and Drug Administration (FDA) is a regulatory agency charged with enforcing the Federal Food, Drug, and Cosmetics Act and several other federal public health laws. It is responsible for the study, regulation, and monitoring of the foods, drugs, cosmetics, and medical devices and the industries that produce them. The FDA regulates over $1 trillion worth of products, which account for 25 cents of every dollar spent annually by American consumers. One of this agency's primary functions is the estimation of risk to the public health from the various products it regulates. The extent of regulation and the regulatory methods employed are based on such estimates. The FDA has extensive consumer information and education activities. One of the most ubiquitous is the FDA's regulation and enforcement of food labeling. Almost any food product one buys now contains basic and consistent nutritional information. The availability of this information to aid individuals in risk reduction activities is a major program of this agency. In 1990, Congress codified the Agency's activities in this area when it passed the Nutrition Labeling and Education Act. This act reaffirmed the FDA's labeling initiatives and set explicit timetables for implementation. These health education activities are now housed in the FDA's Center for Food Safety and Applied Nutrition.

The Administration for Children and Families (ACF) is another of the major organizations under the Secretary of DHHS. The programs within ACF are primarily of a welfare nature and include Child Welfare Services and Aid to Families with Dependent Children (AFDC). The ACF describes its programs as being "at the heart of the Federal effort to strengthen families and give all children a decent chance to succeed" (Administration for Children and Families Homepage, n.d.). In addition to direct cash assistance to families based primarily on need, these programs provide support services such as the Head Start preschool program for children in low income families. The ACF is mentioned in this description of federal level public health activity because of the long-standing role the public health sector has played in reducing risk factors associated with the health of mothers and children. The various social support and direct assistance activities of the ACF are considered by many to be in the public health arena.

There are significant federal programs that attempt to reduce risks to maternal, infant, and child health from a population-based perspective outside of the DHHS. Often, these programs concentrate on proper nutrition as a prevention strategy. Such programs are located in the US Department of Agriculture within its Food, Nutrition, and Consumer Services Division (FNCS). These federal activities are primarily dedicated funding sources for the states to provide nutrition services. The programs include large and well-established activities such as the National School Lunch Program, and the Special Supplemental Food Program for Women, Infants, and Children (WIC). State and local governments administer these programs, and they will be discussed further in a subsequent section of this chapter.

Other agencies within DHHS are less oriented to population-based health promotion and disease prevention activities and more oriented toward individualized therapeutic care. The charge to the Indian Health Service (IHS) has been described as:

> The IHS is charged with providing funding for, or *direct health care services to*, [italics added] Alaskan natives and members of federally qualified Native American Tribes. (Scutchfield & Keck, 1997, p. 323)

Clearly, the IHS focus is health care provided to individuals by practitioners, and is substantially therapeutic in nature. However, this agency provides prevention including health promotion and health education activities, primarily in the context of individualized provision of health care. This demonstrates that the activities of the DHHS go well beyond population-based public health activity. As we stated in the Introduction, the line between population-based public health and individualized preventive medicine is difficult to discern at the level of specific federal agencies. Other program agencies in the DHHS, such as the Health Resources and Services Administration have substantial public health, preventive medicine, and therapeutic activities.

The Environmental Protection Agency (EPA) is an independent agency of the executive branch of the federal government, not within the DHHS, that is primarily public health in its activity. This agency describes its mission in the following way:

> The mission of the U.S. Environmental Protection Agency is to *protect human health* [italics added] and to safeguard the natural environments—air, water, and land—upon which life depends.

Further, the EPA describes its purpose, in part, to be ensuring that:

> All Americans are protected from significant risks to human health and the environment where they live, learn, and work.
> Federal laws protecting human health and the environment are enforced fairly and effectively.
> All parts of society—communities, individuals, state and local governments, tribal governments—have access to accurate information sufficient to effectively participate in managing human health and environmental risks.

In part due to EPA's efforts to reduce risks, communicate risks, and enforce laws, many of the nation's most visible risks from environmental problems have been reduced. Emissions of air pollutants from cars and large industrial facilities have been reduced and, in some cases, like lead emissions from cars, virtually eliminated (Environmental Protection Agency, 1997, p. 16).

Many of the EPA's activities are clearly directed to eliminating or reducing known risks to human health and to using health education methods for such risk reduction. One example of this is in the area of health risks due to exposure to ionizing radiation. The EPA's Radiation Protection Division attempts to identify and evaluate sources of potential radiation exposure and to communicate to the general population the health risks and methods for reducing such risks.

The preceding description of federal public health activities is not a comprehensive delineation of the central government's health promotion programs. Given the extraordinary diversity and dispersion of federal public health activity throughout the various branches of government, this may not be possible at any point in time with any accuracy. For example, we have not discussed any of the extensive public health and health promotion activity undertaken by the Department of Defense. However, the discussion does illustrate the wide-ranging nature of federal attempts to reduce or eliminate risks to the health of the population through health promotion activities. It also illustrates the lack of focus for health promotion at the federal level. No comprehensive evaluation of the effectiveness of federal health promotion programs has ever been undertaken.

State Public Health Activity

Every state and eight US territories have a state health agency (SHA) that is responsible for the administration of public health services within its geographic boundaries. These agencies tend to be independent cabinet-level organizations reporting directly to the governor (64%) or subunits of a state "superagency" for health and welfare. Almost half of the states and the District of Columbia require the head of the SHA to have an MD degree. In 80% of the states, some type of board of health or health council is used for citizen input into the administration of the public health programs of the state. In states with such boards, about half use these bodies in a policy making role (US Department of Health and Human Services, 1991).

The activities of state health agencies are quite varied. While 100% of these organizations are the designated state public health authority, their responsibilities beyond this role are heterogeneous. Table 1 illustrates the heterogeneity of SHA responsibilities.

The relationship between state health agencies and local health agencies also varies among the states. The most common relationships are either decentralized (32%) or a mixture of decentralized and centralized management (34%). Decentralized units are operated directly by local governments such as a county board of supervisors or a city council. In a centralized arrangement, the local health agency reports directly to the state agency or possibly the state board of health. In 20% of the states the system of local health agencies is entirely centralized. In the remaining 14% of the states the jurisdiction over the local health agencies is shared between the state authority and local governments.

A project to delineate how state public health agencies spend their resources was conducted by the Public Health Foundation in 1993 (Public Health Foundation, 1995). The study included data from eight states and attempted to identify core state public health functions and to allocate expenditures within these functional

Table 1. Responsibilities of State Health Agencies[a]

State health agency responsibility	Number of SHAs with this responsibility	Percent of SHAs with this responsibility
State Public Health Authority	51	100
Institutional Licensing Agency	41	80
Institutional Certifying Authority for Federal Reimbursement	40	78
State Agency for Children with Special Health Care Needs	39	77
State Health Planning and Development Agency	22	43
Manager of State Institutions/Hospitals	16	31
Lead Environment Agency for State	15	29
State Professions Licensing Agency	10	20
Medicaid Single State Agency	5	10
State Mental Health Authority	4	8

[a]From US Department of Health and Human Services (1991, p. 7).

areas. One of the ten functional areas was entitled "Public Information and Education and Community Mobilization." This function was defined to include the following programs:

1. Comprehensive school health education
2. Populationwide health promotion/risk reduction programs, including:
   - Injury prevention education and promotion
   - Nutrition education
   - Parenting education
   - Physical activity and fitness
   - Population-based risk reduction programs
   - Seat belts
   - Sexuality education
   - Tobacco use prevention and cessation
3. School campaigns, such as "Say No to Drugs Day"
4. Substance abuse prevention
5. Public education campaigns
6. Work site health promotion

Although there are many definitional and accounting variations from state to state, the study is one of the most rigorous to date in defining and allocating state public health expenditures. The study estimated that 11% of the expenditures on core public health functions in these eight states went to public information, education, and community mobilization.

When extrapolated to the national level, total expenditures on core public health functions by states was estimated to be $11.4 billion in fiscal year (FY) 1993. Hence, this estimate of national expenditures by states for health promotion/health education activities would be approximately $1.25 billion in FY 1993. Of this amount, the study further estimates that 43% of the expenditure is from federal funds and the balance from all other sources.

Although these estimates of health promotion/health education expenditures are conservative and there are such expenditures through other state agencies, these other expenditures are probably not very large. Even if the estimate of $1.25 billion is doubled to include other state and local expenditures, the resultant $2.5 billion expended on health promotion/health education activity by state and local agencies (including the federal contributions) would represent less than three tenths of 1% of total US national health expenditures in 1993 (National Center for Health Statistics, n.d.).

Local Public Health Activity

Variability characterizes the organization and functions of local health departments and is more extensive than that found among SHAs. Depending on which definition one uses, there are between 2850 and 2950 local public health agencies (LPHA) in the United States. The results of a 1992–1993 survey of LPHAs by the National Association of County and City Health Officials (NACCHO) indicates that approximately 44% of LPHAs serve populations of less that 25,000 and nearly 66% of the LPHAs serve populations of less that 50,000 (National Association of County and City Health Officials, 1995).

The scope of activities undertaken by LPHAs appears to be related to the size of the population served. Smaller populations served suggests fewer services from a LPHA, while a large population is likely to be served by an LPHA with a more extensive array of activities. Even public health activities such as Community Outreach and Health Education/Risk Reduction follows this pattern. Table 2 presents data on the percentage of LPHAs that report no activity in Community Outreach and Health Education/Risk Reduction functions by size of jurisdictional population.

Approximately 85% of all LPHAs, regardless of size of population served, reported Community Outreach and Education and Health Education/Risk Reduction activity (either through direct provision or contractual arrangements). This compares with less than 33% of all LPHAs that provided primary care, HIV/AIDS treatment, substance abuse services, radiation control, or occupational safety services (National Association of County and City Health Officials, 1995). A more detailed comparison of local public health activities in health promotion and health education is presented in a later section of this chapter.

The availability of services from local public health agencies is highly variable even within individual states. Table 3 displays data from one state as reported to NACCHO in a 1989 study concerning personal health services provided by LPHAs in that state. All of the local public health agencies in this state provide aids testing, im-

Table 2. Percent of LPHA Reporting No Community Outreach and Education Activity by Population Size Served[a]

Function	Jurisdiction population				
	0 to 24,000	25,000 to 49,000	50,000 to 99,999	100,000 to 499,999	500,000+
No community outreach/education	21%	14%	7%	5%	1%

[a] National Association of County and City Health Officials (1995).

Table 3. Number and Percent of LPHAs Providing a Personal Health Service
an Example from One State

Personal health service provided	Number and percent of LPHAs providing the service in state
1. AIDS testing and counseling	39 (100.0%)
2. Alcohol abuse	2 (5.1%)
3. Child health	38 (97.4%)
4. Chronic diseases	28 (71.8%)
5. Dental health	2 (30.8%)
6. Drug abuse	2 (5.1%)
7. Emergency medical service	1 (2.6%)
8. Family planning	39 (100.0%)
9. Handicapped children	3 (7.7%)
10. Home health care	38 (97.4%)
11. Hospitals	1 (2.6%)
12. Immunizations	39 (100.0%)
13. Laboratory services	19 (48.7%)
14. Long-term care facilities	10 (25.6%)
15. Mental health	2 (5.1%)
16. Obstetrical care	19 (48.7%)
17. Prenatal care	36 (92.3%)
18. Primary care	22 (56.4%)
19. Sexually transmitted diseases	38 (97.4%)
20. Tuberculosis	39 (100.0%)
21. WIC	38 (97.4%)

munizations, TB control, and some family planning services. However, only two local agencies provide drug or alcohol abuse services (CDC, 1991).

Summary

Federal health promotion and disease prevention activity is characterized organizationally by a dispersed, overlapping, and confusing allocation of responsibility among federal agencies. There are also frequent organizational changes. In theory, a federally coordinated effort for population-based preventive interventions should ensure a nationwide availability of these services. The reality at the state and local level is different. Organizational variation within state public health authorities and variation in the organizational relationships between state and local public health agencies reflects significant differences in local perceptions. Local governments and agencies differ markedly in perceptions of the appropriate mix of public health activity, and hence, create substantive differences in the availability of health promotion and health education activity in local communities.

A Brief History of Government Involvement in Health Promotion

As mentioned in the introduction to this chapter, communities, community organization, and hygiene have been intertwined in some manner as far back in history as one can perceive. Clearly, the Old Testament in the chapter Leviticus deals with defilement, uncleanness, and isolation from the community to prevent the spread of contamination. Many scholars considered biblical contamination to be contamination for ritualistic purposes and not for medical or health promotion reasons. However, it is clear that these biblical writing, no matter their original purpose, did become the basis for some very early forms of community health promotion and health education.

An example of the biblical origins of some public health promotion activities can be found in the emergence of quarantine for Hansen's disease. A skin condition designated as *tzara'at* in Leviticus is a reason prescribed for isolation. *Tzara'at* is rendered in Greek translations of the Old Testament as "lepra," meaning, "a scaly condition." This word passed into modern usage via Latin translations and during the Middle Ages was used to identify the disease we now call Hansen's disease or leprosy. In an attempt to combat leprosy in 583, the Church adopted the precepts delineated in Leviticus and restricted association with lepers.

These methods of isolation or "quarantine" were refined and expanded. Communities developed leprosaria, or leper houses for isolation. Lepers were considered a public menace and were expelled from the community to protect healthy citizens. For a community to decide that someone was suffering from leprosy was not a simple matter. Other skin conditions looked similar and no scientific basis for causation was known. A community council of clerics and other citizens was often used to make the significant decision to declare a person a leper and remove them from the community. Essentially, a community decision was made to take a public health measure. For public health reasons, the person was deprived of his or her citizenship. The reasons for taking such steps and the methods to be used were taught through the educational resources of the times, namely, church teachings based on biblical writings. Hence, examples of protection of the public's health through community organization and education date back over 1000 years.

Unless otherwise noted, the discussion of the history of health education in the United States that follows draws on two sources: Pickett and Hanlon's (1990) *Public Health Administration and Practice* and the remarkable *History of Public Health* (1993).

In the United States, health education as a governmental public health activity has much the same beginning as many other governmental actions. It was an adaptation of successful private enterprise that private markets would not continue. Milk distribution centers were a late 19th-century and early 20th-century response to very high rates of infant mortality. The lack of clean cow's milk for mothers who could not breast-feed was recognized as a major contributor to infant deaths. Voluntary action in New York (based on European models) led to the establishment of a system of "milk stations" in the early 1890s. The success of this milk distribution activity led to a governmental response. Similar programs were started under the auspices of the public health department in 1897.

In addition to milk distribution, these centers provided educational interventions to teach mothers sanitary feeding techniques. These were some of the earliest efforts at well-child services provided through governmental public health efforts. Health education for well-child care was a key component of these interventions. It was recognized by the public health community that providing the milk was a way of coming in contact with the mother to teach proper child care.

The success of educational interventions was quickly documented by public health practitioners. In 1908, a public health physician named Josephine Baker intervened in a congested section of the lower East Side of New York with an educational program for mothers of newborns. They were taught how to keep their baby well. After a 2-month intervention, a comparison of death records with the same period 1 year prior showed 1200 fewer deaths in this area during the period of the intervention.

In 1908, the New York City Health Department established the first Division of Child Hygiene. Within a very few years, health education was beginning to differentiate from child health and other public health concerns such as communicable disease control. Health education was developing as a fundamental public health discipline. Organizational recognition within state and local health departments was soon evident. In 1914, the New York City Health Department was the first official health agency to organize a bureau for health education. During the same year a state-level health education bureau was created at the New York State Department of Health. Within the next 15 years, full-time governmental public health positions with titles such as "Director of Health Education" were beginning to emerge.

In 1922, there were enough workers in the field of health education to establish a separate section within the American Public Health Association. However, only a small proportion of these individuals were full-time health educators, and the number of workers in this field grew slowly over the next 20 years. In 1942, an American Public Health Association survey documented only 13 states with a total of 44 workers identified as health educators.

Regardless of the number of public health practitioners devoting full time to health education, this function has been explicitly recognized as fundamental to local public health agency work in the earliest documentation of public health functions in the United States. By the 1920s, local health departments were developing in most larger municipalities. However, there was no information on what the state and local agencies were doing and there was some feeling that there was little logic to their activities. Beginning in the 1920s, a Committee on Administrative Practice of the American Public Health Association began a series of studies to learn about local and state agency functions and to define a mission for official public health agencies. A report of this group, published in 1933, listed two primary goals for public health agencies and four essential aids in pursuing these goals. Among the four essential aids was public health education (Jekel, 1991).

World War II may have provided some of the impetus for increasing demand for professional health educators. The need for a healthy fighting force brought attention to the prevention of communicable diseases and the importance of education as a means to control disease spread. In 1943, schools of public health began to establish programs to train health educators. By 1947, 460 people were employed by governmental and voluntary health agencies as health educators.

Current and accurate figures for employment by federal, state, and local public health agencies in the field of health education are not available. A 1992 publication from the Public Health Foundation using 1989 data indicated less than 1000 health educators employed in noninstitutional professional or technical positions by all state health agencies in the United States (Public Health Foundation, 1992). Pickett and Hanlon (1990), using a 1973 source, reported 25,000 individuals employed in some aspect of health education in the United States. However, they were quick to point out that this figure appeared to be based on some type of organizational affiliation rather than on any type of training and qualifications.

Today, in spite of the difficulty in counting employed health educators, health education in its various forms is perceived to be among the most widely practiced of all public health activities. Even the smallest of local health departments overwhelmingly report they conduct such activity. Table 4 presents information on local public health department activities from a recent National Association of County and City Health Officials survey (National Association of County and City Health Officials, 1995, pp. 78–86). It is useful to note that even the health departments serving the smallest populations report that their personnel provide health education services and that they rarely contract out the provision of such activity. Nearly all local health departments serving larger populations report providing health education activities. This is very different from the case for high blood pressure services where approximately 15 to 20% of local health departments report no activity regardless of the size of the population they serve.

Table 4. Selected Local Health Department Activities

Selected services from local health departments serving populations	Percent directly providing service	Percent contract for service	Percent not providing service
Less than 25,000			
Community outreach and education	73	6	21
Health education/risk reduction	73	5	22
Well child clinic	65	8	27
WIC	61	12	27
Diabetes	56	7	37
High blood pressure	78	8	14
25,000 to 49,999			
Community outreach and education	81	5	14
Health education/risk reduction	91	5	4
Well child clinic	69	9	22
WIC	66	10	24
Diabetes	58	4	38
High blood pressure	82	4	14
50,000 to 99,999			
Community outreach and education	91	2	7
Health education/risk reduction	89	2	9
Well child clinic	80	5	15
WIC	71	12	17
Diabetes	50	6	44
High blood pressure	80	3	17
100,000 to 499,999			
Community outreach and education	92	3	5
Health education/risk reduction	93	2	5
Well child clinic	88	4	8
WIC	80	8	12
Diabetes	52	5	43
High blood pressure	78	3	19
500,000 and above			
Community outreach and education	96	3	1
Health education/risk reduction	99	1	0
Well child clinic	93	1	6
WIC	89	4	7
Diabetes	66	1	33
High blood pressure	77	5	18

Summary

Community-oriented approaches to health promotion and health education are one of the oldest of governmental endeavors. From the earliest efforts at official governmental organization for public health, health promotion and health education have been recognized and conducted activities. Although definitions are inconsistently applied and reporting is poor, it appears that within the United States today nearly all public health agencies undertake to provide some type of health promotion service.

The Legal and Ethical Basis for Governmental Health Promotion Practice

Clearly, federal agencies, state health agencies, and local health departments are involved in the activities of health promotion, health education, and risk reduction. The purpose of these activities is to change the behavior of individuals in ways that will protect or improve their health or the health of their families, and hence improve the overall health status of the community. While federal agencies, through organizations like the Indian Health Service, may undertake health promotion activities directly with individual citizens, the major federal activity is in the arenas of developing information, disseminating information, regulating businesses, and funding health promotion activities of states and local governments. Governmental activities to directly modify individual behavior are primarily undertaken by state and local public health agencies. The purpose of this section is to consider the legal basis on which state and local governments undertake such activity. Also, current debates on ethical issues in the governmental provision of health promotion services will be briefly discussed.

In order to understand the legal basis for state government health promotion activity and the extent of state authority in this area, one needs to consider the basis on which our governments were established. State governments preceded the federal government. The states came together in a convention and formed a constitutionally defined federal government in 1789. Thus, the states are the primary source of federal governmental authority. The federal government only has that authority ceded to it by the states in the United States Constitution. The states were cautious when they ceded power to a central government, and they specifically enumerated those powers in the constitution. Further, they codified this principle in the Tenth Amendment to the Constitution as follows: "The powers not delegated to the United States by the Constitution nor prohibited by it to the States, are reserved to the States respectively, or to the people."

The states also guaranteed certain rights to individual citizens through the federal and state constitutions. These rights also are specifically codified. Therefore, any authority that is not ceded to the federal government nor abridged by rights guaranteed to individual citizens is within the powers of the states to govern. Such authority is collectively referred to as "the police powers of the states."

There is a fundamental difference between the enumerated powers of the federal government, the constitutionally guaranteed rights of individuals, and the police powers of the states. In the case of the federal government or individuals, their authority or rights are circumscribed. There are limits to federal authority and limits to individual rights. The limits to the police powers of the states are less clearly defined. When the states undertake activities to modify individual behavior, they may undertake any such activity that does not interfere with delegated federal authority or infringe on constitutionally guaranteed individual rights. Agencies of the state government, such as state and local health departments, have broad and powerful authority to undertake activities to modify individual behavior.

The extent of this power is best understood by considering some of the legal challenges that have been brought by individuals when the states have exercised the authority to modify personal behavior. One of the most widely cited cases that illustrates the extent of state powers to modify behavior is *Jacobson v. Massachusetts*, 197 US 11 (1905).

The State of Massachusetts had a statute that required each adult to receive a smallpox vaccination. The stature prescribed certain penalties, up to and including criminal penalties, if any individual did not comply. As he asserted in his presentation to the court, Mr. Jacobson believed the following:

> (This law is) hostile to the inherent right of every freeman to care for his own body and health in such a way as to him seems best; and that the execution of such a law against one who objects to vaccination, no matter for what reason, is nothing short of an assault upon his person. (Wing, 1994, p. 24)

The courts did not agree. The decision of the United States Supreme Court is often cited as one of the clearest summaries of the extent of the states police powers in matters relating to the public's health:

> The authority of the State to enact this statute is to be referred to what is commonly called the police power—a power which the State did not surrender when becoming a member of the Union under the Constitution. Although this court has refrained from any attempt to define the limits of that power, yet it has distinctly recognized the authority of the State to enact quarantine laws and "health laws of every description"; indeed, all laws that relate to matters completely within its territory and which do not by their necessary operation affect the people of other States. According to settled principles the police power of the State must be held to embrace at least, such reasonable regulations established directly by legislative enactment as will protect the public health and the public safety. . . . The mode or manner in which those results are to be accomplished is within the discretion of the State, subject, of course so far as Federal power is concerned, only to the conditions that no rule prescribed by a State, nor any regulation adopted by a local government agency acting under the sanction of state legislation, shall contravene the Constitution of the United States or infringe any right granted or secured by that instrument. (Wing, 1995, pp. 24–25)

Although the courts have consistently upheld the states powers to infringe on individual freedoms and, in fact, coerce behavior where the health and safety of populations is at risk, the court's position on coercing individual behavior where the risks are only to the individual is less clear. The courts have suggested that truly "paternalistic" laws may be held to a different standard.

We may not think of health promotion and health education activities as coercive. However, states have resorted to coercive legislation to change individual behaviors even where the risks are only to the individual. Motorcycle helmet laws are one common example of such legislatively mandated behavioral change interventions.

For health promotion and health education as a profession, the more important issue may not be what the courts decide about the use of the states police powers to coerce behavioral change, but rather the resolution of the ethical debate that is ongoing about the appropriate role of government, especially the states, in the provision of health promotion and health education services. There are two central questions that can be delineated within this debate. First, given the enormous power, both legal and financial, of a state, which individual behaviors, if any, should governmental authority and resources seek to modify? Second, which methods are appropriate to employ to produce such behavioral change?

One of the ethical debates about methods raises a series of questions related to the methodological distinction between education and propaganda. The ethics of providing education to allow a better informed individual the opportunity to accurately evaluate risks, and hence assume more healthful behaviors, is rarely questioned. So long as those not assuming the more healthful behavior are not penalized by the state, there is little that is "ethically" questionable in the provision of the service. The ethical issue arises when the health educator presents an intervention with information that is perceived to be from only one side of an issue. Education on only one side of an issue is propaganda (Cole, 1995). Should the state use its power and resources, even with laudable scientific intent, to present a biased educational intervention to an individual? How much discretion do we have as a government to choose the behaviors our citizens should assume and actively attempt to modify individual behavior to conform to our scientific concepts? Can we structure effective behavioral interventions and still present information that all participants in the public policy debates will considered balanced?

Conclusion

The involvement of government in the provision of health promotion and health education services has a long and rich tradition. Public health agencies at all governmental levels are actively involved today in this work. However, we have neither a clear federal focus for the work of health promotion and health education nor a consistent set of services available to all communities through state and local government agencies. States do have the power to intervene to modify individual behavior where the health of the public is at risk. However, the behaviors governmental agencies seek to modify and the methods they choose to employ to achieve such modification are likely to continue to be the subject of litigation and public policy debate.

References

Administration for Children and Families Homepage. (n.d.). http://www.acf.dhhs.gov.
Agency for Toxic Substances and Disease Registry. (n.d.). A primer on health risk communication principles and practices, www Page: atsdr1.atsdr.cdc.gov.8080/HEC/primer.html.
Centers for Disease Control (CDC). (1991). *Profile of state and territorial public health systems: United States, 1990*. Atlanta, GA: Public Health Practice Programs Office, Public Health Service.
Cole, P. (1995). The moral bases for public health interventions. *Epidemiology, 6*(1), 78–83.
Environmental Protection Agency. (1997). *EPA strategic plan*. Washington, DC: US EPA.
Jekel, J. F. (1991). Health departments in the U.S. 1920–1988: Statements of mission with special reference to the role of C.E.A. Winslow. *The Yale Journal of Biology and Medicine, 64*, 467–479.
National Association of County and City Health Officials. (1995). 1992–1993 national profile of local health departments. Washington, DC: NACCHO.

National Center for Health Statistics, DHHS. (n.d.). Health United States 1996–97 (Table 122, p. 259). Hyattsville, MD: DHHS.

Pickett, G., & Hanlon, J. (1990). *Public health administration and practice* (9th ed.). St. Louis: Times Mirror/Mosby College Publishing.

Plaut, W. G., Bamberger, B. J., & Hallo, W. W. (1981). *The Torah, a modern commentary*, New York: Union of American Hebrew Congregations.

Public Health Foundation. (1992, April). State health agency staff, 1989. HRA 240-89-0032. Washington, DC: Public Health Foundation.

Public Health Foundation. (1995). Measuring state expenditures for core public health functions. *American Journal of Preventive Medicine, 11*(6) (Suppl.), 58–73.

Public Health Service. (1995). World wide web home page, updated 5/9/95, Alan Smith.

Rosen, G. (1993). *A history of public health* (expanded edition). Baltimore, MD: The Johns Hopkins University Press.

Scutchfield, F. D., & Keck, C. W. (1997). *Principles of public health practice.* Albany, NY: Delmar Publishers.

Wing, K. R. (1995). *The law and the public's health* (4th ed.). Ann Arbor, MI: Health Administration Press.

CHAPTER 31

Determining the Cost-Effectiveness of Health Promotion Programs

Eli Capilouto

Introduction

Today, new forms of organizing and delivering health care services are emerging. Managed care arrangements are creating more focus on the cost and consequences of health care services. Under many of these managed care plans, providers receive fixed capitated payments regardless of the magnitude of services consumed. The provider assumes more financial risk and is likely to pay greater attention to the costs and benefits of care in this financing arrangement. The managed care movement is creating more emphasis on populations. These populations can be defined by membership in a particular insured group or by membership in a group at risk for a certain disease. In either case, many contend that providers of care will have more incentive to move beyond the delivery of care at the time of illness to more proactive prevention and health promotion programs for these populations. If so, the costs, savings, and health consequences must be measured and compared to alternative interventions.

In a world of limited resources, providers and insurers cannot indiscriminately adopt health promotion programs. The public and elected officials are prone to follow the simple logic of "an ounce of prevention is worth a pound of cure." If only we used more preventive services, fewer people would become ill and require medical services, and consequently health care costs would decrease. Nonetheless, the literature shows that many current preventive programs do not pay for themselves (Leutwyler, 1995) when the program costs are stacked up against the financial benefits of the averted disease. Even so, the program may still be worth doing if the health benefit in the form of extended life or improved quality of life is meaningful or if the program can be done better. Cost analyses of these programs more explicitly reveal the costs and consequences and their inherent trade-offs. Moreover, they can reveal how im-

Eli Capilouto • Department of Health Care Organization and Policy, School of Public Health, UAB Center for Health Promotion, University of Alabama at Birmingham, Birmingham, Alabama 35294.

Handbook of Health Promotion and Disease Prevention, edited by Raczynski and DiClemente. Kluwer Academic/Plenum Publishers, New York, 1999.

provements in effectiveness or changes in the way the program is carried out can make them more attractive. Today's health promotion expert cannot disregard these issues or the methods used to conduct these studies.

This chapter reviews the fundamentals of the methodological approaches to conduct cost-benefit analyses of health care programs or interventions. Basic terminology, measurement of health outcomes, and steps for conducting the analysis are reviewed.

Definitions of Analyses and Use of Terms

Economic evaluations of health care programs compare the cost and outcome of some program to an alternative to determine if it is worth doing. Today's systematic analyses include cost-benefit, cost-effectiveness, and cost-utility analyses. What are the differences in these analyses and when should they be used?

These three types of analyses differ in the way the health benefit is measured. In a cost-benefit analysis, the clinical outcome is measured according to a monetary value. A cost-effectiveness analysis reports health benefits in terms of a clinical, physiological, or effectiveness measures such as lives saved, years of life saved, or cases detected or prevented. The cost-utility analysis, often referred to as a subgroup of cost-effectiveness analysis, is used when the quantity and quality of the lives or life years saved are taken into consideration. In these analyses, preferences are assigned to the health states and reported in such terms as quality-adjusted lives or quality-adjusted-life-years. This is appropriate, for instance, when morbidity is a significant factor. In all of these analyses, the alternative programs being compared measure the resource costs of the programs in monetary terms. Table 1 presents a summary of the characteristics of the three types of studies and the calculation necessary for comparison of alternative programs.

Cost-Benefit Analyses

The conceptual appeal of cost-benefit analysis (CBA) lies in its offer of a common denominator, as all outcomes are measured in dollars. This makes it possible to compare very disparate programs. Respective programs to reduce dental caries, disability days, and mortality can be compared to one another in terms of their respective net benefits. The decision rule is simple. If one were to evaluate a new program to reduce mortality from hypertension, the benefits (in dollars) of the new program would be compared to the benefits (in dollars) of the alternative program or status quo. The net costs of these two alternatives also would be measured in dollars. If the new program produced positive net benefits over the cost of the alternative program, it would be adopted. What does one do if one must choose among several health promotion programs? For disparate programs that address different health care problems, the decision maker adopts all programs that maximize the excess of benefits over costs (Mishan, 1982).

While conceptually appealing, the bane of the CBA rest in determining values for the veritable number of outcomes. How does one value an averted disability day, a life saved, or a pain-free day? Herein lies the major disadvantage of a CBA, the necessity to quantify health outcomes in terms of monetary values.

Table 1. Summary of Characteristics of Economic Analyses of Health Programs

Type of analysis	Cost measure	Health consequences	Measure of health consequence	Calculation for comparison of alternative programs[a]
Cost-benefit	$	Single or multiple effects that may not be common to all interventions and that may be achieved to different degrees by alternative interventions	$	$(B_0-B_1) - (C_0-C_1)$
Cost-effectiveness	$	Single effect common to all alternatives but achieved to different degrees	Natural units (e.g., mg of cholesterol, life-years, disability days)	$(C_0-C_1)/(E_0-E_1)$
Cost-utility	$	Single or multiple effects that may not be common to all interventions and that may be achieved to different degrees by alternative interventions	Healthy life years (e.g., quality-adjusted life-year, or QALY)	$(C_0-C_1)/(QALY_0-QALY_1)$

[a] Subscripts indicate alternative interventions or programs; "B" represents health benefits measured in dollars; "C" represents costs of alternative programs measured in dollars; "E" represents health effectiveness measured in natural units.

The are two primary methods for assessing health benefits in monetary terms for the CBA. The "human capital method" values a therapy, intervention, or health program according to its impact on an individual's lifetime earnings. If a health promotion activity extends the life of someone at high risk for heart disease from 60 to 70 years, then the health benefit is equivalent to the expected earnings of that individual over the period of extended life. While seemingly easy to calculate, many analysts point out that it inherently introduces bias in certain programs. These may include programs that target mostly lesser paid groups (elderly, minorities, women, children) or individuals for whom market wage rates may not discern the values placed upon these roles (e.g., using domestic workers' pay for working-at-home fathers or mothers).

An alternative approach to assigning monetary values on health benefits is the "willingness to pay method," which can directly or indirectly determine values on these health benefits. People are asked directly through a questionnaire or personal survey how much they are willing to pay or how much the government should pay to avoid or reduce the risk of a particular health outcome. Examples of this direct approach are the evaluation of values of life-saving effects created by the availability of mobile coronary care units (Acton, 1973), reduction in arthritic morbidity (Thompson, 1986), and treatments for hypertension (Johannesson, Jonsson, & Borgquist, 1991). Through these hypothetical trade-offs between health and money, the analyst is able to derive a value for a disability-free year of life, a life itself, or an intervention. Willingness-to-pay values can be derived directly from market data. Though seldom used in the medical domain, willingness-to-pay values have been used in product safety and public investment studies (Viscusi, 1979; Olson, 1981; Moore & Viscusi, 1988). In these studies, researchers used wage premiums necessary to induce individuals to work in risky occupations or examined what people did pay for safety devices (e.g., smoke detectors, seat belts). In these cases, the marginal reduction in mortality rates can be applied to the revealed preference of the wage premium or the price of the safety device to derive explicitly the monetary value of extending life.

Pauly (1995) has explored the many criticisms of the direct and indirect approaches to willingness to pay. Many contend that the hypothetical trade-offs in the direct approach are not valid, because we do not know whether people would be willing to pay what they say or whether their answers are positively correlated with wealth. The market-based approach has caveats as well, as markets sometimes do not provide complete information to consumers or by the difficulties encountered in calculating separate estimates of the market value of risk of mortality and morbidity associated with certain jobs and their corresponding wage premiums. Pauly (1995) points out that many conceptual objections to the technique are invalid and advances many ideas to overcome concerns about obtaining valid monetary measures. Even so, the public is most uncomfortable with valuing life in monetary terms. Hence, cost-effectiveness analyses, which measure benefits in the form of a physiological measure, are typically used in analyses of health care interventions.

Cost-Effective Analyses

Cost-effectiveness analysis (CEA) is used to compare several alternative strategies whose health benefits can be measured in a single, common effect which may differ in magnitude (Drummond, Stoddart, & Torrance, 1987). Hence, several alternative approaches to detect a case can be compared in terms of cost per additional case detected for each strategy. For illustration, Table 2 presents the results of a hypothetical CEA of different screening strategies for a particular cancer. [While the data in Table 2 are hypothetical, they do illustrate what is often observed in strategies that become increasingly expensive and yield decreasing incremental gains in health outcomes (Eddy, 1990).] The final column reports a cost-effectiveness ratio, a measure of the incremental change in costs and health effects of one strategy compared with a previous less costly and less effective strategy. Table 2 illustrates, as expected, that life expectancy and costs increase as the intervals between screenings decrease. The incremental costs (cost per additional year of life gained in comparison to the previous strategy) also increase such that an annual screening strategy costs over a $250,000 per additional life year saved (versus screening every 3 years), while an incremental cost of $10,000 for a screening strategy of every 4 years (versus no screening). But, which strategy should one choose? What are the accepted dollar trade-offs for years of life or other health outcomes? Unlike the CBA, no simple criterion exists. Which strategy is "cost-effective"? In the face of this dilemma, it is advised that results of these studies should be reported in a flexible format: "If one is willing to spend ____ dollars per year of life gained, then the most cost-effective strategy is ____" (Doubilet, Weinstein, & McNeil, 1986). A well-endowed society or health care system may choose the annual screening while the less expensive screening strategies may be the choice in financially constrained situations.

Table 2. Estimated Cost-Effectiveness of Different Screening Interval for Hypothetical Cancer Screening for an Average Risk Asymptomatic Cohort

Screening interval	Net costs ($1,000)	Increase in life expectancy (years)	Cost-effectiveness ratio – incremental cost ($) per year of life expectancy gained
No screening	0	0	—
Every 4 years	150	15	10,000[a]
Every 3 years	350	25	20,000[b]
Every 2 years	500	30	30,000[c]
Every year	1,000	32	250,000[d]

[a] Compared with no screening.
[b] Compared with screening every 4 years.
[c] Compared with screening every 3 years.
[d] Compared with screening every 2 years.

Comparisons across diseases can be made as well if the analyses share a single, common effect such as life-years saved. Therefore, programs to save lives from early detection of breast cancer can be compared to programs to save lives through early detection of prostate cancer. A recent investigation reported the cost-effectiveness of 500 life-saving interventions (Tengs *et al.*, 1995). A sample of these analyses are presented in Table 3. The incremental costs per life-year ranges from $\leq$$0 (i.e., a cost-saving strategy) to $34 billion. An intervention that results in a cost savings (e.g., smoking cessation for pregnant women—Table 3) certainly should be adopted. Conversely, programs that cost money and worsen health should be dropped. On the other hand, society or a health care system must confront the question of "what is an acceptable cost per life year?" in those cases where the costs and health benefits are positive.

Weinstein (1995) observes six approaches to arriving at a reasonable cost-effectiveness criterion. He further notes that consensus on their relative roles in decision making is evolving. Complete discussion of these approaches is beyond the scope of this chapter. However, through an example, the problematic nature underlying many of these approaches is revealed. Consider a health maintenance organization (HMO)

Table 3. Life-Saving Interventions and Their Cost-Effectiveness[a]

Life-saving intervention	Cost per life-year[b]
Smoking cessation advice for pregnant women who smoke	$\leq$$0
Pneumonia vaccination for people age 65+	$2,200
Nicotine gum (vs. No gum) and smoking cessation advice for women aged 65–69	$13,000
Colonoscopy for colorectal cancer screening for people age 40+	$90,000
Heart transplantation for patients under age 50 with terminal heart disease	$100,000
Pneumonia vaccination for children aged 2–4	$170,000
Annual mammography (vs. Current screening practices) for women aged 40–49	$190,000
Sickle cell screening for nonblack low-risk newborns	$34 billion

[a] When intervention is compared to a baseline of "the status quo" or "do nothing," the baseline strategy is omitted. Other baseline interventions appear as "(vs.   )."
[b] All costs are in 1993 dollars.

contemplating implementation of the eight interventions in Table 3. This, of course, strongly assumes that the studies listed in Table 3 are generalizable to the HMO population. If the organization values the health benefits (life-years) equally across all groups, then it would implement interventions in Table 3 beginning with the lowest cost per life-year ratio until it meets its budget constraint. Imagine that each of the interventions in Table 3 costs $1 million to implement. With a budget constraint of $3 million, the HMO would adopt the following interventions: smoking cessation advice for pregnant smokers (a costless intervention), pneumonia vaccination for people age 65+, nicotine gum and smoking cessation advice for women aged 65–69, and colonoscopy for colorectal cancer for people aged 40+. Following such a decision rule means that funds are not available for another group of patients or persons in the HMO's population of insured lives that would be affected by the remaining four programs. These distributional issues make it difficult to adopt such a strict cost-effectiveness paradigm.

Detsky and Naglie (1990) point out that many factors may influence the relative values placed on saving life-years. Programs to help children can be more attractive than those targeting other population segments. The heart transplantation program listed in Table 3 may be difficult for the HMO not to implement, because its beneficiaries are highly identifiable compared to programs where recipients are not identified (e.g., many prevention programs). The mission of the organization may influence these decisions. An organization that sees itself as a provider for an underprivilidged segment of the population may focus on raising the health status of this group rather than making marginal improvements in a group that enjoys relatively good health. In contrast, an HMO that sees value in being recognized as a provider of high-tech tertiary care may see advantages to transplant or other sophisticated services. Finally, political and legal factors cannot be discounted. All these factors run counter to the dictates of health maximizing (as measured in life-years in this example) of the strict cost-effectiveness paradigm. Nonetheless, decisions that do not follow this maxim may be rational, as they satisfy other organizational or societal objectives.

Most often, the results of studies such as those in Table 3 are applied in situations where the budget constraint is not as explicit. This is typically the case in decisions at the "societal' level where government or a professional group must approve new drugs, technologies, or treatment guidelines (Weinstein, 1995). While the decision maker must consider cost, there is no specific cost-effectiveness threshold or budget constraint. In this situation, benchmarks are used to guide recommendations. The decision maker can compare the cost-effectiveness ratio for the new interventions against others that have been adopted. This can be most useful in situations where the cost-effectiveness ratio of the new intervention is lower than or much higher than well-accepted interventions. The first four interventions in Table 3 fall within the ranges for well-accepted programs, while the last program (sickle cell screening for nonblack low-risk newborns) is unrealistic against most standards. Most difficult are decisions about new interventions that have cost-effectiveness ratios that fall in the middle of these extremes.

Cost-Utility Analyses

Like CEA, a cost-utility analysis (CUA) determines the incremental costs and incremental health effects of a program compared to an alternative or the status quo. The CEA differs from the CUA in its outcome measure. CEAs measure health effects in units (e.g., cases detected, life-years gained, lives saved) consistent with the objectives of the study. But, what happens if the objectives of the study focus on quality of life? Such was the case of a study of neonatal intensive care for very-low-birth-weight infants, many of whom could have mental and physical deficits (Boyle, Torrance, Sinclair, & Harwood, 1983). In this study, the health improvement was measured in quality-adjusted-life-years, which captured the changes in the quantity and quality of life. Integrating health state values and duration of life is essential in economic analyses in which the improvement of life is an important goal of the intervention.

Descriptive health status measures and valuational or preference-based measures are the two main approaches used to measure health-related quality of life (Bosch & Hunink, 1996). Descriptive health measures ask the respondent to specify the presence and intensity of symptoms and to indicate behaviors, emotions, and social functioning. Perhaps one of the most popular descriptive health status measures is the RAND SF-36 Health Survey (Ware & Sherbourne, 1992), which is designed to summarize a spectrum of core concepts of health and quality of life in a global score on a 0 to 100 scale. Among the dimensions of health assessed through 36 questions are physical functioning, bodily pain, social functioning, mental health, and general health. Question scores in the RAND survey are aggregated and transformed to a global score to describe the individual's overall well-being.

A typical question in the SF-36 asks a respondent to indicate on a scale of 1 to 6 (with 1 being "all of the time" and 6 being "none of the time") whether he or she "has been a very nervous person" during the last 4 weeks. This type of question provides ordinal preferences or simply a rank order of the alternative states from "least preferred" to "most preferred" (Torrance, Furlong, Feeny, & Boyle, 1995). Aggregation of scores on each question into a summated rating assumes that the individual items are monotonically related to the underlying attributes and that the summation of item scores is approximately linearly related to the overall health state. Despite widespread use and the relative ease in which they can be administered, interpretations of the subscores on the various health dimensions, the total scores, and the differences in scores of these measures are unclear (Bergner, 1989).

Valuational or preference-based measures are used in the cost-effectiveness domain. In contrast to the descriptive health status questions, which rank order preferences for health states on an ordinal scale, the numbers or scores of valuational measures represent the strength of preference for those outcomes on an interval scale and are referred to as cardinal preferences (Torrance *et al.*, 1995). Valuational measures are preferred in economic valuations, because preferences can be averaged across individuals and ultimately used in the aggregate as the basis of utilitarian social policy (Kaplan, 1995). Valuational measures obtain "values" and "utilities" on a scale of 0 to 1 where 1 usually is tantamount to perfect health and 0 usually represents death. Values are measured under conditions of certainty, whereas utilities represent preferences measured under uncertainty (Feeny, Torrance, & Furlong, 1996). Utility assessments follow von Neumann's and Morgenstern's (1947) axioms of utility theory in which the decision maker faces trade-offs and probabilities in explicitly weighting the preferences for health states. The three most widely used methods to measure values or utilities for health states are the standard gamble, the time tradeoff, and the visual analogue or rating scale. These techniques are briefly summarized below. However, it should be noted that there is a lack of consensus over which "quality-of-life" measure to use (Kaplan, 1995) and that the choice of any one measure or technique must be consistent with the intent of the study and be undertaken with an understanding of the basic theoretical and conceptual underpinnings (Torrance *et al.*, 1995; Feeny, Furlong, Boyle, & Torrance, 1995).

Standard Gamble

The standard gamble is the classical approach to ascertaining cardinal preferences under conditions of uncertainty. In this technique, an individual is given two choices, as illustrated in Fig. 1. Choice 1 provides the subject two alternatives, a gamble with two possible outcomes: either immediate death, with probability *1 – P* and a value of 0, or normal health, with probability *P* and a value of 1. Choice 2 offers the respondent the certainty of a less preferred or intermediate health state.

For example, an individual could face the choice of a surgical procedure to correct chronic chest pain from an ischemic heart condition. In choice 1 in Fig. 1, this patient faces a probability (*P*) of returning to normal health free of chest pain or probability (*1–P*) of death. In choice 2, the patient can be assured of the chronic chest pain (state C). In this technique, the interviewer typically varies the probabilities of death and normal health beginning with extreme values for each. "If your chance of survival with full health were 98%, would you take choice 1 or 2?" "What if the chance of death was 98%?" You can imagine that one may choose choice 1 with a high probability of survival with normal health, while choice 2 may be the preferred option with a high likelihood of death. The interviewer varies the probabilities for normal health and death until the respondent is indifferent between choices 1 and 2. Let us assume in this example the respondent's indifference point is when the probability of death (*1–P*) is 25% and conversely the probability of normal health is 75%. The utility for state C is:

$$u(\text{state C}) = (P * \text{normal health value}) + ((1 - P) * \text{death value}))$$
$$= (0.75 * 1) + (0.25 * 0)$$
$$= 0.75$$

Visual aids and props (Furlong, Feeny, Torrance, Barr, & Horsman, 1990) have been used to assuage the difficulty that many respondents encounter in considering probabilities inherent in the standard gamble technique. Even so, the standard gamble can be complex and confusing for respondents.

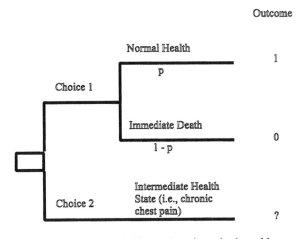

Figure 1. Illustration of standard gamble.

Time Trade-Off

The time trade-off was developed as a more user-friendly technique (Torrance, Sacket, & Thomas, 1972). This method of preference assessment does not incorporate the elements of risk or uncertainty; however, it can be justified by the axioms of utility theory under certain conditions (Pliskin, Shepard, & Weinstein, 1980; Read, Quinn, Berwick, Fineberg, & Weinstein, 1984). In this case, the respondent is offered the choice of living for a specified time in a less preferred or intermediate health state or a variable amount of time in normal or perfect health. This derives what fraction of years in the best health states is equivalent to the same number of years in the less optimal state. For example, a subject facing the same condition in the standard gamble situation is advised he has 12 months to live. He is offered the choice of living these 12 months with chronic chest pain or, alternatively, 2 months in perfect health. He prefers the 12 months, albeit with chest pain. However, when the choice of time in perfect health is increased, this individual is more willing to "trade-off" time. Still facing the choice of 12 months with chronic chest pain, he may accept as a preference 9 months in perfect health instead. In fact, an offer of 9 months in perfect health is his indifference point. Anything less than 9 months in perfect health and his preference switches to 12 months with chronic pain. Again, the "utility" for the chronic health state is 9 months–12 months, or 0.75. Or in other words, 9 out of 12 months in perfect health is equivalent to 12 months in the chronic state. In fact, utility assessments from the different techniques usually are not coincident. This will be discussed subsequently.

Rating or Visual Analogue Scale

The rating scale (including category scaling and visual analogue scales) is the most straightforward of the direct approaches to preference assessment. A scale from 0 to 100 usually is used. The best and worst health outcomes are assigned to the top and bottom of the scale, respectively. The respondent is asked to locate the intermediate health state or states on the scale. This location reflects the individual's value of the intermediate state between perfect health and death. Category rating refers to rating methods in which the scale is divided into discrete points (i.e., 0.1, 0.2, etc.) that must be chosen by the rater. Visual analogue scales contain no internal demarcations. Clearly, the rating scale does not incorporate the theoretical advantages of the previous methods that incorporate the element of risk into the assessment. Its appeal is its simplicity. Researchers have shown mathematical relations between population assessments obtained in the standard gamble and assessments obtained via the standard gamble and time trade-off (Torrance, Boyle, & Horword, 1982; Torrance, 1976). Through power functions, the mean rating scale values can be related to the standard gamble and time trade-off values (Torrance *et al.*, 1995; Feeny *et al.*, 1995).

Steps and Recommendations for Conducting a Cost-Effectiveness Analysis

Recently, a multidisciplinary panel of experts published recommendations and guidelines for conducting cost-effectiveness studies (Gold, Siegel, Russell, & Weinstein, 1996). This publication summarizes the discussions and recommendations of the Panel on Cost-Effectiveness in Health and Medicine, convened by the Public Health

Service. This work represents 2 years of comprehensive research and deliberation designed to produce standard methods to conduct CEAs in policy arenas. Standardization is desired because it permits comparisons of the costs and health outcomes of alternative interventions to improve health. The book provides a detailed discussion of the theoretical and methodological underpinnings that guided the recommendations of the consensus panel. The panel proposed the use of a "reference case" as a standard set of practices that an analyst should follow in conducting these studies. The following section incorporates a review of many of these practices. It is highly recommended that serious analysts consult this important resource before beginning a CEA.

Framing the Analysis

The perspective taken in a CEA determines the costs that are included in the analysis. An insurer, for instance, will be interested in its actual payment for services (e.g., physician and hospital services). The patient receiving these services is interested in the costs he or she incurs. These may include out-of-pocket costs or co-pays for medical services and the time and travel costs associated with receiving treatment, costs which the insurer does not bear. It can seen from these examples that a CEA conducted from these two perspectives—insurer or patient—would collect different cost information and most likely reach different conclusions.

The panel recommends adoption of the societal perspective in studies addressing the broad allocation of resources. Studies conducted from this perspective include all categories of costs and all health effects regardless of who incurs the costs or realizes the health effects. Conducting the analysis from the societal perspective does not preclude another analysis from another viewpoint when this is more important to the party of interest. The preferred approach, when a narrower view is of primary interest, is to conduct the analysis from the broad societal perspective and subsequently from the limited perspective.

Regardless of the perspective taken in the analysis, it is important that a well-defined question be posed in answerable form (Drummond et al., 1987). The alterative treatments or interventions should be identified clearly and completely described as should the target population of the intervention. For example, "From the perspective of the Good Samaritan HMO, is a program of diet and exercise preferable to drug therapies to reduce serum cholesterol (i.e., total cholesterol and low-density and high-density lipoprotein) for adults over the age of 35?" This question compares alternatives that are known to be effective. If either alterative was not know to be effective, then the study would incorporate other relevant strategies including the "status quo" or "do-nothing" alternative. By thoroughly describing alternative strategies, analysts make the study more useful to those who may desire to consider these interventions in their population.

The question also has defined boundaries by designating a target group and specific health consequences. Of course, changes in cholesterol levels are intermediate outcomes. Nonetheless, the changes in the intermediate outcome may be used in models to derive more terminal outcomes such as life-years or lives saved. The use of models for this purpose also has application for the CEA of screening programs. For example, rather than simply determining the cost per additional case detected in a mammography screening program, modeling permits the estimation of the number of lives or life-years gained.

Identifying and Valuing Outcomes

For a reference case analysis, it is recommended that the outcome measure integrate both quantity and quality of life in a single measure such as the quality-adjusted life-years (QALYs). The quality of life weights should be preference-based and interval-scaled. If a direct scaling approach is used, these should be transformed mathematically into an interval scale. The QALY scale should be anchored by a score of 0.0 representing "death" and 1.0 representing "optimal health."

The source of preferences for the relevant health states remains unsettled. Patients, providers, and community samples have been used. The panel concluded, after much consideration of theoretical and practical concerns, that a community sample should serve as the source of preferences for reference case analyses done from the societal perspective. Preferences gathered in this manner are more likely to represent society's judgments about the relative preferences for particular health states. However, this recommendation should be exercised with caution. The panel notes that the community sample must be well-informed about the condition, free of any cognitive impairments, and unbiased. It is recognized that pristine preferences are presently unavailable, primarily because of the necessity of a perfectly informed sample. Nonetheless, it is felt that preferences from a community sample are preferred. Until such time that a broad range of community-based preferences are available, patient preferences may be used. Sensitivity analyses must be used carefully in such circumstances to test the robustness of the findings.

Assessing the Effectiveness of the Health Interventions

The numerator in the cost-effectiveness ratio must reflect the net effect of the differences in health outcomes among those persons subjected to alternative strategies. In most CEAs, a series of events occurs from the point of the intervention (e.g., screening) to the final health effect (e.g., change in QALYs). Many intermediate events are encountered before changes in morbidity and mortality are realized. Models are often used to connect the events along these pathways and estimate the terminal outcomes. The events in these models rely heavily on secondary data from randomized clinical trials, observational sources, descriptive studies, and expert opinion. Secondary data must be scrutinized carefully to ensure that they are derived from well-designed studies and are appropriate for the population under study in the CEA. Expert opinion is reserved for those cases in which data are unavailable and/or when the parameter estimate is not of primary importance.

Estimating Costs

The numerator of the cost-effectiveness ratio must measure the magnitude of the net differences in costs between the alternative interventions. All nontrivial resources used, consumed, and saved in the respective strategies are tabulated in the reference case analysis. These costs include direct costs for health care resources (e.g., provider services, educational materials, and medications) and nonhealth care resources (e.g., time spent in transportation and treatment by the patient and care provided by family members and volunteers). Savings include those resources not consumed as a result of averted disease.

All these resources should be valued according to their opportunity costs (i.e., the value of the foregone benefit, because the resource is not available for its best alternative use). In most cases, prices reflect opportunity costs and may be used as fair values of resources. If market distortions exist, prices do not approximate opportunity costs and should be adjusted. Oftentimes, price estimations are derived from secondary data sources collected at different points in time. To remove the effects of inherent price inflation, all prices should use constant dollars.

Adjusting Costs and Outcomes for Time Differentials

Often, the health consequences of an intervention occur long after the time at which the intervention is delivered. Hence, the savings from an averted disease may occur in the distant future, long after the resources are consumed in delivering the intervention. Allowance must be made for these timing differentials.

In a world of no inflation or interest on savings, it would still be advantageous to have a financial benefit sooner and a cost later. This time preference for money is usually reflected in the rates on risk-free investments or government bonds. The interest rate on these bonds indicates society's willingness to forego consumption today in return for greater consumption in the future. In CEAs, a present value *analysis* is conducted to align in time all resources consumed along the path of an alternative health strategy. A discount rate is used to "present value" in today's dollars those expenditures or savings that occur in the future. The discount rate closely approximates the previously described interest rate. The panel notes that a large number of CEAs have used a discount rate of 5% and recommends that this be used in the base-case analysis. A discount rate of 3% should be used in sensitivity analyses, because it is probably the most real (riskless) discount rate in today's economic climate. This rate should be revised if economic circumstances undergo significant change.

While there seems to be no dispute about discounting resources consumed or saved in a health intervention, there has been some controversy about whether to and at what rate one should discount health effects for differential timing. A complete discussion of this controversy is beyond the scope of this chapter. Coincident discount rates are advised for health effects and costs. It has been shown that nonsensical answers are obtained when health effects and costs are not discounted to present value with the same rate.

Calculating the Results

After the cost and health effects have been tabulated for each alternative strategy, it is time to report results in the form of cost-effectiveness ratios. Basically, the following steps as outlined by Kamlet (1992) are followed. First, the health interventions are ranked in terms of their costs, going from the lowest to the highest cost intervention. If two interventions have coincident costs, the one with the lower health benefits are listed first. Second, any health intervention that costs the same or more than the prior intervention in the list but produces lower health benefits is removed from the list. These interventions are said to be "dominated" or "strongly dominated," because an alternative strategy can yield better health effects at less cost. Third, beginning with the second intervention on the list, each intervention on the list is compared with the preceding intervention in terms of their comparative costs and health effects. Respectively, the net difference in costs and health consequences calculated between these two interventions. This ratio of net costs to net health benefits is the cost-effectiveness ratio. Fourth, the interventions whose cost-effectiveness ratios are greater than that of the next health intervention on the list are eliminated from the list. The eliminated interventions are said to be "weakly dominated" or ruled out by "extended dominance," because a mixed strategy employing a combination of two alternative strategies will be less costly and yield greater health benefits than the eliminated strategy. Finally, the cost-effectiveness ratios of remaining alternatives are recalculates as was done in the third step.

At the conclusion of these steps, the policymaker will face choices similar to the ones in Table 2. Which of these mutually exclusive alternatives would be funded? It depends on the decision maker's values and budget. Referring to Table 2, let us assume that there is an unlimited budget, and this decision maker (e.g., government agency or HMO) has adopted a standard or threshold for cost-effectiveness ratios. If the standard or threshold was lower than $10,000 per year of life expectancy gained, none of the strategies in Table 2 would be adopted. If the threshold was $30,000 per year of life expectancy gained, the "every 2 years" screening strategy would be adopted.

On the other hand, let us assume that this decision maker, facing the same results in Table 2, does not have a cost-effectiveness threshold or standard but does have a limited budget. If the budget limitation was $100,000, a "no screening" policy would be maintained. If $1 million was available, the most intense screening every year could be adopted.

The final assessment also should consider a sensitivity analysis in which the parameter estimates are varied. This is particularly important for estimates that are less certain. Repeating the analysis with wide variances of key parameters reveals the robustness of the analysis and the choice of an optimal decision.

Summary

Cost-effectiveness analysis is not used as a mechanical decision-making tool, but rather a guide. By quantifying the costs and consequences and revealing the trade-offs in choices, it offers the decision maker a much more informed judgment. Nonetheless, judgment is required in the final choice of a strategy. The policymaker, health insurer, or other individual then must weigh other factors not necessarily considered in the analysis. These factors may include ethical considerations of fairness and justice. Armed with explicit revelations of the cost-effectiveness, the decision maker should have the crucial information for better conclusions.

References

Acton, P. (1973). *Evaluating public programs to save lives: The case of heart attacks.* Santa Monica, CA: Rand Corporation (R-950-RC, January).

Bergner, M. (1989). Quality of life, health status, and clinical research. *Medical Care, 27,* S148–S156.

Bosch, J. L., & Hunink, M. G. M. (1996). The relationship between descriptive and valuational quality-of-life measures in patients with intermittent claudication. *Medical Decision Making, 16,* 317–325.

Boyle, M. H., Torrance, G. W., Sinclair, J. C., & Horwood, S. P. (1983). Economic evaluation of neonatal intensive care of very-low-birth-weight infants. *New England Journal of Medicine, 308,* 1330–1337.

Detsky, A. S., &Naglie, I. G. (1990). A clinician's guide to cost-effectiveness analysis. *Annals of Internal Medicine, 113*, 147–154.

Doubilet, P., Weinstein, M. C., & McNeil, B. J. (1986) Use and misuse of the term "cost effective" in medicine. *New England Journal of Medicine, 314*, 253–256.

Drummond, M. F., Stoddart, G. L., & Torrance, G. W. (1987). *Methods for the economic evaluation of health care programmes*. Oxford, England: Oxford Medical Publications.

Eddy, D. M. (1990). Screening for cervical cancer. *Annals of Internal Medicine, 113*, 214–226.

Feeny, D., Furlong, W., Boyle, M., & Torrance, G. W. (1995). Multi-attribute health status classification systems. *PharmacoEconomics, 7*(6), 490–502.

Feeny, D. H., Torrance, G. W., & Furlong, W. J. (1996). Health utilities index. In B. Spiker (Ed.), *Quality of life and pharmacoeconomics in clinical trails* (pp. 239–252). Philadelphia: Lippincott-Raven.

Furlong, W., Feeny, D., Torrance, G. W., Barr, R., & Horsman J. (1990, June). *Guide to design and development of health-state utility instrumentation*. McMaster University Centre for health Economics and Policy Analysis Working paper 90–09,V,141.

Gold, M. R., Siegel, J. E., Russell, L. B., & Weinstein, M. C. (1996). *Cost-effectiveness in health and medicine*. New York: Oxford University Press.

Johannesson, M., Jonsson, B., & Borgquist, L. (1991). Willingness to pay for anti-hypertensive therapy—Results of a Swedish pilot study. *Journal of Health Economics, 10*(4), 461–473.

Kamlet, M. S. (1992). The comparative benefits model. Washington, DC: US Department of Health and Human Services.

Kaplan, R. M. (1995). Utility assessment for estimating quality-adjusted life years. In F. Sloan (Ed.), *Valuing health care* (pp. 31–60). New York: Cambridge University Press.

Leutwyler, K. (1995, April). The price of prevention. *Scientific American*, 124–129.

Mishan, E. J. (1982). *Cost-benefit analysis: An informal introduction* (4th ed.). London: Unwin Hyman.

Moore M. J., & Viscusi, W. K. (1988). The quantity-adjusted values of life. *Economic Inquiry, 26*(3), 369–388.

Olson, C. A. (1981). An analysis of wage differentials received by workers on dangerous jobs. *Journal of Human Resources, 16*(2), 167–185.

Pauly, M. V. (1995). Valuing health care benefits in money terms. In F. Sloan (Ed.), *Valuing health care* (pp. 99–124). New York: Cambridge University Press.

Pliskin, J. S., Shepard, D. S., & Weinstein, M. C. (1980). Utility function for life years and health status. *Operations Research, 28*, 206–224.

Read, J. L., Quinn, R. J., Berwick, D. M., Fineberg, H. V., & Weinstein, M. C. (1984). Preferences for health outcomes. *Medical Decision Making, 4*(3), 315–329.

Tengs, T. O., Adams, M. E., Pliskin, J. S., Safran, D. G., Siegel, J. E., Weinstein, M. C., & Graham, J. D. (1995). Five-hundred life-saving interventions and their cost-effectiveness. *Risk Analysis, 15*(3), 369–390.

Thompson, M. S. (1986). Willingness-to-pay and accept risk to cure chronic disease. *American Journal of Public Health, 76*(4), 392–396.

Torrance, G. W. (1976). Social preferences for health states: an empirical evaluation of three measurement techniques. *Socio-Economic Plan Science, 10*, 129–136.

Torrance, G. W., Sackett, D. L., & Thomas. W. H. (1972). A utility maximization model for evaluation of health care programmes. *Health Services Research, 7*(2), 118–133.

Torrance, G. W., Boyle, M. H., & Horword, S. P. (1982). Application of multi-attribute utility theory to measure social preferences for health states. *Operations Research, 30*, 1043–1069.

Torrance, G. W., Furlong, W., Feeny, D., & Boyle, M. (1995). Multi-attribute preference functions. *PharmacoEconomics, 7*(6), 490–502.

Viscusi, W. K. (1979). *Employment hazards: an investigation of market performance*. Cambridge, MA: Harvard University Press.

von Neuman, J., & Morgenstern, O. (1947). *Theories of games and economic behavior*. Princeton, NJ: Princeton University Press.

Ware, J. E., & Sherbourne, D.C. (1992). The MOS 36-item short-form health survey. *Medical Care, 30*, 473–483.

Weinstein, M. C. (1995). From cost-effectiveness ratios to resource allocation. In F. Sloan (Ed.), *Valuing health care* (pp. 99–124). New York: Cambridge University Press.

PART IX

Future Directions in Health Promotion and Disease Prevention

Promising Theoretical and Methodological Approaches and Future Directions in Health Promotion and Disease Prevention Research and Practice

James M. Raczynski and Ralph J. DiClemente

Introduction

The chapters in this volume outline many promising developments in theory as well as design, evaluation, and implementation methods being applied in the field of health promotion and disease prevention to address different risk behaviors and diseases in varying settings and with different populations. Despite such a heterogeneity of disciplines involved in what is currently most often such a multidisciplinary area of research that convergence of the science of health promotion and disease prevention may be hindered, advances are being made. These advances are most readily made with true interdisciplinary approaches that involve not just individuals who are contributing to a particular project or addressing a particular research question from diverse disciplines, but from active involvement of all disciplines in the research questions and efforts to integrate the disciplines into a science of health promotion and disease prevention.

James M. Raczynski • Behavioral Medicine Unit, Division of Preventive Medicine, Department of Medicine, School of Medicine, Department of Health Behavior, School of Public Health, UAB Center for Health Promotion, University of Alabama at Birmingham, Birmingham, Alabama 35294.   *Ralph J. DiClemente* • Department of Behavioral Sciences and Health Education, Rollins School of Public Health, Emory University, and Emory/Atlanta Center for AIDS Research, Atlanta, Georgia 30322.

Handbook of Health Promotion and Disease Prevention, edited by Raczynski and DiClemente. Kluwer Academic/Plenum Publishers, New York, 1999.

Promising Theoretical Approaches

As in any science, theories are developed to explain phenomena under study. In the case of health promotion and disease prevention, theories of human behavior are useful in explaining why people do or do not engage in certain behaviors that lead to health-related outcomes. Many theories have been used to guide exploratory research designed to identify the antecedents and determinants of health risk behaviors. Likewise, theory has played an integral role in guiding the development of programs designed to eliminate or reduce risk behaviors associated with adverse health outcomes. These theories have been tested and found to be useful in the context of explaining and changing health behavior.

The range of theoretical approaches in health promotion and disease prevention is a reflection of the field itself—eclectic and diverse. Theoretical approaches from a broad spectrum of disciplines have been utilized. And, while the evidence supports the critical role of theory for understanding behavior and designing effective behavior change interventions, there is much more work to be done.

Theory development is not static but rather a dynamic process. Systematic and consistent use of theory across a range of behaviors is necessary to advance the science of health promotion. Also, the theories must be applied to a range of populations, including population groups with different cultural perspectives. Only by constantly reevaluating the explanatory and predictive capacity of theory does the field of health promotion and disease prevention mature. Part of the maturational process involves change. As theories become less useful, that is, they explain an insufficient amount of variance in particular risk behaviors or they are found wanting as a foundation for guiding the design and implementation of behavior change interventions, they are modified or even discarded in favor of potentially more useful theories. This process of development, elimination, and replacement is gradual. New theories are synthesized and embraced. They, too, are subject to empirical validation, and if found lacking, are similarly discarded. This evolutionary process builds on the past as a way of contextualizing the present and predicting the future.

Transtheoretical Model of Change

In the field of health promotion and disease prevention, an emergent theory that has been readily embraced is the transtheoretical model of change (TCM) (see Chapter 3, this volume). The underlying assumption of the TMC is that behavior change is a *process*, not an event, and that individuals are at varying levels of motivational *readiness* for change. The TMC is in stark contrast to many other theories in the field that do not differentiate individuals on the basis of their readiness for changing risk behaviors. Thus, a recent advance in theory has been the ascendancy of the TMC as a model that more accurately captures individual behavior across a range of readiness.

The underlying premise that behavior change is incremental and nonlinear is dependent on an individual's readiness for change and has important implications for understanding behavior and designing interventions. Specifically, individuals at different points on the continuum of change can benefit from different intervention strategies. These strategies are matched to their current level, or stage, of change. For example, rather than offer a unitary intervention to modify an individual's dietary practices, it may be more effective to first assess where on the continuum of readiness the individual is and to tailor the intervention to their acceptability of behavior change and their willingness to adopt new, health-promoting behaviors. Thus, this model offers promise by providing a useful framework for identifying *who* may respond to *what* particular treatment strategies and *when*. Such specificity has been notably lacking in many other theoretical approaches.

The TMC, though having a short history, has had a substantial impact on the ways in which we conceptualize behavior and the ways in which we plan and implement behavior change interventions. This model has been successfully applied across a broad spectrum of risk behaviors, including smoking, lack of exercise, poor diet, inadequate sun protection, to name but a few. Further refinements of the model will continue to enhance its applicability for behavior change.

Importance of Cultural Context in Applying Theory

A cautionary note is warranted about the adoption of a particular theory to guide interventions. Theories should not be utilized without first determining their relevance to a particular population or cultural context (Airhihenbuwa, DiClemente, Wingood, & Lowe, 1992; Burdine & McLeroy, 1992). Theories can and should be modified to be suitable for a particular cultural context. For instance, some constructs may differ in their meaning across cultures and some cultures may not possess a particular theoretical construct. Therefore, it is important to determine the cultural equivalence and relevance of constructs across groups (Berry, 1969). Thus, theories should not constrain interventions, but rather, provide a sound foundation upon which particular cultural elements and environmental constructs can be examined and appropriately integrated into the theoretical framework. It is this broader definition of theory that is most appropriate for designing behavior change interventions.

Promising Methodological Approaches

As theory has evolved over time, so too has methodology. Methodological advances are highlighted in each chapter, with direct relevance to a particular population or intervention venue. However, one emerging cross-cutting methodology issue that is receiving a great deal of attention is that of demonstrating cost-effectiveness. The increasing emphasis on cost containment, the emergence of the managed care environment, and the disproportionate increase in the cost of health care versus other expenditures over the past decade has prompted the examination of cost-effectiveness as one criterion for evaluating health promotion programs.

In our current fiscally constrained environment, it becomes imperative that we not only evaluate program efficacy in terms of impact (changes in behavior, attitudes, norms, knowledge) and outcomes (changes in morbidity, mortality, disability, quality of life) but also assess cost-effectiveness. Such information is vitally important to program planners, policymakers, and other persons involved in the design and implementation of health promotion and disease prevention programs who are responsible for allocating limited financial resources judiciously so as to maximize the number of adverse outcomes [e.g., heart attack, human immunodeficiency virus (HIV) infection] averted through participation or exposure to the intervention program. Particularly as managed care continues to unfold as Bronstein points out in Chapter 29 of this volume, health promotion and disease prevention programs, whether conducted for research or practice purposes, will need to address cost-effectiveness.

Arguably, one might question whether health promotion and disease prevention programs should be held accountable to a standard that a program's economic benefits to society should outweigh its financial costs. This is certainly a debatable issue. However, whether or not one accepts the standard, applications of economic evaluation techniques are as appropriate to behavioral interventions as they are to other health programs.

Unable to sidestep the issue of cost effectiveness, program planners need to become familiar with the underlying theory and methods used to conduct cost effectiveness studies. This methodology represents an entirely different perspective for many in the field of health promotion and disease prevention. Most often, health promotion interventionists have had their philosophical, theoretical, and methodological roots in the social and behavioral sciences. And, while an interdisciplinary perspective is the hallmark of the field, enhancing familiarity with cost effectiveness methodologies is critical for understanding a program's economic impact.

An in-depth discussion, or even a cursory discussion of cost benefit analysis methodology, is beyond the scope of this chapter. It is, however, the intent of this chapter to alert behavior change interventionists and other practitioners of health promotion and disease prevention to the need to become familiar with these methods and to begin to plan their programs with these measures incorporated in the study design. For a concise overview of the fundamentals of the methodological approaches to conduct cost-benefit analyses of health care programs or interventions, we refer the reader to Chapter 31 in this volume. In Chapter 31, Capilouto reviews basic terminology, measurement of health outcomes, and steps for conducting the analysis. As the science of health promotion and disease prevention advances and more interventions are shown to be effective in reducing risk behavior and their adverse health sequelae, it will become increasingly important to establish cost effectiveness of these interventions as well.

Future Directions for Health Promotion and Disease Prevention

Changes are occurring in several different spheres that will affect future directions of health promotion and disease prevention research and practice, including: (1) evolving patterns of traditional epidemiological as well as behavioral and psychosocial epidemiological patterns that may result in shifting priorities for primary, secondary, and tertiary prevention methods and health promotion; (2) innovations in medical care determination of risk for particular diseases that may lead to new behavioral psychosocial issues that emerge related to the screening practices as well as directions for associated behavioral and psychosocial prevention methods; (3) innovations in medical therapies that may lead to new behavioral and psychosocial issues for health promotion and disease prevention; (4) evolutions in the practice of health care and health promotion and disease prevention; (5) changes resulting from technological developments; (6) evolutions in culture, knowledge, attitudes, and beliefs of the population regarding health promotion and disease prevention, diseases, risk factors, and risk reduction methods that may lead to evolving patterns of health promotion and disease prevention priorities; (7) shifts in focus from preventing disease to promoting health; (8) population trends; and (9) newly emerging health threats, particularly in the area of infectious disease. As we discuss below, some directions for health promotion and disease prevention research and practice can be predicted based on trends in some of these nine areas of influence; trends in other areas are not yet so clear to allow confident predictions of future directions. Nonetheless, vigilance to developments and trends in these areas of influence will improve the predictive ability for shifts in research and practice and may allow quicker response to developing research and practice needs.

Evolving Patterns of Traditional as Well as Behavioral and Psychosocial Epidemiological Patterns

As the field of epidemiology evolves in exploring relationships among risk factors and disease outcomes, new knowledge is emerging concerning the role that different risk factors play in determining overall risk. For example, data concerning the independent risk associated with different lipoproteins for coronary heart disease outcomes have led to evolving knowledge concerning the benefits of serum cholesterol treatment through dietary approaches. This evolving risk factor knowledge, of course, impacts on directions for health promotion and disease prevention, influencing the focus on dietary interventions, for instance, for lowering serum cholesterol.

Epidemiological approaches have increasingly incorporated behavioral and psychosocial perspectives that are contributing to identifying behavioral and psychosocial risk factors. As researchers are better trained to assimilate knowledge from both epidemiological and health behavior perspectives in an interdisciplinary manner, it might be anticipated that increased progress will be made in determining the role of behavioral and psychosocial risk factors in different diseases. Good examples of these trends are noted in Chapter 12, this volume. Depression and social isolation appear to be very strong predictors of morbidity and mortality after having a heart attack, suggesting that treatments may be beneficial for patients who show evidence of these psychosocial risk factors.

Innovations in Medical Care Determination of Risk for Particular Diseases

Innovations developed from medical research are leading to new approaches for risk determination. The impact of medical innovations may be evident most prominently in the area of genetic determination of risk. As the human gene is mapped and particular genes are identified as risk factors for particular diseases, it will become increasingly possible to determine individuals' specific risk rather than merely to examine gross estimates of genetic risk based on family histories. These changes in risk identification lead to new behavioral questions that will require research investigation in the next few years, since we are about to experience an explosion in genetic screening. These questions span beyond health behavior issues and include policy and legal issues involved in insurance coverage and rights of access to outcomes of genetic screening. The health behavior issues include matters such as the extent to which genetic information will precipitate fear and anxiety and potentially adversely affect risk reduction efforts. Research that examines methods of communicating genetic risk information and risk reduction recommendations is already beginning to appear, but a great deal of data will soon be needed so that we may be better informed about the means of optimally using genetic risk screening methods to reduce individuals' risk and not threaten their quality of life.

Innovations in Medical Therapies

As mentioned in Chapter 12, innovations in reperfusion therapies to open arteries during a heart attack have led increasingly to recognizing the importance of promoting people's ability to make accurate symptom perceptions and attributions for those symptoms (see Chapter 5) suggestive of a myocardial infarction and to seek prompt health care (see Chapter 6). Patients who delay too long in seeking medical care experience heart damage that cannot be reversed by opening arteries. Thus, there is a clear need to develop effective programs that will encourage people in seeking prompt care. Similar issues are beginning to emerge for stroke, since thrombolytic approaches are beginning to be applied with strokes that result from occlusion of arteries.

In the case of infectious diseases, examples also can be found to demonstrate how evolving medical practice is impacting on applications in health promotion and disease prevention. For example, developing HIV vaccines and pharmacological treatments emphasize the critical importance of adherence to these medical regimens. Particularly in the case of pharmacological treatment for HIV and acquired immunodeficiency syndrome (AIDS), which commonly involve multiple medications administered in a complex regimen, it is essential that patients follow the regimen closely or run the high risk of having the virus mutate to a less treatable form.

Evolutions in the Practice of Health Care and Health Promotion and Disease Prevention

Health care practice is also changing in a manner that may influence health promotion and disease prevention research and practice. As described in Chapter 29, managed care is having influences in the restructuring of health care programs, in general, that may have profound impact on the delivery of health promotion and disease prevention programs. The restructuring of the traditional, small-business physician system into larger managed care organizations can support the implementation of specialized programs such as those for health promotion and disease prevention. Tracking systems can provide an opportunity for early identification of patients with risk factors and repeated opportunities for contact either in the health care setting or with cooperation of the work site. The change in financial incentives so that providers benefit from helping patients stay healthy as much as they benefit from treating them when they are sick, with appropriate physician training, also may create significant changes and new opportunities for research and practice.

As we have discussed above, these changes in managed care also are unquestionably being accompanied by a focus on optimizing the cost-effectiveness of health care programs. Health promotion and disease prevention programs will not escape this focus on cost effectiveness. Hence, it will be essential that both research and practice programs be able to examine costs and outcomes and demonstrate sufficient cost-effectiveness to be attractive to managed care organizations. Even with cost-effective programs, the focus increasingly will be on lowering costs and improving effectiveness. To accomplish this goal of improved cost effectiveness, it will be necessary to focus not just on improving outcomes of programs but also on identifying the individuals who will benefit the most from the efforts and lowering the costs involved in program delivery.

Aside from changes in managed care, legislative and policy changes also are occurring and affecting health promotion and disease prevention. These policies are affecting the practice of health promotion and disease prevention in health department settings. Policy changes in work sites, such as with smoking policies, also are having great influences not only on behaviors of individuals who smoke but in reducing exposure to secondhand smoke and the health of nonsmokers as well. The influence of policy changes on social norms and attitudes and beliefs of those affected is also an important area for research and possible practice. As employers continue to move toward lowering their health care costs attributable to insurance premiums and lost productivity from illness and premature death, other opportunities may emerge for work site policy changes to influence health behaviors. Beyond the work site, important opportunities exist to implement and to examine the benefits of policy changes in communities that affect bicycle lanes and walking and running trails, and other policy changes that may influence physical activity and other health behaviors, increasing the breadth of models for health promotion and disease prevention.

Technological Developments

Developments in computer, television, and communication technologies are beginning to influence the development, implementation, and evaluation of health promotion and disease prevention programs. Interactive computers are allowing some behavioral scientists to begin developing programs to tailor the information to the needs of those using them. Interactive television and other communication technological developments may allow greater access to populations for delivery of interactive programming, including those developed for interactive computers. These developments may allow the development of more complex theories that, for instance, might incorporate an increased number of factors to tailor the intervention to the needs of the observer.

Interactive technologies also might allow the use of improved self-monitoring and feedback methods in the delivery of health promotion and disease prevention programs. For instance, prompts delivered by interactive television, networked computers, or other means might allow for improved methods of prompting people or even direct assessment of health behaviors for feedback purposes.

Evolutions in Culture, Knowledge, Attitudes, and Beliefs of the Population

Unquestionably, the population in the United States is changing as evidenced by the changes in their health behaviors. Secular trends, accounting for population-wide reductions in risk factors over time, in cardiovascular risk factors, for instance, have been acknowledged as a major factor with which community intervention studies must contend (Schooler, Farquhar, Fortmann, & Flora, 1997). This is clearly good news from the perspective of people's health, but these trends create greater methodological challenges for researchers who now not only must demonstrate changes in behavior but changes that will outpace those that are occurring in the general population.

From Preventing Disease to Promoting Health

As discussed in Chapter 1, shifts in the sources of morbidity and mortality attributable to different types of diseases have occurred over time. Infectious diseases were the major sources of mortality at the turn of the 20th century, but changes in medicine and public health accounted for a reduction in mortality attributable to infectious disease and a resultant shift to greater mortality from chronic diseases. Injury, as discussed in Chapters 14 and 15, also emerged as a major source of morbidity and mortality. With the recent emergence of the AIDS epidemic, an increased emphasis has been placed on infectious diseases. However, throughout history, health promotion and disease prevention research probably has emphasized the importance of preventing disease more than it has attempted to promote health. Although clearly preventing disease presumably promotes health, a focus on preventing disease alone detracts from nondisease factors that affect a broad definition of health that includes issues of the quality of life. Promoting quality of life, a component of which is preventing mortality and morbidity from disease, leads to a broader focus for comprehensive health promotion and disease prevention research and practice programs.

Population Trends

Population trends also are occurring. With medical and public health improvements, our population is aging, leading to an increased recognition of the needs of older people and demands for programs to address these needs. As our society becomes increasingly mobile, increasing cultural and ethnic diversity is occurring, requiring health promotion and disease prevention programs that meet the needs of people from different cultural and ethnic backgrounds. These and other population trends will continue to present challenges to those of us who work with human behavior.

Newly Emerging Health Threats: Infectious Diseases

Emerging infectious diseases are those diseases in which the incidence has actually increased in the past two decades or has the potential to increase in the near future. These emerging diseases may include new or known infectious diseases, but clearly will continue to present new challenges for health promotion and disease prevention. Consider, for example, the discovery of the Ebola virus. Ebola virus is a mysterious killer with a frightening mortality rate that reaches 90%; there is no known treatment, and no known reservoir in nature. It appears to be transmitted through direct contact with bodily secretions, and as such potentially can be contained once cases are identified. The reasons for outbreaks, as the recent ones in Sudan and Zaire, are not well understood. Ebola may be an example of a new virus that may appear as civilization broaches the regions of hitherto uninhabited areas, changing the landscape and disturbing the delicate ecosystems that have existed for many years. As movement of people and travel become even easier, distant, previously inaccessible regions of the world become easier to access, creating a "globalization of disease" (Garrett, 1995).

In the United States, the appearance of the Hantavirus and of antibiotic-resistant strains of more common bacterial threats such as staphylococci, streptococcus, and gonorrhea signal both the emergence and persistence of infectious agents as significant health threats. As the reemergence of known, thought-to-be controlled bacterial infectious diseases suggests, treatment may not be a magic bullet. The persistence of sexually transmitted diseases, for example, as a major public health problem, despite the development of effective therapeutic agents, indicates that prevention remains critically important (Yankauer, 1986, 1994).

Interactions between Spheres of Influence: Lessons for the Future

Several converging spheres likely will result in increased attention to health promotion and disease prevention research and practice, but some important caveats must be noted if the result is truly to be an increase in attention to this area of research and practice. First, the science of health promotion and disease prevention is an emerging science of diverse disciplines. Much will be gained by bringing the breadth of perspectives to bear from these different disciplines; however, it is incumbent on both researchers and practitioners in the area not only to embrace the breadth of perspectives but to work toward convergence of theories and methodologies if the goal of achieving a defined science is to be realized. Second, not only will the goal of converging the science of health promotion and disease prevention be advanced by using rigorous, empirically based methodologies, but such methodological rigor will soon be required by managed care organizations and governmental agencies in private and public practice settings as trends toward demonstrable cost effectiveness of service delivery programs continue. Third, these increasing requirements to provide documented cost effectiveness data to support practice programs will require that practitioners in health promotion and disease prevention have adequate research training. This will require the training of scientist–practitioners who are capable of functioning both as practitioners and as scientists to evaluate service programs. In fact, academic researchers who also are trained as scientist–practitioners may be best able to appreciate the barriers of service program implementation and best able to advance the field, while developing empirically validated programs capable of more broad-scale dissemination than at present.

Summary

This handbook has attempted to outline the many promising developments in theory and design, evaluation, and implementation methods being applied in the diverse, emerging field of health promotion and disease prevention that are being used to address different risk behaviors and diseases in varying settings and with different populations. Clearly, the field is rapidly growing in depth and breadth as new health-related behavioral and psychosocial risk factors are identified and as societal, health care, and regulatory influences have increased the focus on health promotion and disease prevention. Despite great diversity in disciplines involved in health promotion and disease prevention research and practice, we believe that at least the beginnings of some convergence of the science of health promotion and disease prevention is occurring as advances are being made in theories and methods. Certainly, there are a variety of spheres of influence that are converging to suggest that future directions of health promotion research and practice will rapidly expand.

References

Airhihenbuwa, C., DiClemente, R. J., Wingood, G. M., & Lowe, A. (1992). HIV/AIDS education and prevention among African-Americans: A focus on culture. *AIDS Education and Prevention, 4,* 251–260.

Berry, J. (1969). On cross-cultural comparability. *International Journal of Psychology, 4,* 207–229.

Burdine, J. N., & McLeroy, K. (1992). Practitioners' use of theory: Examples from a workgroup. *Health Education Quarterly, 19,* 331–340.

Garrett, L. (1995). *The coming plague.* New York: Penguin Books.

Schooler, C. S., Farquhar, J. W., Fortmann, S. P., & Flora, J. A. (1997). Synthesis of findings and issues from community prevention trials. *Annals of Epidemiology, 7* (Suppl.), S54–S68.

Yankauer, A. (1986). The persistence of public health problems: SF, STD and AIDS. *American Journal of Public Health, 76,* 494–495.

Yankauer, A. (1994). Sexually transmitted diseases: A neglected public health priority. *American Journal of Public Health, 84,* 1894–1897.

Index